MALIGNANT MELANOMA
MEDICAL AND SURGICAL MANAGEMENT

NOTICE

MALIGNANT MELANOMA: MEDICAL AND SURGICAL MANAGEMENT

Ferdy J. Lejeune, M.D., Ph.D.

Professor of Oncology
Director, Centre Pluridisciplinaire d'Oncologie
Centre Hospitalie-Universitaire Vaudois
Lausanne, Switzerland

Prabir K. Chaudhuri, M.D.

Professor, Division of Surgical Oncology
Professor of Otolaryngology
Department of Surgery
Medical College of Ohio
Toledo, Ohio

Tapas K. Das Gupta, M.D., Ph.D.

Professor of Surgery
Head, Division of Surgical Oncology
Specialized Center for Cancer Research and Education
University of Illinois
Chicago, Illinois

McGraw-Hill, Inc.

HEALTH PROFESSIONS DIVISION

New York St. Louis San Francisco Auckland
Bogatá Caracas Lisbon London Madrid
Mexico City Milan Montreal New Delhi
Paris San Juan Singapore Sydney Tokyo Toronto

MALIGNANT MELANOMA:
MEDICAL AND SURGICAL MANAGEMENT

1 2 3 4 5 6 7 8 9 0 KGP KGP 9 8 7 6 5 4 3

ISBN 0-07-105421-9

This book was set in Century Schoolbook by J.M. Post Graphics, book division of Cardinal Communications Group Inc.
The editors were Michael J. Houston and Stevin Melvin
the production supervisor was Richard C. Ruzycka
the project supervision was by Tage Publishing Service, Inc.;
the cover designer was Marsha Cohen/Parallelogram
Arcada Graphics/Kingsport was printer and binder.

Library of Congress Cataloging-in-Publication Data

Malignant melanoma : medical and surgical management / [edited by]
Ferdy J. Lejeune, Prabir K. Chaudhuri, Tapas K. Das Gupta.
p. cm.
Includes bibliographical references and index.
ISBN 0-07-105421-9 :
1. Melanoma. I. Lejeune, Ferdy J. II. Chaudhuri, Prabir K.
III. Das Gupta, Tapas K.,
[DNLM: 1. Melanoma--physiopathology. 2. Melanoma--diagnosis.
3. Skin Neoplasms--therapy. WR 500 M2514 1994]
RC280.M37M35 1994
616.99'477--dc20
DNLM/DLC
for Library of Congress 93-31641
CIP

CONTENTS

Color Plates 1–66 appear between pages 114 and 115.

PREFACE

Melanocyte is a truly remarkable cell. Its protective function varies from instantaneous camouflage, as in a chameleon, to the inherited pigmentary characteristics arising from the evolutionary development of a given species. Mammalian melanocytes arise from the precursor melanoblast during embryonic development within the neural crest and migrate throughout the body. Although skin is the most common site of melanocytes, they can be found in other locations (e.g., mucous membranes, central nervous system, and other sundry sites). Thus, melanoma can occur anywhere melanocytes can normally be found. Malignant melanoma has been rare through the ages. In spite of its rarity, interest in the biology of human melanocytes and cutaneous melanoma has always paralleled society's unwholesome interest in the phenomenon of human pigmentation. However, all this has changed since the late 1970s, when the incidence of cutaneous malignant melanoma in the Western world took a leap. Currently, in the United States, melanoma is estimated to be the second fastest growing cancer, eclipsed only by lung cancer in women.

Chapter 1 of this book deals with the epidemiology of malignant melanoma, briefly summarizing the data showing this increase in incidence and delineating the presently available information regarding the reasons for this increase. The reason(s) for this marked rise in incidence could be debated, but there is no doubt that this increase is real, and, by the year 2000, malignant melanoma will pose a major cancer threat in the Western world. Treatment of primary cutaneous melanoma is essentially surgical; thus, a surgeon (surgical oncologist) is always in the first line of attack against this health problem. With this in mind, we developed this treatise on malignant melanoma, focusing on the biology of mammalian melanocytes, the mechanism(s) of development of melanoma, and the therapeutic options presently available for managing malignant melanoma.

The book has been divided into 34 chapters. Chapters 2–7 essentially summarize the salient information on the biological properties and characteristics of mammalian melanocytes, as well as the mechanistic triggers presumedly in operation to transform a melanocyte into a malignant melanoma. In view of the recent advances in research on genetic aspects of melanoma, including the possible identification of putative genes for melanoma, Chapter 6 summarizes the current information on the subject. Recognizing the importance of ultraviolet radiation in the development of melanoma, a chapter (Chapter 8) has been incorporated summarizing the prevailing views on the subject and means of achieving ultraviolet protection. Chapters 9–12 deal with morphologic and morphobiologic aspects of human melanoma, with special emphasis on the recent advances in the histologic techniques being used to diagnose cutaneous melanoma.

Most of the book (Chapters 13–30) deals with the clinical aspects of human melanoma. A group of distinguished authors have summarized their experiences and viewpoints on the diagnosis and treatment of melanoma in both its primary and metastatic forms. For the sake of completeness, Chapters 31 and 32 deal respectively with primary melanoma of the mucosa and the eye. However, the chapter on ocular melanoma does not attempt to answer all of the aspects of melanoma of the eye, which needs a treatise of its own. Finally, in the last two chapters, we have asked the authors to provide an insight on how to make sense of all the clinical trials and studies being reported in the literature.

Although the book was primarily intended for surgical oncologists, anyone interested in the study of melanoma, either in the laboratory or in clinical practice, will find this book invaluable. The authorities who have written the chapters in this book are well-known and extremely well-respected, and indeed constitute a constellation of stars in the melanoma galaxy. We the editors feel extremely fortunate to have worked with these authors, and we sincerely hope our readers will share with us the enthusiasm we feel for this treatise.

CONTRIBUTORS

Karel R. Aigner, M.D. [22]
Leitender Arzt
Sektion Thorax -und Onkologische Chirurgie
Krankenhaus Paulinenstift
Abteilung für Chirurgie
Wiesbaden, Germany

Fritz Wilhelm Anders, M.D. [5]
Em. Professor of Genetics
Genetisches Institut der Justus Liebig-Universität
Giessen, Germany

Philippe Autier, M.D. [1,21]
Oeuvre Belge du Cancer
Institut Bordet
Brussels, Belgium

F. Belli, M.D. [33]
Institute dei Tumori
Division oncologia Chirurgica B
Milano, Italy

Wilma Bergman, M.D., Ph.D. [6]
Department of Dermatology
University Hospital
Leiden, The Netherlands

Eva-Bettina Bröcker, M.D., Ph.D. [11]
Klinik und Poliklinik fuer
Professor
Haut- und Geschlechtskrankheiten
Universität Würzburg
Würzburg, Germany

R. Bufalino [33]
Data Manager
Instituto dei Tumori
Division oncologia Chirurgica B
Milano, Italy

Stefan Carrel, Ph.D. [2]
Institut Ludwig
Chemin dex Boveresses
Epalinges, Switzerland

Natale Cascinelli, M.D. [13,33]
Chairman, WHO Melanoma Program
Instituto dei Tumori
Division oncologia Chirurgica B
Milano, Italy

Devron H. Char, M.D. [32]
Professor of Ophthalmology
University of California
San Francisco Medical Center
Department of Ophthalmology
San Francisco, California

Numbers in brackets refer to contributors' chapters.

Prabir K. Chaudhuri, M.D. [4]
Professor, Division of Surgical Oncology
Professor of Otolaryngology
Department of Surgery
Medical College of Ohio
Toledo, Ohio

Alan S. Coates, M.D., F.R.A.C. [27]
Research Director
Associate Professor in Cancer Medicine
Sydney Melanoma Unit
The University of Sydney
Sydney, Australia

Alistair J. Cochran, M.D. [3,12]
Professor of Pathology and Surgery
Department of Pathology & Laboratory Medicine
University of California, Los Angeles
School of Medicine
Los Angeles, California

Tapas K. Das Gupta, M.D., Ph.D. [18]
Professor of Surgery
Head, Division of Surgical Oncology
Specialized Center for Cancer
Research and Education
University of Illinois
Chicago, Illinois

Jean-François Doré, Ph.D. [2]
Director, Inserm Unit
Centre Leon Berard
Laboratoire d'Immunologie
Lyon, France

Richard Essner, M.D. [17]
Senior Clincal Fellow
Department of Surgical Oncology
John Wayne Cancer Institute
Santa Monica, California

Zohreh Farzad, Ph.D. [3,12]
Professor of Biology
California State University, Northridge
Northridge, California

Ghanem Ghanem, D.Pharm. [21]
Laboratory of Oncology and
Experimental Surgery
Institut Bordet
Brussels, Belgium

Larsolof Hafström, M.D. [23]
Associate Professor
Consultant in Surgical Oncology
Department of Surgery
Gothenburg University
Göteborg, Sweden

Per-Ebbe Jönsson, M.D. [23]
Associate Professor
Consultant in Surgical Oncology
Department of Surgery
University of Lund
Helsingborg, Sweden

Lorenz M. Jost, M.D. [29]
Division of Medical Oncology
University Hospitals
Zürich, Switzerland

Abdul-Ghani Kibbi, M.D. [10]
Professor of Pathology
Department of Dermatology
American University of Beirut
Beirut, Lebanon

John M. Kirkwood, M.D. [29]
Professor, Division of Medical Oncology
University of Pittsburgh
Pittsburgh Cancer Institute
Pittsburgh, Pennsylvania

Ulrick R. Kleeberg, M.D. [26]
Professor of Oncology
Hämatolog.-onkol. Praxis Altona
Hamburg, Germany

Heimen Schraffordt Koops, M.D., Ph.D. [19]
Professor of Surgical Oncology
Head, Department of Surgical Oncology
Groningen University Hospital
Groningen, The Netherlands

Bin B.R. Kroon, M.D., Ph.D. [19]
Department of Surgical Oncology
Netherlands Cancer Institute
Amsterdam, The Netherlands

Ramsay S. Kurban, M.D. [10]
Clinical Associate in Pathology
(Consultant Dermatopathologist)
Massachussetts General Hospital
Boston, Massachusetts
and
Clinical Instructor (Dermatology)
Hershey Medical Center
Pennsylvania State University
Hershey, Pennsylvania

Ana-Maria A. Lana, M.D. [12]
Professor of Pathology
Department of Pathology & Laboratory Medicine
University of California, Los Angeles
School of Medicine
Los Angeles, California

Ferdy J. Lejeune, M.D., Ph.D. [19,20,21]
Professor of Oncology
Director, Centre Pluridisciplinaire d'Oncologie
Centre Hospitalier
Universitaire Vaudois
Lausanne, Switzerland

Danielle Liénard, M.D. [20,21,24]
Instructor
Centre Pluridisciplinaire d'Oncologie
University Hospital
Centre Hospitalier Universitaire Vaudois
Lausanne, Switzerland

David M. Mahvi, M.D. [16]
Assistant Professor of Surgery
Section of Surgical Oncology
University of Wisconsin Clinical Science Center
Madison, Wisconsin

Michael J. Mastrangelo, M.D. [28]
Professor, Department of Medicine
Chief, Division of Medical Oncology
Thomas Jefferson University
Philadelphia, Pennsylvania

William H. McBride, D.Sc. [3]
Professor of Radiation Oncology
University of California, Los Angeles
School of Medicine
Los Angeles, California

William Henry McCarthy, M.D. [14]
Professor (Melanoma and Skin Oncology)
The Sydney Melanoma Unit
Royal Prince Alfred Hospital
Camperdown, Australia

G. Roderick McLeod, M.D. [15]
Chairman, Division of Surgery
Director Queensland Melanoma Project
Princess Alexandra Hospital
Brisbane, Australia

Martin C. Mihm, Jr., M.D., Ph.D. [10]
Professor of Pathology
Dermatopathology Division
Massachusetts General Hospital

Donald L. Morton, M.D., Ph.D. [12,17,31]
Medical Director
Surgeon-In-Chief
John Wayne Cancer Institute
Santa Monica, California

H. Müller, M.D. [22]
Sektion Thorax -und Onkologische Chirurgie
Krankenhaus Paulinenstift
Abteilung für Chirurgie
Wiesbaden, Germany

Brian O'Sullivan, M.D., F.R.C.P. [30]
Staff Radiation Oncology
Assistant Professor, Department of Radiation Oncology
The Ontario Cancer Institute
Toronto, Ontario, Canada

Jean-Paul Ortonne, M.D. [7]
Chairman
Department of Dermatology
Centre Hospitalier Régional et Universitaire de Nice
Hôpital Pasteur
Nice, France

Jean-Claude Pector, M.D., Ph.D. [25]
Service de Chirurgie
Institut Bordet
Brussels, Belgium

Arthur R. Rhodes, M.D., M.PH. [9]
Professor of Dermatology
University of Pittsburgh School of Medicine
Pittsburgh, Pennsylvania

P. Rocmans, M.D., Ph.D. [24]
Department of Thoracic Surgery
Erasme Hospital
University of Brussels
Brussels, Belgium

Dirk J. Ruiter, M.D. [11]
Professor of Pathology
Instituut voor Pathologie
Academisch Ziekenhuis St. Radboud
Nijmegen, The Netherlands

Philip Rümke, M.D., Ph.D. [27]
Honorary Professor of Immunology
Department of Immunology
Antoni van Leeuwen Hoekhuis
Amsterdam, The Netherlands

François Sales, M.D. [21]
Institut Bordet
Service de Chirurgie
Tumor Center of the University of Brussels
Brussels, Belgium

M. Santinami, M.D. [33]
Instituto dei Tumori
Division oncologia Chirurgica B
Milano, Italy

P. I. Schrier, Ph.D. [6]
Department of Clinical Oncology
University Hospital
Leiden, The Netherlands

Helen Maureen Shaw, M.D. [14]
Senior Research Fellow
The Sydney Melanoma Unit
Royal Prince Alfred Hospital
Camperdown, Australia

F. Kristian Storm, M.D. [16]
Professor of Surgery and Human Oncology
Chairman, Section of Surgical Oncology, and Associate
Director of the Comprehensive Cancer Center
University of Wisconsin Clinical Science Center
Madison, Wisconsin

Lars-Göran Strömblad, M.D. [23]
Consultant in Neurosurgery
Department of Neurosurgery
University Hospital
Lund, Sweden

Stefan Suciu, M.Sc. [34]
Statistician
EORTC Data Center
Brussels, Belgium

Richard Tsang, M.D., F.R.C.P. [30]
Staff Radiation Oncologist
Princess Margaret Hospital
The Ontario Cancer Institute
Toronto, Ontario, Canada

Rex M. Tyrrell, Ph.D. [8]
Head, Physical Carcinogenesis Unit
Swiss Institute for Experimental Cancer Research
Lausanne, Switzerland

Laura J. van't Veer, Ph.D. [6]
Division of Molecular Pathology
Netherlands Cancer Institute
Amsterdam, The Netherlands

Michael A. Warso, M.D. [18]
Assitant Professor of Surgery
University of Illinois
Specialized Cancer Center
Chicago, Illinois

Duan-Ren Wen, M.D. [12]
Staff Research Oncologist
Department of Pathology & Laboratory Medicine
University of California, Los Angeles
School of Medicine
Los Angeles, California

Jan H. Wong, M.D. [31]
Assistant Professor of Surgery
Division of Surgical Oncology
University of California, Los Angeles
School of Medicine
Los Angeles, California

Christina Sabina Zechel, M.D. [5]
wiss. Assistentin
Genetisches Institut
der Justus Liebig-Universität
Giessen, Germany

Qing-Si Zeng, M.D. [12]
Staff Research Assistant
Department of Pathology & Laboratory Medicine
University of California, Los Angeles
School of Medicine
Los Angeles, California

Stefano Zurrida, M.D. [13]
Instituto dei Tumori
Division oncologia Chirurgica B
Milano, Italy

MALIGNANT MELANOMA
MEDICAL AND SURGICAL MANAGEMENT

Chapter 1

EPIDEMIOLOGY OF MELANOMA

Philippe Autier

THE RISING INCIDENCE OF CUTANEOUS MELANOMA

In the European community, the average annual cutaneous melanoma incidence between 1978 and 1982 was 4.2 per year for 100,000 men, and 6.2 for 100,000 women.[1] This malignancy represents 1 percent of all cancers among men and 1.8 percent among women. The worldwide variations in the incidence ranges from about 1 per 100,000 per year in the noncaucasian populations to 30 per 100,000 per year for fair-skinned people living in the Queensland Province of Australia.

Table 1-1 displays the incidence rates for selected countries.[2,3] Although by epidemiologic standards, cutaneous melanoma remains an uncommon disease, it is the most rapidly increasing malignancy in the industrialized countries. Some authors do not hesitate to speak of an epidemic phenomenon.[4] The average yearly cutaneous melanoma increase in Denmark is of 6 percent per year, 7 percent in New Zealand, 7.4 percent in Scotland, and 7 percent in the United States. This phenomenon has been known since the fifties[5] and although it affects principally the caucasian populations, it is also observed in Japan.[6] This increase in incidence encompasses all age groups and both genders; but the increase seems more rapid among young people. In very sunny areas (Australia and the southwestern part of the United States), it is the most frequent malignancy among fair-skinned people between the ages of 20 and 40. Primarily, the increase involves the superficial spreading histopathologic type, and cannot merely be attributed to better detection and diagnosis.[7]

In the absence of an efficient treatment for advanced stages, it is expected that an increasingly larger number of fair-skinned people will die of cutaneous melanoma. Hence, this cancer becomes a disease of primary public health importance.

In spite of this grim picture, the overall prognosis of cutaneous melanoma is improving, principally because patients are seeking treatment at an earlier stage of the disease.[8,9]

Table 1-2 summarizes the estimated relative risk for development of cutaneous melanoma according to the most frequently studied risk factors. Since the risk estimates may differ from one study to another, ranges of relative risks are displayed.

HOST RISK FACTORS

Familial atypical multiple mole melanoma (FAMMM) syndrome or hereditary dysplastic nevus syndrome (HDNS) is a hereditary disease transmitted by an autosomal dominant gene characterized by an inherited predisposition to dysplastic nevi and to cutaneous melanoma.[10] The gene has a variable penetrance and the phenotype can be limited to expression of only one dysplastic nevus and a normal number of other acquired nevi. The cumulative lifetime incidence of cutaneous melanoma in subjects with dysplastic nevus *and* with familial history of cutaneous melanoma approaches 100 percent.[11] However, cutaneous melanoma developing among people with hereditary predisposing factors represent only a small fraction of all cutaneous melanoma, probably less than 5 percent.

Sporadic dysplastic nevi (in the absence of hereditary disease) is a frequent skin lesion. Two to eight percent of the general population carry one dysplastic nevus or more, and it is present in about one third of all melanoma patients. The risk of cutaneous melanoma associated with the presence of one or more dysplastic nevi ranges from 2 to 8,[12–14] and some studies report relative risks of 27.[15] The differences in risk estimates lies probably in the disparities in the definition of the risk factors (i.e., the number of lesions considered, the clinical and/or his-

TABLE 1-1
INCIDENCE RATES OF CUTANEOUS MALIGNANT MELANOMA IN SELECTED COUNTRIES

COUNTRIES	AREA OR SUBPOPULATION	CRUDE RATE FOR ALL AGES* 1967–1971	1979–1982
Canada	British Columbia	4.0	7.6
	Quebec	1.3	2.8
United States of America	San Francisco white	7.0	12.7
	Connecticut	4.9	10.4
Australia	Queensland	n.a.[a]	33.3[b]
	South Australia	n.a.[a]	15.5
New Zealand	Non-Maori	7.5	17.0
Israel	All country	3.3	5.8
Japan	Miyagi Prefecture	0.3	0.6
	Osaka Prefecture	0.3	0.2
Czechoslovakia	Slovakia	n.a.[a]	3.2
Denmark	All country	3.5	7.4
Finland	All country	2.9	5.3
France	Bas-Rhin	n.a.[a]	3.6
	Doubs	n.a.[a]	3.4
Germany	Saarland	2.5	4.7
Italy	Varese Province	n.a.[a]	4.0
Netherlands	All country	n.a.[a]	4.3
Norway	All country	6.3	10.9
Sweden	All country	5.4	10.0
Switzerland	Geneva	4.6	11.8
United Kingdom	South Western Region	2.2	4.5
	Oxford Region	2.5	3.1

*(Per 100,000 person/years—adapted from references 2 and 3)
[a]n.a. = figure not available
[b]For 1982 only

tological characteristics of dysplastic nevi, etc.). The risk of cutaneous melanoma is increased 2 to 8 times among persons who have one child, or parent or sibling with cutaneous melanoma.[16]

Among the commonly encountered host risk factors, the density of benign nevi is strongly linked to melanoma.[17–19] Studies report estimates of relative risk as high as 20 when more than 10 nevi (any type) are counted on both arms.[20] Other host risk factors usually associated with cutaneous melanoma are a high propensity to freckle, red or blond hair, and a light complexion. Also, individuals prone to sunburns and with a low ability to tan seem more at risk. An intriguing observation made in several studies is the independence of effect of the number of raised nevi, the degree of freckling, and the tendency to sunburn: one indicator is not a surrogate for the other, but rather, they seem linked to different aspects of cutaneous melanoma development and biology.[18,19]

ENVIRONMENTAL AND BEHAVIORAL RISK FACTORS

Constitutional factors cannot explain the rising incidence of cutaneous melanoma in caucasian populations. Hence, the causes must be sought in the environment or in changing behavior patterns.

Sunlight

Nonmelanoma skin cancers are directly related to the total sun exposure and their frequency is augmenting in caucasian populations. Ultraviolet radiations have a plethora of effects on the skin (immunological, pharmacological, etc.), and experimentally, ultraviolet radiations B (UVB) are able to trigger cutaneous malignant lesions.[21,22] Migrants from European origin in Australia and Israel experience an increase in the incidence of cutaneous melanoma proportional to the duration of residence in the new country.

Hence, it appears that there could be a simple relationship between the cumulative exposure to sunlight and the occurrence of cutaneous melanoma. However, many epidemiologic researchers have failed to demonstrate such a relationship. Furthermore, some studies found a lower risk for outdoor workers than for indoor workers,[23,24] suggesting that chronic exposure to sunlight may induce deep tanned skin, able to filter the UVB better, and hence, confer a certain degree of protection against their detrimental effects. In men, the increase in cutaneous melanoma incidence is particularly important for the trunk, a part of the body generally covered by clothes, while the cutaneous melanoma incidence on head and neck has not increased in the same propor-

TABLE 1-2
RISK OF CMM OCCURRENCE ESTIMATED FOR VARIOUS FACTORS

	ESTIMATE OF RELATIVE RISK[a]
Host risk factors	
History of previous CMM	9
Presence of dysplastic mole(s) and familial history of CMM	148
Presence of dysplastic nevus without history of CMM in first degree relatives	2 to 8
CMM in first degree relatives	2 to 8
Depressed immunity (e.g., in renal transplants, leukemias, lymphomas)	4
High-nevi density	5 to 20
High degree of freckling on arms	2 to 4
Sunburn easily, tan rarely (versus tan easily and never burn)	2 to 5
Blond or red hair	1.5 to 5
Blue eyes	0.8 to 2.5
Socioeconomic status (highest versus lowest)	2 to 3
External risks factors	
Intense intermittent sun exposures	2 to 3
A history of sunburn (at least one versus never)	1.5 to 3
Five or more painful sunburns before age 15	2 to 6
Outdoor leisure (boating, skiing, etc., at some time versus never)	1 to 2
Factors not proven to be risk factors	
Fluorescent lamps	
Use of oral contraceptives	
Factors still under study	
Sunlamps and sunbeds	

[a]The relative risk linked to a given factor informs about the degree of increased risk for persons with the risk factor compared with persons without the risk factor. A relative risk of 1.0 implies no difference in risk.

tions.[9,25] If cumulative dose of solar radiations was the pivotal event, then one would expect at least an equivalent increase of cutaneous melanoma incidence on usually uncovered parts of the body.

These puzzling observations indicate that the relationship of cutaneous melanoma to the sun is more complex than one of total exposure. Other concepts like the "intensity of exposure"[25] were advanced, and studies started to explore in depth the habits and patterns of exposure to the sunlight.[26–28] It appeared that intermittent overexposure to sunlight and the sunburns could be the critical factors for cutaneous melanoma, rather than total lifetime exposure to sunlight. To model this factor, scientists forged the concept of "repeated intermittent exposure to sunlight."[29] However, it must be mentioned that all epidemiologic studies done so far have not yielded results consistent with this concept. A critical inconvenience is the difficulty to decode the multiple forms of exposure to sunlight (i.e., chronic, intermittent, continuous, cumulative, intense, repeated, etc.). Furthermore, this exposure (in terms of the level of UV on the ground and of individual habits) differs considerably between Australia, North America, and northern Europe.

The etiologic processes giving raise to cutaneous melanoma seems more active during childhood or adolescence. Virtually all studies demonstrate that intensive exposure to sunlight during the infancy or early adolescence is more hazardous than exposure during adult life. The increasing incidence of cutaneous melanoma among migrants coming from less sunny areas of the world is mostly true for migrants arriving at young ages.[30] A history of blistering sunburns seems more meaningful if occurring during childhood.[31,32]

Importance of Recreational Exposure to Sunlight

To exemplify the probable key role of recreational exposure in occurrence of melanoma, we present some preliminary results of a multicentric case-control study in progress in Belgium, Germany, and France (note 1). Its main objective is to assess the relationship between exposure to artificial UV light sources (sunlamps and sunbeds) and melanoma. The results presented here are not related to the main study endpoint (exposure to artificial UV sources), but to factors related to recreational sun exposure.

The study started in October 1991. By the end of 1992, 800 cases and controls are expected. Cases are histologically confirmed cutaneous melanoma diagnosed from January 1990 on. They must be 20-years-old or older. Controls were randomly selected from the same municipality as the case, with a frequency matching on sex and age. Because the access to general population registries is extremely difficult in the participating countries, the random selection of controls was performed using a quota sampling method. All interviews were performed at home. Charts were used to assess the constitutional factors such as the degree of freckling.

Up to March 1992, 197 eligible cases and 205 controls were registered. Among the cases, 12 were not interviewed (6 refusals and 6 not reachable). Five controls did refuse the interview.

The study found the usual associations with the host factors, (the ability to tan, the nevi density, the freckling index, or the eye color). The results displayed in Table 1-3 show that cutaneous melanoma is associated with most variables linked to recreational sun exposure. Adjustment by logistic regression for nevi density (on both forearms) and for the skin phototype did not notably modify the results,

TABLE 1-3
CMM AND RECREATIONAL EXPOSURE TO SUNLIGHT. NUMBERS AND (% OF COLUMN)

	CASES N = 185	CONTROLS N = 200	ODDS RATIO[a] 95% CI	CHI-SQ. p VALUE
Has ever suffered from sunburns in his/her life				
Yes	142 (77)	119 (59)	2.25 (1.41–3.59)	0.0003
No	43 (23)	81 (41)		
Painful sunburns before age 15				
None	133 (72)	163 (81)	1.00 —	0.025[b]
1	14 (8)	13 (7)	1.31 (0.56–3.11)	
2–4	12 (7)	6 (3)	2.45 (0.83–7.55)	
>4	26 (14)	18 (9)	1.77 (0.89–3.54)	
Painful sunburns after age 15				
None	72 (39)	108 (54)	1.00 —	0.027[b]
1	49 (26)	33 (17)	2.23 (1.26–3.33)	
2–4	27 (15)	30 (15)	1.35 (0.71–2.57)	
>4	37 (20)	29 (14)	1.91 (1.04–3.52)	
Average number of holiday weeks in sunny resorts (per year)				
None	30 (16)	53 (26)	1.00 —	0.0002[b]
1–2	55 (30)	76 (39)	1.28 (0.70–2.34)	
>2	100 (54)	71 (35)	2.49 (1.40–4.44)	
Sunbathing during hot hours of the day				
Yes	25 (14)	16 (8)	1.80 (0.89–3.67)	0.08
No	160 (86)	184 (92)		
Ever done nudism				
Yes	17 (9)	8 (4)	2.43 (0.96–6.31)	0.039
No	168 (91)	192 (96)		
Was aware of the hazards due to unconsidered exposure to sunlight[c]				
Yes	117 (63)	176 (88)	4.26 (2.45–7.47)	<0.0001
No	68 (37)	24 (12)		

[a]The odds ratio is an estimate of the relative risk linked to a given factor: It informs about the degree of increased risk for persons with the risk factor compared with persons without the risk factor. An odds ratio of 1.0 implies no difference in risk.
[b]Mantel Chi-square for trend.
[c]Before diagnosis of melanoma in cases.

but for nudism, whose odds ratio rose to 3.06 (95% CI: 1.19–7.90, p = 0.015).

So far, those trends are found in all three countries, which underlines the ubiquitous nature of these risk factors. To estimate the presence of recall bias, two "distracting" questions[33] were introduced, one asking if the interviewee had experienced skin wounds (and how many) during childhood, and one concerning childhood food allergies (e.g., to cow milk). Both items are not statistically associated with the presence of cutaneous melanoma suggesting that recall bias is not likely to influence the observed associations.

Artificial Sources of Ultraviolet Radiations

Fluorescent lamps seem not to represent risk factors for cutaneous melanoma.[34] Tanning under sunlamps or sunbeds is becoming more of a prevalent fashion, principally among young people. Given the high-exposure rate, even if sunlamps and sunbeds were small risk factors for cutaneous melanoma, their public health importance would be considerable, with their long term possible consequences on cutaneous melanoma incidence. Most epidemiologic studies done in the eighties did not find any link between cutaneous melanoma and exposure to sunlamps and sunbeds. Modern sunbeds, which generate only ultraviolet A radiation (UVA), are considered to be harmless. Psoriasitic patients treated by PUVA do not display higher frequencies of cutaneous melanoma. However, recent publications started to question the innocence of UVA, urging the development of sunscreens able to protect against them.[35] Two epidemiologic studies, one done in the United Kingdom[36] and the other in Canada[32] found a significant relationship between cutaneous melanoma and exposure to sunlamps and sunbeds. Other descriptive studies underline the possible correlation between cutaneous melanoma and those sources of UV radiations.[37] But people attracted by sunlamps and sunbeds are also more attracted to recreational exposure to sunlight.[37] Hence, voluntary exposure to artificial sources of ultraviolet radiations could simply be a surrogate for intermittent exposure to sunlight.

Studies are in progress to better evaluate the risk linked to sunlamps and sunbeds. A difficulty resides in the fact that exposures to sunlamps and sunbeds in the sixties and seventies were infrequent compared to the fashion in the western countries at present.

OTHER RISK FACTORS

Many studies have reported an increasing cutaneous melanoma incidence with the increase of socioeconomic status.[24,38] But when taking into account the exposure to sunlight during leisure and vacations, the socioeconomic gradient tend to reduce, indicating that high socioeconomic status is associated with more time spent in sunny recreational activities.[39]

Cutaneous melanoma is slightly more frequent among women than among men, but its prognosis is better among women. Biological researches have indicated the possible link with hormonal and reproductive factors. The use of oral contraceptive has been widely studied, without evidence of an association with occurrence of cutaneous melanoma (see Chapter 4 Endocrine Influence on Melanoma). Tobacco, alcohol consumption, food habits, and infectious diseases do not appear to be related to frequency of cutaneous melanoma.

DISCUSSION

To summarize, three factors appear to combine their effects on occurrence of cutaneous melanoma: (1) intermittent and repeated intense exposure to sunlight; (2) a fair skin with a high density of nevi and/or dysplastic nevi; and (3) aggressive exposures to sunlight during childhood or early adolescence with associated sunburns. This conceptual frame is mostly valuable for the superficial spreading melanoma. The nodular melanoma seems less concerned, and the lentigo form remains dependent on the chronic exposure to sunlight, like the nonmelanoma skin cancers.

If the intermittent exposure hypothesis holds, then the increase in cutaneous melanoma is essentially due to the augmentation of intense recreational exposure to sunlight. This concept is tightly connected to a profound change in the behaviors in sun exposure that appeared after World War II. It fits well with the evolution of holidays and cosmetic fashions in the industrialized societies. It is in agreement with the south-north gradient of cutaneous melanoma incidence seen in Europe: people living north have a lighter skin complexion than people living on the mediterranean coast, and they have a greater temptation to go uncovered in sunny areas. It partly explains the most marked increase of cutaneous melanoma incidence on the trunk and the limbs.

Acute exposure to UV light sources for tanning purposes is more prevalent among higher socioeconomic strata,[37] the social gradient where melanoma is concentrated on the anatomic sites normally covered by clothing,[38] and outdoor workers are more likely to pertain to lower socioeconomic classes.

Some scientists indicated the possibility that the depletion in the ozone layer could be responsible for an elevation of UVB radiations on the surface of the earth. If true, this phenomenon could be crucial for the cutaneous melanoma incidence. But to date, there exists no proper international monitoring of the UVB radiation level.[40] However, a recent study in Norway[41] attributes most of the increase in skin cancer incidence to the changing sun exposure habits, and discard the ozone depletion as a possible cause.

Complex questions remain to be studied. It is still unclear whether dysplastic nevi and common nevi are true precursors of cutaneous melanoma, or if those lesions are markers of high-risk patients, like the skin type or the hair color. Answering these questions could have many implications in clinical practice and screening programs: could cutaneous melanoma be prevented through the surveillance of nevi and to what extent? Or does a high-nevi density just represent an indication that skin examinations should be periodically performed? The same question holds for the sunburns: do they act as causal factors, or do they signal warnings against predisposition to cutaneous melanoma?

Another question concerns the possible interaction between some genetic predisposition to cutaneous melanoma and the environmental factors: do genetic trait lead to an enhanced susceptibility to UV light? So far the results of epidemiologic studies do not support the existence of such interaction. In the Danish study,[31] the constitution factors and the factors linked to exposure to the sunlight appeared as having independent and additive effects.

PREVENTION AND SCREENING FROM AN EPIDEMIOLOGIC PERSPECTIVE

There is a strong relationship between survival from cutaneous melanoma and the depth of tumor invasion at diagnosis. The overall prognosis of cutaneous melanoma has improved essentially because patients are seeking treatment at an earlier stage of the disease.[8,9] This suggests that cutaneous melanoma may be considered as a disease suitable for screening programs.

Most cutaneous melanoma are detected by the patients themselves.[42] However, cutaneous melanoma patients are less informed of the danger of excessive exposure to sunlight than healthy controls

(Table 1-3). These observations advocate for putting the emphasis on public awareness on the dangers of sunlight, and on the self-surveillance of skin lesions.

The systematic screening of the healthy subjects by physicians in order to detect early suspicious skin lesions is appealing. In North America, this policy has been recommended by the American Cancer Society,[43] and by several dermatologists,[44] but not by other institutions such as the Canadian Task Force on Periodic Health Examination. General screening by professionals might be very costly and time consuming, and there is no current evidence that this procedure is actually cost-effective.[45]

It is also proposed to promote screening in high-risk subjects.[14] Members of melanoma-prone families having acquired dysplastic nevus and cutaneous melanoma patients are usually aware of the importance of regular skin examinations. But cutaneous melanoma developing in those individuals represent only a small fraction of all cases. Hence, other criteria must be defined to identify the high-risk subjects. This remains largely unsolved and the most appropriate exposure index for predicting melanoma risk has not been discovered.[6] There exists a considerable interobserver variation for the recognition of the relevant skin lesions (e.g., the dysplastic nevus). The definition of several risk factors is not straightforward (e.g., "overexposure to sunlight"), with the danger of inappropriately labeling many people as being "at risk for cutaneous melanoma."

Most important, the risk factors useful for the definition of causal relationships may not perform well as markers of the disease, especially if the disease is rare.[46] If a factor has a relative risk around 2 to 4, most cases will not display it, and hence, will not be identified for possible preventive efforts. On the other hand, the predictive value of positive screening may be low, with the possibility for numerous costly biopsies for nonmelanoma lesions, and to overtreat borderline lesions that would perhaps never evolve in cutaneous melanoma.

Recently, several studies have tried to better identify the indicators (and their combination) that are able to identify individuals at greater risk for cutaneous melanoma.[11,44] The use of host-risk factors (e.g., number of raised nevi, history and tendency to sunburn, degree of freckling) as markers of high-risk subjects seems able to identify a sizable part of cutaneous melanoma. Now, the relevant indicators should be studied as clinical predictors, that is in terms of sensitivity, specificity, predictive value, likelihood ratio, reproductibility, and costs. Their application should be carefully evaluated in prospective studies.

CONCLUSION

In 1982, John A. Lee wrote: "Much is known about the epidemiology of malignant melanoma, but as yet the pieces of the puzzle do not connect."[8] During the past decade, a wide effort has been made by the scientific community to better understand why the cutaneous melanoma incidence is rising at such a pace in industrialized countries. In 1992, it is felt that the pieces connect better.

At present, besides improving the treatment for cutaneous melanoma, efforts should be directed towards preventive programs aiming at reducing the risk from environmental factors (with the evaluation of their impact on cutaneous melanoma incidence) and towards the recognition of the host factors indicating high-risk patients for screening purposes (with the evaluation of their impact on cutaneous melanoma mortality).

Note 1: The following institutions participated in the study: J. Bordet Institute, Brussels (Belgium); Universitad Göttingen, Göttingen (Germany); H.O. P.A, Hamburg (Germany); Saint Louis Hospital, Paris (France); INSERM, Lyon (France). The study is supported by a grant of the "Europe against Cancer" program.

REFERENCES

1. Moller Jensen O, Estève J, Moller H and Renard H. Cancer in the European Community and its member states. *European J. of Cancer* 26:1167–1256, 1990.
2. International Agency for Research on Cancer. Cancer Incidence in Five Continents. Vol. III. IARC Publication No 15, Lyon, 1976.
3. International Agency for Research on Cancer. Cancer Incidence in Five Continents. Vol. V. IARC Publication No 88, Lyon, 1987.
4. Glass A and Hoover R. The emerging epidemic of melanoma and squamous cell skin cancer. *JAMA* 262:2097–2100, 1989.
5. Lancaster HO. The mortality in Australia from cancer. *Med J Aust* 2:93–97, 1954.
6. Tomatis L, et al. Cancer: Causes, occurrence and control. IARC Scientific Publications No 100, Lyon, 1990.
7. Van Der Esch EP, Muir CS, Nectoux J, et al. Temporal changes in diagnostic criteria as a cause of the increase of malignant melanoma over time is unlikely. *Int J of Cancer* 47:483–490, 1991.
8. Lee JAH. Melanoma. In: Schottenfeld D, Fraumeni JF, (eds.) *Cancer Epidemiology and Prevention.* Philadelphia; WB Saunders Co, 1982.
9. MacKie RM, Hunter JAA, Aitchison TC, et al. Cutaneous malignant melanoma, Scotland 1979–1989. *Lancet* 339:971–975, 1992.
10. Lynch HT and Fusaro RM. Genetic epidemiology of the familial atypical multiple mole melanoma syndrome. In: Lynch HT, Tautu P (eds.) *Recent Progress in the Genetic Epidemiology of Cancer.* New York; Springer-Verlag, 1991, 114–131.
11. Greene MH, Clark WH, Tucker M, et al. Acquired precursors of cutaneous malignant melanoma. *NEJM* 312:91–94, 1985.

12. Kraemer KH, Greene MH, Tarone R, et al. Dysplastic naevi and cutaneous malignant melanoma. *Lancet* ii:1076–1077, 1983.
13. MacKie R, Freudenberger T and Aitchison TC. Personal risk-factor chart for cutaneous melanoma. *Lancet* ii:487–490, 1989.
14. Halpern AC, Dupont G and Elder DE. Dysplastic nevi as risk markers of sporadic (non familial) melanoma. *Arch Dermatology* 127:995–1000, 1991.
15. Rhodes AR, Weinstock MA, Fitzpatrick TB, Mihm M and Sober AJ. Risk factors for cutaneous melanoma. *JAMA* 258:3146–3154, 1987.
16. Duggleby WF, Stoll H, Priore RL, Greenwald P and Saxon G. A genetic analysis of melanoma: Polygenic inheritance as a threshold trait. *Am J Epidemiology* 114:63–72, 1981.
17. Holman CAJ and Armstrong B. Pigmentary traits, ethnic origin, benign nevi, and family history as risk for cutaneous malignant melanoma. *JNCI* 257–266, 1981.
18. Grob JJ, Gouvernet J, Aymar A, et al. Count of benign melanocytic nevi as a major indicator of risk for nonfamilial nodular and superficial spreading melanoma. *Cancer* 66:387–395, 1990.
19. Elwood JM, Williamson C and Stapleton PJ. Malignant melanoma in relation to moles, pigmentation, and exposure to fluorescent and other lighting sources. *Br J Cancer* 53:65–74, 1986.
20. Green A, MacLennan R and Siskind V. Common acquired naevi and the risk of malignant melanoma. *Int J Cancer* 35:297–300, 1985.
21. Kripke ML. Effects of UV radiations on tumor immunity. *JNCI* 82:1392–1396, 1990.
22. International Agency for Research on Cancer. Monographs on the evaluation of the carcinogenic risk of chemicals to humans. Vol. 40, Lyon, 1990.
23. Gallagher RP, Elwood JM and Yang P. Is chronic sunlight exposure important in accounting for increases in melanoma incidence? *Int J Cancer* 44:813–815, 1989.
24. Graham S, Marshall J, Haughey B, et al. An inquiry into the epidemiology of melanoma. *Am J Epidemiology* 122:606–619, 1985.
25. Magnus K. Habits of sun exposure and risk of malignant melanoma. *Cancer* 48:2329–2335, 1981.
26. Sober AJ, Lew RA, Fitzpatrick TB and Marvell R. Solar exposure patterns in patients with cutaneous melanoma—A case control series. *Clin Res* 27:536A, 1979.
27. Mackie RM and Aitchison T. Severe sunburns and subsequent risk of primary cutaneous malignant melanoma in Scotland. *Br J Cancer* 46:955–960, 1982.
28. Elwood JM, Gallagher RP, Davison J and Hill GB. Cutaneous melanoma in relation to intermittent and constant sun exposure—The Western Canada Melanoma study. *Int J Cancer* 35:427–433, 1985.
29. Armstrong BK. Epidemiology of malignant melanoma: Intermittent or total accumulated exposure to the sun? *J Dermtol Surg Oncol* 14:835–849, 1988.
30. Holman CDJ, Armstrong BK and Heenan RJ. A theory of the etiology and pathogenesis of human cutaneous malignant melanoma. *JNCI* 71:651–656, 19?.
31. Osterlind A, Tucker MA, Stone BJ and Jensen OM. The Danish cage-control study of cutaneous malignant melanoma. II. Importance of UV-light exposure. *Int J Cancer* 42:319–324, 1988.
32. Zanetti R, Franceshi S, Rosso S, Colonna S and Bidoli E. Cutaneous melanoma and sunburns in childhood in a southern European population. *EJC* 28A:1172–1176, 1992.
33. Walter SD, Marrett LD, From L, et al. The association of cutaneous malignant melanoma with the use of sunbeds and sunlamps. *Am J Epidemiology* 131:232–243, 1990.
34. Elwood JM. Could melanoma be caused by fluorescent light? A review of relevant epidemiology. In: Recent Results in Cancer Research, 102:127–136, 1986.
35. Hawk JLM. Ultraviolet A radiation: Staying within the pale. *BMJ* 302:1036–1037, 1991.
36. Swerdlow AJ, English JSC, MacKie RM, et al. Fluorescent lights, ultraviolet lamps, and risk of cutaneous melanoma. *BMJ* 297:647–650, 1988.
37. Autier P, Joarlette M, Lejeune F, et al. Cutaneous malignant melanoma and exposure to sunlamps and sunbeds: A descriptive study in Belgium. *Melanoma Research* 1:69–74, 1991.
38. Kirkpatrick CS, Lee JAH and White E. Melanoma risk by age and socio-economic status. *Int J Cancer* 46:1–4, 1990.
39. Gallagher RP, Elwood JM, Threfall WJ, Spinelli JJ, Finchman S and Hill GB. Socioeconomic status sunlight exposure, and risk of malignant melanoma—The Western Canada Melanoma Study. *JNCI* 79:647–652, 1987.
40. Editorial. *Lancet* 337:1132–1133, 1991.
41. Moan J and Dahlback A. The relationship between skin cancers, solar radiation and ozone depletion. *Br J Cancer* 65:916–921, 1992.
42. Koh HK, Geller AC, Miller DR and Lew RA. Screening for melanoma/skin cancer in the United States. In: Miller AB, Chamberlain J, Day NE, Hakama M, Prorock PC, (eds.) *Cancer Screening*. New York, Cambridge University Press, 1990.
43. Hayward RSA, Steinberg EP, Ford DE, Roizen MF and Roach KW. Preventive care guidelines: 1991. *Annals of Internal Medicine* 114:758–783, 1991.
44. Friedman RJ, Rigel DS, Silverman MK, Kopf AW and Vossaet KA. Malignant melanoma in the 1990s: The continued importance of early detection and the role of physician examination and self-examination of the skin. *CA* 41:201–226, 1991.
45. Elwood JM. Screening and early diagnosis for melanoma in Australia and New Zealand. In: Miller AB, Chamberlain J, Day NE, Hakama M, Prorock PC, (eds.) *Cancer Screening*. New York, Cambridge University Press, 1990.
46. Baron JA. The clinical utility of risk factors data. *J Clin Epidemiol* 42:1013–1020, 1989.

Chapter 2

BIOLOGY OF MELANOMA DIFFERENTIATION AND PROGRESSION

Jean-François Doré and Stefan Carrel

INTRODUCTION

Malignant melanoma belongs to the few cancers whose incidence and mortality is increasing every year. The incidence of cancer has increased nearly 15 percent for all cancer sites between 1973 and 1987 and melanoma tops the list with an 85 percent increase and during the same period of time the mortality due to malignant melanoma has increased by 29.8 percent.[1] In 1983 melanoma represented the second cause of death among all cancers for Americans under 35 years of age. In addition, nothing has modified the outcome of malignant melanoma in the past 70 years. Metastatic melanoma still represents one of the most difficult tumors to treat, the actual objective response rate of melanoma to chemotherapy being less than 25 percent[2] and the cure rate being virtually 0 percent, while the treatment of early melanoma results in a better prognosis.[3] Accurate early diagnosis of precursor lesions and of primary tumors is therefore of crucial importance.

Malignant melanoma can be considered as a disorder of cell differentiation and proliferation. While normal melanocytes, stemming from precursor melanoblasts, usually undergo a series of differentiation events before reaching the final end-cell differentiation state,[4] they can be arrested in their differentiation process at any given state of maturation, without loss of their proliferation capacity.

Early primary melanomas characterized by radial growth and with limited vertical thickness (<0.75 mm) show a little tendency to metastasize, while the potential for metastasis formation is associated with the onset of a vertical growth phase and correlates with increasing vertical thickness.[5] In addition to morphological features which characterize these stages, a series of monoclonal antibodies (mAbs) have been described which possibly identify surface markers on melanocytic lesions whose expression correlates with defined stages of tumor progression.[6–11] Recent experimental studies of cultured melanoma cells have helped in the definition of the successive steps in tumor development, in terms of nonrandom chromosomal abnormalities, expression of specific antigens, requirements for growth factors, production of endogenous growth factors and expression of growth factors receptors.[12] Furthermore, the transformation of melanocytes or nevus cells with viral oncogenes,[13,14] and the isolation of human melanoma metastatic variants through selection in animal hosts[15,16] will now enable a thorough characterization of the mechanisms of tumor development and progression in the melanocytic system.

MELANOCYTE DIFFERENTIATION

Normal adult melanocytes originate from a precursor melanocyte (e.g., melanoblast) that undergoes a series of differentiation events before reaching the final end-cell differentiation state, as illustrated in Fig. 2-1.[4,17]

Malignant melanoma can be considered as a disorder of cell proliferation.[18] At any given state of maturation, melanoblasts can be arrested in their differentiation process without loss of their proliferative capacity. As schematically outlined in Fig. 2-2 under normal conditions, proliferation and maturation are regulated by specific compounds: such growth factors (GF) and differentiation factors (DF), respectively, induce their target cells to proliferate and to differentiate. The primary event responsible for freezing the neoplastic cell in its proliferation mode is the accumulation of a proliferation factor or factors (PF). Such an over accumulation of PF(s) completely inhibits the differentiation program of the target cells. This arrest at a given immature stage of differentiation is however not necessarily an irreversible event. Thus, PF-mediated activity appears to be subject to regulation by specific exogenous signals including GF and DF. A number of substances have been reported to induce differentiation such as retinoic acid, corticosteroids, prednisolone, some prostaglandins, phorbol esters, DMSO, and cyclic AMP.[19–25] At sufficiently high concentration, DF are capable of interrupting the proliferative cycle by curtailing the transcription of mRNA required for the synthesis of PF and by reinducing the differentiation program. The deactivated neoplastic cell has then the possibility to mature to a nonproliferative end state of differentiation.

Based on the concept that in vitro induction of differentiation in tumor cells is similar to in vivo maturation of the normal counterpart, it is believed that the induction, in vitro, of differentiation of melanoma cells can be a useful model to study differentiation of this cell lineage at the clonal level.

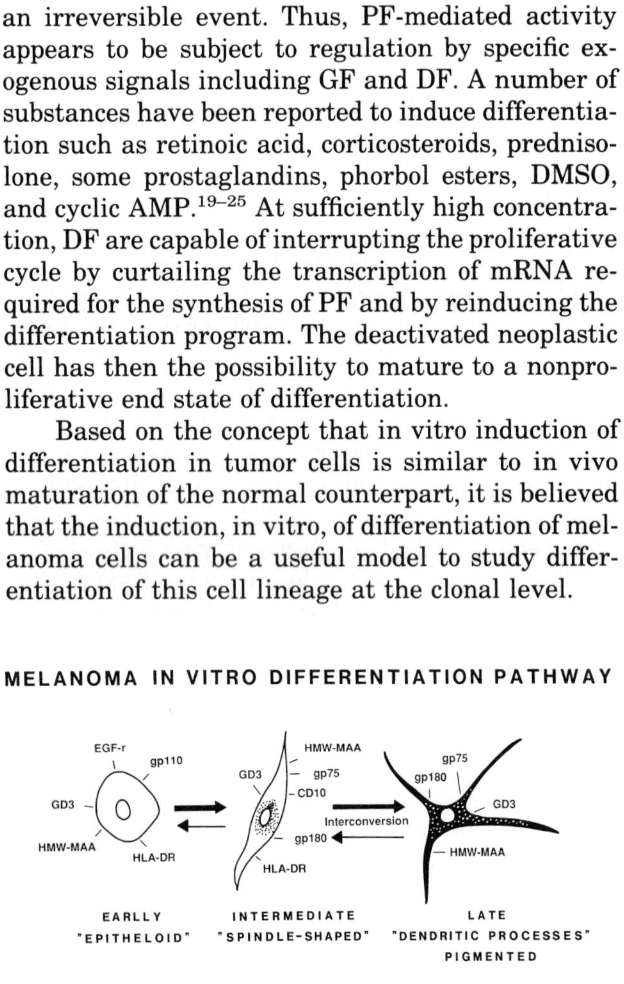

FIG. 2-1. *Pathway of normal melanocyte differentiation based on morphology and on the surface antigenic phenotype.*[4]

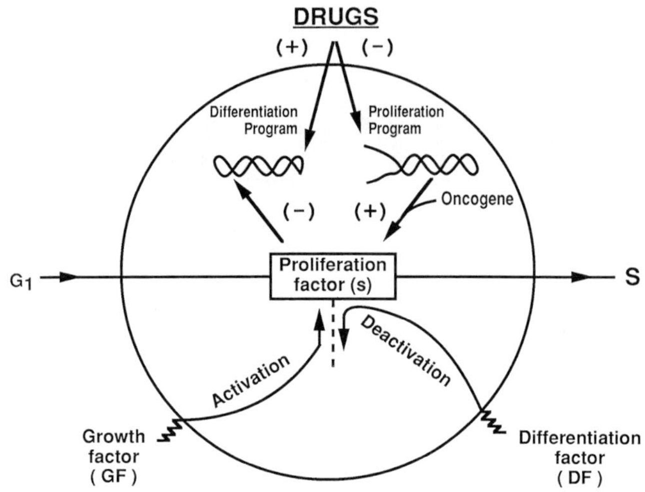

FIG. 2-2. *Schematic outline of cellular events considered to participate in melanoma cell differentiation.*[18]

From previous work, it appears that antimelanoma monoclonal antibodies (mAbs) are able to define a number of antigenic systems expressed by melanoma cells. The expression of some of these antigenic systems seems to be related to a given differentiation state of the tumor cell.[4,17] In addition, the study of membrane antigens on malignant melanoma using a panel of mAbs has shown that these cells express at least three types of antigens.

1. Antigens preferentially expressed by melanomas and other tumors of neuroectodermal origin such as gliomas, neuroblastomas, and retinoblastomas.[26,27]
2. Antigens normally expressed by lymphoid cells (T- and B-cells) such as HLA-DR, -DC, the common acute lymphoblastic leukemia antigen CALLA, and the T-cell antigens T101, LAU-A1, and Thy-1.[28,29]
3. Antigen of which expression can be modulated by interferons, retinoic acid, cyclic AMP as, for example, HLA-DR, -DC, and several melanoma associated antigens.[30]

As illustrated in Fig. 2-3, melanoma cells in culture can be classified into three different categories based on their morphological appearence: early "epitheloid," intermediate "spindle shaped," and late "dendritic." Preliminary experiments showed that interconversion between these very distinct morphological types of melanoblasts can be induced by several drugs. These changes in morphology (i.e., the appearance of cellular projections) seem to be accompanied by consistent changes in the expression of a wide range of antigenic systems, suggesting a transition between distinct differentiation phenotypes.

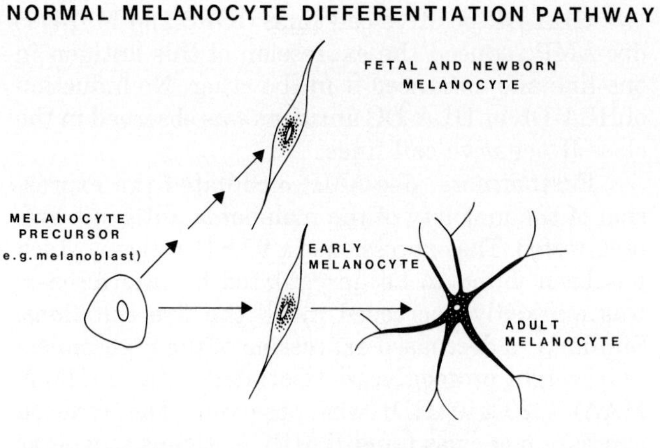

FIG. 2-3. Melanoma in vitro differentiation pathway based on surface antigenic phenotype and morphology.

Cyclic AMP Induces In Vitro Differentiation of Human Melanoma Cells

Several investigators have shown that in vitro differentiation of human melanomas reflects the in vivo maturation of normal melanocytes. Hubermann et al.[21] reported that treatment of human melanoma cells with the tumor promoter phorbol-12-myristate-13 acetate (PMA) resulted in growth inhibition, enhancement of melanin synthesis, and formation of dendrite-like structures. Changes in cell surface membrane antigens associated with morphological differentiation were observed more recently by Ziegler-Heitbrock et al.[24] after treatment of four human melanoma cell lines with the same agent. The effect of retinoids on melanoma cells is more controversial and depends mainly on the particular cell line studied. In some cases[22] retinoids decreased the rate of proliferation and increased melanogenesis; in others, they acted as inhibitors of differentiation.[23]

In vitro studies on mouse melanomas have shown that N^6, O^2-dibutyryladenosine 3′;5′-cyclic monophosphate (dbc-AMP) might act as a regulator of cellular morphology and proliferation.[31]

Treatment of human melanoma lines with the cAMP analog resulted in morphological changes associated with altered expression of cell surface antigens. As shown in Fig. 2-4, cells developed long cellular projections, characteristic of mature melanocytes and electron microscopy analysis showed the

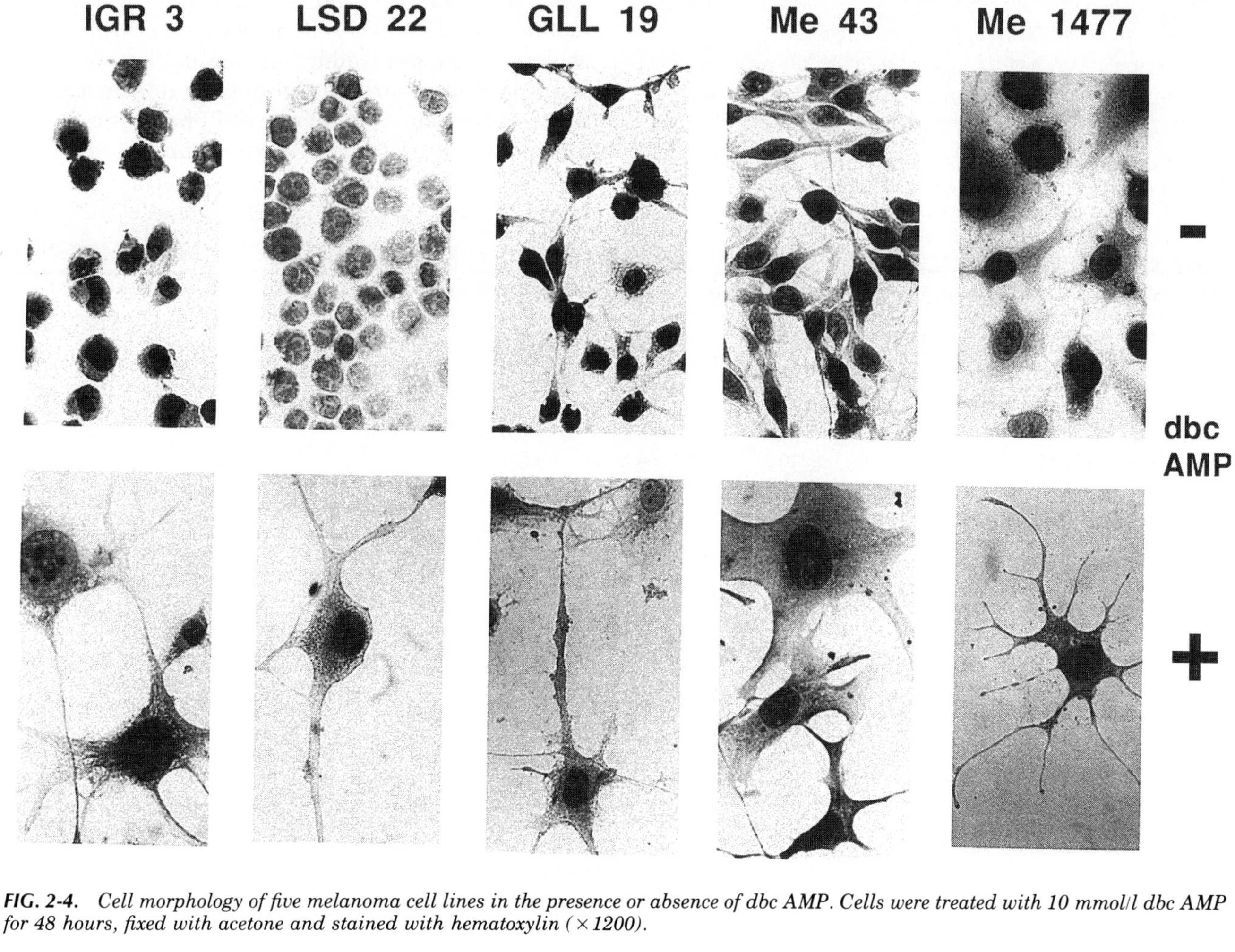

FIG. 2-4. Cell morphology of five melanoma cell lines in the presence or absence of dbc AMP. Cells were treated with 10 mmol/l dbc AMP for 48 hours, fixed with acetone and stained with hematoxylin (×1200).

presence of an increased number of Stage II premelanosomes. In addition, induction of melanin synthesis, detected as brown perinuclear pigmentation, was observed (Table 2-1). Furthermore, dbc-AMP drastically reduced the growth rate of all melanoma cell lines tested.[25] These effects were completely reversible 3 days after removal of the agent from the culture medium (interconversion). Table 2-2 shows the antigenic phenotype of five melanoma lines before and after dbc-AMP treatment, using monoclonal antibodies directed against MHC class I and II antigens and six monoclonal antibodies défining different melanoma-associated antigenic systems. The dbc-AMP treatment reduced the expression of HLA-ABC antigens in 5/5 melanoma lines, while in the two HLA-DR positive cell lines (IGR3 and Me1477) dbc-AMP reduced the expression of this antigen in one line and enhanced it in the other. No induction of HLA-DR or HLA-DC antigens was observed in the class II negative cell lines.

Furthermore, dbc-AMP modulated the expression of the majority of the melanoma antigenic systems tested. The expression of a 90 KD antigen, which has been found to be upregulated by interferon-γ, was markedly decreased in all the five cell lines. Similarly, a decreased expression of the high-molecular weight proteoglycan-associated antigen (HMW MAA) (220-240 KD) was observed. The reduced expression of class I and II MHC antigens as well as the altered expression of the melanoma-associated antigens studied were shown to be reversible after removal of dbc-AMP.

The decrease in class I expression observed in five melanoma cell lines is in slight opposition with the results of a previous study by Hougthon et al.,[4] which have shown that HLA-ABC were expressed on cell lines established from newborn and adult melanocytes. This discrepancy could, however, be explained by the fact that in order to induce normal melanocytes to proliferate, phorbol ester (PMA) and cholera toxin were added to the culture medium. Both compounds are known to alter cell surface antigen expression. Therefore, the phenotype of melanocytes cultured under these conditions, does not necessarily reflect the phenotype of normal skin melanocytes. And indeed, Berthier-Vergnes et al.[32] have

TABLE 2-1
EFFECT OF dbc AMP ON THE MELANIN PRODUCTION IN MELANOMA CELL LINES

CELL LINE	CELLS TREATED FOR 4 DAYS WITH dbc AMP 10 mM	CONTROL UNTREATED CELLS
IGR3	95%[a]	11%
Me1477	92%	3%
LSD-22	90%	9%
Me43	88%	10%
GLL-19	91%	6%

[a]For each cell line, three coverslips of dbc AMP treated and untreated cells were analyzed and a total of 300 cells per coverslip was counted. The results are expressed as percent of cell showing a brown perinuclear pigmentation following dopa treatment.

TABLE 2-2
EFFECT OF dbc AMP ON THE EXPRESSION OF MELANOMA-ASSOCIATED ANTIGENS AND HLA CLASS I AND II MOLECULES

CELL LINE	Me1-14[b] HMWMAA	Me1-12[b] gp97	Me14/D12[b] ICAM-1	Me14/F12[b] 40KDa	Me14/G12[b] 70KDa	Me15/B3[b] 90KDa	B9.12.1[c] HLA-ABC	D1-12[c] HLA-DR	PX63[d]
IGR3[a]									
control	1195	4030	1200	890	1530	2070	1130	1720[a]	220
dbc AMP	920 ↓	1670 ↓	2240 ↑	1500 ↑	1470	540 ↓	610 ↓	870 ↓	190
Me1477									
control	1950	2170	1620	4100	745	2140	2610	1140	100
dbc AMP	900 ↓	950 ↓	1970	5170 ↓	1885 ↑	1080 ↓	1830 ↓	1940 ↑	125
LSD22									
control	460	570	2230	1520	3300	2870	3620	500	310
dbc AMP	340	400	2370	630 ↓	6810 ↑	1550 ↓	1820 ↓	660	240
Me43									
control	790	240	255	1100	2640	3180	3640	140	250
dbc AMP	1130 ↑	440	1350 ↑	1250	3400 ↑	2210 ↓	2600 ↓	160	110
GLL19									
control	890	360	250	1010	1745	3025	3430	550	200
dbc AMP	600	360	310	990	1680	2340 ↓	750 ↓	500	170

[a]Cells were grown for 8 days in the presence of 10 mM dbc AMP. Results (mean value of duplicate) are expressed as CPM of ^{125}I-labeled rabbit antimouse F(ab')$_2$ antibodies bound to 10^5 target cells incubated with the various culture fluids. The highest values are underlined and the changes in antigen expression indicated by arrows.
[b]Antimelanoma monoclonal antibodies (mAbs)
[c]Anti-MHC mAbs
[d]PX63: control culture fluid

recently shown that the addition of the phorbol ester TPA (12-O-tetradecanoylphorbol 13-acetate) to primary cultures of normal adult human melanocytes results in growth inhibition, formation of dendrites, and alters surface glycoprotein expression. TPA-treated melanocytes bind the lectins PNA (peanut agglutinin) and *Bauhinia purpurea,* while normal melanocytes in the skin do not bind PNA. An alternative explanation could be that the reduction of HLA-ABC expression on more differentiated melanoma cells is just one effect of cAMP.

Normal newborn and adult melanocytes do not express class II antigens[4,33] while these are, however, constitutively expressed by a number of melanoma cell lines. It was of interest to note that when IGR3 melanoma cells were induced to differentiate with dbc-AMP, a marked decrease in DR expression was observed. These data are consistent with the observation made by Ziegler-Heitbrock et al.,[24] that treatment of IGR3 cells with the phorbol ester PMA induced a strong decrease in DR expression. These results are in agreement with the idea that class II antigen expression on melanoma cells is inversely correlated with the stage of differentiation. The fact that dbc-AMP treated IGR3 cells still express some DR antigens might indicate that these cells undergo only a certain degree of differentiation but do not reach full maturation. Surprisingly, when Me1477 cells were treated with dbc-AMP, an upregulation of DR expression was observed. Events occurring during the initial process of malignant transformation might be responsible for the constitutive expression of class II antigens. Induction of class II antigen expression by normal melanocytes after the introduction of the *ras* oncogene supports this hypothesis.[13] Both transformation events and induction of differentiation might, therefore, regulate class II expression, which could explain this somehow confusing result.

Individual melanoma cell lines established in culture appear to be arrested at different stages of differentiation and may have a different type of resistance to the induction of differentiation. This might explain why each cell line displays a slightly different surface phenotype and why dbc-AMP treatment did not induce a uniform antigenic phenotype on each cell line treated. Some general tendencies could however be observed. For example, on all cell lines, the expression of the 90 KD antigen defined by mAb Me15/B3 was markedly decreased. Likewise, the high-molecular weight antigen seen by mAb, Mel-14 was also drastically decreased on two cell lines. These results are in agreement with a previous report that shows TPA-treated melanoma cells have a reduced reactivity for mAb 225.28.S, which is another antibody directed against the high-molecular weight antigen.[24] Collectively, these data suggest that a number of mAbs define molecules that are linked to differentiation and could provide useful tools in designing a scheme of differentiation of the melanocyte lineage.

Changes in antigen expression would further allow the classification of malignant melanoma cells to an early, intermediate, or late stage of the differentiation pathway, which would be a diagnostic aid for both prognosis and therapy.

Characterization of Receptors for α-Melanocyte-Stimulating Hormone on Human Melanoma Cells

The α-melanocyte-stimulating hormone (α-MSH) induces melanogenesis in melanocytes and melanoma cells by interaction with specific membrane receptors coupled to adenylate cyclase which in turn activates tyrosinase, the rate-limiting enzyme of melanin formation.[34] The α-MSH also affects the proliferation of cultured melanoma cells; various cell lines have been isolated responding to α-MSH treatment either with increased, unaltered[35] or with decreased[36,37] growth rate. In vivo, α-MSH is thought to have a proliferative effect on both melanocytes and melanoma cells.[34] Since elevated plasma α-MSH levels have been found in many melanoma patients[38] and several MSH-responsive human melanoma cell lines have been established,[39] α-MSH and its receptor are receiving considerable interest at present. The hormone can be regarded as a potential tool in the diagnosis and therapy of melanoma, for example, in the form of an antagonistic α-MSH analog,[34] as an α-MSH-cytotoxin conjugate,[40] or as an α-MSH-antibody conjugate which is directed to T-cell receptors of cytotoxic lymphocytes thus serving as an agent for focusing these killer cells onto melanoma cells.[41]

Such studies, however, require a broad knowledge of the expression and characteristics of MSH receptors on human melanoma cells. Because of the lack of a reliable binding assay for the MSH receptor on human melanoma cells, very little information on its characteristics is available. Recently, α-MSH, ACTH, and peptide analogues have been studied extensively in a mouse melanoma tyrosinase[34–42] and a melanin assay[43] as well as in a radioreceptor assay established for mouse B16 cells.[37] In addition, the mouse MSH receptor has recently been identified by photoaffinity labeling.[44] More recently convincing evidence for the existence of MSH receptors on various human melanoma cell lines by using a new receptor binding assay developed for human cells has been reported.[45] In addition, the expression of receptors for α-MSH on human malignant melanoma cell lines was investigated with a specific binding assay, a structure-activity study, and photoaffinity crosslinking of the hormone-receptor complex.[46] As summarized in Table 2-3 in our study, 10 out of 12 human cell lines showed specific binding sites for α-MSH with K_Ds ranging from 0.195 to 2.87 n*M* and the sites per cell being ~400 to ~1600. Two human melanoma lines (S7 and RPMI 7951) did not display specific binding of [^{125}I]α-MSH. In contrast, the mouse B16-F1 and Cloudman S19 melanoma cells used as positive controls exhibited ~10,000 sites per cell with a K_D of 1.3 n*M* and 4660 sites per cell with a K_D of 0.8 n*M*, respectively. Structure-activity studies with the D10 cell line and α-MSH/ACTH peptides showed (Table 2-4) that oxidized α-MSH had a ~40-fold lower affinity than α-MSH whereas [Nle^4, *D*-Phe^7]-α-MSH displayed a three-fold and the ACTH fragments a 20- and 8-fold higher affinity.

The finding that 10 out of 12 human melanoma cell lines (see Table 2-3) contain high-affinity binding sites for α-MSH indicates that a majority of melanoma lines express MSH receptors. Whether these receptors are expressed continuously during all stages of the cell cycle and in a majority of the cells of a solid tumor will only be resolved when MSH-receptor autoradiography for human melanoma becomes available.

The physiological significance of the expression of MSH receptors by human melanoma cells is not clear at present. As mentioned, some of the cell lines tested (LSD 22, IGR3, Me1477, Me43, and GGL 19) were shown to differentiate when incubated with dibutyryl cyclic AMP; they responded with dendrite formation, reduced growth, an increase in the number of premelanosomes (Stage 2) and a modulation of the expression of various surface antigens.[10] However, a marked pigmentary effect of α-MSH or [Nle^4, *D*-Phe^7]-α-MSH has not yet been observed for the cell lines previously listed. Nevertheless, the presence of MSH receptors on human melanoma cells is of considerable interest for the specific targeting of toxins, other pharmaceuticals or even cytolytic lymphocytes to the melanoma.

TABLE 2-3
CHARACTERISTICS OF [^{125}I]α-MSH BINDING TO HUMAN AND MOUSE MELANOMA CELL LINES

CELL LINE	*B_{max}[a] (sites/cell ± SD)[c]*	*K_D[b] (pM ± SD)[c]*
Human melanoma		
D10	1590 (± 510)	195 (± 42)
LSD22	1518 (± 729)	1040 (± 614)
Me8	1281 (± 500)	2870 (± 1091)
IGR3	704 (± 232)	850 (± 349)
A375	608 (± 134)	410 (± 123)
Me1477	574 (± 304)	420 (± 319)
Me43	478 (± 306)	280 (± 216)
GLL19	467 (± 229)	460 (± 331)
Mel Juso	391 (± 160)	770 (± 370)
S7	no specific binding	
RPMI 7951	no specific binding	
Mouse melanoma		
B16-F1[d]	9570 (± 1750)	1310 (± 310)
Cloudman S91	4660 (± 120)	820 (± 120)

The capacity for [^{125}I]α-MSH binding of the different cell lines and the dissociation constant were determined from competition binding data, using a Scatchard analysis performed with the iterative nonlinear regression program Ligand.
[a]Binding capacity
[b]Dissociation constant
[c]The values are the mean of $n = 10$ experiments with D10 cells and $n = 2$ experiments for all other cell lines.
[d]The dissociation constant was calculated from saturation binding experiments performed with monoiodinated [Nle^4]α-MSH.

TABLE 2-4
POTENCIES OF α-MSH AND ACTH ANALOGS AND FRAGMENTS IN THE BINDING ASSAY

PEPTIDE	*K_D[a] (pM ± SD)*	*RELATIVE POTENCY*
α-MSH	195 ± 42	1.0
Desacetyl-α-MSH	2040 ± 410	0.096
[Tyr(I)^2]-α-MSH	153 ± 8	1.28
[Nle^4,D-Phe^7]-α-MSH	62.5 ± 5.2	3.12
[Nle^4]-α-MSH	1460 ± 608	0.134
[Met(O)^4]-α-MSH	8665 ± 785	0.023
human $ACTH_{1\text{-}39}$	487 ± 253	0.40
$ACTH_{1\text{-}24}$	26.5 ± 5.3	7.4
[Phe^2,Nle^4]-$ACTH_{1\text{-}24}$	48.1 ± 9.8	4.1
$ACTH_{1\text{-}17}$[b]	8.9 ± 1.2[c]	21.9

The dissociation constants for the different peptides were determined in a competition binding study using human D10 melanoma cells and the iterative nonlinear regression program Ligand for Scatchard analysis.
[a]Dissociation constant. The value for α-MSH is the mean of $n = 10$ experiments and those for all other peptides are the means of $n = 2$ experiments.
[b][β-Ala^1]-$ACTH_{1\text{-}17}$-*N*-$(CH_2)_4$-NH_2.
[c]When iodinated [β-Ala^1]-$ACTH_{1\text{-}17}$-*N*-$(CH_2)_4$-NH_2 was used as tracer, the mean K_D was 15.6 ± 1.7 p*M*.

Effect of Interferon-γ on the Antigenic Phenotype of Melanoma Cell Line

Several authors have shown that interferons enhance the expression of the major histocompatibility class I (HLA-ABC) antigens on a wide variety of both murine and human cells,[47–50] while their effect on the expression of class II antigens (HLA-DR) was more controversial. Imai et al.[51] reported that incubation of cultured melanoma cells with partially purified human leukocyte interferon-γ significantly increased the expression of HLA-ABC and B2-microglobulin but did not alter the expression of HLA-DR, and of two melanoma associated antigens. Similar results were observed by Liao et al.[52] with interferon-γ (IFN-γ) using another melanoma line. However, they tested only one melanoma associated antigen of which the expression was enhanced in equal extent as β2-microglobulin. Likewise, no change in HLA-DR antigen expression was observed. Basham and Merigan[53] showed that IFN-γ, but not IFN-α, increases the expression of HLA-DR on HLA-DR positive melanoma cells. Later, several authors reported that recombinant IFN-γ, not only enhances the expression of HLA-DR on DR positive cells, but also induces the synthesis of HLA-DR by melanoma, glioma and colon carcinoma cell lines which did not express this antigen.[30,54] Furthermore, it was shown that IFN-γ also induces the expression of HLA-DQ, another class II histocompatibility antigen in melanoma cells.[30]

Recombinant IFN-γ induces the expression of HLA-DR, when added to the culture medium of melanoma cell lines which did not express these antigens. It enhances HLA-DR expression on melanoma cells already expressing HLA-DR. In addition, IFN-γ also enhances the expression of HLA-ABC and β2 microglobulin, as well as HLA-DR on DR positive melanoma cells. In contrast, IFN-α and IFN-β did not induce expression of HLA-DR on DR negative melanoma lines, while it did enhance the expression of HLA-ABC and of β2 microglobulin. In a study with Me43 melanoma cells, the expression of six out of seven melanoma associated differentiation antigens in addition to HLA-ABC and HLA-DR were enhanced by IFN-γ treatment. Interestingly, none of these molecules, except HLA-ABC, were either induced or enhanced by IFN-α or IFN-β (see Table 2-5).

The modulation of antigens by IFN-γ was both dose and time dependent. A minimum incubation time of 48 hours was necessary for the appearance of HLA-DR on the two HLA-DR negative melanoma lines (Me43 and GLL-19); whereas HLA-ABC and β2 microglobulin were already increased after 24 hours. A dose of 20 U/ml induced a detectable increase of HLA-DR and DQ expression on melanoma cells GLL-19 and Me43 and a plateau of maximum antigen expression was reached with 100 U/ml. Analyses of IFN-γ treated Me43 cells by flow microfluorometry showed a homogeneous distribution of increased staining intensity rather than the appearance of two cell populations (Fig. 2-5). Treatment of HLA-DR negative GLL-19 cells with IFN-α showed no induction of HLA-DR but a slight enhancement of HLA-ABC expression (Fig. 2-5). The induction or enhancement of HLA-antigens or melanoma-associated molecules was reversible when IFN-γ was removed. Eight days after removal of interferon, the HLA-DR level was reduced by more than 90 percent and the induced level of ICAM-1 (Me14/D12) by more than 80 percent (Fig. 2-6).

The observation that a number of melanoma cell lines can be induced to express HLA-DR and HLA-DC antigens by IFN-γ treatment, raises at least one basic question. Namely, whether the enhancement or induction of expression of HLA class I and II molecules and tumor-associated antigens plays a role in the antitumor effect of interferons, since the appearance of tumor-associated antigens in the context of class I or class II molecules may trigger the induction of cytolytic or helper T-lymphocytes, respectively. However, it remains to be demonstrated that in vivo IFN-γ is able to induce or enhance the expression of MHC class I and II molecules and other tumor associated antigens.

Conclusion

Melanoma cell lines treated with either dbc-AMP or IFN-γ were tested with a panel of monoclonal antibodies, defining several different surface antigenic

TABLE 2-5
EFFECT OF INTERFERON TREATMENT OF THE EXPRESSION OF SURFACE ANTIGENS ON Me43 MELANOMA CELLS

		CELLS TREATED WITH			
mAbs	ANTIGEN	UNTREATED	INTERFERON-γ	INTERFERON-α	INTERFERON-β
Me1-12	gp97	810	1600[a]	1100	940
Me1-14	HMWMAA	490	510	520	470
Me4-F8	Glycolipid	300	1500	280	340
Me6-C8	130 KDa	1700	2830	1570	1810
Me14/F12	40 KDa	1100	3040	1200	1220
Me14/D12	ICAM-1	500	2900	630	480
Me15/B3	90 KDa	2070	3250	2100	2030
D1-12	HLA-DR	120	2040	140	110
B9-21	HLA-ABC	1950	3860	2630	4200
Control		130	210	120	140

Cells were grown for 4 days in the presence of 500 U/ml IFN-γ, 1000 U/ml IFN-α, or 1000 U/ml IFN-β.
[a]Results (mean value of duplicate) are expressed as CPM of ^{125}I-labeled rabbit antimouse F(ab')2 antibodies bound to 10^5 target cells incubated with the various culture fluids.

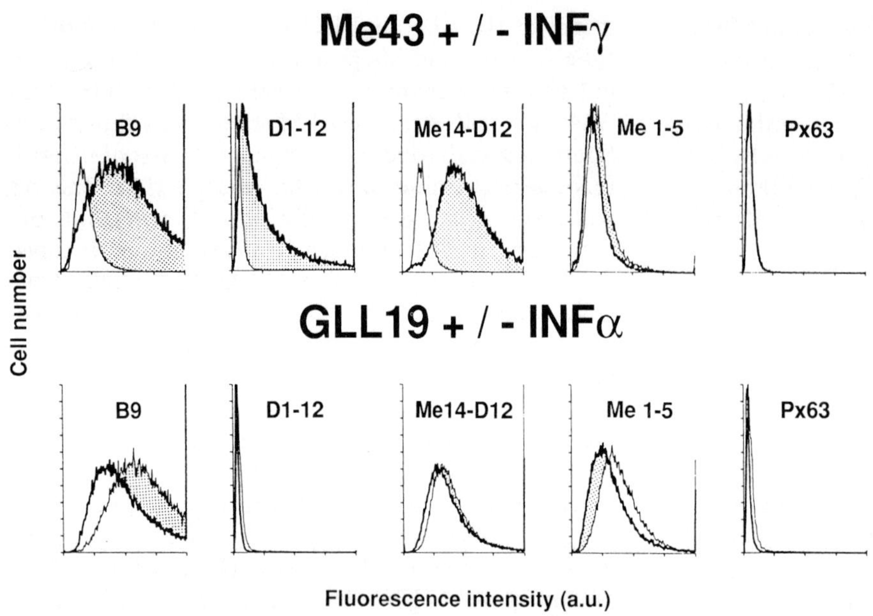

FIG. 2-5. *Treatment of Me43 melanoma cells with IFN-γ and of GLL-19 melanoma cells with IFN-α. Cells were treated for 4 days with 500 U/ml of IFN-γ or with 1000 U/ml of IFN-α. Expression of antigens was tested by 1 hour incubation at 4°C with the relevant mAb followed by FITC-GaMIg. The results are depicted as FACS histograms plotting fluorescence intensity versus vell number. Untreated control cells were tested in parallel. B9, anti-HLA-ABC; D1-12, anti-HLA-DR; Me14/D12 anti-ICAM-1; Mel-15 anti-HMW-MAA; PX63, control culture fluid.*

systems, before and after treatment. Both compounds appeared to modulate the surface expression of the majority of the antigens recognized by these mAbs. For IFN-γ the modulation was mostly in the sense of an enhanced expression, while for dbc-AMP treated cells, the majority of antigens showed a marked decrease or suppression of the expression (Table 2-6). Every melanoma cell line tested appeared to be arrested at a slightly different stage of differentiation and, therefore, may have a different type of resistance in the induction of differentiation. This may explain why each cell line displays a slightly different surface phenotype and why IFN-γ or dbc-AMP treatment did not induce a uniform antigenic phenotype on each cell line.

MELANOCYTE MALIGNANT TRANSFORMATION

Melanoma results from the malignant transformation of skin melanocytes or may alternatively arise from the transformation of a pre-existing nevocellular nevus.[55]

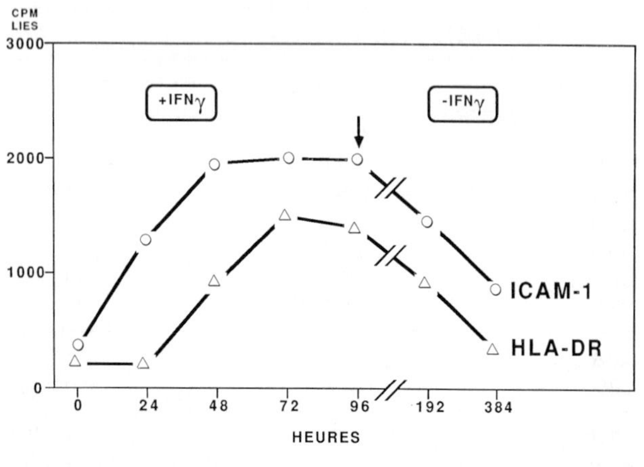

FIG. 2-6. *Reversibility of HLA-DR and ICAM-1 induction by IFN-γ on Me43 melanoma cells. Cells were treated for 4 days with 500 U/ml of IFN-γ and from there are cultured in the absence of IFN-γ.*

TABLE 2-6
MELANOMA ASSOCIATED DIFFERENTIATION ANTIGENS MODULATED BY INTERFERON-γ AND CYCLIC-AMP

		MODULATED BY	
Mab	*ANTIGEN*	*INTERFERON-γ*	*CYCLIC-AMP*
Mel-14	HMW-MAA	unchanged	suppressed
M1-12	gp97	enhanced	suppressed
Me4-F8	glicolipid	enhanced	suppressed/ enhanced
Me6/C8	130 KD	enhanced	suppressed
Me14/F12	40 KD	enhanced	suppressed
Me14/D12	ICAM-1	enhanced/induced	enhanced/ induced
Me14/G12	100 KD	enhanced	enhanced
Me15/B3	90 KD	enhanced	suppressed
D1-12	HLA-DR	enhanced/induced	supressed
Tu312	HLA-DQ	enhanced/induced	suppressed
B9-81	HLA-ABC	enhanced	suppressed

Nevocellular nevus is nothing but a benign proliferation of melanocytes,[56–58] which can be either congenital or acquired. Nevi are rare in children; they appear during childhood and their prevalence reaches a peak by the end of the teenage period or in young adults. Their number then slowly decreases during the adult life. They appear to be more frequent on sun-exposed body areas than on sun protected areas, and are hence, currently thought to reflect sun exposure during childhood.[57] According to the skin layer where the nevus is being localized, one can distinguish epidermal and dermal nevi. But there are also intermediate varieties such as the junctional nevus, localized at the junction between the dermis and the epidermis and which can show intraepidermal "junctional activity," and the compound nevus made from both dermal and epidermal elements.

Nevi do normally evolve during the lifetime: initially epidermal, they show a tendency to embed themselves deeper and deeper into the dermis, which results in their disappearance with increasing age. In most cases, the nevus remains a benign lesion, but in some instances, it can transform into a malignant proliferation. Melanoma frequently develops from a nevocellular nevus[55] (up to 70% of melanoma were shown to originate from a pre-existing nevus in a recent study of 800 melanoma cases—Avril, personal communication). A limited number of nevi may present cytological and/or architectural atypia and are known as dysplastic nevi and regarded as potential direct precursors of melanoma.[58,59]

Factors involved in the malignant transformation of skin melanocytes are still a matter of high controversy. The causes of melanoma and of its increase remain obscure. Epidemiological data gathered over the last decade indicate that melanoma in people is related to both host factors and to sun exposure habits (see refs. 60–63 for review) and fail to indicate any relationship with known carcinogens or promoters (see refs. 63, 64 for review), with the possible exception of polychlorinated biphenyls and benzoyl peroxide.[65] However, the relationship of melanoma to the sun seems more complex than one of simple total exposure, and has therefore been questioned.[66,67] By contrast to epidemiological data in humans, experimental studies have failed to demonstrate the ability of ultraviolet (UV) irradiation to induce melanomas in rodents but have documented the induction of melanomas and precursor lesions by chemical carcinogens (see ref. 68 for review).

Skin carcinomas and fibrosarcomas can readily be induced in mice following ultraviolet irradiation, but melanoma, a rare tumor in rodents, has hardly been induced in mice following UV irradiation. In an experiment designed to test the effect of intermittent exposure to UV radiation, Kripke,[69] almost 12 years ago, obtained the induction of a melanoma in a C3H/HeN mouse that had received over a period of 2 weeks 10 1-hour irradiations ($10^4 J/M^2$) with UV of 280 to 340 nm wavelength, followed 2 weeks later by twice weekly topical applications of croton oil. Under these circumstances, a melanoma developed in 92 weeks in one mouse out of 40 animals treated. This melanoma (K1735 melanoma) was subsequently serially transplanted to syngeneic mice. This experiment has apparently never been reproduced.

On the other hand, melanomas have been induced in mice and other rodents (guinea pigs, hamsters) following initiation by single or repeated applications of dimethylbenz(*a*)anthracene (DMBA) and eventual promotion with croton oil or other promoters.[70–76] It is worth noting that in most of these experiments, the apparition of melanomas was preceded by the apparition of nevi (Table 2-7).

In people, Rampen et al. have postulated that nevi and melanoma could result from exposure to a yet unidentified chemical xenobiotic.[66,77] As a support to such an hypothesis, they have recently reported that nevocytic nevi are more frequent in children following chemotherapy for childhood cancer than in normal children of comparable age.[78]

In mice, Epstein et al. have shown that UV irradiation of blue nevi induced by DMBA in hairless mice could lead to their transformation into malignant melanomas.[79] Romerdahl et al. have recently utilized the initiation-promotion protocol described in 1982 by Berkelhammer and colleagues for the induction of skin melanomas in C57Bl/6 mice,[70] to determine whether UV irradiation can contribute to the induction or subsequent growth of melanomas in C3H mice. The incidence of melanomas in C3H mice treated with DMBA and croton oil was 30 percent. Ultraviolet irradiation of the carcinogen-treated site dramatically accelerated the appearance of the melanomas, although their final incidence was not significantly increased. Exposure of the skin to UV radiation prior to implantation of K1735 melanoma cells also caused an accelerated outgrowth of the transplanted tumors, this effect being rather specific for melanoma cells since it was not observed when fibrosarcoma or hepatoma cells were implanted in a UV preirradiated site. Additional experiments showed that in vitro irradiation of mouse skin induced the release in the incubation medium of factor(s) able to enhance in vitro growth of melanoma cells.[80] Furthermore, Blog and Szabo have shown in mice that the addition of UV-A or UV-B irradiation to a topical treatment with DMBA or psoralens triggers the multiplication of cutaneous melanocytes.[81,82]

Thus, at least in experimental models, mela-

TABLE 2-7
CHEMICALLY INDUCED MELANOMAS IN EXPERIMENTAL ANIMALS

SPECIES	INDUCTION INDUCER/PROMOTER	RESULTS	REFERENCES
Mouse (C57BL/6)	Single application of DMBA[a] in 4-day old mice, followed by bi-weekly applications of croton oil for 7 months	Induction of melanomas in 10–15% mice in 16–40 weeks. Presence of precursor lesions (nevi)	70, 71
Mouse	Single application of DMBA in 7-week old mice, followed 2 weeks later by croton oil applications 3 times a week for 2 years	Induction of melanomas following 25 weeks promotion. Frequency of melanomas varies with strain: 80% in BDF1, 30% in C57BL/6, 0% in DBA2	72
Guinea pig (Mapple-Weisel)	Repeated applications of DMBA	Induction of intraepidermal melanocytic hyperplasia giving rise to melanoma in 4–5% of the animals	73
Guinea-pig (Hartley)	Repeated applications of DMBA in acetone	Induction of nevi in 196 days in most animals, and of invasive melanomas in 214 days in 40% of the animals	74
Syrian Hamster	Intragastric inoculations (×2) of DMBA, followed by topical applications (3 times a week) of TPA[b]	Induction in 40–60 days of multiple melanomas in 50% of the animals	75
Syrian Hamster	Single intragastric inoculation of DMBA, followed by topical applications (3 times a week) of benzoyl peroxide	Induction in 6–16 months of numerous dermal melanocytic foci and melanomas	76

[a]DMBA = dimethylbenz(*a*)anthracene
[b]TPA = 12-O-tetradecanoylphorbol-13-acetate (active constituent of croton oil)

nomas can be induced following exposure to carcinogens such as DMBA, and UV irradiation appears to exert promotion effects. In people, melanoma, as any other tumor, is likely to result from multiple causes and malignant transformation of melanocytes proceeds through multiple sequential steps.

TUMOR PROGRESSION IN MALIGNANT MELANOMA

Histological as well as clinical studies have shown that the evolution of melanomas proceeds through sequential steps of local invasion, and that their malignancy is linked to the invasion level in the skin[83] or to the thickness of the primary tumor.[84] Superficial spreading melanoma (the most frequent histological variety), as well as Lentigo maligna and acral lentiginous melanomas, have no competence for metastasis in their early stages and are examples of indirect tumor progression, while nodular melanoma, with competence for metastasis, is an example of direct tumor progression.

STAGES OF TUMOR PROGRESSION IN HUMAN MELANOMA

On purely histological grounds, one can distinguish melanocytic lesions corresponding to five stages of tumor progression in human melanomas (Table 2-8). The first two stages correspond to benign melanocytic lesions, while the three further stages correspond to the development of melanoma of increasing malignancy and to the final step of metastasis.

With the recent progress in melanocyte culture techniques,[85–87] the obtention of numerous monoclonal antimelanoma antibodies,[88–90] and the identification of growth factors and of their receptors, these progression stages could be studied, either directly on histological sections[11,91] or using melanocytes isolated from normal skin or from premalignant and malignant lesions and cultured in vitro as primary or long term cultures.[17,92–95] Melanocytes have thus been characterized in terms of in vitro growth abilities, caryotype abnormalities, expression of growth factor receptors, susceptibility to growth factors, and expression of antigens.[96]

Characterization of the Progression Steps

The *normal melanocyte* is a cell, which, in the skin usually shows little tendency to divide. In vitro, cultures have been derived from newborn melanocytes, and less frequently from adult melanocytes.[32,86,87] Such cultures require the presence of growth factors: phorbol esters,[85] basic fibroblast growth factor (bFGF),[86] but also insulin-like growth factor (IGF-1) α-MSH and calcium.[96] Their lifespan is limited

TABLE 2-8
SEQUENTIAL STEPS OF TUMOR PROGRESSION IN MELANOMAS

STEP	CORRESPONDING MELANOCYTIC LESION
0	Normal skin melanocyte
1	Nevocellular nevus (common acquired nevus) (programmed differentiation, may present architectural atypia)
2	Dysplastic nevus (architectural atypia and foci of cytologically atypic cells) Marker of individual risk of melanoma? Melanoma precursor?
3	Primary melanoma (early stage) Radial growth phase, low malignancy, no competence for metastasis (invasive tumor of low thickness)
4	Primary melanoma (advanced stage) Vertical growth phase, high malignancy, competence for metastasis (new cell populations appearing as cell foci in step 3 lesion, greater thickness, similarities with metastatic nodules)
5	Metastatic melanoma

See ref. 91

and they do not form colonies in semisolid agar (anchorage dependant growth). Their caryotype is diploid, and they do not produce tumors when grafted to athymic nude mice. The normal melanocyte express receptors for growth factors: nerve growth factor (NGF), and, to a lesser extent, epithelial cell growth factor (EGF) and platelet-derived growth factor (PDGF). It also expresses antigenic markers such as Class I histocompatibility antigens (but not Class II), and adenosine deaminase binding protein, the expression of this latter antigen being lost in malignant transformation.[97] Finally, normal melanocyte do not significantly express in situ the high-molecular weight melanoma-associated antigen (proteoglycan),[11] but this antigen can be expressed by normal melanocytes or nevus cells in culture.

Nevus cells can grow in vitro, this growth being stimulated by growth factors. The lifespan of such cultures is limited, but they have a 1 percent ability to grow in semisolid agar. Some random chromosomal aberrations have been evidenced. As normal melanocytes, nevi grafted onto nude mice do not produce tumors, but they can maintain their characteristic architecture for up to 4 to 6 weeks; it is worthy of note that following topical treatment with a carcinogen (DMBA) some of these nevi may develop cytological atypia.[92] In vivo, nevus cells only rarely express Class II histocompatibility antigens and the intercellular adhesion protein ICAM-1,[91,98] but express the high-molecular weight melanoma-associated antigen. It is not unlikely that some antigenic markers may distinguish common acquired nevocellular nevi from dysplastic nevi.[91]

Primary melanomas can grow autonomously in vitro, but cells from the *radial growth phase* are stimulated by phorbol esters, while cells from the *vertical growth phase* do not respond to such factors. There is only a limited number of cell strains derived from the radial growth phase and the lifespan of such culture is not precisely known, but cells from the vertical growth phase have an infinite lifespan. The typical features of malignant transformation do appear at this stage and are more pronounced at the vertical growth phase. The ability to grow in semisolid agar (anchorage independence) is low (1%) for cells from the radial growth phase, and more marked for vertical growth phase cells (6%); moreover, both clinicopathological arguments and analysis of in vitro growth abilities lead to think that the competence for metastasis is being acquired with the onset of the vertical growth phase.[95] Nonrandom abnormalities of chromosomes 1, 6, and 7 have been described in cell lines derived from primary melanoma in the vertical growth phase. Grafted to nude mice, two-cell lines derived from melanoma in the radial growth phase have not produced tumors, while most of the cell lines from the vertical growth phase are tumorigenic.[95] Cells from primary melanoma strongly express NGF and EGF receptors but have lost the expression of the PDGF receptor. Cells from primary melanoma express GD2 ganglioside and the high-molecular weight antigen. The cell adhesion protein ICAM-1 is only slightly expressed in primary melanomas of low thickness (<.75 mm), but its expression increase in frequency with increasing thickness of the primary tumor.[11,91]

Several features, including the expression of the vitronectin receptor,[99] of ICAM-1,[91] of GD2 ganglioside and of the EGF receptor,[96] tend to demonstrate that cells from the vertical growth phase differ from cells in the radial growth phase and are similar to cells in melanoma metastases.

At the *metastasis* stage, malignacy features are overt. Melanoma metastases can grow autonomously in vitro, they are much less dependent on growth factors. Their lifespan is illimited and they show high ability to grow in semisolid agar (30%). Numerous nonrandom abnormalities of chromosomes 1, 6, and 7 have been evidenced in melanoma metastases. The transplantation of fragments of metastases in nude mice produces tumors with an appreciable frequency, and that of metastasis-derived cell lines produces tumors in most instances, the tumorigenicity of melanoma cell lines being related to the number of copies of chromosome 7 contained in tumor cells.[100] Cells from metastases express NGF and EGF receptors; the EGF-receptor gene is localized to human chromosome 7, and only cells with multiple copies of this chromosome do express high amounts of EGF receptor.[101] Finally, cells from metastases do noticeably express the high-molecular weight proteoglycan, GD2 ganglioside, histocompatibility Class II antigens, and ICAM-1; most of them express histocompatibility Class I antigens, but this expression can be quantitatively diminished.[11]

Antigenic Markers of Tumor Progression

More than 60 different antigenic systems have been identified on human melanoma cells with monoclonal antibodies (see refs. 90, 102 for review) (Table 2-9).

The expression of some among these antigens depends on the progression stage of the tumor cells, and they may help in identifying progression steps in human melanomas (Table 2-10). In this respect, the expression of the ME 491 antigen is remarkable: it is not expressed in normal melanocytes, but is strongly expressed by dysplastic nevus cells and by tumor cells in primary melanomas in the radial growth phase, its expression declines in vertical growth phase primary melanomas and in melanoma metastases.[103–105]

Among molecules belonging to the integrin family of receptor molecules, human melanomas express at least six integrins (VLA 1-6), and the $\alpha_V\beta_3$ vitronectin receptor which may be of importance in the development of tumor invasiveness.[99,106,107]

TABLE 2-9
ANTIGENS EXPRESSED ON MELANOMA CELLS

ANTIGENIC GROUP	*ANTIGEN*
Histocompatibility antigens	HLA-ABC
	HLA-DR
Gangliosides	GD3
	O-acetyl GD3
	GD2
	OFA-I-1 (GM2)[a]
	N-glycolyl[a]
Oncofetal antigens	Proteoglycan
	p120
	p150/95
	p130/105
Growth factor receptors	R-NGF
	R-EGF
Pigmentation antigens	p75
	p50/18/17
Cation binding and transport proteins	p97 (melanotransferrin)
	S-100
	ceruloplasmin
Highly glycosylated proteins	p30–50
Basal membrane proteins	p230
Cell adhesion proteins (and receptors)	ICAM-1 (p89)
	Vitronectin receptor
	VLA 1–6 integrins
Melanocyte and nevus antigens	p110
	p98
	p145
	ADAbp (gp 120)
Cytoplasmic antigens	p94/75/70/25
	p80

[a]Human mAbs

TABLE 2-10
ANTIGENIC MARKERS OF TUMOR PROGRESSION IN MELANOMA

High molecular weight proteoglycan (mAbs Mel-14, G7A5)
 nonexpressed (or slightly) by normal melanocytes in situ, expressed by most of nevi and melanomas
Class I histocompatibility antigens
 expression quantitatively diminished in metastases
Adenosine deaminase binding protein
 expressed only by melanocytes and nevus cells, lost with malignant transformation
ME 491 antigen
 nonexpressed by normal melanocytes, strongly expressed by dysplastic nevi cells and melanoma cells in the radial growth phase, its expression declines in advanced melanomas
GD2 ganglioside
 expressed by primary melanomas, strongly expressed by metastatic melanomas
Class II histocompatibility antigens
 nonexpressed by normal melanocyte or nevus cells, expressed by some primary melanoma and by most metastases
Cell adhesion protein ICAM-1 (MAb P 3-58)
 hardly expressed by normal melanocytes, nevi, dysplastic nevi and low thickness primary melanomas; frequency of expression increases with increasing thickness in primary melanomas; expressed by most of the metastases

See ref. 11,91.

The Malignant Melanoma Cooperative Group of the European Organisation for Research and Treatment of Cancer (EORTC) undertook a large multicentric monoclonal antibody (mAb) study. Fourteen laboratories of seven European countries tested a mAb Panel of 23 antibodies for their immunohistological staining reactivity for malignant and nonmalignant lesions of the melanocytic lineage. A standardized immunoperoxydase procedure was used and the results were evaluated according to a protocol form developed in collaboration with the EORTC Data Center and statistically analyzed. According to this analysis, the antibodies in the Panel could be classified into three main groups. The first group of mAbs includes those antibodies that stained the majority (more than 80%) of all primary tumors irrespective to their Breslow thickness and the majority of metastatic lesions. In addition, these mAbs stained a high percentage of cells within a given lesion. Several antibodies of Group I were also reactive for the majority of nevoblasts and of normal melanocytes. The second group of mAbs included antibodies reacting with a limited number of primary melanomas and metastatic lesions. Antibodies of Group II were only weakly if ever reactive for normal melanocytes or nevoblasts. The percentage of cells within a lesion stained by these mAbs was always rather low. The third group of mAbs consists of antibodies detecting surface structures whose expression seems to be related to tumor progression. Antibodies of Group III were almost non or only weakly reactive with nevi,

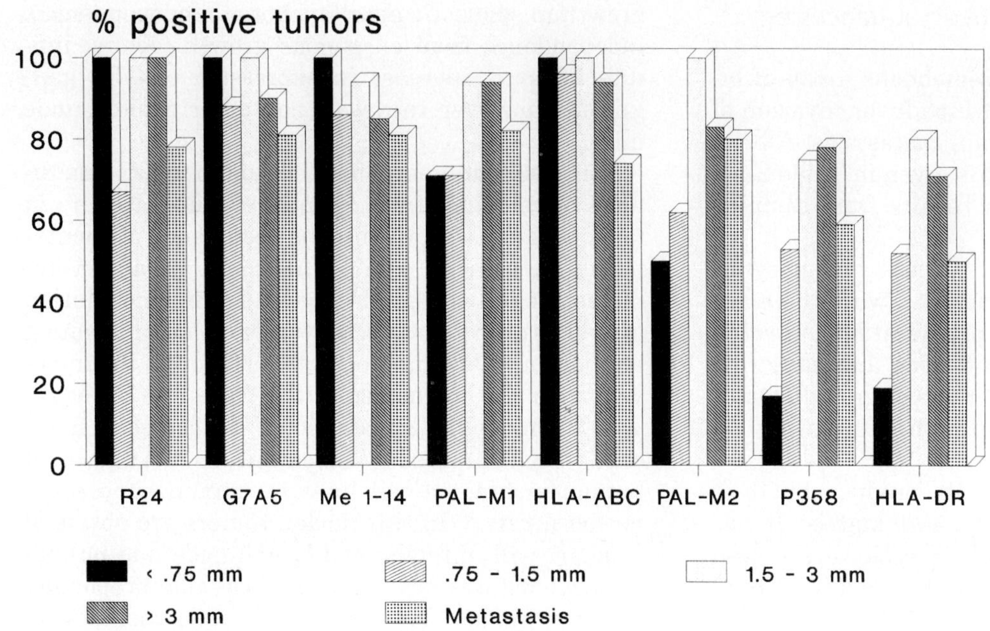

FIG. 2-7. Expression of antigens by primary melanomas of increasing thickness and melanoma metastases in a multicentric monoclonal antibody study.[11] *Specificity of the monoclonal antibodies: R24 = GD3, G7A5 and Mel-14 = high molecular weight proteoglycan, PAL-M1 = gp 185 (CD71), PAL-M2 = gp 95, P358 = ICAM-1.*

they all reacted with a small number of early primary melanomas (<75 mm). With increasing Breslow thickness, the number of lesions stained augmented gradually (Fig. 2-7). This multicentric mAb study showed that the use of a Panel of well-defined mAbs might be of a diagnostic aide.[11]

BIOCHEMICAL MECHANISMS OF TUMOR PROGRESSION

The different steps in tumor progression are likely to result from the activation of genetically determined functions of tumor cells. For instance, in experimental models, the transfection of tumor cells with oncogenes from the *ras* gene family confers the metastatic ability.[108] The production of proteolytic enzymes by tumor cells[109] and the interactions between tumor cells and the extracellular matrix,[110] and with endothelial cells and platelets[111] are of crucial importance in the mechanisms of local invasion and distant metastasis.

Invasion and Metastasis

Invasion is the first step in a complex process finally leading to the formation of metastases. Metastatic cells must locally invade adjacent normal tissues, then penetrate blood or lymphatic vessels, survive in the bloodstream to the mechanical trauma and to host defenses, arrest in small vessels of the target organ (as embols or through direct adherence to endothelial cells), and finally extravasate to reach the organ parenchyme and settle to produce a metastasis.

A three-step hypothesis has been proposed to describe the invasion of the extracellular matrix.[112] The first step involves attachment of tumor cells through specific surface receptors to components of the matrix such as laminin (basal lamina) or fibronectin (stroma). The tumor cell then secretes proteolytic enzymes (or may alternatively induce their production by host cells) which degrade the matrix in the near vicinity of tumor cells. The third step is a forward move of the tumor cell. The cyclic repetition of these steps leads to continuous invasion of the matrix.

Human melanomas express receptors for attachment to the extracellular matrix, release proteolytic enzymes, and a tumor cell motility stimulating factor.

It has been shown that human melanoma cells express a surface receptor for laminin, a high-molecular weight glycoprotein which is the major component of basal lamina.[112] And experimental studies in mouse melanoma have shown that tumor cells are more especially metastatic as they express such a receptor, and that the occupation of the receptor by a laminin fragment inhibits metastasis.[112]

In a series of murine melanomas with different metastatic abilities, the metastasis rate was correlated to the release of type IV collagenase.[113]

Finally, from a human melanoma, an autocrine motility factor (AMF) was isolated which stimulates as well random cellular movements (chimiokinesis) as oriented movements (chimiotactism).[114]

Secretion of Biologically Active Substances by Human Melanoma Cells

Melanoma cells produce a tremendous array of biologically active substances which favor invasion of surrounding tissues and distant metastasis. A brief summary of these substances is given in Table 2-11. Tumor growth and invasion results from complex interactions.

Melanoma cells, but not normal melanocytes, produce a variety of growth factors. Two of these are of special importance in the proliferation control of melanoma cells, acting as autocrine and paracrine growth factors: the basic fibroblast growth factor (bFGF) and the melanoma growth stimulating activity (MGSA).

Nevus and melanoma cells produce bFGF[122] which is found in the extracellular matrix. It has been demonstrated that anti-bFGF antibodies as well as antisense deoxynucleotides of bFGF inhibit melanoma cell growth.[123,124]

MGSA, first identified by Richmond and Thomas,[116] is produced by most nevus and melanoma cells. In normal skin, MGSA, as bFGF, is also produced by keratinocytes.

TABLE 2-11
PRODUCTION OF BIOLOGICALLY ACTIVE SUBSTANCES BY HUMAN MELANOMA CELLS

Growth factors
Transforming growth factors (TGF)
TGFα/EGF[115]
TGFβ[115]
Melanoma growth stimulating activity (MGSA/IL-8)[116]
Autocrine motility factor[114]
Proteases and protease inhibitors
Plasminogen activators (tPA and uPA)
Type IV Collagenase[109,113]
α-2-macroglobulin[117]
Cell adhesion proteins
Host response modifiers
Tumor derived chemotactic factor (TDCF) and inhibitor[118]
Factors interfering with hemostasis mechanisms[111]
Soluble antigens[119]
Gangliosides[120]
Interleukin-1[121]

EXPERIMENTAL STUDY OF TUMOR PROGRESSION IN HUMAN MELANOMA

The direct study of the successive steps in tumor progression in human melanoma will be greatly facilitated by the successful in vitro transformation of normal human melanocytes and the isolation of human melanoma metastatic variants.

Normal melanocytes and common-acquired nevus cells have recently been transformed in vitro by infection with an adenovirus 12-simian virus 40 hybrid.[14] The transformed cells acquired several of the characteristics of spontaneously transformed cells: growth in semisolid agar (anchorage independence), independence from exogenous growth factors, infinite lifespan, increase in expression of GD2 ganglioside; however, they were not tumorigenic in nude mice.

The subcutaneous graft of human melanoma tumors or cell lines in nude mice produces tumors in most occasions. However, the occurrence of spontaneous metastasis in this situation is a rare event; metastases have been obtained following inoculation of in vitro or in vivo selected tumor cells[96] or in young animals or following inoculations through the intravenous or the intrasplenic route (see ref. 15 for review). A model of "spontaneous" metastases has recently been obtained by subcutaneous inoculation of human melanoma cell lines in immunosuppressed newborn rats.[16] In this model, tumors are obtained in nearly all animals, and lymph node and pulmonary metastases develop in a noticeable proportion of the animals. Using this new model, variants selected in vivo and clones selected in vitro have been developed, the study of which has shown an increase in genetic instability of the metastatic cells,[125] and the preferential expression of nonsialylated galactoglycoproteins binding the lectin PNA by the metastatic cells.[126] Further study of these metastatic human melanoma cells will enable the approach of the host-tumor interactions in the metastatic process, and more especially the molecular mechanisms governing organ specific metastasis.

CONCLUSION

Malignant melanoma can be considered as a disorder of cell differentiation and proliferation. Normal melanocytes stem from precursor melanoblasts and undergo a series of differentiation events. In the course of malignant transformation, they can be arrested at any given state of maturation.

Under normal conditions proliferation and maturation are regulated by specific growth and differentiation factors. The primary event responsible for freezing the neoplastic cell is held to be the accumulation of proliferation factors, which inhibit the differentiation program of the target cells. This arrest is not an irreversible event, and substances such as phorbol esters, cyclic-AMP, and IFN-γ induce melanoma cell differentiation: the neoplastic cell has then the possibility to mature to a nonproliferative state. The in vitro induction of differentiation in melanoma cells can be a model to study differentiation of this cell lineage at the clonal level.

We have presented data that clearly illustrate that a number of mAbs define molecules linked to differentiation thus suggesting that such antibodies might help in designing a scheme of differentiation of the melanocyte lineage. Changes in antigen expression would allow to relate the malignant melanoma cells to an early, intermediate, or late stage of the differentiation pathway, which could be a useful tool for both prognosis and therapy. Finally, a better understanding of in vitro cell differentiation and a search for specific agents capable of bypassing the differentiation block which occurs in malignant cells could open alternative possibilities of controlling the growth of melanoma, a tumor which is resistant to most conventional chemotherapeutic regimens.

Melanoma results either from the malignant transformation of skin melanocytes or from the transformation of a pre-existing nevocellular nevus. Some nevi, that is, dysplastic nevi, with cytological and/or architectural atypia are regarded as potential direct precursors of melanoma.

In rodents, melanoma can be experimentally induced following exposure to chemical carcinogens such as DMBA, and UV irradiation can act as a promoter. In most experiments, the apparition of melanomas is preceded by the apparition of nevi.

In people, factors involved in the malignant transformation of skin melanocytes are still not fully understood. Epidemiological data indicate that melanoma is related to both host factors and to sun exposure habits, but do not support the possible role of known carcinogens (the prevalence of melanoma is independant of tobacco smoking or alcohol consumption). However, it has recently been postulated that exposure to chemotherapy for childhood cancer may increase the number of nevi. Obviously, there is a need for experimental models of melanoma induction in people that would enable to directly test the possible role of the multiple factors likely to be involved in melanoma induction.

Malignant transformation of melanocytes proceeds through multiple sequential steps. These steps have been identified according to histopathological criteria and characterized in terms of growth abilities. Antigenic markers of tumor progression have been identified among the 60 different antigenic systems described in human melanoma; a striking feature is that a number of them are cell adhesion-related molecules, such as ICAM-1, possibly emphasizing the role of such molecules in tumor cell motility.

Melanoma cell, but not normal melanocytes secrete a variety of growth autocrine and paracrine factors, such as bFGF and MGSA.

The direct study of the characteristics linked to tumor progression is now feasible, since normal melanocytes could be partially transformed following infection with an adenovirus 12-simian virus 40 hybrid, and since human melanoma metastatic variants have been isolated using new models for metastasis of human tumors in experimental animals. Further study of these selected cells will certainly prove to be of utmost interest in the study of the molecular mechanisms underlying cell differentiation and tumor progression in the human melanocytic system.

REFERENCES

1. New cancer statistics, show, losses, gains. *J Natl Cancer Inst* 82:138–140, 1990.
2. Voigt H and Kleeberg U. Systemisch chemotherapie malignen melanome. In: Voigt H, and Kleeberg U, (eds.), *Malignant Melanoma.* Berlin: Springer, 1986, 235–298.
3. De Vita VT, Hellmann S, and Rosenberg SA (eds.). *Cancer, Principles and Practice of Oncology,* 3d ed. Philadelphia: Lippincott, 1989.
4. Houghton AN, Eisinger M, Albino AP, Cairncross JG, and Old LJ. Surface antigens of melanocytes and melanomas. Markers of melanocytes differentiation and melanoma subset. *J Exp Med* 156:1755–1766, 1982.
5. Breslow A. Thickness, cross-sectional areas and depth of invasion in the prognosis of cutaneous melanoma. *Ann Surg* 172:902–908, 1970.
6. Holzmann B, Bröcker EB, Lehmann JM, Ruiter DJ, and Sorg C. Tumor progression in human malignant melanoma: Five stages defined by their antigenic phenotypes. *Int J Cancer* 39:466–471, 1987.
7. Lehmann JM, Holzmann B, Breitbart EW, Schmiegelow P, Riethmüller G, and Johnson JP. Discrimination between benign and malignant cells of melanocytic lineage by two novel antigens, a glycoprotein with a molecular weight of 113,000 and a protein with a molecular weight of 76,000. *Cancer Res* 47:841–845, 1987.
8. Johnson JP, Demmer-Dieckmann M, Meo T, Hadam MR, and Riethmüller G. Surface antigens of human melanoma cells defined by monoclonal antibodies. I. Biochemical characterization of two antigens found on cell lines and fresh tumors of diverse tissue origin. *Eur J Immunol* 75:3405–3409, 1981.
9. De Vries JE, Keizer GD, Te Velde AA, Voordouw A, Ruiter DJ, Rümke Ph, Spits H, and Figdor CG. Characterization of melanoma-associated surface antigens involved in the adhesion and motility of human melanoma cells. *Int J Cancer* 38:465–473, 1986.
10. Brüggen J, and Sorg C. Detection of phenotypic differences on human malignant melanoma lines and their variant sublines with monoclonal antibodies. *Cancer Immunol Immunother* 15:200–205, 1983.
11. Carrel S, Doré JF, Ruiter DJ, Prade M, Lejeune FJ, Kleeberg UR, Rümke P, and Bröcker EB. The EORTC Melanoma Group exchange program: Evaluation of a multicenter monoclonal antibody study. *Int J Cancer* 48:836–847, 1991.
12. Heerlyn M. Human melanoma: Development and progression. *Cancer Metastasis Rev* 9:101–112, 1990.
13. Albino AP, Houghton AN, Eisinger M, Lee JS, Kanter RS, Oliff AI, and Old LJ. Class II histocompatibility antigen expression in human melanocytes transformed by harvey murine sarcoma virus (Ha-MSV) and Kirsten MSV Retrovirus. *J Exp Med* 164:1710–1722, 1986.
14. Jambrosic J, Mancianti ML, Ricciardi R, Sela BA, Koprowski H, and Heerlyn M. Transformation of normal human melanocytes and nonmalignant nevus cells by adenovirus 12-SV 40 hybrid virus. *Int J Cancer* 44:1117–1123, 1989.

15. Doré JF, Bailly M, and Bertrand S. Metastases of human tumours in experimental animals. *Anticancer Res* 7:997–1002, 1987.
16. Bailly M, and Doré JF. Human tumor spontaneous metastasis in immunosuppressed newborn rats. II: Multiple selections of human melanoma metastatic variants. *Int J Cancer* 49:750–757, 1991.
17. Houghton AN, Real FX, Davis LJ, Cordon-Cardo C, and Old LJ. Phenotypic heterogeneity of melanoma. Relation to the differentiation program of melanoma cells. *J Exp Med* 164:812–829, 1987.
18. Bloch A. Induced cell differentiation in cancer therapy. *Cancer Treat Reports* 68:199–205, 1984.
19. Prasad KN, and Hsie AW. Morphologic differentiation of mouse neuroblastoma cells induced *in vitro* by dibutyryl adenosine 3′;5′-cyclic monophosphate. *Nature* (New Biol) 233:141–142, 1971.
20. Waris T, Rechardt L, and Waris P. Differentiation of neuroblastoma cells induced by nerve growth factor in vitro. *Experientia* 29:1128–1129, 1973.
21. Hubermann E, Heckman C, and Langenbach R. Stimulation of differentiated functions in human melanoma cells by tumor promoting agents and dimethyl sulfoxide. *Cancer Res* 39:2618–2624, 1979.
22. Lotan R, and Lotan D. Stimulation of melanogenesis in a human melanoma cell line by retinoids. *Cancer Res* 40:3345–3350, 1980.
23. Hoal E, Wilson EL, and Dowdle EB: Variable effects of retinoids on two pigmenting human melanoma cell lines. *Cancer Res* 42:5191–5195, 1982.
24. Ziegler-Heitbrock HWL, Munker R, Johnson J, Petersmann I, Schmoeckel Ch, and Riethmüller G. In vitro differentiation of human melanoma cells analyzed with monoclonal antibodies. *Cancer Res* 45:1344–1350, 1985.
25. Giuffrè L, Schreyer M, Mach J-P, and Carrel S. Cyclic AMP induces differentiation in vitro of human melanoma cells. *Cancer* 61:1132–1141, 1988.
26. Carrel S, Accolla RS, Carmagnola AL, and Mach J-P. Common human melanoma-associated antigens detected by monoclonal antibodies. *Cancer Res* 40:2523–2528, 1980.
27. Carrel S, Schreyer M, Schmidt-Kessen A, and Mach J-P. Reactivity spectrum of 30 monoclonal antimelanoma antibodies to a panel of 29 melanoma and control cell lines. *Hybridoma* 1:387–397, 1982.
28. Carrel S, Schmidt-Kessen A, Mach JP, Heumann D, and Girardet C. Expression of common acute lymphoblastic leukemia antigen (CALLA) on human malignant melanoma cell lines. *J Immunol* 130:2456–2460, 1983.
29. Carrel S, Gross N, Heumann D, Sekaly RP, Girardet C, Schmidt A, and Mach J-P. Monoclonal antibody against a "Pan-T-cell" antigen expressed by thymocytes peripheral T lymphocytes and T-cell leukemias. *Mol Immunol* 21:831–840, 1984.
30. Carrel S, Schmidt-Kessen A, and Giuffrè L. Recombinant interferon-γ can induce the expression of HLA-DR and -DC on DR-negative melanoma cells and enhance the expression of HLA-ABC and tumor-associated antigens. *Eur J Immunol* 15:118–124, 1985.
31. Kreider JW, Rosenthal M, and Lengle N. Cyclic adenosine 3′,5′-monophosphate in the control of melanoma cell replication and differentiation. *J Natl Canc Inst* 50:555–558, 1973.
32. Berthier-Vergnes O, Berrux V, Réano A, and Doré JF. Expression of cell surface sialic acid and galactose by normal adult human melanocytes in culture. *Pigment Cell Res* 3:55–60, 1990.
33. Real FX, Houghton AN, Albino AP, Cordon-Cardo C, Melamed MR, Oettgen HF, and Old LJ. Surface antigens of melanomas and melanocytes defined by mouse monoclonal antibodies: Specificity analysis and comparison of antigen expression in cultured cells and tissues. *Cancer Res* 45:4401–4411, 1985.
34. Eberle AN. *The Melanotropins; Chemistry, Physiology and Mechanism of Action.* Basel: S. Karger, 1988.
35. Pawelek JM, Sansone M, Koch N, Christie G, Halaban R, Hendee J, Lerner AB, and Varga J. Melanoma cells resistant to inhibition of growth by melanocyte-stimulating hormone. *Proc Natl Acad Sci U S A* 72:951–956, 1975.
36. Cobb JP, and McGrath A. *In vitro* effects of melanocyte stimulating hormone, adrenocorticotropic hormone, 17b-estradiol, or testosterone propionate on Cloudman S91 mouse melanoma cells. *J Natl Cancer Inst* 52:567–570, 1974.
37. Siegrist W, Oestreicher M, Stutz S, Girard J, and Eberle AN. Radioreceptor assay for α-MSH using mouse B16 melanoma cells. *J Receptor Res* 8:323–343, 1988.
38. Ghanem G, Liénard D, Hanson P, Lejeune F, and Frühling J. Increased serum α-melanocyte stimulating hormone (α-MSH) in human malignant melanoma. *Eur J Cancer Clin Oncol* 22:535–536, 1986.
39. Fuller DD, and Meyskens FL. Endocrine responsiveness in human melanocytes and melanoma cells in culture. *J Natl Cancer Inst* 66:799–802, 1981.
40. Murphy JR, Bishai W, Borowski M, Miyanohara A, Boyd J, and Nagle S. Genetic construction, expression, and melanoma-selective cytotoxicity of a diphtheria toxin-related α-melanocyte-stimulating hormone fusion protein. *Proc Natl Acad Sci U S A* 83:8258–8262, 1986.
41. Liu MA, Nussbaum SR, and Eisen HN. Hormone conjugated with antibody to CD3 mediates cytotoxic T cell lysis of human melanoma cells. *Science* 239:395–398, 1988.
42. Eberle AN, de Graan PNE, Baumann JB, Girard J, van Hees G, and van de Veerdonk FCG. Structural requirements of α-MSH for the stimulation of MSH receptors on different pigment cells. In: Bagnara J, Klaus SN, Paul E, and Schartl M (eds.), *Pigment Cell* Tokyo, University of Tokyo Press, 1985, 191–196.
43. Siegrist W, and Eberle AN. In situ melanin assay for MSH using mouse B16 melanoma cells in culture. *Anal Biochem* 159:101–197, 1986.
44. Scimonelli T, and Eberle AN. Photoaffinity labelling of melanoma cell MSH receptors. *FEBS Lett* 226:134–138, 1987.
45. Ghanem GE, Comunale G, Libert A, Vercammen-Grandjean A, and Lejeune FJ. Evidence for α-melanocyte-stimulating hormone (α-MSH) receptors on human malignant melanoma cells. *Int J Cancer* 41:248–255, 1988.
46. Siegrist W, Solca F, Stutz S, Giuffrè L, Carrel S, Girard J, and Eberle AN. Characterization of receptors for α-melanocyte-stimulating hormone on human melanoma cells. *Cancer Res* 49:6352–6358, 1989.
47. Lindahl P, Leary P, and Gresser I. Enhancement by interferon of the expression of surface antigens on murine leukemia L1210 cells. *Proc Natl Acad Sci U S A* 69:721–723, 1972.
48. Heron I, Hokland M, and Berg K. Enhanced expression of β2-microglobulin and HLA antigens on human lymphoid cells by interferon. *Proc Natl Acad Sci U S A* 75:6215–6219, 1978.
49. Fellows M, Kamoun M, Gresser I, and Bono R. Enhanced expression of HLA antigens and β2 microglobulin on interferon-treated human lymphoid cells. *Eur J Immunol* 9:446–449, 1979.
50. Kelley VE, Fiers W, and Strom TB. Cloned human inter-

feron-γ but not interferon-α or β induces expression of HLA-DR determinants by fetal monocytes and myeloid leukemia cell lines. *J Immunol* 132:240–245, 1984.
51. Imai K, Ng AK, Glassy MC, and Ferrone S. Differential effect of interferon on the expression of tumor-associated antigens and histocompatibility antigens on human melanoma cells: Relationship to susceptibility to immune lysis mediated by monoclonal antibodies. *J Immunol* 127:505–508, 1981.
52. Liao S-K, Kurong PC, Khosravi M, and Dent PB. Enhanced expression of melanoma-associated antigens and β2-microglobulin on cultured human melanoma cells by interferon. *J Natl Cancer Inst* 68:19–25, 1982.
53. Basham TY, and Merigan TC: Recombinant interferon-increases HLA-DR synthesis and expression. *J Immunol* 130:1492–1494, 1983.
54. Houghton AN, Thomson TM, Gross D, Oettgen HF, and Old LJ. Surface antigens of melanoma and melanocytes. Specificity of induction of Ia antigens by human-γ interferon. *J Exp Med* 160:255–269, 1984.
55. McGovern VJ. *Malignant Melanoma: Clinical and Histological Diagnosis.* New York: Wiley, 1976, 47–54.
56. Achten G, and Ledoux-Corbusier M. Naevus mélanocytaires et mélanomes malins. In: Saurat JM, Grosshans E, Laugier P, and Lachapelle JM (eds.), *Précis de dermatologie et de vénéréologie.* Paris: Masson, 1986, 441–453.
57. Armstrong BK, and English DR. The epidemiology of acquired melanocytic naevi and their relationship to malignant melanoma. In: Mackie RM (ed.), *Pigment Cell,* vol 9 Basel: Karger, 1988, 27–47.
58. Greene MH, Clark WH, Tucker MA, Elder DE, Kraemer KH, Guerry DP, Witmer WK, Thomson J, Matozzo I, and Frazer MC. Acquired precursors of cutaneous malignant melanoma. The familial dysplastic nevus syndrome. *N Engl J Med* 312:91–97, 1985.
59. National Institutes of Health: Precursors to malignant melanoma. National Institutes of Health Consensus Development Conference Summary 4:1–6, 1984.
60. Armstrong BK, and Holman CDJ. Malignant melanoma of the skin. *Bull World Health Organ* 65:245–252, 1987.
61. Mackie RM, Elwood JM, and Hawk JLM. Links between exposure to ultraviolet radiation and skin cancer. *J Royal Coll Phys London* 21:91–96, 1987.
62. Longstreth J. Cutaneous melanoma and ultraviolet radiation: A review. *Cancer Met Rev* 7:321–333, 1988.
63. Doré JF, Muir CS, and Clerc F (eds.). *Soleil et Mélanome. Analyse des Risques de Cancers Cutanés. Moyens de Prévention.* Paris: INSERM, 1990, 186.
64. Gallagher RP (ed.). *Epidemiology of Melanoma. Recent Results in Cancer Research Series* no. 102. Berlin: Springer-Verlag, 1986.
65. Wright WE, Peters JM, and Mack TM. Organic chemicals and malignant melanoma. *Am J Int Med* 4:577–581, 1983.
66. Rampen FHJ, and Fleuren E. Melanoma of the skin is not caused by ultraviolet radiation but by a chemical xenobiotic. *Med Hypotheses* 22:341–346, 1987.
67. Cascinelli N, and Marchesini R. Increasing incidence of cutaneous melanoma, ultraviolet radiation and the clinician. *Photochem Photobiol* 50:497–505, 1989.
68. Beattie CW, Tissot R, and Amoss M. Experimental models in human melanoma research: A logical perspective. *Seminars Oncol* 15:500–511, 1988.
69. Kripke ML. Speculations on the role of ultraviolet radiation in the development of malignant melanoma. *J Natl Cancer Inst* 63:541–548, 1979.
70. Berkelhammer J, Oxenhandler RW, Hook RR, and Hennessy JM. Development of a new melanoma model in C57Bl/6 mice. *Cancer Res* 42:3157–3163, 1982.
71. Berkelhammer J, and Oxenhandler RW. Evaluation of premalignant and malignant lesions during the induction of mouse melanomas. *Cancer Res* 47:1251–1254, 1987.
72. Takizawa H, Sato SI, Kitajima H, Konishi S, Iwata K, and Hayashi Y. Mouse skin melanoma induced in two stage chemical carcinogenesis with 7,12 dimethylbenz(*a*)anthracene and croton oil. *Carcinogenesis* 6:921–923, 1985.
73. Clark WH, Min BH, and Klingman LHL. The developmental biology of induced malignant melanomas in guinea pigs and a comparison with other neoplastic systems. *Cancer Res* 36:4079–4091, 1976.
74. Pawlowski A, Haberman HF, and Menon IA. Skin melanoma induced by 7,12 dimethylbenzanthracene in albino guinea pigs and its similarities to skin melanoma of humans. *Cancer Res* 40:3652–3660, 1980.
75. Goertler K, Loehrke H, Schweizer J, and Hesse B. Two-stage tumorigenesis of dermal melanocytes in the back skin of the syrian golden hamster using systemic initiation with 7,12 dimethylbenz(a)anthracene and topical promotion with 12-O-tetradecanoylphorbol 13-acetate. *Cancer Res* 40:155–161, 1980.
76. Schweizer J, Loehrke H, Edler L, and Goertler K. Benzoyle peroxide promotes the formation of melanotic tumors in the skin of 7,12 dimethylbenz(a)anthracene-initiated syrian golden hamsters. *Carcinogenesis* 8:479–482, 1987.
77. Rampen FH, Fleuren BA, De Boo TM, and Lemmens WA. Prevalence of common "acquired" naevi and dysplastic naevi is not related to ultraviolet exposure. *J Am Acad Dermatol* 18:679–683, 1988.
78. De Wit PE, De Vaan GA, De Boo TM, Lemmens WA, and Rampen FH. Prevalence of naevocytic naevi after chemotherapy for childhood cancer. *Med Pediatr Oncol* 18:336–338, 1990.
79. Epstein JH, Epstein WL, and Nakai T. Production of melanomas from DMBA induced blue nevi in hairless mice with ultraviolet light. *J Natl Cancer Inst* 38:19–30, 1967.
80. Romerdahl CA, Donawho C, Fidler IJ, and Kripke ML. Effect of ultraviolet-B radiation on the in vivo growth of murine melanoma cells. *Cancer Res* 48:4007–4010, 1988.
81. Blog FB, and Szabo G. The effects of psoralen and UVA (PUVA) on epidermal melanocytes of the tail of C57BL mice. *J Invest Dermatol* 73:533–537, 1979.
82. Blog FB, and Szabo G. The effects of UVB and 7,12-dimethylbenz(a)anthracene (DMBA) on epidermal melanocytes of the tail of C57BL mice. *J Invest Dermatol* 73:538–544, 1979.
83. Clark WH. A classification of malignant melanoma in man correlated with histogenesis and biological behaviour. In: Montagna W and Hu F (eds.), *The Pigmentary System.* New York: Pergamon Press, 1967, 621–647.
84. Breslow A. Thickness, cross-sectional areas and depth of invasion in the prognosis of cutaneous melanoma. *Ann Surg* 172:902–908, 1970.
85. Eisinger M, and Marko O. Selective proliferation of normal human melanocytes *in vitro* in the presence of phorbol ester and cholera toxin. *Proc Natl Acad Sci U S A* 79:2018–2024, 1982.
86. Gilchrest BA, Vrabel MA, Flynn E, and Szabo G. Selective cultivation of human melanocytes from newborn and adult epidermis. *J Invest Dermatol* 83:370–377, 1984.
87. Medrano EM, and Nordlund JJ. Successful cultures of adult human melanocytes obtained from normal and vitiligo donors. *J Invest Dermatol* 95:441–445, 1990.

88. Houghton AN, Eisinger M, Albino AP, Cairncross JG, and Old LJ. Surface antigens of melanocytes and melanomas. Markers of melanocyte differentiation and melanoma subsets. *J Exp Med* 156:1755–1766, 1982.
89. Koprowski H, Steplewski Z, Herlyn D, and Herlyn M. Study of antibodies against human melanoma produced by somatic cell hybrids. *Proc Natl Acad Sci U S A* 75:3405–3408, 1978.
90. Reisfeld RA. Antigen repertoire of human melanoma. In: Bagnara JT (ed.), *Advances in Pigment Cell Research*. New York: Alan R. Liss, 1988, 343–360.
91. Holzmann B, Bröcker EB, Lehman JM, et al. Tumor progression in human malignant melanoma: Five stages defined by their antigenic phenotypes. *Int J Cancer* 39:466–471, 1987.
92. Herlyn D, Helder DE, Bondi E, et al. Human cutaneous nevi transplanted onto nude mice: A model for the study of lesional steps in tumor progression. *Cancer Res* 46:1339–1343, 1986.
93. Herlyn M, Balaban G, Benicelli J, et al. Primary melanoma cells of the vertical growth phase: Similarities to metastatic cells. *J Natl Cancer Inst* 74:283–290, 1985.
94. Herlyn M, Clark WH, Rodeck U, Mancianti ML, Jambrosic J, and Koprowski H. Biology of tumor progression in human melanocytes. *Lab Invest* 56:461–474, 1987.
95. Herlyn M, Thurin J, Balaban G, et al. Characteristics of cultured human melanocytes isolated from different stages of tumor progression. *Cancer Res* 45:5070–5076, 1985.
96. Herlyn M. Human melanoma: Development and progression. *Cancer Met Rev* 9:101–112, 1990.
97. Houghton AN, Albino AP, Cordon-Cardo C, Davis LJ, and Eisinger M. Cell surface antigens of human melanocytes and melanoma. *J Exp Med* 167:197–212, 1988.
98. Johnson JP, Stade BG, Hupke U, Holzman B, and Riethmuller G. The melanoma progression associated antigen P3-58 is identical to the intercellular adhesion molecule ICAM-1. *Immunobiol* 178:275–279, 1988.
99. Albeida SM, Mette SA, Elder DE, Stewart RM, Damjanovich L, Herlyn M, and Buck CA. Integrin distribution in malignant melanoma: Association of the β_3 subunit with tumor progression. *Cancer Res* 50:6757–6764, 1990.
100. Bertrand S, Jacubovich R, Cabrillat H, Thomasset N, Doré JF. Karyotype and tumorigenicity in nude mice of human melanoma cell lines. In Sordat B (ed.), *Immune Deficient Animals*. Bâle: Karger, 1984, 220–223.
101. Koprowski H, Herlyn M, Balaban G, Parmiter A, Rose AH, and Nowell PC. Expression of the epidermal growth factor receptor correlates with increased dosage of chromosome 7 in malignant melanoma. *Somatic Cell Genet* 11:297–302, 1985.
102. Herlyn M, and Koprowski H. Melanoma antigens: Immunological and biological characterization and clinical significance. *Ann Rev Immunol* 6:283–308, 1988.
103. Atkinson B, Ernst CS, Ghrist BFD, et al. Identification of melanoma-associated antigens using fixed tissue screening of antibodies. *Cancer Res* 44:2577–2581, 1984.
104. Atkinson B, Ernst CS, Ghrist BFD, et al. Monoclonal antibody to a highly glycosylated protein reacts in fixed tissue with melanoma and other tumors. *Hybridoma* 4:243–255, 1985.
105. Hotta H, Ross AH, Huebner K, et al. Molecular cloning and characterization of an antigen associated with early stages of melanoma tumor progression. *Cancer Res* 48:2955–2962, 1988.
106. Boukerche H, Berthier-Vergnes O, Bailly M, Doré JF, Leung LK, and McGregor JL. A monoclonal antibody (LYP18) directed against the blood platelet glycoprotein IIb/IIIa complex inhibits human melanoma growth *in vivo*. *Blood* 74:909–912, 1989.
107. McGregor B, McGregor JL, Weiss LM, Wood GS, Hu CH, Boukerche H, and Warnke RA. Presence of cytoadhesins (IIb/IIIa-like glycoproteins) on human metastatic melanomas but not on benign melanocytes. *Am J Clin Pathol* 92:495–499, 1989.
108. Nicolson GL. Tumor oncogene expression and the metastatic phenotype. *Cancer Met Rev* 3:25–57, 1986.
109. Liotta LA, Thorgeirsson UP, and Garbisa S. Role of collagenases in tumor cell invasion. *Cancer Met Rev* 1:277–279, 1982.
110. Liotta LA, Guirguis R, and Stracke M. Biology of melanoma invasion and metastasis. *Pigment Cell Res* 11:5–15, 1987.
111. Weiss L, Orr FW, and Honn KV. Interactions of cancer cells with microvasculature during metastasis. *FASEB J* 2:12–21, 1988.
112. Liotta LA. Tumor invasion and metastases—Role of the extracellular matrix. *Cancer Res* 46:1–7, 1986.
113. Liotta LA, Guirguis R, and Stracke M. Biology of melanoma invasion and metastasis. *Pigment Cell Res* 1:5–15, 1987.
114. Liotta LA, Mandler R, Murano G, Katz DA, Gordon RK, Chiang PK, and Schiffmann E. Tumor cell autocrine motility factor. *Proc Natl Acad Sci U S A* 83:3302–3306, 1986.
115. Roberts AB, and Sporn MB. Transforming growth factor β. *Adv Cancer Res* 51:107–145, 1988.
116. Richmond A, and Thomas HG. Melanoma growth stimulatory activity. *J Cell Physiol* 129:375–380, 1986.
117. Bizik J, Lizonova A, Grofova M, Bertrand S, and Doré JF. Clonal variation in the production of α2-macroglobulin in a malignant human melanoma and association with growth stimulation. *Cancer Res* 49:983–990, 1989.
118. Benomar A, Ming WJ, Taraboletti G, Ghezzi P, Mantovani A, and Doré JF. Chemotactic factor and P15E-related inhibitor in human melanoma cell lines with different macrophage content and tumorigenicity in nude mice. *J Immunol* 138:2372–2379, 1987.
119. Jacubovich R, and Doré JF. Tumor associated antigens in culture medium of malignant melanoma cell strains. *Cancer Immunol Immunother* 7:59–66, 1979.
120. Portoukalian J. Immunoregulatory activity of gangliosides shed by malignant tumors. In Oettgen HF (ed.), *Gangliosides and Cancer*. Weinheim: VCH Publishers, 1989, 209–216.
121. Benicelli JL, Elias J, Kern J, and Guerry D. Production of interleukin 1 activity by cultured human melanoma cells. *Cancer Res* 49:930–935, 1989.
122. Scott G, Stoler M, Sarkar S, and Halaban R. Localization of basic fibroblast growth factor mRNA in melanocytic lesions by in situ hybridization. *J Invest Dermatol* 96:318–322, 1991.
123. Halaban R, Kwon BS, Ghosh S, Delli Bovi P, and Baird A. bFGF as an autocrine growth factor for human melanoma. *Oncogene Res* 3:177–186, 1988.
124. Becker D, Meier CB, and Herlyn M. Proliferation of human malignant melanoma is inhibited by antisense oligodeoxynucleotides targeted against fibroblast growth factor. *EMBO J* 8:3685–3691, 1989.
125. Bailly M, Bertrand S, and Doré JF. Increased spontaneous mutation rates and prevalence of karyotype abnormalities in highly metastatic melanoma cell lines. *Melanoma Res* 3:51–61, 1993.
126. Berthier-Vergnes O, Zebda N, Bailly M, Bailly C, Doré JF, Thomas L, and Cochran AJ. Expression of peanut agglutinin-binding glycoconjugates in primary melanomas with high risk of metastases. *Lancet* 341:1292, 1993.

Chapter 3

IMMUNOLOGY OF MELANOMA

Zohreh Farzad, William H. McBride, and Alistair J. Cochran

INTRODUCTION

The incidence of human cutaneous melanoma in the United States is increasing. It is estimated that one out of every 100 persons born today will develop melanoma[1] and that, by virtue of its metastatic tendencies, melanoma will continue to account for the vast majority of deaths from cutaneous neoplasms. The predictors that a patient with Stage I malignant melanoma will develop metastases remain the measured thickness and depth of invasion of the primary tumor. In Stage II the number of lymph nodes that contain metastatic melanoma index likely outcome.[2] Spread to the regional lymph nodes is a preferred route for this neoplasm.

Immune factors appear to be more involved in the progression of melanoma than in many other cancers. Although malignant melanoma represents less than 1 percent of cancer deaths, it accounts for 11 percent of cases of spontaneous cancer regression.[3] A number of different tumor antigens have been defined on melanoma cells by the use of monoclonal antibodies of both human and murine origin. Humoral and cellular responses by patients to melanoma associated antigens have been described, and clonal analysis of tumor infiltrating lymphocytes has demonstrated the presence within the tumor of potentially cytotoxic lymphocytes that can show a degree of tumor-selective lysis. Transfusions of blood from patients with spontaneous regression have been reported to induce regressions of malignant melanoma in transfusion recipients.[4] All of this immunological evidence, taken together with the finding that melanoma appears to show more frequent responses to immunotherapy regimes than other solid tumors, has fostered belief that melanoma is one of the more immunogenic human tumors. Despite this, many melanomas grow progressively, metastasize, and eventually kill the host. Several mechanisms have been described whereby tumor cells may evade the host's defense and grow progressively. These include reduction in frequency, changes in or loss of expression of antigens at the cell surface (antigenic modulation), immunologic tolerance, and immunosuppression.[4] The exact importance of any particular escape mechanism has not been determined and may vary at different stages of tumor evolution.

In his short review we will use only selected experimental observations to highlight points that we believe to be pertinent to the immunology of melanoma. We are mindful that we are not citing numerous excellent publications on this subject that have been instrumental in developing these concepts, but space considerations dictate that this cannot be an exhaustive review.

SPONTANEOUS IMMUNE REACTION

The spontaneous regression of established melanomas is a rare but well-documented phenomenon. More common is the focal regression found in primary melanomas. This histologic regression is associated with an infiltrate predominantly consisting of T lymphocytes, but with scattered B lymphocytes, macrophages, and Langerhans cells. Later there is tumor replacement by fibrovascular scarring.[5] T cells in early melanoma lesions express IL2R and HLA-DR antigens indicating that they are activated.[6] Histologic regression is most frequently associated with the radial growth of superficial spreading melanoma and is less evident in vertically growing tumor. There is an ongoing controversy about the prognostic significance of regression. Most recent studies conclude that histologic regression within the primary tumor has no significant correlation with survival for patients if other major prognostic indicators are equivalent[7–9] or that the prognosis is worse.[10] However, it is generally considered that a histologic infiltrate is evidence of an attempt by the host to keep tumor in check. The isolation of tumor infiltrating lymphocytes from melanoma that can be stimulated in vitro to display selective tumor cytotoxicity lends support to this belief. However, it should be remembered that cells can be attracted to a site by a wide variety of nonspecific factors some of which may be produced by tumor cells, and that an infiltrate *per se* does not necessarily reflect an ongoing immune response. Also the interaction of tumor and infiltrate is as likely to result in enhanced tumor growth as tumor growth inhibition due to the release of growth factors to which the tumor can respond.

MELANOMA ASSOCIATED ANTIGENS (MAA)

There has been considerable debate as to whether human cancers ever express unique "neoantigens" as are found on some chemically induced murine tumors. Most of the immune responses that have been demonstrated in humans are against tumor cell surface molecules that are altered in a quantitative rather than a qualitative way or that are expressed at an inappropriate time in development.[11] A series of different steps in the malignant transformation of melanocytes and evidence of antigenic changes that accompany this complex process are well reviewed by Parmiani et al.[12] and Ferrone et al.[13] The major question in attempts to develop active immunotherapy is how best to stimulate "autoimmune" responses against these antigens.

Several classes of melanoma associated antigens (MAA) have been identified. MAA were first identified in melanoma cell membrane and cytoplasm using sera of patients suffering from malignant melanoma[14,15] and from spent culture medium of human malignant melanoma cell lines.[16,17] A murine monoclonal antibody (JSI) raised against a fetal antigen purified from the spent serum-free culture medium of a human melanoma cell line, UCLA-SO-M14, identified a molecule of 31 kDa to 42.7 kDa[18] present on melanoma, carcinoma, and sarcoma cell lines, but not on cell lines derived from normal skin or lung. Experiments have indicated the presence of a common MAA which is excreted in the patients' urine.[19] The urines of 68 percent of melanoma patients were also found to contain a high molecular weight glycoprotein (590-620 kDa), which was expressed by melanoma cells. This antigen reacted with autologous antibody[20] and has been termed urinary tumor-associated antigen (U-TAA).

Of particular interest in melanoma are the ganglioside antigens. The oncofetal antigen (OFA-I), a tumor-associated fetal antigen, described by Irie and coworkers,[21] was later identified as a ganglioside. The OFA-1 antigen is present on a variety of malignant cells in addition to melanoma.[4] Tumor tissues of malignant melanoma have a high content of gangliosides compared to other tumors, and their ganglioside profile is different from that of normal tissues. Normal melanocytes express predominantly GM3, whereas melanomas express mainly GD3. The expression of other molecules such as GM2, GD2, O-acetyl GD3 and *N*-glycolyl-containing gangliosides is also changed, with different tumors having individual profiles.[22] Melanoma-associated gangliosides are shed into the tumor microenvironment and into the circulation, and thereby can affect immune responses. There is evidence that circulating gangliosides may induce immune suppression in tumor-bearing hosts.[23] They are capable of binding to lymphokines, such as interleukin 2,[24] and have inhibitory effects on both B and T cell proliferation in vitro[25] and on macrophage functions.[26]

Other antigens that have been described on melanoma cells include high molecular weight antigens (HMW-MAA),[27,28] neuroglandular antigen (NGA),[29] and Hanganutziu-Deicher (H-D) antigen.[30] A seemingly unique antigenic epitope (FD) of human melanoma has been identified on the common glycoprotein gp95/p97 that is detectable in sera of melanoma patients.[31] Another antigen, P3.58, which is homologous to intercellular-adhesion molecule 1 (ICAM-1), appears to be associated with tumor progression. This antigen is consistently expressed on advanced malignant melanoma, but rarely found on early melanomas or benign nevi.[32] Most recently recombinant DNA technology has been used to produce a M_r 100,000 human MAA cell surface glycoprotein,[33] which is perhaps indicative of the future of this field.

Quantitative alterations in the expression of molecules from superfamilies that have known immunological functions have been described in melanoma. HLA-Class II antigens are frequently expressed on melanoma cells as they are on melanocytes in the early phases of differentiation.[34] Class II HLA-DR, ICAM-1, and MUC18 (a molecule that shows homology to NCAM) are only rarely expressed on melanocytic nevi and thin melanomas, but such molecules are found on 70–80 percent of metastatic melanomas.[32] The known functions of these cytokine-inducible cell adhesion molecules in immune responses and the clear association between the expression of these molecules and the development of metastatic disease suggests a role for the immune system in disease progression. The functional link has, however, yet to be forged. HLA-DR expression on primary melanomas is associated with antigen presenting function as measured by proliferation of autologous lymphocytes[35] while, on the contrary, the presence of DR on metastatic melanoma cells appears to have a negative immunoregulatory role[36] for reasons that are unknown.

MURINE MONOCLONAL ANTI-MELANOMA ANTIBODIES

A large number of murine monoclonal antibodies (MoAb) have been raised to MAA[25] and are finding increasing usage in the diagnosis and therapy of melanoma. The list is too extensive to cover here but in our own division several MoAbs have been produced and characterized that serve as examples. A 250 kDa antigen defined by one of these MoAbs, designated 34.1, is similar to a high molecular weight proteoglycan and an excellent tumor marker for human melanoma.[37] A murine MoAb of the subclass IgG2b, designated JSI, produced against the fetal antigen that had been extracted from culture media of melanoma cell line, reacts with several tumor types but not with equivalent normal tissues.[18] A MoAb 202 produced by immunization with human melanoma cell line UCLA-SO-M14 was reactive with a number of ganglioside species.[38] Kageshita et al.[27] produced an anti-HMW-MAA (225.28) and an anti-96K MAA (CL207.14) MoAb and have used them in clinical trials for passive immunotherapy. They further developed a murine anti-idiotype MoAb (MF11-31) by immunization with syngeneic anti-HMW-MAA. This anti-id competes with antigen in binding assays and is currently being utilized in active specific immunotherapy of patients with advanced melanoma. Two mouse MoAb to human melanoma, NKI/C-3[39] and HMB45/50[40] are in daily use in our laboratory for diagnosis of malignant melanoma.

HUMAN MONOCLONAL ANTI-MELANOMA ANTIBODIES

Human MoAb to melanoma-associated gangliosides were first produced by Irie and co-workers in our division at UCLA.[41] They developed B lymphoblastoid cell lines from lymphocytes of melanoma patients by Epstein-Barr virus transformation. Two clones (L55 and L72) were obtained which secreted MoAb to two oncofetal antigens designated originally OFA-I-1 and OFA-I-2, respectively. These antigens are GM2 (L55) and GD2 (L72). MoAb L72 reacts preferentially with tumors of neuroectodermal origin.[42] MoAb L55 is very specific in its reactivity with GM2, but shows a wider pattern of reactivity with cultured cells, and reacts with a variety of human cancers. This antibody is cytostatic in vitro to both biopsy and cultured melanoma cells and has been used in treatment of melanoma.[38,43] Many other human anti-ganglioside MoAb have been produced either by EBV transformation alone or by fusing EBV transformed cells with a mouse myeloma cell line to produce heterohybridomas which are more stable.[44] Human MoAb (3-207) with dual GM2/GD2 specificity has been generated by EBV transformation of lymphocytes from GM2-immunized patients. This antibody is reactive with a range of tumor cells including melanoma.[45] All reported human MoAb reactive gangliosides are of the IgM class.[25] More recently a chimeric human/mouse MoAb specific to GD2 was engineered using recombinant DNA technology. The second constant region domain (CH2) was deleted, to maintain its antigen binding capacity while removing its Fc receptor binding capacity thus making it a useful reagent for the radioimaging of tumors.[46]

HUMORAL RESPONSE TO MELANOMA

Melanoma-directed antibodies were first found by Morton et al.[14] Antibodies were detected in the sera of patients with malignant melanoma by indirect immunofluorescence that bound to both intracellular and cell membrane antigens. The demonstration provided early direct experimental evidence of immunologic factors in malignant melanoma. The sera of melanoma patients contained antibodies that were not only reactive to their autologous melanoma cells, but were cross reactive with melanomas from other patients. This was indicative of the presence of common antigens shared by most malignant melanomas.[4,14] Lewis and co-workers[47] found two types of MAA, a cell-surface antigen that was individually distinct for each melanoma, and a cross-reactive cytoplasmic antigen. Patients' sera have been shown also to react with H-D antigen expressed on melanoma cells as measured by flow cytometry. The sera were found to be cytotoxic to melanoma cells in a complement-dependent cytotoxicity assay.[30] Natural anti-H-D antibodies have been detected in man with or without malignancies, but in this study elevated anti-H-D antibody levels were found more frequently in melanoma patients. A significantly higher level of IgG and IgM anti-H-D antibody was demonstrated in those patients who were free of disease for more than five years after surgery, than in those who relapsed within two years.

That MAA could be immunogenic in humans was demonstrated by immunizing patients with the common tumor ganglioside antigen (OFA-I).[21,42] Anti-OFA-I (anti-GM2) was cytotoxic to cancer cells in vitro, inhibiting tumor colony formation, and in the presence of complement lysing melanoma cells. Specificity was indicated by the lack of reactivity of these antibodies with normal autologous tissues. The level of existing antimelanoma antibodies, such as anti-GM2[48,49] or anti-U-TAA,[17] in melanoma patients can be increased by active specific immunotherapy using melanoma cell vaccine (MCV) or by immunization with GM2.[50]

The relevance of the humoral response to melanoma is unclear. The presence of antimelanoma antibodies in the sera of melanoma patients seems to correlate with the clinical status of the patient. In some patients the antibody was found to disappear from the serum as the disease progressed.[15] This could be due to formation of anti-idiotype antibody directed against the antimelanoma antibody, increased circulation of soluble tumor antigens that may saturate all antibody combining sites,[51] increased levels of immunosuppression, or absorption of the antibodies to the tumor mass. Evidence for in vivo binding of specific antitumor antibodies to human melanoma comes from the finding that tumor-reactive antibodies can be eluted from tumor cells obtained at surgery.[52] Binding of antibodies to Fc receptor-bearing cells and the killing of melanoma cells by antibody-dependent cellular cytotoxicity (ADCC) is one possible effector mechanism for humoral antibodies.[51] In melanoma patients, ADCC varies with tumor stage and burden,[53] with high levels of ADCC being associated with better prognosis in patients with primary melanoma. Direct intralesional injection of antibodies has been shown to cause tumor regression.[42] The mechanism of this effect is unknown, but it may be brought about by complement-mediated lysis as the MoAb was of the IgM isotype.

CELL-MEDIATED IMMUNE RESPONSES

Although there are proponents of the view that humoral effector mechanisms may be important in controlling metastases, in recent years more emphasis has been placed on the role of cell-mediated immune responses, and considerable effort and resources have been put into the in vitro assessment of cell-mediated immunity to tumor antigens. Detection of such responses in vitro has proved to be more difficult than the detection of antibody responses. The major problems are defining specificity and increasing sensitivity. Even in murine systems, in vitro responses to highly immunogenic chemically induced solid tumors are difficult to demonstrate with lymphoid cells taken directly from the animal. Usually some form of in vitro activation/amplification step or in vivo adoptive transfer step is required to demonstrate tumor-specific cellular responses. Recent major technical advances have, however, allowed progress to be made. These are (1) the availability of IL2 to propagate T cells and to allow clonal expansion of lymphocytes and limiting dilution assays to be performed, (2) the ability to phenotype cell populations, and (3) the recognition of the molecules involved in MHC-restricted specific lymphocyte-tumor interactions, which set these responses apart from those involving natural killer/cytotoxic cells. There are excellent reviews on cell-mediated immune responses to melanoma[54] and the immunological relationship between melanoma and host[12] by Parmiani et al. Only certain issues will be raised here.

IN VITRO ANALYSIS OF CELLULAR REACTIVITY TO MELANOMA

Vose and Bonnard[55] and Vanky and Klein[56] were among the first to use the new techniques to study cell-mediated responses to human tumors. They detected T lymphocytes reactive to autologous tumor in 70 percent of patients with primary cancers of various types. These findings were confirmed by Fossati et al.[35] and Parmiani et al.[57] in melanoma; however, they found reactions with tumor cells in only 10 percent of individuals with metastatic lesions. The lack of reaction to metastatic cells could be due to many factors such as the loss of MAA, functionally different antigens, the release of suppressive products by melanoma cells, low levels of expression of Class I MHC molecules, and lack of involvement of HLA-DR antigens on metastatic cells.[54] Studies on the correlation between cell-mediated immune responses of melanoma patients to autologous tumor cells and disease progression indicate that stage I patients show an immune response to autologous melanoma cells and that this response drops with the appearance of metastases.[35]

In recent years, the clonal analysis of cytotoxic T lymphocytes (CTL) has been carried out by several groups.[54,58–60] The basic strategy is to culture lymphocytes with autologous tumor, expand them in IL-2, and then clone them in the presence of feeder cells with occasional restimulation with autologous tumor. As with all extended cultures of this type, the frequencies of the eventual phenotypes and the functions probably reflect the culture conditions; however, the results do appear to demonstrate the degree of heterogeneity expected from an antitumor response and are in many ways similar to the results from short-term limiting dilution assays. Mukherji et al.[61] described three different functional classes of T cell clones derived from melanoma patients using this technique. Class 1 clones are bona fide $CD3^+$,$CD8^+$ cells which are cytotoxic only for autologous tumor cells. They kill in an MHC Class 1-restricted fashion and use their CD3-α/β TCR complex for cognate recognition. Another feature of these cells that distinguishes them from lymphokine-activated killer (LAK) cells may be that they are not inhibited by IL-4.[62] Class 1 type clones are present in low frequency, which might reflect a restricted range of antigens that they recognize. The nature of these antigens has not been elucidated, but preliminary data suggest that different clones from one individual can respond to different antigens.[61,63] Class 2 clones have the same phenotype as Class 1 clones but exhibit broad reactivity to a variety of tumors. As with LAK and natural killer (NK) cells the structures responsible for tumor cell recognition are not well defined and may be diverse and multiple with more reliance on cell adhesion molecules than on T cell receptors for tumor cell recognition. Class 3 molecules are $CD4^+$ or $CD8^+$ clones that are α/β TcR^+. They exhibit no cytotoxicity but can be immunoregulatory, possessing the ability to help or suppress the cytotoxic clones.

The question of whether the specific CTLs are functionally as active in vivo as they are in vitro remains to be answered. It is also unclear whether clones with restricted specificity are more efficient than those with broader specificity or LAK cells. In animal experiments, specific cell-mediated responses are most effective in inducing tumor regression, require minimal amounts of IL-2, obtain ready access to tumor, and display lasting tumor immunity. The use of specific T cell clones for immunotherapy may have problems, in that there appears to be strong intratumoral heterogeneity with respect to susceptibility to lysis, which could result from loss of antigen or adhesion molecules and could permit tumor to escape from the antitumor effects of restricted clones. The requirement of these clones for helper cells remains unclear. However, the advantage of tumor specificity will most likely outweigh the disadvantages.

TUMOR INFILTRATING LYMPHOCYTES

Tumor-infiltrating lymphocytes (TIL) have shown both in vivo and in vitro antitumor reactivity. Initial studies by Vose and Bonnard[55] suggested that the frequency of precursors of responsive cells was higher in tumor than in peripheral blood. More recent studies suggest that TIL also contain a higher frequency of mature tumor-specific lymphocytes than do lymphoid population from other sources. This, together with evidence from murine models that TIL were more effective than LAK cells in IL-2-based immunotherapy protocols[64–66] and could localize better in tumor,[67] led to the first clinical trials of TIL plus IL-2 by Rosenberg's group. It is still not clear whether TIL are clinically more effective than LAK cells, or sufficiently so to warrant the extra uncertainty and expense involved in their preparation. The results from the first clinical trial with various forms of cancer were disappointingly similar to earlier studies with LAK cells.[68] However, in a more recent study with 20 melanoma patients, a high (60 percent) response rate was achieved.[69] Further studies to determine the frequency of precursor cells, optimal culture conditions, and relative efficacy of TIL populations compared to LAK are necessary before any conclusions can be drawn.

LNL-MEDIATED IMMUNE RESPONSE AND TUMOR-PROXIMAL IMMUNE SUPPRESSION

There is a substantial body of evidence to show that regional lymph nodes can act as the outposts of the immune system and their response can greatly influence the development of the primary tumor and the secondary spread of malignant cells.[2,70] Nodal responses to tumor are not always protective, and there is evidence that under certain circumstances the immunological responses of lymph nodes regional to tumor may be suppressed by the tumor burden.[71–73] In human melanoma, lymphocytes from tumor-involved nodes have been shown to be suppressive for PBL-mediated cytotoxic responses against autologous tumor.[60,74,75]

The majority of studies on LNL function have been done using lymphoid cell from a pooled group of nodes rather than individual nodes. Our studies[2,76] on the spatial orientation of immunoreactivity of regional nodes were performed on single nodes individually oriented relative to the nearest melanoma. Histologic and immunohistological studies indicating reduced reactivity in tumor-proximal nodes are discussed in detail in Chap. 12. Our functional studies have shown that LNL from nodes near tumor show reduced responses to mitogens such as PHA, Con A, IL-2, and alloantigens,[77] and contain more Con A-inducible suppressor cells than nodes further from tumor.[78] In more recent studies (Farzad Z, unpublished data), we examined nodes from 62 melanoma patients for their ability to inhibit the in vitro growth of allogeneic melanoma cell line (UCLA-So-M14). We found that while LNL from the majority of lymph nodes (67 percent) inhibited M14-proliferation, the opposite effect, an increase in M14-growth, was seen in 33 percent of the nodal populations. This was more often (in 90 percent of cases) observed with LNL derived from nodes near to tumor, than with cells from more remote nodes,[79] indicating that proximal nodes are not only suppressed but may in fact be tumor stimulatory. The nature of the effector cells responsible for in vitro tumor cell cytostasis was investigated by panning out potentially responsive lymphocyte subpopulations. The data show that $CD8^+$ T cells and to a lesser extent $CD4^+$ cells are responsible for most of the cytostatic effects of LNL against the tumor cells.[79] This is consistent with the observations that cytotoxic T cell clones can be isolated from LNL that are CD8$^+$ CD4$^-$ and that display varying degrees of specificity in their killing of autologous melanoma.[60] NK cells do not appear to be active, as M14 is an NK resistant cell line and LNL have little functional NK activity.[72,80,81] Lymph nodes also show only a low percentage of cells expressing the NK marker Leu 19 (CD56) as analyzed by flow cytometry.[82] However, it should be noted that the number of CD56 positive NK cells increased progressively in nodes near tumor, and such cells were more numerous in uninvolved nodes from stage II patients compared to nodes from stage I patients.[82] It is not clear which cells are responsible for stimulation of the target cell growth. Macrophages in certain states of activation have been reported to promote growth of tumor cells in vitro.[83,84] Our depletion studies (Farzad Z, unpublished) suggest macrophages are not major participants as cytotoxic or stimulatory effector cells in our system.

Our phenotypic studies showed that, compared with stage I melanoma patients, LNL from stage II patients had a significant decrease in helper/inducer (CD4$^+$) T cells ($p < .001$), with a corresponding increase in cytotoxic/suppressor (CD8$^+$) cells ($p < .001$). In some stage II patients, the presence of tumor within a node was associated with a large decrease in CD3$^+$ cells in the total T cell population.[82] The mechanism is unknown, but it may be associated with the appearance of an immunologically inert T cell population. Alternatively, they may belong to the recently described CD3$^-$CD20$^-$CD16$^-$ LNL-subset that appears to be responsible for most of the LAK cell activity following IL-2 stimulation of nodal cells.[85]

Clearly, there are important changes in T cell populations within tumor draining nodes that point to a prominent role for these cells as determinants of the progression or regression of melanoma and support our view that lymph nodes draining melanoma are immune suppressed as a result of contact with tumor cells or their products. This may be an important mechanism that facilitates metastatic growth.

CONCLUSION

There is strong evidence that patients who develop melanoma can generate humoral and cell-mediated immune responses to their tumor.

A number of melanoma-associated antigens have been identified. Murine and human monoclonal antibodies to these antigens are proving useful for the detection of minimal tumor deposits. Certain antibodies to melanoma have been shown to cause regression of localized disease.

The reasons for progression of melanoma in the face of immunity are not clear. A number of tumor products such as gangliosides have been shown to have immunosuppressive properties and their shedding may lead to blocking or inactivation of locoregional responses. Changes in certain cell-adhesion molecules that can participate in the generation of immune responses appear to correlate well with tumor progression and may be functionally relevant to the ability of the tumor to metastasize. Class II molecules on metastatic cells seem unable to generate the same lymphocyte responses as they can when expressed on primary tumors. The mechanisms of this apparent paradox have not been elucidated. There is evidence that regional lymph node responses are depressed in melanoma, and this may facilitate the development of metastases. Clonal analysis of T cells from within tumor mass have demonstrated the presence of immunoregulatory suppressor T cells in co-existence with cytotoxic T cells. Further work is necessary to define the temporal and spatial development of these cells to establish their role in the development of metastases.

Attempts at immunotherapeutic intervention in melanoma have been more successful than in other cancers, at least in dealing with individual tumor deposits. IL-2 based LAK and TIL immunotherapy protocols have concentrated on this disease with some success. The in vitro generation of tumor-specific T cells against melanoma will provide an opportunity to test the relative efficacy of these cells compared to nonspecific LAK cells in immunotherapy regimens. Other approaches to specific immunotherapy that are ongoing include specific immunization with tumor antigens, anti-idiotype antibodies, and the use of tumor-specific monoclonal antibodies.

It is to be hoped that such efforts at tumor-specific immunotherapy are not thwarted by those same mechanisms that allow the melanoma to escape native host defenses and which make it such a deadly disease.

REFERENCES

1. Bystryn JC. Vaccine immunotherapy of melanoma. In: Ferrone S. ed. *Human Melanoma: From Basic Research to Clinical Application.* Berlin: Springer-Verlag, 1989:514–530.
2. Cochran AJ, Wen D-R, Farzad Z, Stene MA, McBride WH, Lana AM, Hoon DB, and Morton DL. Immunosuppression by melanoma cells as a factor in the generation of metastatic disease. *Anticancer Res* 9:859–864. 1989.
3. Everson TC and Cole WM. In: *Spontaneous Regression of Cancer.* Philadelphia: WB Saunders; 1966:560.
4. Morton DL and Wells SA. Immunobiology of neoplastic disease; melanoma; soft tissue sarcomas. In: Sabiston DC, ed. *Textbook of Surgery: The Biological Basis of Modern Surgical Practice.* Philadelphia: WB Saunders; 1981:577–604.
5. Cochran AJ and Hoon DB. Immunological aspects of malignant melanoma. In: Veronesi U, Cascinelli N, Santinami M (eds.), *Cutaneous Melanoma: Status of Knowledge and Future Prospective.* London: Academic Press; 1987, 47–61.
6. Whiteside TL. Tumor-infiltrating lymphocytes: Phenotype

and functional characteristics. *J Cancer Res Clin Oncol* 116:785, 1990.

7. Kelly JW, Sagebiel RW, and Blois MS. Regression in malignant melanoma: A histologic feature without independent prognostic significance. *Cancer* 56:2287–2291, 1985.
8. McGovern VJ, Shaw HM, Milton GW. Prognosis in patients with thin malignant melanomas: Influence of regression. *Histopathology* 7:673–680, 1983.
9. Trau H, Kopf AW, Rigel DS, Levine J, Rogers G, Levenstein M, Brat RS, Mintzis MM, and Friedman RJ. Regression in malignant melanoma. *J Am Acad Dermatol* 8:363–368, 1983.
10. Ronan SG, Han MC, Das Gupta TK. Histologic prognostic indicators in cutaneous malignant melanoma. *Semin Oncol* 15:558–565, 1988.
11. Greiner JW, Horan P, Colcher D, Weeks M, Thor A, Noguchi P, Pestka S, and Schlom J. Modulation of human tumor antigen expression. *J Lab Clin Med* 109:244–261, 1987.
12. Parmiani G, Mortarini R, and Castelli C. Immunological relationship between melanoma and host. In: Cascinelli N, Santinami M, Veronesi U (eds.), *Cutaneous Melanoma: Biology and Management.* Milan: Masson S.p.A.; 1990, pp 139–151.
13. Ferrone S and Natali PG. Immunological relationship between melanoma and host. In: Cascinelli N, Santinami M, Veronesi U (eds.), *Cutaneous Melanoma: Biology and Management.* Milan: Masson S.p.A.; 1990:193–203.
14. Morton DL, Malmgren RA, Holms EC, and Ketcham AS. Determination of antibodies against human malignant melanoma by immunofluorescence. *Surgery* 64:233–240, 1968.
15. Lewis MG, Ikonopisov RL, Nairn RC, Phillips TM, Hamilton G, Bodenham DC, and Alexander P. Tumor-specific antibodies in human malignant melanoma and their relationship to the extent of the disease. *BMJ* 3:547–552, 1969.
16. Gupta RK, Irie RF, Chee DO, Kern DH, and Morton DL. Demonstration of two distinct antigens in spent tissue culture medium of a human malignant melanoma cell line. *J Natl Cancer Inst* 63:347–356, 1979.
17. Gupta RK and Morton DL. Studies of a melanoma tumor-associated antigen detected in the spent culture medium of a human melanoma cell line by allogeneic antibody. II. Immunological characterization. *J Natl Cancer Inst* 72:75–82, 1984.
18. Wong JH, Xu SH, Saxon RE, Gupta RK, and Morton DL. Immunological characterization of a tumor-associated antigen defined by a monoclonal antibody. *J Surg Res* 48:539–546, 1990.
19. Carrel S and Theilkaes L. Evidence for a tumour-associated antigen in human malignant melanoma. *Nature* 242:609–610, 1973.
20. Euhus DM, Gupta RK, and Morton DL. Detection of a tumor-associated glycoprotein antigen in serum and urine of melanoma patients by murine monoclonal antibody (AD1-40F4) in enzyme immunoassay. *J Clin Lab Anal* 3:184–190, 1989.
21. Irie RF, Giulliano AE, Morton DL. Oncofetal antigen: A tumor-associated fetal antigen immunogenic in man. *J Natl Cancer Inst* 63:367–373, 1979.
22. Ravindranath MH and Irie RF. Gangliosides as antigens of human melanoma. In: Nathanson L (ed.), *Malignant Melanoma: Biology, Diagnosis and Therapy* Boston: Kluwer Academic Publishers; 1988, 17–43.
23. Marcus CM. A review of the immunogenic and immunomodulatory properties of glycosphingolipids. *Mol Immunol* 21:1083–1091, 1984.
24. Hoon DB, Irie RF, and Cochran AJ. Gangliosides from human melanoma immunomodulate response of T cells to interleukin-2. *Cell Immunol* 111:1–10, 1988.
25. Furukawa K and Lloyd KO. Gangliosides in melanoma. In: Ferrone S ed. *Human Melanoma: From Basic Research to Clinical Application.* Berlin: Springer-Verlag; 1989, 15–30.
26. Hoon DB, Jung T, Naungayan J, Cochran AJ, Morton DL, and McBride WH. Modulation of human macrophage functions by gangliosides. *Immunol Lett* 20:269–276, 1989.
27. Kageshita T, Temponi M, Kekish U, Chen ZJ, Mittelman A, Matsui M, and Ferrone S. Active specific and passive immunotherapy of melanoma: Clinical and experimental investigations with murine monoclonal antibodies. In: Ferrone S (ed.), *Human Melanoma: From Basic Research to Clinical Application* Berlin: Spring-Verlag, 1989, 15–30.
28. Schlingemann RO, Rietweld FJ, de Waal RM, Ferrone S, and Ruiter DJ. Expression of the high molecular weight melanoma associated antigen by pericytes during angiogenesis in tumors and in healing wounds. *Am J Pathol* 136:1393–1405, 1990.
29. Dixon WT, Demetrick DJ, Ohyama K, Sikora LK, and Jerry LM. Biosynthesis, glycosylation and intracellular processing of the neurograndular antigen, a human melanoma associated antigen. *Cancer Res* 50:4557–4565, 1990.
30. Nakarai H, Chandler PJ, Kano K, Morton DL, and Irie RF. Hangannutziu-Deicher antigen as a possible target for immunotherapy of melanoma. *Int Arch Allergy Appl Immunol* 91:323–328, 1990.
31. Furukawa KS, Furukawa K, Real FX, Old LJ, and Lloyd KO. A unique antigenic epitope of human melanoma is carried on the common melanoma glycoprotein gp95/p97. *J Exp Med* 169:585–590, 1989.
32. Johnson JP, Lehmann JM, Stade BG, Rothbacher U, Sers C, and Riethmuller G. Functional aspects of three molecules associated with metastatic development in human malignant melanoma. *Invasion Metastasis* 9:338–350, 1989.
33. Rosenburg CD, Ferrone S, Hamby CV, Mancino V, and Graf LH Jr. Interspecific DNA-mediated transfer and amplification of a gene specifying a M_r 100,000 human melanoma-associated cell surface glycoprotein. *Cancer Res* 50:1559–1565, 1990.
34. Houghton AN, Real FX, Davis LJ, Cordon-Cardo C, and Old LJ. Phenotypic heterogeneity of melanoma. Relation to the differentiation program of melanoma cells. *J Exp Med* 164:812–829, 1986.
35. Fossati G, Anichini A, Taramelli D, Balsari A, Gambacorti-Passerini C, Kirkwood JM, and Parmiani G. Immune response to autologous human melanoma: Implication of class I and II MHC product. *Biochim Biophys Acta* 865:235–251, 1986.
36. Taramelli D, Fossati G, and Balsari A. The inhibition of lymphocyte stimulation by autologous human metastatic melanoma cells correlates with the expression of HLA-DR antigens on the tumor cells. *Int J Cancer* 34:797–806, 1984.
37. Saxon RE, Burke MW, Torbett B, Fairhurst M, Morton DL, and Cochran AJ. Detection of malignant melanoma with monoclonal antibodies. *Dis Markers* 6:97–108, 1988.
38. Tai T, Sze L, Kawashima I, Saxon RE, and Irie RF. Monoclonal antibody detects monosialogangliosides having a sialic acid 2-3-galactosyl residue. *J Biol Chem* 14:6803–6807, 1986.
39. Van Duinen SG, Ruiter DJ, and Hageman PH. Immunohistochemical and histochemical tools in the diagnosis of amelanotic melanoma. *Cancer* 53:1566–1573, 1984.
40. Gown AM, Vogel AM, Hoak D, Gough F, and McNutt MA. Monoclonal antibodies specific for melanocytic tumors distinguish subpopulations of melanocytes. *Am J Pathol* 123: 195–203, 1986.
41. Irie RF, Sze LL, and Saxon RE. Human antibody to OFA-I, a tumor antigen, produced in vitro by Epstein-Barr virus transformed human B-lymphoid cell lines. *Proc Natl Acad Sci U S A* 79:5666–5670, 1982.

42. Irie RF and Morton DL. Regression of cutaneous metastatic melanoma by intralesional injection with human monoclonal antibody to ganglioside GD2. *Proc Natl Acad Sci U S A* 83:1242–1246, 1986.
43. Irie RF, Takasumi M, and Morton DL. Human monoclonal antibody to ganglioside GM2 for melanoma treatment. *Lancet* 1 (8641):786–787, 1989.
44. Yamaguchi H, Furukawa K, Fortunato SR, Livingston PO, Lloyd KO, Oettgen HF, and Old LJ. Cell-surface antigens of melanoma recognized by human monoclonal antibodies. *Proc Natl Acad Sci U S A* 84:2416–2420, 1987.
45. Old LJ. Human monoclonal antibody with dual GM2/GD2 specificity derived from an immunized melanoma patient. *Proc Natl Acad Sci U S A* 87:3333–3337, 1990.
46. Mueller BM, Reisfeld RA, and Gilles SD. Serum half-life and tumor localization of a chimeric antibody deleted of the CH domain and directed against the disialogangliosides GD2. *Proc Natl Acad Sci U S A* 87:5702–5705, 1990.
47. Lewis MG and Phillips TM. The specificity of surface membrane immunofluorescence in human malignant melanoma. *Int J Cancer* 10:105–111, 1972.
48. Jones PC, Sze LL, Liu PY, Morton DL, and Irie RF. Prolonged survival for melanoma patients with elevated IgM antibody to oncofetal antigen. *J Natl Cancer Inst* 66:249–254, 1981.
49. Morton DL, Foshang LJ, Nizze JA, Gupta RK, Famatiga E, Hoon DS, and Irie RF. Active specific immunotherapy in malignant melanoma. *Semin Surg Oncol* 5:420–425, 1989.
50. Livingston PO, Ritter G, Srivastava P, Padavan M, Calves MJ, Oettgen HF, and Old LJ. Characterization of IgG and IgM antibodies induced in melanoma patients by immunization with purified GM2 gangliosides. *Cancer Res* 49:7045–7050, 1989.
51. Golub SH. Host immune response to human tumor antigens. In: Becker, FF, ed. *Cancer: Comprehensive Treatise*. Vol. 4 New York: Plenum Press; 1975, 259–300.
52. Gupta RK and Morton DL. Suggestive evidence for in vivo binding of specific antitumor antibodies of human melanoma. *Cancer Res* 32:58–62, 1975.
53. Plain MJ, Whitehead RH, and Jose DJ. Immunity to melanoma-associated antigens detected by leucocyte adherence inhibition and antibody dependent cellular cytotoxicity assays. *Pathology* 15:177–182, 1983.
54. Parmiani G, Anichini A, and Fossati G. Cellular immune response against autologous human malignant melanoma: Are in vitro studies providing a framework for a more effective immunotherapy? *J Natl Cancer Inst* 82:361–370, 1990.
55. Vose BM and Bonnard GD. Human tumour antigens defined by cytolytic and proliferative responses of cultured lymphoid cells. *Nature* 296:359–361, 1982.
56. Vanky F and Klein E. Specificity of auto-tumor cytotoxicity exerted by fresh, activated and propagated human T lymphocytes. *Int J Cancer* 29:547–553, 1982.
57. Parmiani G, Anichini A, Castelli C, and Fossati G. HLA class II antigens on melanoma cells. In: Ferrone S, ed. *Human Melanoma, from Basic Research to Clinical Application*. Berlin: Springer-Verlag; 1989, 197–211.
58. Vose BM and White W. Tumor-reactive lymphocytes stimulated in mixed lymphocyte and tumor culture. Clonal analysis of effector cells in cytotoxic and proliferative assay. *Cancer Immunol Immunother* 15:227–236, 1983.
59. Mukherji B, Guha A, Loomis R, and Ergin MT. Cell-mediated amplification and downregulation of cytotoxic immune response against autologous human cancer. *J Immunol* 128:1987–1991, 1987.
60. Mukherji B, Guha A, Chakraborty NG, Sivanandham M, Nashed AL, Sporn JR, Ergin MT. Clonal analysis of cytotoxic and regulatory T cell responses against human melanoma. *J Exp Med* 169:1961–1976, 1989.
61. Mukherji B, Chakraborty NG, and Sivanandham M. T-cell clones that react against autologous human tumors. *Immunol Rev* 116:33–62, 1990.
62. Yamada T, Holmes EC, and Golub SH. Differential regulation by interleukin-4 and interferon-gamma of an autologous melanoma specific cytotoxic T-cell clone and the tumor-infiltrating lymphocytes from which it was established. *Cancer Commun* 2:113–121, 1990.
63. Notter M and Schirrmacher V. Tumor-specific T-cell clones recognize different protein determinants on autologous human malignant melanoma cells. *Int J Cancer* 45:834–841, 1990.
64. Riddel S, Cheever MA, and Greenberg PD. Interleukin-2 in cancer immunotherapy. *ISI Atlas Sci Immunol* 1:175–183, 1988.
65. Mule JJ, Jones FR, Hellstrom I, and Hellstrom KE. Selective localization of radiolabelled immune lymphocytes into syngeneic tumors. *J Immunol* 123:600–606, 1979.
66. Hamaoka T and Fujiwara H. Phenotypically and functionally distinct T-cell subsets in antitumor responses. *Immunol Today* 9:267–269, 1987.
67. Mukherji B, Arnbjarnarson O, Spitznagle LA, Kalish, Hoffman J, Ergin MT, and Spencer RP. Imaging pattern of previously in vitro sensitized and interleukin-2 expanded autologous lymphocytes in human cancer. *Nucl Med Biol* 15:419–427, 1988.
68. Topalian S, Solomon D, Avis FP, Chang AE, Freerkson DL, Linehan WM, Lotze MT, Robertson CM, and Seipp CA. Immunotherapy of patients with advanced cancer using tumor-infiltrating lymphocytes and recombinant interleukin-2: A pilot study. *J Clin Oncol* 6:839–843, 1988.
69. Rosenberg SA, Packard BS, Aebersold PM, Solomon CD, Topalian S, Toy ST, Simon P, Lotze MT, Yang JC, and Seipp CA. Use of tumor-infiltrating lymphocytes and interleukin-2 in the immunotherapy of patients with metastatic melanoma. *N Engl J Med* 319:1676–1680, 1988.
70. Cochran AJ, Wen D-R, and Hoon DB. Immunobiology of the regional lymph nodes in cutaneous malignant melanoma. In: Ferrone S, ed. *Human Melanoma: From Basic Research to Clinical Application*. Berlin: Springer-Verlag; 1989, 180–196.
71. Hawrylko E. Tumor bearer T cells suppress BCG-potentiated anti-tumor responses. I. Requirement for their effect. *Cell Immunol* 66:121–138, 1982.
72. Anderson TM, Wasylyshyn ML, Moy PM, and Golub SH. Local and regional immune function in cancer patients. In: Moloy PJ and Nicolson GL, eds. *Occult Nodal Metastasis in Solid Carcinoma*. New York: Praeger 1987, 49–59.
73. Mickel RA, Kessler DJ, Taylor JMG, and Lichtenstein A. Natural killer cell cytotoxicity in the peripheral blood, cervical lymph nodes, and tumor of head and neck cancer patients. *Cancer Res* 48:5017–5022, 1988.
74. Mukherji B, Wilhelm SA, Guha A, and Ergin MT. Regulation of cellular immune response against autologous human melanoma. *J Immunol* 136:1888–1898, 1986.
75. Koba F, Akiyoshi T, Tsuji H. Depression of the generation of cell-mediated cytotoxicity in regional lymph nodes of patients with gasteric carcinoma. *J Clin Lab Immunol* 22:181–184, 1987.
76. Cochran AJ, Wen D-R, Hoon DB, Pihl E, Fairhurst MV, and Korn, EL. Tumor proximate immune suppression of regional lymph nodes in patients with malignant melanoma. In: Hellmann and Eccles SA, eds. *Treatment of Metastasis* London: Taylor & Francis; 1985, 69–72.
77. Hoon DB, Korn EL, and Cochran AJ. Variations in func-

tional immunocompetence of individual tumor-draining lymph nodes in humans. *Cancer Res* 28:1740–1744, 1987.

78. Hoon DB, Bowker RJ, and Cochran AJ. Suppressor cell activity in melanoma-draining lymph nodes. *Cancer Res* 47:1529–1533, 1987.

79. Farzad Z, Cochran AJ, McBride WH, Oghbechi H, Osnog C, and Morton DL. Variation in immunoreactivity of human lymph nodes located at different distances from tumor. In Preparation

80. Vose BM, Vanky F, Argov S, and Klein E. Natural cytotoxicity in man: Activity of lymph node and tumor-infiltrating lymphocytes. *Eur J Immunol* 7:753–757, 1977.

81. Golub SH, Niitsuma M, Kawate N, Cochran AJ, and Holmes EC. NK activity of tumor infiltrating and lymph node lymphocytes in human pulmonary tumors. In: Herberman RB, ed. *NK Cells and Other Natural Effector Cells.* London: Academic Press; 1982, 1113–1118.

82. Farzad Z, Cochran AJ, McBride WH, Gray JD, Wong V, and Morton DL. Lymphocyte subset alterations in nodes regional to human melanoma. *Cancer Res* 50:3585–3588, 1990.

83. Norbury KC: In vitro stimulation and inhibition of tumor cell growth mediated by different lymphoid cell populations. *Cancer Res* 37:1408–1415, 1977.

84. Mantovani A, Peri G, Polentarutti N, Bolis G, Mangioni C, and Spreafico F. Effects on in vitro tumor growth of macrophages isolated from human ascitic ovarian tumor. *Int J Cancer* 23:157–164, 1979.

85. Yano T, Murata M, Ishida T, Mitsodomi T, Kimura G, Sugimachi K, and Nomoto K. Phenotypic characterization of lymphokine-activated killer cells from human lymph node lymphocytes. *Cell Immunol* 122:578–584, 1989.

Chapter 4

ENDOCRINE INFLUENCE ON MELANOMA

Prabir K. Chaudhuri

INTRODUCTION

Endocrine influence on melanocyte and melanoma have been studied for many decades. Although human melanoma and melanomas in other animal models have some morphologic, genetics, and biological similarities, effect of hormones on biology of melanoma is quite variable in different species. The influence of hormones on melanocyte and melanoma have been studied extensively in animal models. In comparison studies on human melanoma has been less extensive and primarily restricted in the field of steroid hormones. In this review, we will evaluate the current status of the influence of both peptide and steroid hormones on biology of melanoma.

PEPTIDES AND GROWTH FACTOR

Melanotropin

Melanotropins are peptide hormones secreted from pituitary gland (pars intermedius). Although vertebrate pituitary secrete both α-MSH and β-MSH, in human, α-MSH is considered as the primary melanotropin for pigmentary effect on epidermal melanin unit.[1,2] MSH exerting its influence through specific cell membrane receptor, increases the tyrosine activity in a calcium dependent cyclic AMP protein kinase system.[3,4] The responsiveness of the cells to MSH may depend on factors such as numbers of available MSH receptor. L-DOPA can increase the number of membrane receptors for MSH and enhance the melanin synthesis activity of cells.[5]

In animal model both in vitro and in vivo, MSH has shown to modulate growth and metastatic potential of melanoma.[6,7,8] Others have demonstrated no specific growth related activity of melanoma in response to MSH.[9] Clinical observation of increased α-MSH secretion by the melanoma patients suggests that higher plasma α-MSH levels in advanced cases may be due to either a positive feedback mechanism or of hormone paraneoplastic production.[10] It is of interest to know that there is a marked increase in expression of α-MSH receptor in human melanoma cells compared to benign nevi cells.[11] Lejeune et al. have demonstrated higher delivery of melphalan to tumor cells through α-MSH receptor in both human and B-16 mouse melanoma cells, when melphalan was conjugated with α-MSH.[12] However, whether the effect of MSH on melanoma cells can be exploited to gain clinical advantages by targeting treatment through this metabolic axis, remains to be seen.

Melatonin

Melatonin, a peptide hormone secreted from pineal gland, has shown to modulate growth of malignant tumors including melanoma.[13,14,15] Although, the actual mechanism of action is not well-defined, it has been proposed that activity of melatonin is through adrenal or gonadal axis, or indirectly through MSH. In a B-16 murine melanoma model, inhibition of the growth of the tumor by melatonin was associated with decrease in gonadal and adrenal weights.[16] In hamster melanoma, under long photoperiod, melatonin decreases growth rate.[17] We have demonstrated a biphasic growth pattern of hamster melanoma in vitro in response to melatonin.[18]

An in vitro study performed by Bartsch demonstrated decrease in growth of human melanoma by crude pineal extract. However, melatonin, pyridines, arginine, vasotocin, and others, did not influence the growth of melanoma. Thus, yet unrecognized factors in crude pineal extract is thought to be responsible for growth inhibition.[19] Recently, the effect of melatonin has been studied in melanoma patients. In this study, melatonin with dose ranging from 5 mg/m^2/day to 700 mg/m^2/day showed objective partial response in 15 percent of the cases. There appeared to be some dose response relationship. Median duration of response was 33 weeks with minimal toxicity. Further studies will be required to evaluate the effect of melatonin in human melanoma.[20]

Growth Factors

A number of growth factors are implicated to modulate the biology of melanoma in vitro and also thought to have effect on tumor transformation and progression in animal model. The clinical importance of these growth factors are yet undetermined. Goustin et al.[21] and Bradshaw and Rubin[22] have elucidated the general principles on mechanism of actions of some polypeptide growth factors and their molecular structures.

Epidermal Growth Factors

The influence of epidermal growth factors (EGF) has been studied on a large variety of tumors including melanoma.[23] The physical and chemical properties of EGF have been described earlier.[24] EGF is a 53 amino acid polypeptide containing six cystine residue forming three interchain disulfide bonds.[25] The receptor for EGF has been characterized and a close similarity of protein sequence of EGF receptor to v-*erb* β-oncogene has been demonstrated.[26] Expression of EGF receptors were found only in melanoma cell lines that have an extra copy of chromosome 7.[27] (See Chap. 6, section on chromosome 7 for EGF receptors.) The EGF receptor was detected in epithelioid nonpigmented melanoma cells.[28] Elder has reported EGF receptor in metastatic melanomas but not in benign nevi and primary melanoma.[29] Rodeck et al. also reported mitogenic activity of EGF in 56 metastatic melanomas in culture but not in the primary melanomas corroborating the finding of the EGF receptors only in metastatic melanomas.[30]

The effect of EGF on melanoma may be through EGF receptor. However, the presence of EGF receptor in melanoma has been questioned.[31] EGF receptors and EGF could mediate the effect of estrogen and glucocorticoid on melanoma. It has been proposed that glucocorticoid may have an effect on EGF receptor level and conversely EGF may mediate glucocorticoid receptor level.[32]

Nerve Growth Factor

Nerve growth factor (NGF) is a polypeptide exerting its activity through specific receptors.[33,34] The receptor for NGF encoded on chromosome 17 is expressed on normal melanocyte and melanoma cells.[35] Metastatic cells have higher expression of the receptor.[36] The biological activities of NGF is thought to be due to the β subunit that has amino acid sequence similar to pro insulin and insulin like growth factors I and II.[33] The main effect appears to be trophic and not mitogenic. Despite demonstration of high level of NGF receptor in melanoma, no growth regulating effect of NGF on this tumor has been demonstrated.[29]

Melanoma Growth Stimulatory Activity Factor

The melanoma growth stimulatory activity (MGSA) factor is present in acid, ethanol extract of human melanoma tissue, and in media from established melanoma culture.[37,38] MGSA is 14 KDa to 16 KDa protein which stimulates proliferation of cell line at concentration from 0.3 to 30 pM.[38,39,40] MGSA was shown to be present in most melanomas, majority of benign nevi, and some keratinocyte.[41] The effect of MGSA could not be altered by other growth factors such as platelet derived growth factors, TGF, EGF, or combination of these growth factors.[42] Richmond et al. have reported chromosomal abnormality and MGSA production in 6 of 8 benign nevi raising speculation that MGSA may have some role on sequence of malignant transformation from benign nevi to melanoma.[42] However, direct evidence is lacking. Recently, MGSA has been demonstrated to be similar to platelet derived thromboglobulin and the gene for MGSA has been mapped to chromosomes 4 (region q 13-q 21).[43]

Transforming Growth Factors

Recently, transforming growth factor (TGF) has raised interest due to its effect on a variety of malignant tumors such as squamous cell ca, breast ca, hepatomas, and melanoma.[44] The TGF may directly mediate the mitogenic effects or act as a second messenger for estrogen and other steroids in melanoma.[32] Two subtypes, α-TGF and β-TGF, have been studied.[44] Alpha-TGF is a 5.6 KDa species consisting of 50 amino acid with resemblance to EGF and has the ability to bind to EGF receptor.[45,46,47,48] Increased level of mRNA for α-TGF has been demonstrated in human melanoma tissue. Beta-TGF subunit, on the other hand is a 25 KDa disulfide linked homodimer[49] and its effect on melanoma, like many other hormones, is species specific. In B-16 mouse melanoma β-TGF stimulates colony formation and increases thymidine incorporation. In human melanoma, however, β-TGF inhibits colony formation.[50,51,52] In an interesting paper, Ellis et al. have speculated on the role of α-TGF in production of cutaneous paraneoplastic syndrome, such as acanthosis nigricans and multiple acrochordons in a melanoma patient.[53]

Platelet Derived Growth Factor

Platelet derived growth factor (PDGF) was isolated from culture media of melanoma cell lines but not melanocyte.[54] The c-*sis* gene is considered to be a structural gene for PDGF. The human c-*sis* is a single copy gene that has been isolated and mapped to chromosome 22.[55] The mitogenic influence of PDGF has been speculated.[56,57] Melanoma cells in culture can incorporate PDGF in absence of receptor for PDGF.[54] The role of PDGF on biology melanoma remains unclear at this time.

Fibroblastic Growth Factor

Fibroblastic growth factors (FGF) have been detected in a wide spectrum of normal and neoplastic cells including melanoma.[58,59] Two different types of FGF have been identified. The basic type appears to have wider tissue distribution.[58] Basic FGF, a 146 amino acid polypeptide, is a potent angiogenic factor. It is considered essential for growth of melanocyte in vitro in serum free media.[57] Although FGF is considered mitogenic for both melanoma and melanocyte,[57,60] its exact influence on growth and spread of melanoma in vivo remain unclear.

Prostaglandins

Recently, the effect of various types of prostaglandins on melanoma has been evaluated.[61,62,63,64] Most of these studies were performed in vitro. Prostaglandin E_1 and E_2 increased tyrosinase activity of Cloudman S91 melanoma cell line, but inhibited cell proliferation raising speculation that melanogenious and proliferation are regulated by different mechanisms probably independent of cyclic AMP.[65] Prostaglandin A_1 and E_1 reduced plating efficiency and inhibited proliferation although both these agents raised cAMP and CGMP levels.[66] Prostaglandin D_2 was found to be a better inhibitor of B-16 melanoma cell growth compared to prostaglandin A_2 and E_2.[67] Using human melanoma cell lines, protaglandins D_2 was found to be more potent inhibitor compared to A_1 and A_2. The primary effect of prostaglandin appear to be blockade of cell progression from G_1 to S phase.[68] Using an althymic mice model, Bregman et al.[69] have shown growth inhibitory effect of 15 deoxy-16-hydroxyl-16 vinyl prostaglandin A_2 administered subcutaneously. The inhibitory effect was dose dependent. The therapeutic role of prostaglandin on treatment of human melanoma remains largely unexplored at this time.

STEROID HORMONES

The influence of steroid hormones on melanocyte, benign nevi, and melanoma has long been speculated and remains a subject of controversy.[70,71] Changes of pigmentation and size of benign nevi during pregnancy or estrogenic therapy along with reports of melanoma during puberty and pregnancy and intermittent reports in the literature on adverse outcome of melanoma during pregnancy have lent credence to a possible role of steroid hormone such as estrogen on biology of melanoma. However, the actual role of these hormones remain unclear. Not only the effect of these hormones appears to be species specific, variable and often conflicting evidence of function within same species is noted.[72,73,74,75,76,77,78] It is generally accepted that presence of intracellular steroid hormones receptor is a prerequisite for direct effect of these hormones on cells. Demonstration of estrogen receptor in melanoma renewed interest on studies of influence of steroid hormones on melanoma.[79,80,81,82,83,84,85,86,87] Voluminous literature on the effect of such hormones on initiation, progression, and therapeutic modalities in melanoma have been published.

Influence of Steroid Hormones on Benign Nevi

Change of morphology of nevi including size and color during pregnancy is a common observation. The possibility of a direct effect of hormones on benign nevi as on other steroid hormone target organs has been raised by demonstration of estrogen receptor in subset of such nevi of both congenital and acquired origin.[87] The similarity in incidence of detectable estrogen receptor in benign nevi from melanoma patients and melanoma tissue (see Table 4-1) raised speculation of possible effect of estrogen on initiation of melanoma. However, the direct evidence is lacking. Although possibility of influence of estrogen on multisteps complex process of transformation of benign melanocyte (possibly genetically predisposed or environmentally altered) to melanoma exists, the extent of such influence and the sequence of such events is unknown. The possibility of other steroid hormonal influence such as progesterone and androgen on nevi are much less studied and appreciated.

Influence of Steroid Hormones on Melanoma

Excess steroid hormones, either endogenous such as during pregnancy or exogenous have been incriminated either in increased incidence or in altered outcome of melanoma patient. Again, demonstration of intracellular estrogen receptor in melanoma strengthen the possiblity of direct effect of such hormones on biology of melanoma. We will briefly evaluate the influence of these hormones on melanoma.

Influence of Pregnancy on Melanoma

The effect of pregnancy on melanoma patients is controversial. Approximately one-third of all female patients with melanoma are in child bearing age. With trend toward first pregnancy at older age, this number may increase. Melanoma also comprises a sizeable number of all cancer associated with pregnancy. Potter and Schoeneman estimated the incidence of melanoma among all cancer associated with pregnancy is approximately 8 percent.[88] Smith and Randall reported an incidence of melanoma at 2.8 per 1000 delivery.[89] Several questions regarding association of melanoma and pregnancy have been raised including influence of pregnancy on prognosis, risk

TABLE 4-1
ESTROGEN BINDING TO CYTOSOL RECEPTOR IN HUMAN MELANOMA AND BENIGN NEVI

HISTOLOGIC DX	NUMBER	RECEPTOR	PERCENT	AMOUNT BOUND (femtomole/mg cytosol protein)	AFFINITY (Kd)
Benign nevi, normal individual	17	0	0	—	—
Benign nevi, no clinically active melanoma	22	9	41[a] (21–238)	86[b] (0.27–3.1)	1.79×10^{-9}M
Melanoma tissue	35	12	34[b] (4.3–250)	75 (0.12–4.0)	1.43×10^{-9}M
Bathing trunk nevi	2	1	50	42.0	5.6×10^{-9}M
Highly active junctional nevus	1	1	100	21.3	2.8×10^{-9}M

[a] $p < 0.05$ versus benign nevi normal individual.
[b] $p < 0.001$ versus benign nevi normal individual. Fisher's exact probability test was used to determine statistical difference in receptor incidence among the different groups. (Reproduced with permission from Chaudhuri et al., *JAMA* 244:791, 1980.)

of transplacental spread, effect of termination of pregnancy on course melanoma, and influence of prior pregnancy on melanoma. Pack and Scharnagel[90] in a review of 32 melanoma patients during pregnancy noted poor prognosis. Subsequently, several case reports supported this observation. In contrast, George et al.[91] reported 5 and 10 years survival in 115 patients with melanoma during pregnancy to be similar to control group of 337 patients. When the control group was further divided into child bearing age and older, the survival among pregnant patients was very similar to nonpregnant patients of childbearing age. The older patient had a poorer prognosis. George however noted a higher incidence of lymph node metastasis among pregnant patients, but ultimate survival in both groups were comparable. A number of other investigators also reported somewhat higher incidence of truncal lesion and Stage II disease associated with pregnancy.[92,93] However, when patients were compared by age, site, and staged matched control, no difference was observed. From analysis of a group of 18 patients diagnosed to have melanoma during their pregnancy, including 12 patients who became pregnant following diagnosis of melanoma, they found similar distribution of stage. Patients diagnosed to have melanoma during pregnancy were found to have worse prognosis. The authors suggested that a subgroup of patients in whom melanoma is stimulated by pregnancy may have worse prognosis. In a large retrospective study, Reintgen and colleagues[94] compared outcome of 58 patients with melanoma diagnosed during pregnancy to 585 patients who were not pregnant during diagnosis or at least 5 years thereafter. The mortality rate from melanoma was statistically indifferent in these two groups. Interestingly, multivariate analysis showed disease-free interval significantly shorter in pregnancy group although overall all survival were similar. This may be due to the fact that although pregnancy results in earlier relapse, the disease becomes more indolent following recurrence. Such explanation is supported by experimental evidence.[95] Alternatively, a longer follow up may actually show a survival advantage in nonpregnant group. In general, it appears that pregnancy either during diagnosis of melanoma or shortly thereafter does not influence the ultimate survival. The recommendation of avoidance of pregnancy in high-risk group is probably based mostly on avoidance of stress of concurrent pregnancy and fatal disease.[96] Also, termination of pregnancy to alter the course of the disease in melanoma patient is not indicated.

Influence of Prior Pregnancy on Melanoma

The influence of prior pregnancy on melanoma also remains controversial. All reported studies are retrospective making proper analysis difficult. Shaw et al.[97] reported favorable outcome among patients with more than two pregnancies compared to nulliparous women (81.6 versus 73.8%). Others reported survival advantage in women who had five or more pregnancies.[98] The 8-year survival among multiparous women was 90 percent compared to 73.4 percent for nulliparous women. Hersey et al.[99] reported better survival among parous women compared to nulliparous women both for age group below 50 (83 versus 73%) and above 50 years (73 versus 53%). This survival advantage was more prominent among Stage I patients. The survival advantage among higher stage patients was much less. In contrast, Elwood and

Coldman,[100] Lederman and Sober,[101] and Shiu et al.[93] showed no difference in survival based on parity. Currently, parity is not considered to be an independent prognostic variable among melanoma patients.

Transplacental Metastasis

The rarity of reported cases of transplacental metastases compared to the incidence of melanoma during pregnancy suggest that fetus and placenta are uncommon sites for metastases. Potter and Schoeneman[88] in a review of metastases of maternal cancer to fetus reported eleven cases involving melanoma. In six of the eleven cases, placental metastases were noted. Seven of the children died before 10 months, two without evidence of metastatic disease. Of the other four children, two had no detectable fetal metastases (both had placental metastases) and two children had complete regression of metastatic tumor and were alive up to 2 years at the time of report. This is probably due to homograft rejection. However, the influence of altered hormonal milieu cannot be totally discarded. Subsequently, several other cases of fetal or placental metastases have been reported. Sokol et al.[102] reported a case of amelanotic melanoma metastatic to placenta without fetal metastases. Russell and Laverty[103] and Moller et al.[104] also reported only placental involvement without metastases to children. Campbell et al.[105] reported a fetal malignant melanoma detected by ultrasound. Such congenital melanomas may be truly congenital in nature. On the other hand, unknown primary from maternal source cannot be ruled out.

Effect of Oral Contraceptive on Melanoma

The influence of exogenous hormones, specifically, oral contraceptive on causation of melanoma has been speculated. Coor et al.[106] reported hyperpigmentation of skin as a side effect of oral contraceptive. In a study reported by Jelinek[107] on cutaneous manifestation of oral contraceptive melasma was noted to be one of the commonest side effects. Recently, we demonstrated the presence of high affinity receptors for estrogen in benign acquired and congenital nevi. Schwartz et al.[108] also demonstrated the presence of progesterone receptor in benign nevi and suggested hormonal stimulation increases the receptor sites in nevi cells. Ellerbrock[109] reported a case of melanoma arising in a pre-existing nevus in a 25-year-old female following use of oral contraceptives for 3 months. In this report he mentioned, "I am not implying a necessarily causal relationship. But I do feel that the event deserves reporting." Sadoff et al.[110] reported melanoma in male patients following diethylstilbestrol therapy for prostatic cancer. Subsequently, Lerner et al.[111] reported three additional cases of melanoma developing in women following oral contraceptives. In two of these three reported cases, malignant changes were noted in pre-existing congenital nevi.

Beral and coauthors[112] examined the association between oral contraceptive use and melanoma. They noted that the use of oral contraceptive for more than 4 years was associated with higher incidence of melanoma. However, the same group had an overall higher incidence of other skin cancer. Thus, it is possible that this increased incidence of melanoma among oral contraceptive users may be due to other factors such as excess exposure to sunlight.

Similarly, in a larger study, Holly et al.[113] observed a higher risk of superficial spreading melanoma among users of oral contraceptive for 5 years or more. Holman et al.[114] reported a nonstatistically significant trend toward higher risk for superficial spreading melanoma among long-term users of exogenous unopposed estrogen. However, the review of several studies on the effect of oral contraceptive on causation of melanoma showed the combine incidence rate ratio was 1.12 with a 95 percent confidence limit of 0.94 to 1.33. Thus, it appears that among oral contraceptive users, the risk is increased, if any, only slightly. In another study, Stevens et al.[115] observed lack of increase in the age-specific incidence of melanoma among female patients compared to male patients 10 years before and after introduction of oral contraceptive. Adams et al.[116] also failed to observe an increased risk of melanoma among users of oral contraceptive. In another study reported by Bain et al.,[117] relationship between the use of oral contraceptives and the development of melanoma was studied by postal survey among 2961 nurses in the United States. No increased risk for development of melanoma was detected among users of oral contraceptives. Thus, it appears that oral contraceptive may have little influence, if any, on malignant transformation of melanocyte. However, several important questions remain unresolved. These include the risk among long-term users of oral contraceptive (over 10 years or longer) and outcome following a long latent period (over 10 years or longer).

Estrogen Receptor in Nevi and Melanoma

As mentioned previously, several clinical observations support a possible direct effect of steroids such as estrogen on benign nevi and melanoma.[118] In women, pigment pattern in nevi parallels changes in hormonal status such as pregnancy and menopause.[119] There is an increase in number of nevi after puberty, and also an increase in the incidence of melanoma in childbearing age.[120,121] However, for a direct cellular effect of estrogen, intracellular receptors for estrogen in target tissue is necessary.

Several investigators have demonstrated estrogen receptors in nevi and melanoma.[79,80,82,85,86,87] These receptor assays were done by radio-receptor methods and were characterized regarding their specificity, affinity, binding sites, and molecular weight and were found to be similar to receptors for estrogen in breast cancers.[76,77,86,87] Using cell culture systems[73] and athymic mice model,[95] we demonstrated that these receptors are functionally active and growth of receptor-positive cells could be altered by manipulation of hormones. However, the presence of true receptors in melanoma has been questioned.[122]

The presence of estrogen and progesterone receptors also have been demonstrated in benign nevi.[87] In congenital nevi, there were detectable intracellular receptors. Schwartz et al.[108] demonstrated increase in receptor binding in nevi in response to hormonal stimulations. The incidence of detectable estrogen receptors in benign nevi from melanoma patients (41%) was similar to that of incidence of estrogen receptors in melanoma tissue (34%).[86] However, in benign nevi from normal population, no receptor was demonstrated. (See Table 4-1). These receptors were high affinity, low capacity, saturable, and similar to estrogen receptor in other hormonal dependent tissue.[86] The high incidence of estrogen receptor in benign nevi from disease-free melanoma patients and in melanoma tissue itself compared to absence of estrogen receptor in nevi from normal population leads to the speculation that estrogen receptor in benign nevi from melanoma patients probably represents a molecular alteration associated with neoplastic changes. However, direct evidence is lacking.

The influence of estrogen on growth of melanoma has been evaluated both in vitro and in vivo using a number of animal melanoma models. The effects are species specific. Significant alteration of growth is commonly observed in animal melanoma.[123] Also, sex of host animal has been found to be a significant factor in growth rate.[124,125]

In human melanoma cell lines, the influence of estrogen is more dose specific. In estrogen receptor containing cell lines, low-dose estrogen stimulates the growth and high-dose estrogen inhibits the growth.[72] In the experimental model,[95] the sex of host was also a factor in growth rate of receptor-positive tumor. In female athymic mice, the growth rate of receptor-positive tumor was significantly lower than observed in male athymic mice suggesting a beneficial effect of estrogenic hormonal milieu. There was no apparent difference in growth rate in male and female athymic mice when injected with receptor-negative melanoma cell line (see Table 4-2).

In athymic mice model, the growth of an estrogen receptor-positive human melanoma cell line was significantly inhibited by administration of estradiol.[86] However, growth of receptor-negative tumor showed no alteration with estradiol treatment. Interestingly, although receptor-negative tumor had longer latent period, once the tumor growth was initiated, it showed accelerated growth rate compared to growth of tumor from receptor-positive cell line. This may suggest that estrogen may have two separate effects on initial tumor take and subsequent growth rate (see Table 4-3). Others have found estrogen growth inhibitory effect on receptor negative cell lines raising speculation that the effect of estrogen is not mediated through specific receptors.[126]

The influence of estrogen and antiestrogen in melanoma patients have been detailed in the section on therapeutic effect of hormone manipulation.

Effect of Progesterone on Melanoma

Similar to estrogen, progesterone also increases melanin pigmentation although to a lesser extent.[71] The most pronounced pigmentary effect was when both estrogen and progesterone were given together. Also as previously mentioned, receptors for progesterone were detected in benign nevi.

Progesterone receptors also have been demonstrated in melanoma tissue and cell lines.[72,127] However, these receptors have not been well-characterized. Bojar and Fabry[128] have suggested that progesterone influence on a cell may be mediated directly through its intracellular receptors or through glucocorticoid receptors. Estrogen also has been shown to induce progesterone receptor in melanoma.[78] In hamster melanoma cell lines, we did not observe any growth inhibitory or stimulatory effect of progesterone.[18] Similarly, no progesterone effect was noted on B-16 cell lines. However, progesterone reduced the number and size of pulmonary metastasis in B-16 melanoma in C57BL/G mice without significant prolongation of life.[129] The influence of progesterone on receptor-positive and receptor-negative human melanoma cell lines were evaluated in our laboratory. All three receptor-positive cell lines showed growth inhibition by progesterone. There was no effect on receptor-negative cell lines.[72]

The effect of progesterone on melanoma patients has been reported in several studies. In two other trials, Beretta et al.[130] and Rose et al.[131] observe extremely low incidence of objective response (3%). Thus, it appears progesterone has only minimal activity on metastatic human melanoma.

Effect of Androgen on Melanoma

The influence of androgen has been more thoroughly studied on animal models than in human. In the animal model, influence of androgen appears to be variable. Lipkin[125] and Walker et al.[18] reported growth inhibition of hamster melanoma cell lines by testos-

TABLE 4-2
INFLUENCE OF HOST SEX ON GROWTH OF RECEPTOR POSITIVE AND RECEPTOR NEGATIVE CELL LINE IN ATHYMIC MICE

TUMOR	NUMBER OF MICE	SEX	TREATMENT	TUMOR INCIDENCE (%)	TUMOR LATENCY (days)	TUMOR WEIGHT (g)	INCIDENCE OF METASTASIS (%)
RNeg	7	F	—	100	6.3 ± 0.6[a,b]	8.9 ± 2.1[c]	43
	7	M	—	100	6.5 ± 0.6[d]	7.3 ± 1.6	26
RPos	8	F	—	100	3.8 ± 0.5	3.7 ± 1.0[e]	13
	8	M	—	100	4.5 ± 0.3	9.6 ± 1.8	17

Growth data were analyzed by ANOVA. Differences between groups were tested for significance by student-Neuman-Keuls sequential range test. Fisher's exact probability test was used to determine the significance of sex and treatment on tumor and metastatic incidence.
[a]Mean ± SE
[b]$p < 0.01$ tumor RNeg versus tumor RPos (female mice).
[c]$p < 0.05$ tumor RNeg versus tumor RPos (female mice).
[d]$p < 0.02$ tumor RNeg versus tumor RPos (male mice).
[e]$p < 0.05$ tumor RPos (female mice) versus tumor RPos (male mice).
Reproduced with permission from Walker et al., *Proc Soc Exp Biol Med* 165:96–99, 1980.

terone. In male hamster, castration increased the growth rate of melanoma. On the other hand, castration had either no effect or increased effect on the growth rate of B-16 melanoma in male mice. Androgenic influence on biology of human melanoma also has been speculated for a long time. Initially, Herbst[132] reported partial response of widespread metastatic choroidal melanoma to orchiectomy. Shortly thereafter, Howes[133] raised caution against use of orchiectomy as a treatment of metastatic melanoma without further research. Also, ablative therapy has failed to produce any significant palliation for melanoma.[134] Recently, Rampen[135] and Rampen and Mulder[136] proposed that malignant melanoma may be an androgen dependent tumor. This hypothesis was derived from the finding that median survival in men is significantly shorter than in women following detection of systemic metastases. The result was more pronounced when premenopausal women were compared to men less than 50 years ago. Demonstration of receptor for androgen in melanoma rekindled interest for androgenic manipulation for metastatic melanoma.[79,83] However, overall incidence for detectable receptors is low and biochemical characterization of these "receptor protein" is not sufficient to evaluate the exact nature. In our laboratory,[72] high-dose androgen (10^{-6}M) suppressed the growth of an androgen receptor negative but estrogen receptor-positive cell line. The exact mechanism is unclear but may be from aromatization of androgen to estradiol by tumor cells or may be from translocation of estrogen receptor to the cell nucleus by pharmacologic dose of androgen. Physiologic dose of testosterone had no effect on growth of other cell lines. Others also showed no effect of testosterone on receptor-negative cell line.[137,138] In a phase II trial using antiandrogen (Cyproterone acetate), Rose et al.[131] did not see any objective response in 18 treated patients. Thus, it appears that the androgenic influence on growth of human melanoma is probably not significant.

Effect of Glucocorticoid on Melanoma

The mechanism of action of glucocorticoid on cells is more complex. It may have a direct influence; however, the influence may be mediated through other growth factors.

Weinberger et al.[139] found similarity of glucocorticoid receptor structure to the v-*erb*-a oncogene product of avian erythroblastosis virus suggesting steroid receptor gene and c-*erb*-a proto-oncogene are derived from a common primordial regulatory gene. As mentioned previously, growth factors such as EGF may mediate the glucocorticoid receptors in cells.

Animal models have been used frequently to study the influence of glucocorticoid on growth of melanoma. Tyrosinase activity was shown to be enhanced in melanoma under influence of glucocorticoid.[140] A pharmacological dose of glucocorticoid also inhibited growth of hamster and mouse melanoma cell lines.[141,142,143] Receptors for glucocorticoid were demonstrated in both tumor tissue and cloned cell lines.[144,145,146] In hamster melanoma, the glucocorticoid receptor is well-characterized regarding its specificity, binding characteristic, and molecular weight.[145,146] Adrenalectomy also altered the growth of the hamster melanoma.[147] However, Hawkins et al. indicated that the presence of receptor for glucocorticoid did not correlate to a biologic response.[148]

Glucocorticoid receptors have been demonstrated and well-characterized in human melanoma tissue. The incidence of such a receptor in human melanoma varies widely (19 to 86%).[49,149] Receptors for glucocorticoid also have been shown in human

TABLE 4-3
RESPONSE OF ESTROGEN RECEPTOR-POSITIVE AND NEGATIVE MELANOMA CELL LINES TO INCREASING DOSES OF ESTRADIOL (E2)[a] IN VIVO IN MALE ATHYMIC MICE

RECEPTOR STATUS	TREATMENT	NUMBER	PERCENT TUMOR INCIDENCE	TUMOR LATENCY (days)[b]	FINAL TUMOR WEIGHT (g)[b]	INCIDENCE OF METASTASIS
Positive	control	13	100	4.5 ± 0.2	3.9 ± 0.3	8.3
Positive	0.01 μE_2	10	100	4.4 ± 0.4	1.0 ± 0.1[c]	0
Positive	0.1 μE_2	5	80	5.0 ± 0.6	0.1 ± 0.2[c]	0
Negative	control	13	100	6.5 ± 0.6	7.58 ± 1.0[d]	38.0[c]
Negative	0.01 μg	5	100	6.8 ± 0.2	11.7 ± 2.6	40.0[c]
Negative	0.1 μg	8	100	5.7 ± 0.2	7.51 ± 0.4	50.0[c]

[a]E_2 administered s.c. in corn oil every other day.
[b]Mean ± SE
[c]$p < 0.01$ from vehicle control; analysis of variance (ANOVA) followed by Student-Neuman-Keuls discrimination test.[11]
[d]$p > 0.05$ by Fisher's exact probability test[11] from receptor-positive control.
Reproduced with permission from Chaudhuri et al. *Phenotypic Expression in Pigment Cells.* Mokoto Seiji ed., Tokyo: Tokyo Press.

melanoma cell lines.[137,138,150] The growth of such cell lines could be manipulated by glucocorticoid suggesting a possible direct influence of the hormone through its receptor.[151] Also, following stimulation of glucocorticoid receptor-positive human cell line by the hormone, enhanced cytotoxicity to melphalan was noted.[152] The exacerbation of growth of metastatic melanoma by dexamethasone in patients with glucocorticoid receptor-positive melanoma has been reported.[153] In phase I, clinical trials with NSC 17256 (6α-methyl-pregn-4-ene-3,11,20 trione), a controversial synthetic hormone with both glucocorticoid and progestational activity, 11 percent partial and complete response rate was noted.[154] In a phase II, only 6 out of 111 patients (5.4%) had objective response[155] to the same hormone.

Therapeutic Effect of Hormone Manipulation in Melanoma

The therapeutic implications of steroid hormones receptor in melanoma have been limited. Majority of the studies reporting presence of estrogen receptor demonstrate low receptor content which may partly account for lack of estrogen responsiveness. Some investigators have questioned the presence of true estrogen binding protein in melanoma. Several reports have been published on the effect of DES and antiestrogen (Tamoxifen) on metastatic melanoma in patient population.[156,157,158,159,160,161,162,163] Fisher et al.[156] reported that among 18 patients treated with DES at a dose of 5 mg p.o. t.i.d. showed objective response in two patients and prolong tumor stabilization in one patient. Furthermore, both responses were in receptor-negative tumors. Nesbit et al.[157] and Meyskens and Voakes[158] reported an encouraging response rate of 40 percent using tamoxifen in advanced melanoma. The number of patients treated in both series was limited. Southwest Oncology Group[163] reported only one complete response and no partial response among 28 patients treated with tamoxifen. This response was noted in a patient with receptor-negative tumor. Using two different dose schedules, Creagan reported only one minor response of soft tissue lesion among 42 patients treated with tamoxifen.[159,160] An overall partial and complete response rate of approximately 10 percent have been reported. Accumulated response rate, duration of response and correlation to receptor status, and sex has been compiled by Hodgins.[84] It appears that female patients have a higher response rate than male. Also, there is a higher incidence of complete response in female patients compared to male patients. The response rate is higher among patients who had receptor-positive tumor, (4/18) than the overall group. However, other investigators have demonstrated an objective response following tamoxifen therapy in receptor-negative patients, raising speculation that the effect of tamoxifen may not be mediated through estrogen receptor. (See Chap. 28 for combination of chemotherapy and tamoxifen.)

The influence of progesterone is more difficult to assess since synthetic progestational agents also have androgenic, synandrogenic, and glucocorticoid activity. Beretta et al.[130] reported a 25 percent response rate following treatment of melanoma patients with medroxyprogesterone acetate. Similarly, in phase I and phase II studies, 6α-methyl-pregn-4-ene-3,11,20 trione (NSC 17256) was shown to have an 11 percent and a 6 percent response rate, respectively, in unselected patients.[154,155]

Clinical trials of testosterone on melanoma patients are sparse. Bodenham and Hale noted partial

TABLE 4-4
COMPARISON OF DISEASE-FREE INTERVAL BETWEEN RECEPTOR-POSITIVE AND RECEPTOR-NEGATIVE PATIENTS (MALE AND FEMALE COMBINED) WITH CUTANEOUS MELANOMA (LEVEL IV AND V; STAGE I AND II)

RECEPTOR STATUS	NUMBER	NUMBER STAGE II	DFI (MONTHS) MEAN ± SEM
Positive	23	14	39.5 ± 6.31
Negative	42	16	17.56 ± 2.23

$p < 0.05$; ANOVA followed by Student's t test.
Reproduced with permission from Chaudhuri et al. Proc. XIIth International Pigment Cell Conference 7:595–599, 1983.

TABLE 4-5
COMPARISON OF DISEASE-FREE INTERVAL BETWEEN RECEPTOR-POSITIVE AND RECEPTOR-NEGATIVE FEMALE PATIENTS WITH CUTANEOUS MELANOMA (LEVEL IV; STAGE I AND II)

RECEPTOR STATUS	NUMBER	NUMBER STAGE II	DFI (MONTHS) MEAN ± SEM
Positive	9	5	55.11 ± 11.33
Negative	16	7	21.40 ± 7.56

$p < 0.01$; ANOVA followed by Student's t test.
Reproduced with permission from Chaudhuri et al. Proc. XIIth International Pigment Cell Conference 7:595–599, 1983.

response in male patients treated with testosterone.[164] However, Rose et al.[131] observed no significant response with cyproterone acetate for metastatic melanoma.

Prognostic Influence of Sex and Steroid Receptor in Melanoma Patients

Although there is not significant sex predilection for melanoma, the female population appears to have a better prognosis. In a study reported from Norway, Magnus[165] found that overall, female patients have a better survival than male patients at 5 years (70.5% versus 50.5%) and at 10 years (60% versus 40%). In this study, superior survival was noted irrespective of anatomic location. Improved outcome in female, however, was noted in patients with localized disease. When metastasis was detected, no survival difference was noted from detection of metastases to death according to sex. Correlation between age and sex on survival of melanoma patients has been reported by Olsen.[166] In the Norwegian study, the female superiority was more pronounced in older patients. On the contrary, Olsen reported a better outcome in the younger age group. Shaw et al.[167,168] attributed the female superiority in survival in Stage I disease to early lesions in females compared to males. Later on, the same group reported no difference in survival among different sex for clinical Stage II lesions. Danforth et al.,[169] Blois et al.,[170] and Griffel[171] also indicated better outcome in female patients. In a large study from Duke University[172] consisting of 1489 melanoma patients, better survival in females was found to be independent of anatomic site, histologic, and morphologic type or Clark level of invasion. Contrary to this finding, Shaw et al.[173] and Weidner[174] did not find any improved survival rate in female patients based on sex as a sole discriminatory factor.

The influence of sex on response to chemotherapy also has been postulated. Comis and Carter[175] reported a better response rate to chemotherapy in female patients. However, this difference in response to chemotherapy may be due to difference in tumor growth rate between male and female patients.[176] The presence of estrogen and progesterone receptor to the prognosis in melanoma has been evaluated. Initial demonstration of improved prognosis in patients with receptor-positive tumor[177] was supported by another report in a larger group of patients.[85] The improved survival in the receptor-positive group was more prominent among female patients as compared to males. This receptor-positive group enjoyed a better survival in spite of the fact that a large proportion of patients were in Stage II at the time of initial treatment (see Table 4-4 to Table 4-6). This improved survival in receptor-positive patients is also paralleled in experimental model.[95] The growth rate of receptor-positive human melanoma was significantly less in athymic mice model than the growth rate of receptor-negative tumors. The receptor-negative tumor had a much higher incidence of metastasis. Presence of progesterone receptors has not shown to be a prognostic discriminator.[161]

CONCLUSION

The endocrine effects on biology of melanocytes and melanomas have long been speculated. The influence of various peptides and steroid hormones are to a great extent species specific. It is clear at this time

TABLE 4-6
COMPARISON OF DISEASE-FREE INTERVAL BETWEEN RECEPTOR-POSITIVE AND RECEPTOR-NEGATIVE MALE PATIENTS WITH CUTANEOUS MELANOMA (LEVEL IV AND V; STAGE I AND II)

RECEPTOR STATUS	NUMBER	NUMBER STAGE II	DFI (MONTHS) MEAN ± SEM
Positive	14	9	29.42 ± 6.36
Negative	26	9	17.83 ± 3.11

p < N.S. ANOVA followed by Student's t test.
Reproduced with permission from Chaudhuri et al. Proc. XIIth International Pigment Cell Conference 7:595–599, 1983.

that the therapeutic benefit of hormonal manipulation of melanoma is very little. However, detailed study of the mechanism of action of various hormones may open avenues for development of new therapeutic approach. Synchronization of cell cycles by hormone manipulation for better antitumor effect of chemotherapeutics or targeting cells by conjugation of chemotherapeutic and hormones may be more beneficial.

At present neither oral contraceptive nor pregnancy is thought to exert adverse effect on nevi and melanoma. Termination of pregnancy in melanoma patients is not indicated to alter the outcome of the disease. Although several cases of transplacental metastasis to fetus have been reported, the overall risk appears to be very small. Recommendation to avoid pregnancy in newly diagnosed melanoma patients is based more on social implication than medical reason in poor risk patients.

REFERENCES

1. Hadley ME. In: Hadley ME (ed.), *The Melanotropins: in Endocrinology*. Englewood Cliffs, N.J.: Prentice Hall, 1988, 160–181.
2. Pawelek JM. Factors regulating growth and pigmentation of melanoma cells. *J Invest Dermatol* 66:201–209, 1976.
3. Gerst JE, Sole J, and Mather JP. Regulation of adenylate cyclase by β melanotropin in M2R melanoma cell line. *Mol Cell Endocrinol* 46:137–144, 1986.
4. Gerst JE, and Solomon Y. Inhibition by mellition and fluphenarim of melatropin receptor function and adenylate cyclase in M2R melanoma cell membranes. *Endocrinol* 121:1766–1772, 1978.
5. McLane J, Orber N, and Pavelek JM. Phosphorylated isomer of L-DOPA stimulate MSH binding capacity and responsiveness to MSH in cultured melanoma cells. *Biochem et biophysics.* Research communication 145:719–725, 1987.
6. Cobb JP, and Willetts N. Response of clondman S91 melanoma cells to melanocyte stimulating hormone: Enhancement by cytochalasin B. *J Natl Cancer Inst* 56:1079–1081, 1976.
7. Halaban R, and Lerner A. Dual effect of a melanocyte stimulating hormone in the growth of melanoma cell. *Exp Cell Res* 108:118, 1977.
8. Maleh ZA, Hadley ME, and Bregman MD. Action of melanotropin on mouse melanoma cell growth in vitro. *J Natl Cancer Inst* 76:857–863, 1986.
9. Nordlund JJ, Collins Ce, and Rheirs LA. Prostaglandin E_2 and D_2 but not MSH stimulate the proliferation of pigmented cells in pineal epidermis of DBA/2 mouse. *J Invest Dermatol* 86:433–437, 1986.
10. Ghanem G, Lienard D, Hanson P, Lejeune F, and Fruhling J. Increased serum alpha-melanocyte stimulating hormone (Alpha-MSH) in human malignant melanoma. *Eur J Cancer Clin Oncol* 22:535–536, 1986.
11. Libert A, Ghanem G, Gebski MJ, and Lejeune F. Inability of detecting αMSH binding cells in normal human cultured melanocyte. *Proc 3rd Ann Meeting of the Eur Soc Pg Cell Res,* Sept 1991, Amsterdam.
12. Ghanem GE, Libert A, Arnould R, Varcammen A, and Lejeune F. Human melanoma targeting with αMSH melphalan conjugate. *Melanoma Research* 1:105–114, 1991.
13. DasGupta TK, and Terz J. Influence of pineal gland on the growth and spread of melanoma in hamster. *Cancer Res* 27:1306–1311, 1967.
14. Barone RM, and DasGupta TK. Role of pinealtectomy in Walker 256 carcinomas in rats. *J Surg Oncol* 2:313–322, 1970.
15. El-Domeiri AA, and DasGupta TK. Reversal by melatonin of the effect of pinealectomy on tumor growth. *Cancer Res* 33:2830–2833, 1973.
16. Mariita J, and Kudo H. Effect of melatonin on B16 melanoma growth in athymic mice. *Cancer Res* 45:4175–4177, 1985.
17. Stanberry LR, DasGupta TK, and Beattie CW. Photoperiodic control of melanoma growth in hamster influence of pinealectomy and melatonin. *Endocrinology* 113:469–475, 1983.
18. Walker MJ, Chaudhuri PK, Beattie CW, et al. Neuroendocrine and endocrine correlates to hamster melanoma. *Surgical Forum* 151–152, 1979.
19. Bartsch H, Bartsch C, and Notebarn H. Growth inhibiting effect of crude pineal extracts in human melanoma cells in vitro is different from that of known synthetic pineal substances. *J Neural Trans* 69 (3–4):299–311, 1987.
20. Gonzalez R, Sanchez A, Ferguson JA, Balmer C, Daniel C, Cohn A, and Robinson W. Melatonin therapy of advanced human malignant melanoma. *Melanoma Research* 1:237–243, 1991.
21. Goustin AS, Leof EB, Shipley GD, and Moses HL. Growth factors and cancer. Perspectives in cancer research. *Cancer Res* 46:1015–1029, 1986.
22. Bradshaw RA, and Rubin JS. Polypeptide growth factors: Some structural and mechanistic considerations. *J Supramolecular Structure* 14:183–199, 1980.
23. Singletary SE, Baker FL, Spitzer G, Tucker SL, Tomasovic B, Brock WA, Ajani JA, and Kelly AM. Biological effect of epidermal growth factor on the in vitro growth of human tumors. *Cancer Res* 47:403–406, 1987.
24. Taylor JM, Mitchell WM, and Cohen S. Epidermal growth factor. *J Biol Chem* 247:5928–5934, 1972.
25. Gray A, Dull TJ, and Ullrich A. Nucleotide sequence of epidermal growth factor cDNA predicts a 128,000-molecular weight protein precursor. *Nature* 303:722–725, 1983.
26. Downward J, Yarden Y, Mayes E, Scrace G, Totty N, Stockwell P, Ullrich A, Schlessinger J, and Waterfield MD. Close similarity of epidermal growth factor receptor and v-erb-B oncogene protein sequences. *Nature* 307:521–527, 1984.
27. Koprowski H, Herlyn M, Balaban G, Parmiter A, Ross A, and Nowell P. Expression of the receptor for epidermal growth factor correlates with increased dosage of chromosome 7 in malignant melanoma. *Somat Cell Mol Genet* 11:297–302, 1985.
28. Real FX, Wolfgang JR, Chesa PG, Melamed MR, Old LJ, and Mendelsohn J. Expression of epidermal growth factor receptor in human cultured cells and tissues: Relationship to cell lineage and stage of differentiation. *Cancer Res* 46:4726–4731, 1986.
29. Herlyn M, Clark WH, Rodeck U, Mancianti ML, Jambrosic J, and Koprowski H. Biology of disease: Biology of tumor progression in human melanocytes. *Lab Invest* 56:461–474, 1987.
30. Rodeck U, Herlyn M, Menssen HD, Furlanetto RW, and Koprowski H. Metastatic but not primary melanoma cell lines grow in vitro independently of exogenous growth factors. *Int J Cancer* 40:687–690, 1987.
31. Kudlow JR, Khosravi MJ, Kobrin MS, and Mak WW. Inability of anti-epidermal growth factor receptor monoclonal

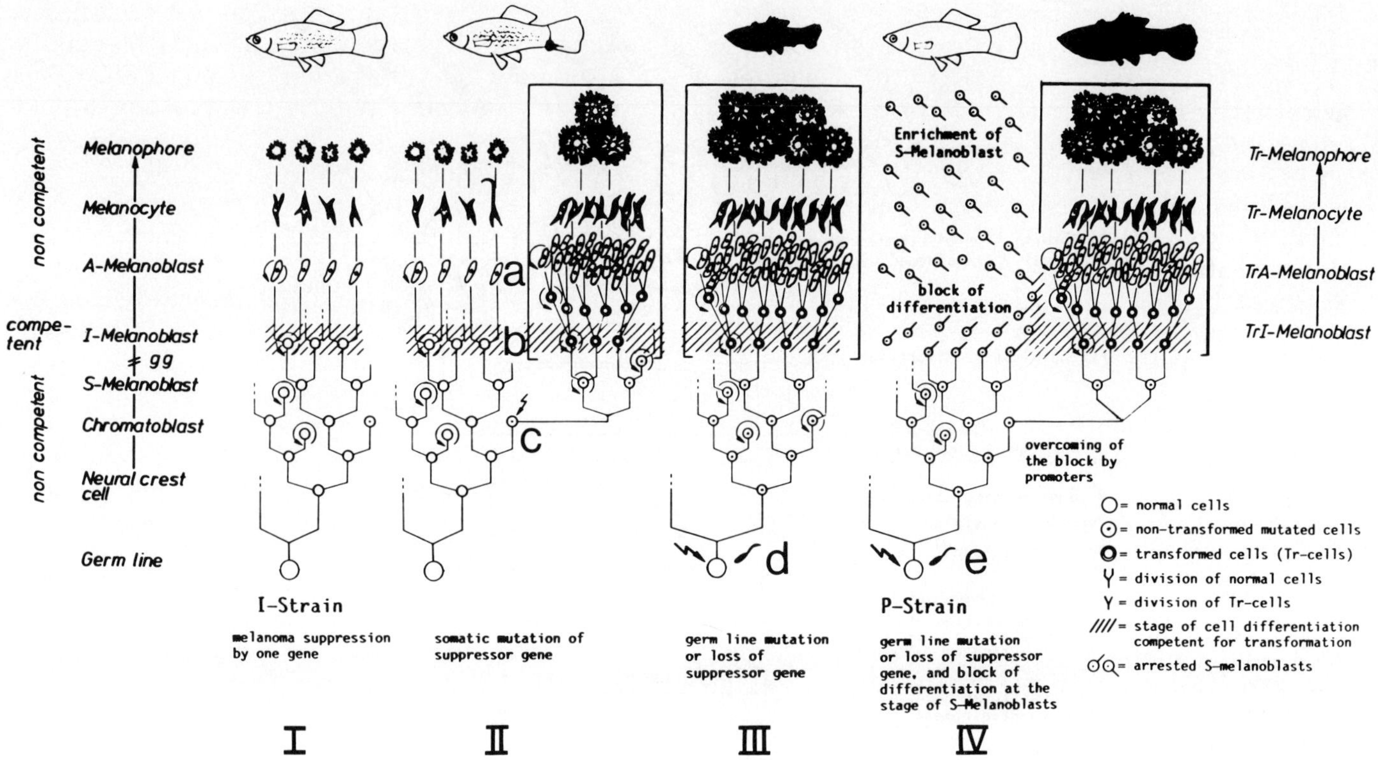

FIG. 5-2. Normal and melanomatous pigment cell differentiation. I. I-strain (sensitive to initiators, i.e., mutagenic carcinogens), protected from melanoma by one suppressor gene. II. I-strain developing somatic mutation-conditioned melanoma: a, if the suppressor gene is hit at this place of cell differentiation no melanoma develops; b, melanoma of unicellular origin develops (following complete removal there is no relapse); c, melanoma of oligicellular origin develops (if all chromatoblasts, S-melanoblasts, and I-melanoblasts are removed there is no relapse). IIId. Animals developing melanoma "spontaneously," that is, provoked by selective matings (elimination or "loss" of suppressor genes), or induced by germ-line mutation (loss or impairment of suppressor genes). These melanomas are of multicellular origin. Complete removal does not remove the source of the I-melanoblasts, therefore, is followed by relapse. IVe. P-strain developing promoter-provoked melanoma. Pigment cell differentiation is blocked between S- and I-melanoblasts by g/g ("golden" gene). A boost of cell differentiation by tumor promoters is required for melanoma formation. Melanomas are of multicellular origin. Complete removel is difficult; relapse is expected.[17]

the development of malignant melanoma. However, in the presence of the differentiating gene *Diff* in the system, the majority of the *Tr*-melanocytes branch out to terminally differentiating *Tr*-melanophores which stop dividing, achieve a fixed life span, and are removed by machrophages following cell death. These cells determine the final stage in the development of benign in differentiation melanoma. The chronology of the cell differentiation in the genuine malignant and benign melanomas clearly indicates that both neoplasms start with an indistinguishable malignant stage. The melanoma lacking *Diff* (differentiating gene) continues a malignant course while the melanoma containing *Diff* changes to a more benign or differentiated course. The generally accepted sequence of tumor development from normal tissues to benign, and thereafter, to malignant neoplasia could not be confirmed on the basis of the chronology of pigment cell differentiation in our model. Neoplastic transformation, although composed of a long chain of different events on the molecular level, appears in total as an all-or-nothing process of malignancy which later on may be modified to a more benign or differentiated stage.

Most of the cellular activities of normal and transformed pigment cells comprising proliferation, enzymes, maturation of melanosomes, and so on, were found in the different stages of melanoblasts and melanocytes. Thereafter these activities terminate.

The Differentiation Gene Diff

Differentiation of both normal and transformed pigmented cells is encoded in several genes which include the differentiation gene *Diff*. In melanoma development this gene acts posttransformationally in transposition, and therefore, is considered as an oncostatic gene. If both copies of *Diff* are lost in the course of selective breeding or treatment with

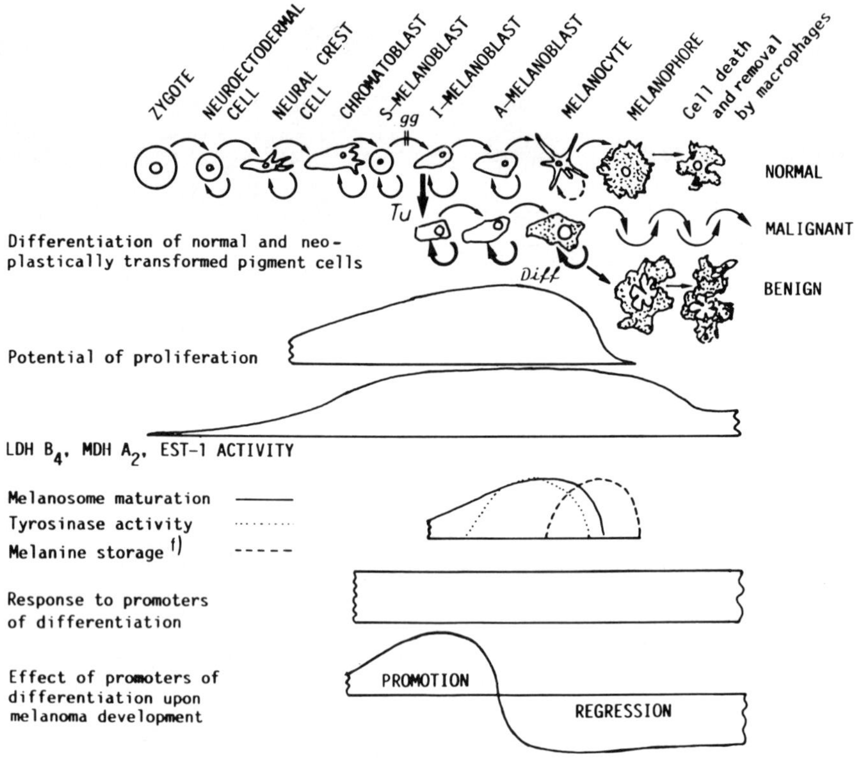

FIG. 5-3. Chronology of typical and atypical pigment cell differentiation.[17]

carcinogens, malignant melanomas develop. Loss of one copy results in a more benign or differentiating melanoma. If *Diff* is present in the homozygous state, spots develop.

Diff is linked to several isozyme genes,[18,19,20] which are functionally independent from *Diff;* they serve as markers for *Diff* in all tumorous and normal tissues. Besides this linkage, *Diff*-congregates with the appearance of a family of modified tRNAs including $tRNA^{Asn}$, $tRNA^{Asp}$, $tRNA^{His}$, and $tRNA^{Tyr}$ that contain queuosine (Q) instead of guanosine (G) in the first position (position 34) of the anticodon.[21,22] Evidence for the possible involvement of this tRNA modification in the process of cell differentiation comes from other laboratories working with eubacteria, slime molds, and normal and neoplastic mammalian cells and tissues in vitro.[23] The more the cells are differentiated, the more replacement of guanosine by queuosine is observed. Similarly, the tRNA family of the malignant melanoma (no *Diff*—low differentiation) is G-rich while that of the benign melanoma (one copy of *Diff*—almost always terminal differentiation) is Q-rich.[24] The cosegregation of *Diff* and the appearance of the modified tRNAs is not only observed in the melanoma but also in the normal tissues (skin, brain) of the melanoma-free segregant. This kind of tRNA modification, therefore, might be related to the oncostatic *Diff*-effect rather than to secondary processes in benign melanomas.

The differences in the functional properties of Q-containing and Q-lacking tRNAs require further elucidation. The (Q)-tRNAs are suggested to prefer codons NAU over NAC, whereas the Q-lacking tRNAs recognize NAC and NAU equally well. This may be an important mechanism in the regulation of translation.

ETIOLOGICAL TYPES OF MELANOMA

Human neoplasms can be classified into five groups according to etiology: (1) a large group that is carcinogen-dependent, for example, melanoma, basal cell carcinoma, lung cancer; (2) another large group which is promoter-dependent, that is, endocrine and ingestion-related, for example, breast, prostatic, and colon cancer; two smaller groups; (3) familial spread, and (4) Mendelian inherited, in which genes are supposed to be the critical factors, for example, certain melanomas and colon cancers, retinoblastoma, meningioma, neuroblastoma, xeroderma pigmentosum; and (5) a probably small group that is virus-dependent, for example, leukemia and papilloma.[1,25] These groups are often considered completely independent from each other.

Additional types of tumor etiology are conceivable. For instance, neoplasia following the deficiency of repair of damage to DNA or following the deficiency of immune surveillance. These and other deficiencies, however, are involved in control of tumor growth rather than in the actual process of neoplastic transformation.

The same groups were identified in *Xiphophorus*. They provide an excellent material for studies on the biology of tumor etiology. We shall focus on four types (see Fig. 5-2 and Table 5-1).

Carcinogen-Dependent Melanoma

Fish collected from wild populations and inbred in the laboratory are insusceptible to melanoma. Certain interpopulational and interracial hybrids, however, are susceptible. Studies on the genetic aspect of this phenomenon revealed that, the more suppressor genes are lost or eliminated in the course of selective breeding, the more susceptibility emerges. Complete loss results in whole body-melanoma, that starts developing in the early embryo and kills the fish at the time of birth. Melanoma development finally depends on the release of a formally identified tumor gene-complex (*Tu*-complex, or *Tu*) from its control, normally accomplished by controller genes, that is, suppressor genes.

Fishes were bred lacking the suppressor genes except for the one type that is capable of compensating the deficient controllers. None of the thousands of these animals bred developed melanoma spontaneously. However, 8 to 10 months after treatment with "tumor initiators," for example, directly acting mutagenic agents such as X rays, MNU (N-methyl-N-nitrosourea), and ENU (N-ethyl-N-nitrosourea), or the indirectly acting carcinogen dethylnitrosamine, and the adduct-forming IQ (2-amino-3-methylimidazo[4.5-f] quinoline), depending on the mode of application, the majority of these individuals may develop melanoma and a large variety of other kinds of neoplasms. The melanomas may develop at any place of the body where a pigment cell precursor is released from control by mutation of the only crucial controller present in the system (Fig. 5-4). The carcinogen may affect a pigment cell at several stages of its differentiation (Fig. 5-2 I, II, a, b, c).

a. The mutagenic carcinogen may influence the controller gene, for instance, in an A-melanoblast. This mutation cannot be expressed and is, therefore, undetectable.
b. The genetic change may be induced in an I-melanoblast. This cell is competent and becomes neoplastically transformed to a *TrI*-melanoblast. After division and differentiation, this cell gives rise to an easily detectable clone consisting of transformed cells. The smallest clones observed so far consisted of 8 *Tr*-melanocytes indicating that there were three cell divisions between the mutation event and the occurrence of the *Tr*-melanocytes. These *Tr*-cells may continue to divide, and give rise to a slowly growing melanoma. The origin of a melanoma of this kind is clear-cut unicellular, and its growth proceeds only by proliferation. After complete removal, relapse does not occur.
c. The change may also occur in an S-melanoblast. This cell is not yet competent and, therefore, remains still nontransformed and may multiply over a long period as a normal stem cell. Later on, those descendants reaching the stage of competence by normal differentiation, are transformed simultaneously. After some cell divisions, paralleled by cell differentiation, they become visible as a large cell clone consisting of hundreds or thousands of dividing *TrA*-melanoblast and *Tr*-melanocytes which give rise to the melanoma. Those melanoma cells, which are located at the margin of the clone, may differentiate to *Tr*-melanophore and are removed by macrophage. Those S-melanoblast, however, which do not further differentiate, may reproduce identically throughout the life of the fish and may serve as a permanent source of I-melanoblast, which then become neoplastically transformed. The origin of such a melanoma is multicellular or oligocellular at the morphological level, although it can be traced back to a single mutational event in a somatic cell. After complete removal of the melanoma there may or may not be a relapse. We assume that relapse occurs if some mutated stem cells escape removal and differentiate to the competent I-melanoblast which become neoplastically transformed. No relapse has been observed after extirpation of entire fins or large parts of the skin that carry the localized clonal melanomas.

The majority of the mutagenic carcinogen-dependent neoplasms induced in somatic cells of different genotypes is probably always due to a single mutational event in a particular controller gene. This is derived from the fact that these neoplasms appear as foci of cells in the tissues of the fish. The susceptibility of the fish to this etiological type of neoplasms is hereditary, while the neoplasms themselves are nonhereditary (see first column of Table 5-1).

Germ Line-Conditioned Melanoma

The genealogy of the germ line-conditioned melanoma induced by mutagenic carcinogens or provoked by crossings, is basically the same as that of the somatic mutation conditioned neoplasms (Fig. 5-2, III, d). As a consequence of the inheritance of the genetic defect or loss of controllers, the *Tu*-complex

TABLE 5-1
MELANOMA CONDITIONED BY

	SOMATIC MUTATION (TYPE I)	GERM LINE MUTATION (TYPE IIa)	CROSSINGS (TYPE IIb)	ALTERED DIFFERENTIATION (TYPE III)
Precondition	*Tu* predominantly repressed by not more than one suppressor	*Tu* predominantly repressed by not more than one supressor (suppressor was found to be always linked to *Tu*)	*Tu* predominantly repressed by suppressor nonlinked to *Tu*	*Tu* derepressed; delay of *Tu* target cells in a diffentiation stage noncompetent to *Tu* activity
Induction	Mutagens-carcinogens	Mutagens-carcinogens	Selective matings (interspecific and interpopulational)	BrdUrd, cAMP, UV, ACTH, low temperature, etc.: mutagens-carcinogens
Determination	In a somatic cell: mutation or deletion of the suppressor	In a germ-line cell: mutation or deletion of the suppressor	In the fertilized egg: replacement of suppressor containing by suppressor-lacking chromosomes	In somatic cells: promotion of delayed cells from noncompetence to competence
Transformation	a. Transformation of a single mutated competent cell b. Simultaneous transformation of the descendants of a single mutated noncompetent cell after getting competent	Continuous transformation of competent cells	Continuous transformation of competent cells	Simultaneous transformation of cells after getting competent
Origin	a. Unicellular b. Oligo- to multicellular	Multicellular	Multicellular	Multicellular
Occurrence	In treated animals ("induced")	In the descendant generations of a treated animal ("spontaneously")	In the offspring of specific matings ("spontaneously")	In treated animals ("induced")
Localization	Site of the mutated cell	Depends on the location of the competent cells	Depends on tissue- and compartment specificity of R	Site of altered cells
Growth	a. Only proliferation b. Permanent transformation and proliferation of the descendants of a single mutated cell	Permanent transformation and proliferation	Permanent transformation and proliferation	New transformation, followed by proliferation
Complete removal	a. No relapse b. No relapse, if mutated stem cells are also removed c. Relapse, if mutated stem cells are not removed	Relapse	Relapse	Theoretical no relapse (no complete removal possible)
Inheritance	Nonhereditary; genetically conditioned susceptibility	Dominant Mendelian trait	a. Hereditary if suppressors remain lacking b. Nonhereditary, if suppressors are reintroduced into genome	Nonhereditary; genetically conditioned susceptibility

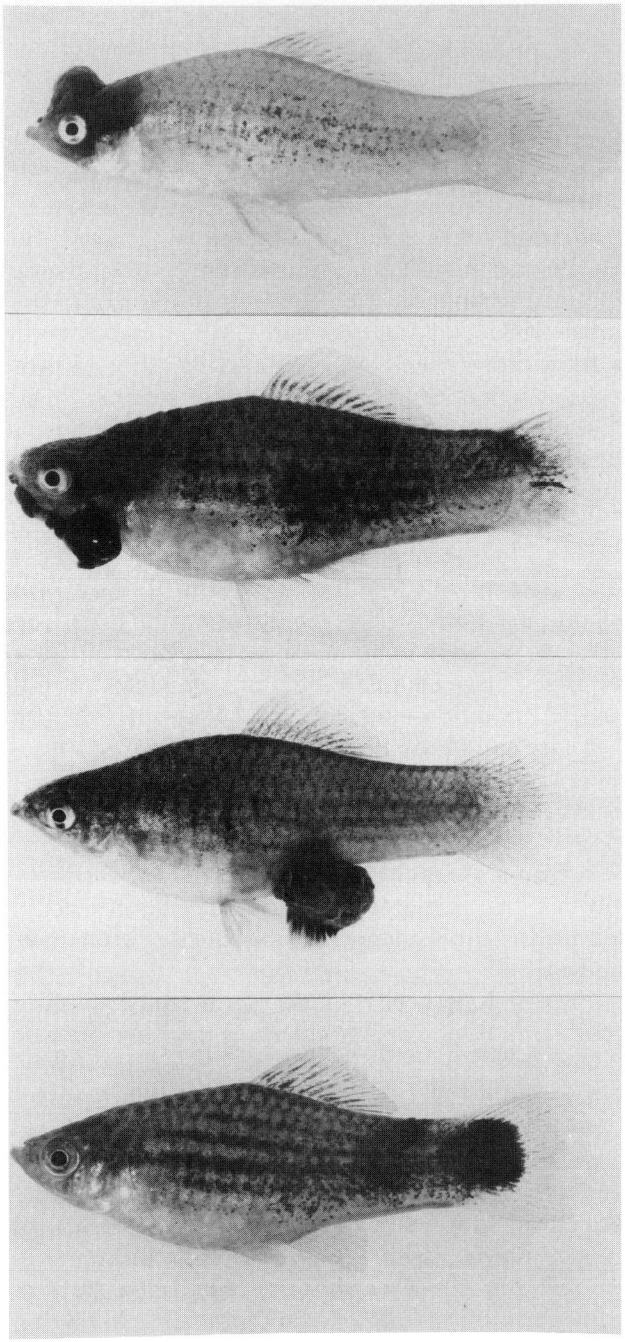

FIG. 5-4. *Clonal melanomas induced by MNU in initiator-dependent fish (I-strain, according to Fig. 5-2, II, b and c). Development of this etiological type of melanoma depends on somatic mutation of the only suppressor gene for the* Tu-complex *present in the system. Note that the melanomas develop 8 to 10 months after treatment. No relapse after complete removal. See Table 5-1, first column.*

becomes active in the developing progeny as soon as the melanophore precursor cells differentiate to the competent I-melanoblast. Sometime later some single dividing *Tr*-melanocytes appear at the peduncle of the tail fin. Neoplastic transformation continues in all areas of the developing fish where the pigment cell precursors become competent, thus reflecting the genuine effect of the completely derepressed tumor determinant in the melanophore system.

Hereditary melanomas of the fish and probably most of the other hereditary neoplasm of other species are of multicellular origin and grow, depending on the supply of stem melanoblast, by both transformation and proliferation. After removal it shows relapse, because stem cells remain available for differentiation to the competent cells, which become transformed (see second and third column of Table 5-1).

Promoter-Dependent Melanoma

Actually the cell genealogy of the promoter-dependent melanoma is the same as that of the hereditary conditioned melanomas induced by germ-line mutation or provoked by selective breeding (see Fig. 5-2, IV. e: compare with III. d). The difference is that promoter-dependent, that is, promoter-sensitive fish contain a genetic block of cell differentiation in the stage of stem melanoblast, and therefore, are normally melanoma free.

However, 6 to 8 weeks after treatment with authentic "tumor promoters" such as TPA (12-0-tetradecanoylphorbol-13-acetate)[26] or questionable agents such as betel nut extracts[27] almost all of these fish developed melanoma (Fig. 5-5 and Table 5-1, column 4). A large variety of compounds such as the DNA-hypomethylating 5-azacytidine, the adduct-forming safrole, androgens (testosterone, 5-dihydortestosterone, 19-nortestosterone, 17-methyltestosterone, trenbolone), estrogens (ethinylestradiole), antiestrogens (tamoxifen), or even the second messenger cyclic AMP that altogether are not truly mutagenic and were known as inert, were found to have tumor promoting effect. On the other hand, x rays, MNU, and ENU, besides being confirmed as mutagenic-carcinogenic agents, displayed promoting effects on melanoma growth.

In a paradoxical and perplexing manner, certain therapeutic and preventive measures were found to have tumor provoking effect. Contradictory effects in the fish were observed after treatment with all 13 reliable tumor promoters so far tested[2]: We consider the arrest of pigment cell differentiation at the stem-cell stage by the controller gene, as a Janus face. The face that occurs after the boost of differentiation of the arrested pigment cells at the stem-cell stage by tumor promoters shows transformation and

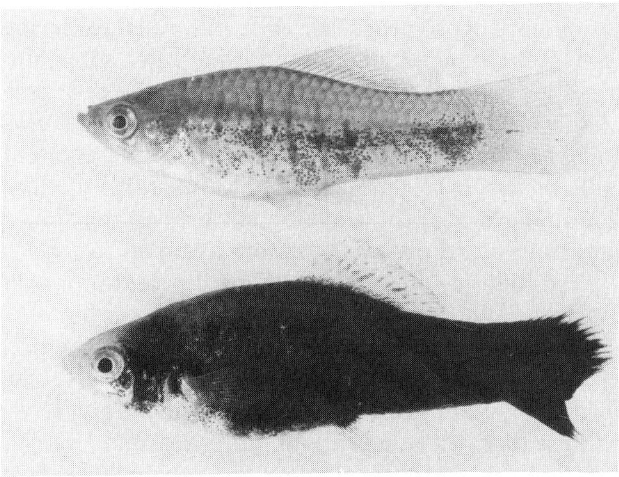

FIG. 5-5. *Melanoma of multicellular origin provoked by the tumor-promoter diethylstilbestrol in an extremely sensitive P-strain, according to Fig. 5-2, IV and Fig. 5-3 (promotion). Note that the melanomas develop within 6 to 8 weeks after treatment. Complete removal is difficult; relapse is expected. See Table 5-1, fourth column.*

melanoma promotion. The other face, however, that occurs after the boost of differentiation of the incompletely differentiated melanoma cells by the same tumor promoters shows terminal differentiation, removal of the old tumor cells by macrophage and finally, regression of melanoma. Even candidates of death due to melanoma could be cured by tumor promoters and raised up to maturity (Fig. 5-6). Their offspring, however, develop melanoma according to their genetic constitution.

Tumor promoters as previously mentioned did not initiate melanoma or any kind of neoplasia in the fish that require somatic mutation for melanoma formation.

Since sunlight and artificial UV exposure is considered as the important etiologic factor for melanoma in human, via thymidine dimerization and somatic mutation, some remarks in the view of our model are pertinent. UV is a powerful mutagen in microorganisms. Our irradiation experiments, however, suggest that melanoma of the fish cannot be initiated by mutation but may be promoted by a UV-induced boost of cell differentiation. As shown in irradiation experiments performed by Setlow and Woodhead,[28] melanoma of the fish develops following exposure to filtered radiation from sunlamps in the wavelengths ranging between 290 nm and 304 nm in their strains which are phenotypically and genotypical comparable to our promoter-sensitive fish. The induced neoplasms look like our promoter-induced melanomas which are different from the initiator-induced ones. The background rate of "spontaneous" melanoma (2 to 12%) indicates that the authors eliminated most of the crucial controller genes before treatment by selective breeding and thus set the preconditions for melanoma formation in the ancestry as we have done when we developed our promoter-sensitive strains. The promoting effect of UV in the promoter-sensitive xiphophorine strains, therefore can easily be replaced by other tumor promoters including hormonal or dietary factors.

It has been argued for a long time that melanoma in human is due to overexposure to the sun. This simple assumption, based on statistics, is probably not the whole truth, and so far nobody could explain the rapid increase of melanoma throughout the world.[29]

Taken together, it appears that regardless of what actually provokes spontaneous development of susceptibility to initiator and promoter-dependent melanoma, the end result of a transformed cell is the same. Namely, the unrestrained growth associated with atypical cell differentiation and cell accumulation to the neoplasm. These genetic and cytological statements imply that the process of transformation itself, as well as the maintenance and somatic inheritance of the neoplastic state of pigment cells, are also genetic problems involving disorders at the biochemical and molecular levels.

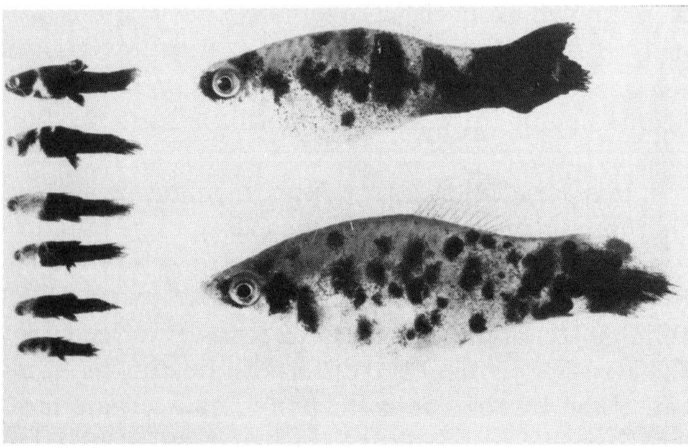

FIG. 5-6. *Melanoma of candidates of death (left) is suppressed (right) by the tumor promoter diethylstilbestrol. Treated fish reach maturity and can be propagated.*

ONCOGENES IN MELANOMA DEVELOPMENT

Coinheritance of x-erb*B**[a] and Susceptibility to Melanoma

Among 20 oncogenes for which we have probes available to us, the *Xiphophorus* genome contains all except *ros* and *mos*. There is no difference in platyfish and sword-tails which, by genetic reasons are actually different races.

Platyfish and swordtails were crossed and those hybrids which were susceptible to melanoma were back-crossed with the swordtail. By consequent application of this selective crossing procedure it turned out that the chromosome carrying the information for "spontaneous" melanoma formation or susceptibility to melanoma, respectively, is derived from the platyfish. Fish were bred, in which this chromosome is the only platyfish chromosome in the diploid set of 48 chromosomes. The critical question was to find oncogene sequences that are inherited along with the inheritance of spots of purebred platyfish or with the inheritance of melanoma in BC-segregants containing the platyfish-derived *Tu*-complex-carrying chromosome and 47 swordtail-derived chromosomes. Restriction fragment lengths polymorphisms (RFLP) was used for distinction of platyfish-specific oncogenes from swordtail-specific oncogenes and for tracing the inheritance of these genes (x-*oncs*) through the fish generations.[30,31] An oncogene fragment, determined by its length, which is independently inherited from the inheritance of spots or melanoma suggests that the oncogene in questions is not "critical" for melanoma formation. Only the gene or genes, that are inherited along with the *Tu*-complex in purebred and hybrids may code for a "critical" link of the chain leading to spots or melanomas, respectively. This does not imply that swordtail-derived oncogenes are not involved in melanoma formation at all; x-*erb*A, x-*src,* x-*sis,* x-*pdgf-r,* x-*ras,* x-*myc,* x-*myb,* certain v-*erb*B related x-*erb*B-genes, and probably other oncogenes that are contributed by the swordtail to the genome of the highly backcrossed melanoma developing fish are expressed, and some of them are even overexpressed in the melanomas.[30–33] They are apparently involved in the molecular, biochemical, and morphological processes leading to melanoma formation but are not involved in the genetically based platyfish-derived processes that actually start the selfish productive power of the pigment cell system.[1,25] So far, the only oncogene restriction fragment that is coinherited with spot and melanoma formation represent an oncogene which, as shown by sequencing of the subcloned fragments, refers to putative exons that probably encode the kinase domain of a growth factor receptor. This x-*onc* is related to the v-*erb*B from the erythroblastosis virus, to the *neu*-gene of the rat and to h-*egf-r* which is the human epidermal growth factor (EGF) receptor gene. The homology of these genes on both nucleotide and amino acid level comprises about 85 percent. Because of the high homology of this gene to the viral prototype v-*erb*B, it was designated as x-*erb*B*.[30,31] Sequencing was extended by means of this gene derived of a melanoma cell line[34] and it was shown that x-*erb*B* is not only expressed in the melanoma but also in certain fibrosarcomas and thyroid tumors.[33,35]

According to the assignment of a large variety of neurogenic, epithelial, and mesenchymal neoplasms to the platyfish-derived *Tu*-complex,[36] it is however unlikely that this gene is melanoma-specific. We could not identify a gene that alone may make a tumor, or what one would term a "melanoma gene," "neuroblastoma gene," "liver-cell carcinoma gene," and so on, while others working with other systems have thought they did. The widely held hypothesis of one gene—one tumor type is untenable for neoplasia in *Xiphophorus* and in this view, requires re-examination in the other systems.

More information about x-*erb*B* came from 15 mutational and phenotypical different purebred and hybridized xiphophorine fishes (Fig. 5-7): wherever initiator or promoter-induced or spontaneous melanomas (differentiated and undifferentiated) developed, a restriction fragment was found comprising 4.9 (X-chromosomal), 6.7 (T- and Z-chromosomal), or 11.5 (X-chromosomal) kb.[30,31] On the other hand, wherever these restriction fragments were found, we could evoke spontaneous melanoma formation, or sensitivity to mutagenic carcinogens or tumor promoters by appropriate selective matings. These fragments are clearcut genetic markers indicating a risk for melanoma of any type of etiology. They are the accessories in the genome. If they are lacking or lost there is almost no risk but also no harm for the fish.

Besides these fragments representing different melanoma-associated copies of the same gene which are accessories, a melanoma-nonassociated fragment comprising 7.5 kb (see Fig. 5-7) was identified. This fragment is present in all individuals, platyfish, and swordtail, and is therefore, not involved in the inheritance, that is, the very beginning of or susceptibility to the melanoma. The x-*erb*B* represented by this fragment is probably indispensable in the fish. We, therefore, distinguish between x-*erb*B*ᵃ copies that are accessory, and the x-*erb*B*ⁱ copy that is indispensable. The xiphophorine EGF-receptor gene (x-*egf*-r, x-*erb*B) itself appears to be represented by a *Tu*-complex nonlinked fragment comprising 5.5 kb. (Fig. 5-6). The platyfish-derived x-*erb*B*ᵃ and the swordtail derived x-*erb*B*ⁱ and x-*erb*B are expressed in melanoma and other kinds of tumors.[33] Their transcripts are of different lengths.

Oncogenes, Growth Regulation, and Inositol Lipid Turnover in Melanoma

The observation that most of the oncogenes including the "critical" x-*erb*B*ᵃ are expressed in the melanomas prompted us to examine the inositol lipid turnover in the melanomas. Other laboratories have demonstrated in mammalian and human cell types that an activation of the EGF-receptor enhances phosphoinositide metabolism[37] which appears to be causally involved in cell proliferation (see Fig. 5-8). The need to investigate the inositol lipid turnover was reinforced by our detection of highly elevated x-

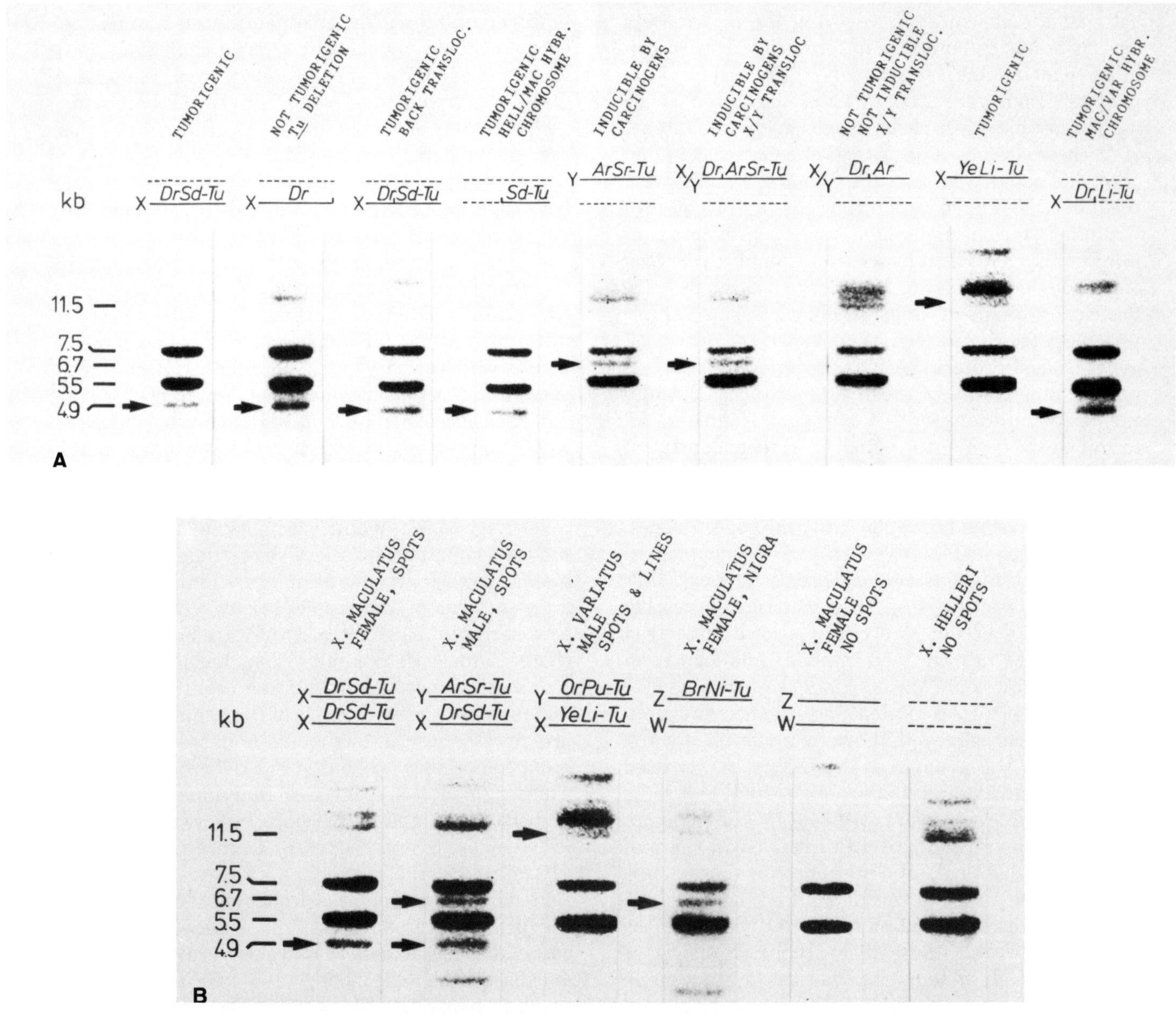

*FIG. 5-7. Assignment of v-*erb*B homologous Eco R1 fragments to the melanoma determining accessory* Tu*-complexes (Southern blot) in BC hybrids and purebred fish. Hybridization of v-*erb*B-specific probe against Eco R1 digested genomic DNA. X,Y,W,Z, sex chromosomes of the platyfishes; dashes, homologous chromosomes or chromosome fragments of the swordtail. Arrows indicate x-*erb*B^{*a}-specific fragments. The 7.5 kb fragment indicates x-*erb*B^{*i}, and the 5.5 kb fragment probably x-*erb*B (the xiphophorine EGF receptor gene). For color prints of the respective fish, see Ref. 30.*

src expression (measured by $pp60^{x\text{-}src}$ kinase activity in the xiphophorine melanoma,[38,39] based on the demonstration[40] that a potential substrate for $pp60^{c\text{-}src}$ kinase activity in mammalian systems is phosphatidyinositol kinase (PI-KINASE). One form of this enzyme initiates the pathway for the synthesis of polyphosphoinositides. Other forms of kinase phosphorylate phosphatidylinositol (PI) to phosphatidylinositol 4-monophosphate (PIP) which then, in turn, can be phosphorylated to phosphatidylinositol 4.5-biphosphate (PIP_2) which can be degraded by phospholipase C (PLC). PLC is activated by the platelet-derived growth factor (PDGF) via PDGF-receptor. This pathway is important because x-*sis* and x-*pdgf-r*, that is, the respective genes coding for the xiphophorine PDGF and PDGF-receptor, are expressed in melanomas.[33] PLC creates diacylglycerol (DG) which is an endogenous promoter acting on protein

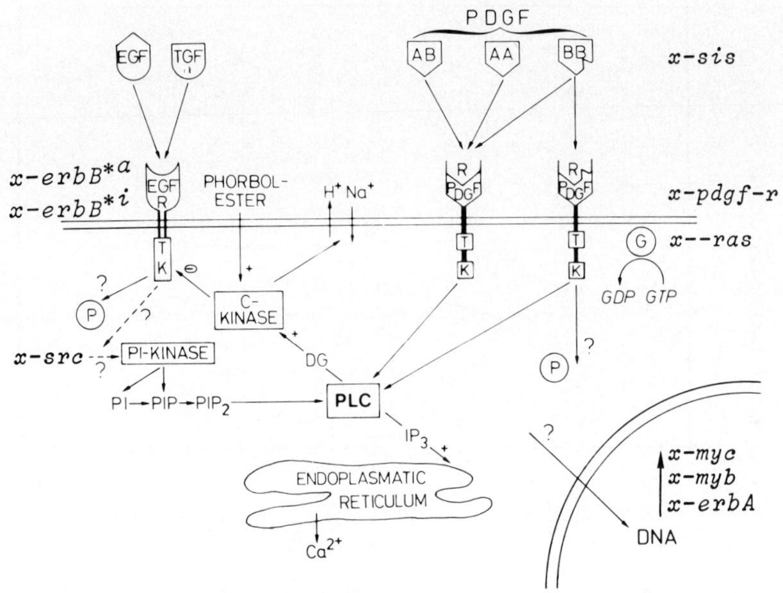

FIG. 5-8 Scheme of phosphoinositide response and oncogenes involved in xiphophorine melanoma formation (based on Ref. 46, modified).

kinase C (C-KINASE) comparable to 12-0-tetradecanoylphorbol-13-acetate (Phorbolester) which is an exogenous tumor promoter not only in mammalian systems but also in *Xiphophorus* hybrids. Activation of protein kinase C by diacylglycerol may, in turn, elevate the activity of the EGF-receptor which may enhance phosphoinositide metabolism (for review see Ref. 41). Phosphoinositide metabolism is classically reflected by increased levels of inositol phosphate intermediates which accumulate in the presence of Li^+. Thus, turnover of (^3H) inositol into phosphoinositides was measured, by means of in vitro assays of melanomas of different etiology. A considerable elevation of phosphatidyl inositol lipid turnover was found without any differences among the different types of melanoma based on etiology. However, incorporation of (^3H)-inositol into phosphoinositides in benign or differentiated melanoma was about three times and in malignant or less differentiated melanoma about 10 times elevated over that of the brain of purebred platyfish and swordtail which served as the controls.[42]

The expression of several oncogenes, and the elevation of phosphatidylinositol lipid turnover in the melanomas as studied so far suggest that tumor development in *Xiphophorus* depends on a foreign command on a molecular and biochemical system composed of a large number of genes which control normal pigment cell patterns. Out of these genes, so far, only one gene, x-*erb*B*^{a}, could be assigned to the platyfish *Tu*-complex where the command for melanoma comes from. x-*erb*B*^{a} appears as a master gene which, if it gets rid of control by loss, elimination, or dysfunction of suppressor genes, becomes carcinogenic through the power of its slaves.[43]

Approach to Predict Susceptibility and Insusceptibility of Healthy Individuals to Develop Melanoma in the Xiphophorine Model

A highly unsolved problem concerns the possibilities to determine the genetic risk of an individual to develop neoplasia. Our results possibly might show how to approach this problem.

Backcross individuals developing spontaneously melanoma do not only show an elevated pp60$^{x\text{-}src}$ kinase activity in their melanoma (and other tumors) but also in their healthy tissues, particularly in brain tissues.[44] pp60$^{x\text{-}src}$ activity in the brain of the tumorous segregants was increased three folds over that of the melanoma-free segregants. The activity in the melanoma itself was also found to be increased three-fold above that of the already elevated activity in the brain. The parallel elevation in melanoma and brain possibly reflects the neurogenic origin of both tissues.

The levels of (^3H) inositol in phosphatidylinositol of the brain were plotted against the activity of pp60$^{x\text{-}src}$ kinase, and thus, an excellent correlation was observed (Fig. 5-9). Two groups of genotypes can be discerned.[1,42,43] The first group showing low levels of inositol incorporation and x-*src* kinase activity in the brain, concerns genotypes that are either insusceptible to melanoma or require somatic mutation

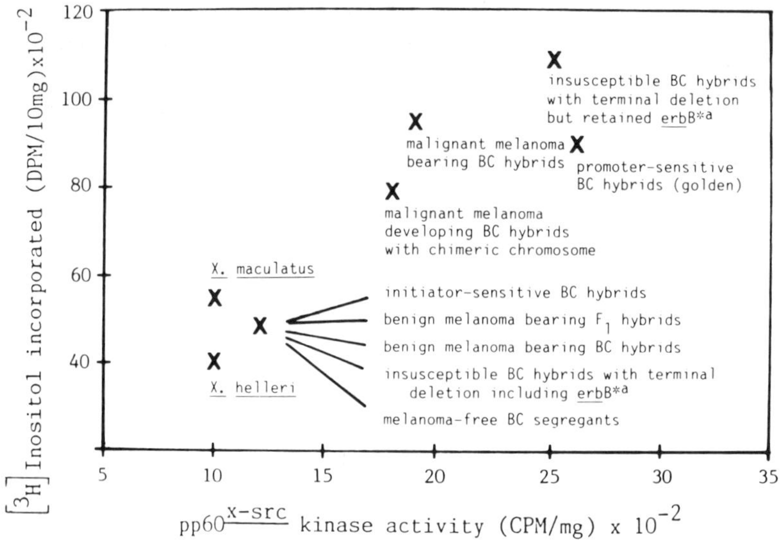

FIG. 5-9. Incorporation of (^{3}H)inositol in phosphatidylinositol in brain extracts, plotted against activity of pp60$^{x\text{-}src}$ kinase. Note the excellent correlation of both parameters, and the distinction of genotypes showing low or high susceptibility to melanoma. Data from Ref. 42, extended.

thus permitting development of malignant melanoma. This group covers purebred platyfish (x-*erb*B^{*a} is under perfect control), purebred swordtails as well as melanoma-free BC hybrids and a deletion mutant (all are free of x-*erb*B^{*a}), differentiated melanoma bearing fish (they contain x-*erb*B^{*a}, but are partly under control of *Diff*), and the BC hybrids of an initiator-sensitive strain (x-*erb*B^{*a} is well controlled by one suppressor gene). In contrast, the second group, displaying high levels of inositol incorporation and x-*src* kinase activity in the brain, represents animals capable of developing malignant melanoma spontaneously or following treatment with tumor promoters. Extremely high values were found in BC hybrids that have lost the melanophore-specific gene but retained x-*erb*B^{*a} (see Fig. 5-7, upper part, lane 2); these animals are insusceptible to melanoma because pigment cells are not available for transformation. The biochemical and molecular biological machinery of melanoma formation, however, appears to be running by genetic reasons.[42,43]

Parallelism similar to that of x-*src* expression and phosphoinositide turnover were found also in other laboratories in cell lines of other species including humans.[40,45] However, to our knowledge, no one has described the highly complex results that the healthy tissue and the malignant neoplasm show elevated phosphoinositide turnover and cellular *src* expression, and that this correlation parallels the capacity of healthy individuals to develop neoplasia "spontaneously" or after treatment with tumor promoters.

CONCLUSIONS

Our efforts to understand the melanoma of the *Xiphophorus* model on the genetic, systemic, cellular, and molecular levels showed new possibilities to interfere in the processes preceding the outburst of morphologically detectable de novo melanoma formation and relapse.

Individuals detectable by their uniformity in low inositol incorporation and low x-*src* kinase activity in their brains (the representative of probably all tissues), require at least one, mostly many somatic mutations of controller genes for activation of the ubiquitous oncogenes. Melanoma formation including the biochemical and molecular processes starts in one focus with a long latent period, and is of unicellular origin. Following complete removal, no relapse takes place if all mutated stem cells are also removed.

In contrast, individuals detectable by their more or less uniform high parameters, do not require genetic changes, neither somatic nor germinal. Their genetic requirements for melanoma formation including biochemical and molecular features are anticipated in both germ line and somatic cells and are detectable before the onset of melanoma. Melanoma formation may finally start according to minor factors of the genome either "spontaneously" or following tumor promotion by a large variety of endogenous or exogenous influences. The latent period is short, and the appearing tumor is of multicellular origin. This altogether explains why relapse takes place immediately after removal of germ line-conditioned spontaneous occurring or promoter-provoked melanoma; all pigment cell precursors of these animals are prospective melanoma cells.

ACKNOWLEDGMENTS

This work has been generously supported for many years by the Justus-Liebig-Universität Giessen, the Deutsche Forschungsgemeinschaft, by the Bundesminister für Forschung and Technologie, and by the Umweltbundesamt. Thanks are due to Sybill Lenz and Kristine Krüger for their help in the preparation of the manuscript.

REFERENCES

1. Anders F. Contributions of the Gordon-Kosswig melanoma system to the present concept of neoplasia. *Pigment Cell Res.* 3:7–29, 1991.
2. Anders A, Zechel Ch, Schlatterer B, Gröger H, Schmidt D, Smith A, and Anders F. Genetic and molecular approach for breeding and use of laboratory fish for the detection of agents with carcinogenic and/or promoting activity. *Bull Cancer Radiother.* 78:415–433, 1991.
3. Gordon M. The melanoma cell as an incompletely differentiated pigment cell. In: Gordon M (ed.), *Pigment Cell Biology.* New York: Academic Press, 1959, 215–239.
4. Sobel H, Marquet E, Kallman KD, and Corley GJ. Melanoma in *Xiphophorus.* In: Ribelin WE, and Migaki G (eds.), *The Pathology of Fishes.* Madison: University of Wisconsin Press, 1975, 945–981.
5. Vielkind U, and Paul E. Normal and malignant melanin-containing pigment cells of xiphophorine fish as studied with formaldehyde-induced fluorescence. *J Invest Dermato* 70:80–83, 1978.
6. Riehl R, Schartl M, and Anders F. An ultrastructural study of melanoma in *Xiphophorus.* In: Bagnara J, Klaus SN, Paul E, and Schartl M (eds.) *Pigment Cell 1985. Biological, Molecular and Clinical Aspects of Pigmentation.* Tokyo: University of Tokyo Press, 1985, 457–464.
7. Clauss G, Lohmeyer J, Hamby CV, Ferrone S, and Anders F. Melanoma-associated antigens in *Xiphophorus* fish. In: Ferrone S (ed.), *Human Melanoma.* Berlin-Heidelberg-New York-London-Paris-Tokyo-Hong Kong: Springer-Verlag, 1990, 74–86.
8. Clauss G, Winkler Ch, Lohmeyer J, Anders F, and Schartl M. Oncofetal antigen in *Xiphophorus* detected by monoclonal antibodies directed against melanoma-associated antigens. *Int J Cancer* 45:136–142, 1990.
9. Felding-Haberman B. Glykolipide in Tumoren und extraneuralen Geweben von *Xiphophorus.* University of Giessen, thesis, 1983.
10. Dippold WG, Knuth A, and Meyer zum Buschenfelde KH. Monoclonal anti-GD3-ganglioside antibody: Blocking of melanoma growth and T-cell cytotoxicity. In: Bagnara J, Klaus SN, Paul E, and Schartl M (eds.) *Pigment Cell 1985 Biological, Molecular, and Clinical Aspects of Pigmentation.* Tokyo: University of Tokyo Press, 1985, 291–302.
11. Felding-Haberman B, Anders F, Dippold WG, Stallcup WB, and Wiegandt H. Melanoma-associated gangliosides in the fish genus *Xiphophorus. Cancer Res* 48:3453–3460, 1988.
12. Peter RU, Schartl M, Anders F, and Duncker HR. Pigment pattern formation during embryogenesis in *Xiphophorus.* In: Bagnara J, Klaus SN, Paul E, and Schartl M (eds.), *Pigment Cell 1985. Biological, Molecular, and Clinical Aspects of Pigmentation.* Tokyo: University of Tokyo Press, 1985, 291–302.
13. Anders A, Diehl H, and Anders F. Differentiation of normal melanophores and neoplastically transformed melanophores in the skin of fishes of genus *Xiphophorus.* In: Spearman RIC, and Riley PA (eds.), *The Skin of Vertebrates.* Linnean Society Symposium Series 9:211–224, 1980.
14. Vielkind U, Schlage W, and Anders F. Melanogenesis in genetically determined pigment cell tumors of platyfish and platyfish-swordtail hybrids: Correlation between tyrosinase activity and degree of malignancy. *Z Krebsforschung* 90:285–299, 1977.
15. Schmidt H, and Anders A. Phenoloxidase (EC 1.14.18.1) und präformiertes Melanin als mögliche Marker zur Unterscheidung genetisch bedingter melanomfreier und melanombildender Rückkreuzungs-Segreganten bei *Xiphophorus. Biologisches Zentralblatt* 108:463–475, 1989.
16. Vielkind U. Genetic control of cell differentiation in platyfish-swordtail melanomas. *J Exp Zool* 196:197–205, 1976.
17. Anders A, and Anders F. *Xiphophorus* als Modell der Krebsforschung. In: Zellenergetik and Zelldifferenzierung, Marburg. *Jahresberichte des SFB 103.* 1980–1988, 8 volumes.
18. Siciliano MJ, and Wright DA. Biochemical genetics of the platyfish-swordtail melanoma system. *Prog Exp Tumor Res* 20:398–411, 1976.
19. Ahuja MR, Schwab M, and Anders F. Linkage between a regulatory locus for melanoma cell differentiation and an esterase locus in *Xiphophorus. J Heredity* 71:403–407, 1980.
20. Valentin P. Esterase-Isoenzyme bei *Xiphophorus* (Poeciliidae). University of Giessen, thesis, 1985.
21. Dess G. Das übermodifizierte Nukleosid Queuosin in Transfer-Ribonukleinsäuren aus Melanomen von *Xiphophorus.* University of Giessen, thesis, 1981.
22. Kersten H. Involvement of tRNA and the modified nucleoside Queuosine in cell development and differentiation. In: Jaenicke J (ed.), *Biochemistry of Differentiation and Morphogenesis.* Berlin-Heidelberg-New York: Springer-Verlag, 1982, 117–119.
23. Nass G (ed.), *Recent Results in Cancer Research. Modified Nucleosides and Cancer.* Berlin-New York: Springer-Verlag, 1983.
24. Anders A, Dess G, Nishimura S, and Kersten H. A molecular approach to the study of malignancy and benignancy in melanoma of *Xiphophorus.* In: Bagnara J, Klaus SN, Paul E, Schartl M (eds.), *Pigment Cell 1985. Biological, Molecular, and Clinical Aspects of Pigmentation.* Tokyo: University of Tokyo press, 1985, 314–324.
25. Anders F. The Mildred Scheel memorial lecture. A biologist's view of human cancer. In: Neth R, Gallo RC, Greaves MF, Gaedicke G, Gohla S, Mannweiler K, and Ritter J (eds.), *Modern Trends in Human Leukemia VIII.* Berlin-Heidelberg-New York-London-Paris-Tokyo-Hong Kong: Springer-Verlag, 1989, 23–45.
26. Schwab M. How can altered differentiation induced by 12-0-tetradecanoylphorbol-13-acetate be related to tumor promotion? In: Hecker E, Kunz W, Fusenig NE, Marks F, Thielmann HW (eds.), *Carcinogenesis.* New York: Raven Press, 1982, 7:417–426.
27. Stich HF, and Anders F. The involvement of reactive oxygen species in oral cancers of betel quid/tobacco chewers. *Mutat Res* 214:47–61, 1989.
28. Setlow RB, Woodhead AD, and Grist E. Animal model for ultraviolet radiation-induced melanoma: Platyfish-swordtail hybrid. *Proc Natl Acad Sci U S A* 86:8922–8926, 1989.
29. Marshal E. Experts clash over cancer data. *Science* 250:900–902, 1990.
30. Zechel Ch, Schleenbecker U, Anders A, and Anders F. v-*erb*B related sequences in *Xiphophorus* that map to mela-

noma determining Mendelian loci and overexpress in a melanoma cell line. *Oncogene* 3:605–617, 1988.

31. Zechel Ch, Schleenbecker U, Anders A, Pfütz M, and Anders F. Search for genes critical for the early and/or late events in carcinogenesis: Studies in *Xiphophorus* (Pisces, Teleostei). In: Neth R, Gallo RC, Greaves MF, Gaedicke G, Gohla S, Mannweiler K, and Ritter J (eds.), *Modern Trends in Human Leukemia VIII*. Berlin-Heidelberg: Springer-Verlag, 1989, 366–385.
32. Mäueler W, Raulf W, and Schartl M. Expression of proto-oncogenes in embryonic, adult, and transformed tissues of *Xiphophorus* (Teleostei: Poeciliidae). *Oncogene* 2:421–430, 1988.
33. Zechel Ch, Peters H, Schleenbecker U, and Anders F. Expression of genes related to the human *erb*B, *erb*A, *pdgf* and *pdgf*-2 in tumors of different etiology in *Xiphophorus*. *Int J Cancer* 52:66–75, 1992.
34. Wittbrodt JA, Malitscheck B, Mäueler W, Raulf F, Telling A, Robertson SM, and Schartl M. Novel putative receptor tyrosine kinase by the melanoma inducing *Tu* locus in *Xiphophorus*. *Nature* 341:415–421, 1989.
35. Adam D, Mäueler W, and Schartl M. Transcriptional activation of the melanoma inducing *Xmrk* oncogene in *Xiphophorus*. *Oncogene* 6:73–80, 1991.
36. Schwab M and Anders A. Carcinogenesis in *Xiphophorus* and the role of the genotype in tumor susceptibility. In: Kaiser E (ed.) *Neoplasms, comparative pathology of growth in animals, plants, and man*. Baltimore-London: Williams and Wilkins, 1981, 451–459.
37. Ullrich A, and Schlesinger J. Signal transduction by receptors with tyrosine kinase activity. *Cell* 61:203–212, 1990.
38. Barnekow A, Schartl M, Anders F, and Bauer H. Identification of a fish protein associated with a kinase activity and related to the Rous sarcoma virus transforming protein. *Cancer Res* 42:2429–2433, 1982.
39. Schartl M, Barnekow A, Bauer H, and Anders F. Correlations of inheritance and expression between a tumor gene and the cellular homolog of the Rous sarcoma virus-transforming gene in *Xiphophorus*. *Cancer Res* 42:4222–4227, 1982.
40. Courtneidge SA and Heber A. An 81 kd protein complexed with middle T antigen and $pp60^{c\text{-}src}$: A possible phosphatidylinositol kinase. *Cell* 50:1031–1037, 1987.
41. Cantley LC, Auger KR, Carpenter Ch, Duckworth B, Graziani A, Kapeller R, and Soltoff St. Oncogenes and signal transduction. *Cell* 64:281–302, 1991.
42. Smith AD, Gronau Th, Pröfrock A, Zechel Ch, Bird IM, Lane PA, Barnekow A, and Anders F. EGF-receptor gene, x-*src* oncogene and inositol lipid turnover in key processes preceding melanoma in *Xiphophorus* model. In: Lynch HT, and Fusaro RM (eds.), *Hereditary Malignant Melanoma*. Boca Raton, Fla.: CRC Press, 1991, 97–108.
43. Anders A, Anders F, Zechel Ch, Schleenbecker U, and Smith A. Ansätze zur Analyse der Initiation von Initialprozessen der Krebsbildung am Melanom-Modell von *Xiphophorus*. *Arch Geschwulstforsch* 60:249–263, 1990.
44. Schartl M, Schmidt CR, Anders A, and Barnekow A. Elevated expression of the cellular *src* gene in tumors of differing etiologies in *Xiphophorus*. *Int J Cancer* 36:199–207, 1985.
45. Kaplan DR, Whitman M, Schaffhausen B, Pallas DC, White M, Cantley K, and Roberts TM. Common elements in growth factor stimulation and oncogenic transformation: 85 kd phosphoprotein and phosphatidylinositol kinase activity. *Cell* 50:1021–1029, 1987.
46. Berridge MJ, and Irwine RF. Inositol triphosphate, a novel second messenger in signal transduction. *Nature* 312:315–321, 1984.

Chapter 6

HUMAN MELANOMA GENETICS

Involvement of Oncogenes and Tumor Suppressor Genes

Peter I. Schrier, Laura J. van't Veer, and Wilma Bergman

INTRODUCTION

It is now well established that cancer has a genetic basis and is accompanied by structural alterations in the chromosomal DNA. Often, these alterations occur in genes playing an important role in the regulation of proliferation and differentiation. The function of these genes is directly related to the process of oncogenic transformation, and therefore these genes are often referred to as oncogenes.[1,2] More than a hundred of these oncogenes have presently been characterized. Apart from the biochemical and molecular evidence for altered genes in cancer cells, also classical genetic studies hint at genetic defects that correlate with the development of cancer: a number of human cancers are occurring either frequently in families (familial cancer) or have an unambiguous hereditary basis (hereditary cancer).[3,4] An example of the latter is hereditary retinoblastoma, which is, in carriers, unequivocally linked to the inactivation of one (recessive) allele of a gene localized on chromosome 13, the *Rb* gene.[5] The disease becomes manifest when the other (intact) *Rb* gene is inactivated by a somatic mutation. The precise function of the protein encoded by the *Rb* gene is not known, but it is most likely involved in the control of genes or proteins involved in DNA replication and cell proliferation. Also in the nonhereditary (sporadic) form of retinoblastoma, the *Rb* alleles are inactivated, pointing to an important role of the *Rb* protein in suppressing the occurrence of that form of cancer. This is the reason why this class of genes is usually referred to as tumor suppressor genes, although sometimes they are also called recessive oncogenes.[5]

A serious complication in establishing the genetic defect segregating in familial cancer is that, in general, the development of cancer is a multistep process involving more than one gene.[6] So far, no consistent combinations of gene defects have been found in almost any form of human cancer, which makes it difficult to ascertain one particular gene defect that is associated with transmission of the disease. In cutaneous melanoma (CM), around 10 percent of the disease occurs in families,[7] and in that case the disease is associated with an inherited cutaneous phenotype, the familial atypical multiple mole melanoma (FAMMM) syndrome, also called familial dysplastic nevus syndrome.[8] The atypical nevi can be considered as a precursor lesion for melanoma,[9,10] and therefore, the development of melanoma, at least in FAMMM patients, is likely to take place in discrete steps. One step leads to an atypical melanocyte, a subsequent step is correlated with the transition to melanoma. One possibility is that, analogous to other familial cancer syndromes like retinoblastoma, Wilms tumor, and colorectal cancer, the first step involves inactivation of a tumor suppressor gene. In that case, the second step may consist of the activation of an oncogene. The latter alteration may be, for instance, caused by UV exposure.[11] Interestingly, about half of the patients with sporadic melanoma have atypical moles[12,13] in contrast to only 2–9 percent of the overall population,[14,15] suggesting that sporadic and familial melanoma have similar genetic defects determining the precursor stage. Also in clinical and histological respect, no differences have been found between the two,[16] indicating that the subsequent genetic alterations leading to melanoma are similar in sporadic melanoma and the FAMMM syndrome. In this chapter, we will briefly exemplify the hereditary features of FAMMM and summarize the cytogenetic defects associated with FAMMM and CM. Finally, we will review the activation of oncogenes in melanoma and discuss the tentative role of UV exposure on the activation of one of these genes.

THE FAMMM SYNDROME

It was as early as 1820 that a family history of cutaneous melanoma was reported by William Norris.[17,18] The tumor originated in a mole, and Norris noted that many family members of the proband, including his children, father, and his father's brothers, had many moles. Now, it is well established that melanoma may occur in families and is always associated with the occurrence of the multiple atypical nevi called dysplastic nevi.[8,16] In pedigrees, it is apparently inherited as an autosomal dominant trait.[19,20] Figure 6-1(a) shows a characteristic example of such a patient. The pedigree of this proband is shown in Fig. 6-1(b) (arrow). This family is one out of 10 FAMMM families located near Leiden, The Netherlands, five of which are from a single coastal fishing village, suggesting a "founder effect." It has not been proven, however, that a common ancestor is involved in the FAMMM trait in this restricted area. Putting together the data of the families, we could evaluate 428 of the 540 individuals that were affected or at risk[21]: 37 developed a melanoma; 123 had multiple atypical nevi; and 27 were obligate gene carriers, who did not have suspicious nevi themselves but had affected children. The data clearly indicated that an autosomal dominant gene with variable expression and incomplete penetrance (nonpenetrance rate of 0.16) was responsible for the FAMMM syndrome in these families.[21] These findings are in line with earlier reports on the FAMMM syndrome.[19,20]

A number of features of the FAMMM syndrome further corroborate its hereditary properties:

1. The melanomas are much earlier manifest than in the nonfamilial cases.[22,23] One should, however, interpret these data with some care because usually the lesions are thinner,[23,24] indicating that the tumors are earlier diagnosed probably due to the alertness of the individuals at risk.
2. Often more than one primary melanoma develops,[23] which is characteristic for familial cancer (compare retinoblastoma and breast cancer, where the tumors often occur in paired organs).
3. Multiple forms of cancer have been found in FAMMM patients, indicating that the genetic defect does not only allow neoplastic transformation of the melanocyte in these families. This is well illustrated in Fig. 6-1, showing that 8/27 of the individuals in generations I and II developed cancer of some sort in addition to 5/27 with melanoma.

Recently, nine of the ten Dutch families were surveyed for secondary tumors, and an unexpected preponderance of digestive tract cancers, in particular pancreatic carcinoma, was observed.[25] In fact, from 21 gastrointestinal tumors, nine were pancreatic and none were colorectal, which is in sharp contrast to Dutch incidence data, that is half of the digestive tract cancers being colorectal and only 10 percent pancreatic. Also, in another report an excess of gastrointestinal cancers was observed in a group of examined blood relatives with dysplastic nevi.[26]

Interestingly, the high frequency of gastrointestinal tumors is confined to a subset of three of the nine families, while in the remaining six no significant excess of systemic cancer was found. This indicates that the FAMMM families are largely heterogeneous with respect to susceptibility to systemic cancer, which in part may reconcile the data with those of earlier reports stating that the frequency of systemic cancer was not increased in FAMMM patients.[24] This would mean that at least two different gene defects may be associated with the FAMMM syndrome.

More Than One Gene Involved?

Other findings have hinted at the involvement of more than one gene defect in the development of melanoma, which probably also holds for melanoma occurring in the FAMMM syndrome. First, the risk to develop a melanoma is not constant but depends greatly on the total count of the nevi, in particular the dysplastic nevi.[27,28] Second, not only the nevus count but also the total nevus area determines the risk.[29] This may allow a two-locus model: a common recessive locus determining the high nevus count and another (co-dominant) determining the proliferative capacity of the nevus.[29] Third, other hereditary factors have been implied in the etiology of melanoma like hair color[27,30] and skin phototype.[19,31–34] Moreover, in patients with xeroderma pigmentosum, a recessively inherited disorder as-

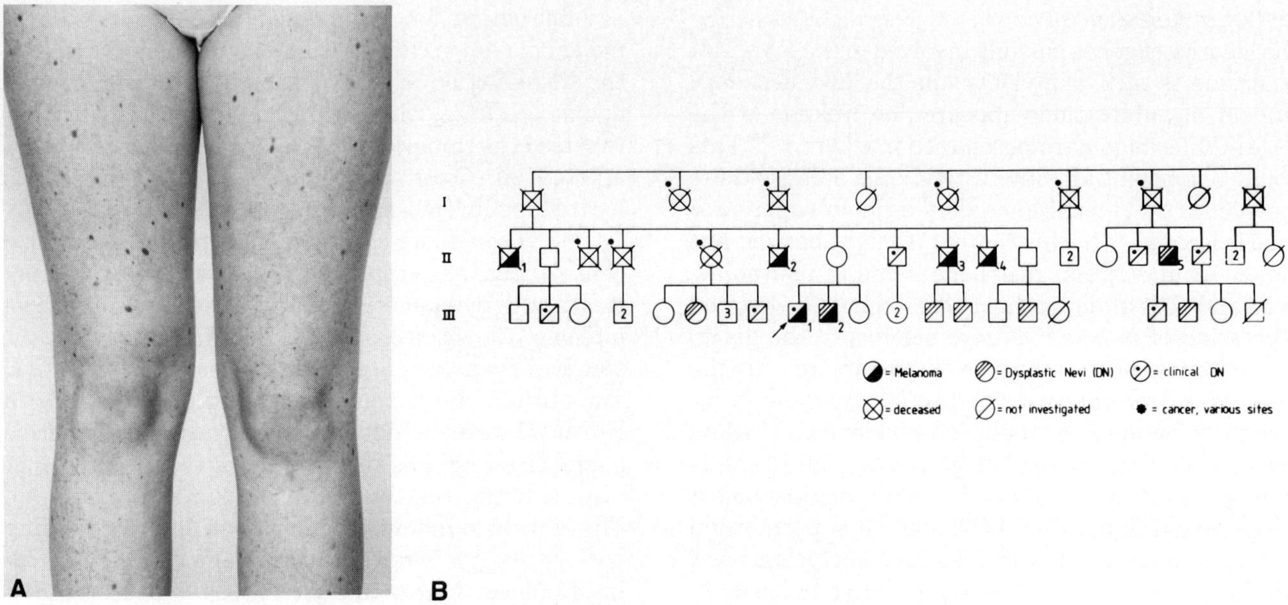

FIG. 6-1. The FAMMM syndrome. A. Typical patient with the FAMMM syndrome. B. Pedigree of a FAMMM family. This pedigree represents one out of the 10 Dutch families with the FAMMM syndrome under investigation. Note the high frequency of non-melanoma cancer. This family, by chance, comprises more males than females. Clinical DN is defined by the presence of multiple clinically recognizable dysplastic nevi without histological verification.

sociated with DNA repair deficiency, an increased frequency of melanoma has been observed.[35,36] These findings altogether point to more than one genetically determined factor capable of contributing to the FAMMM syndrome and support the polygenic concept.[37]

In our opinion, however, the polygenic concept does not argue against a "major" autosomal dominant inheritable gene or gene defect predisposing to the FAMMM syndrome. Such a gene defect might be recessive as in the case of hereditary retinoblastoma, where the tumor becomes only manifest after loss of heterozygosity (LOH) due to a somatic mutation in the unaffected allele. In the case of the FAMMM syndrome, LOH would lead to the induction and proliferation of atypical melanocytes in the dysplastic nevi. This could be due to the loss of suppressor activity allowing the expression of one or more growth stimulating (onco)genes. One has to postulate that another somatic mutation in this or a distinct dominant oncogene will transform the preneoplastic melanocyte to a melanoma (Fig. 6-2). In an alternative model given in Fig. 6-2, the FAMMM gene is represented as a dominantly inheritable activated oncogene. In this case, one has to assume that the activity of the oncogene is rigorously suppressed in the non-penetrant carrier by the counteracting activity of two tumor suppressor alleles. This suppression is released in the preneoplastic melanocytes through inactivation of one of the two suppressor alleles resulting in a decreased dose of suppressor activity. In the next step, the melanoma will develop through the inactivation of the second suppressor allele.

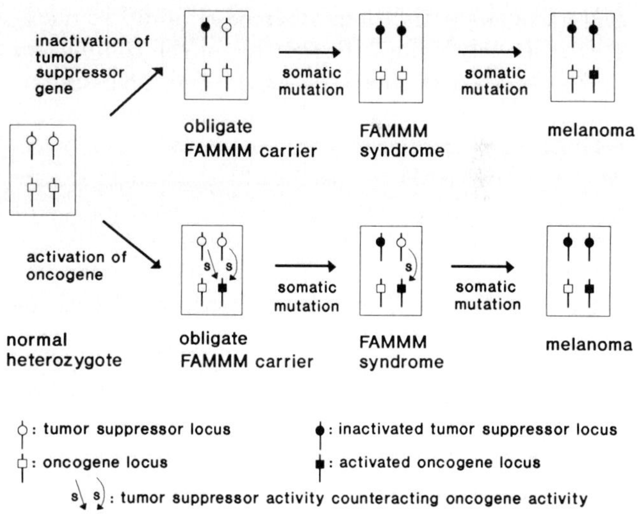

FIG. 6-2. Development of melanoma in patients with the FAMMM syndrome. A hypothetical genetic model. Circles: tumor suppressor locus. Squares: oncogene locus. The open symbols represent normal loci, the closed symbols affected loci. S→ : Activity of the tumor suppressor gene repressing the activity of the activated oncogene. See text for further details.

Loss of Heterozygosity

The identity of genes possibly involved in the FAMMM syndrome is still a mystery. In the last decade a number of publications appeared on linkage of the FAMMM locus to chromosome 1p markers.[38,39] This would be a potentially interesting locus because there is evidence that on chromosome 1 a tumor suppressor gene is located.[40] In this context it might be relevant that LOH at #1p has also been found in neuroblastoma and goes along with amplification and elevated expression of N-*myc*.[41] N-*myc* belongs to the group of *myc* oncogenes playing an important role in the onset of cell proliferation.[42] The N-*myc* gene is incidentally found to be amplified in melanoma,[43] while the expression of the homologous c-*myc* oncogene is often elevated in melanoma.[44,45] This would suggest a tentative link between LOH at #1 and permission of (elevated) *myc* expression. Authors analyzing other families, however, could exclude a linkage between the FAMMM syndrome and the chromosome 1 marker.[46,47,48] Diagnostic and genetic heterogeneity might account for the discrepancy between the various data. Genetic diversity is very possible because of the complexity of the situation with respect to the different steps in tumor progression, as mentioned before. Moreover, a vast number of genetic defects and oncogene activations have been found in melanoma (see following). Illustrative of the complexity are several reports that describe frequent loss of heterozygosity in melanoma patients at numerous informative loci at different chromosomes.[49,50] The LOHs were not restricted to specific chromosomes. In one report,[51] six independent metastases of one patient were analyzed and LOH was detected at 8 of 16 autosomes with at least one informative locus and at three informative X-linked loci. On the basis of these LOHs, a genealogy of tumor progression in this particular patient was permitted and showed a complex development of various subclones of an originally clonal tumor.[51]

Chromosomes Involved in LOH

The biological significance of the LOHs is not clear. One may speculate on loss of tumor suppressor genes in at least some of the steps. Of interest in this context is the finding that members of retinoblastoma families (carriers as well as patients cured of their eye tumor) do often develop melanoma,[52] indicating that deletion of a tumor suppressor gene (in this case the *Rb* gene, see above) may contribute to the formation of a melanoma. Anecdotal is the case report[53] of a melanoma on the trunk of a black individual (which is very uncommon) suffering from neurofibromatosis (von Recklinghausen's disease). This disease is strongly associated with inactivation of a tumor suppressor gene at chromosome 22.[54]

Searching for a biological significant LOH in melanoma, an exciting result was recently obtained[55]: the introduction of chromosome 6 into human melanoma cell lines, which are tumorigenic in nude mice, reversed the tumorigenic phenotype, suggesting that a potential tumor suppressor gene for melanoma is located on chromosome 6.[55]

An even more complex situation arises when considering the recent finding[82] that melanoma patients with cytogenetic abnormalities in either chromosome 7 or chromosome 11 had significantly shorter survival than patients without these abnormalities. The authors did not mention whether patients with FAMMM were included in their study. An attractive possibility would be that the changes in #7 and #11 are occurring relatively late in tumor progression. The defects found on chromosome 7 are overlapping with the region where the oncogene c-*erbB1*, encoding Epidermal Growth Factor (EGF), is located. Remarkably, an oncogene locus activated in fish melanomas harbors a gene with high homology to the human c-*erbB1*,[56,57] suggesting that this gene might be activated in fish as well as in human melanomas. The activation of other oncogenes in melanoma will be further discussed (Section "Oncogenes").

Further Evidence for Tumor Suppressor Genes

An intriguing observation, stressing the importance of tumor suppressor genes in melanoma, is the strongly increased incidence of melanoma in the mixed South American population, when compared with the ancestral races, the American Indians and the Spanish. The latter two have a low melanoma incidence.[31,37] As noticed by Traupe,[37] this peculiar finding resembles the situation with respect to the pattern of inheritance when crossing the platyfish *Xiphophorus maculatus* (low pigmentation) and swordtail fish *Xiphophorus helleri* (no pigmentation) (see also Chap. 5). The F1 is a hybrid with increased pigmentation. When the F1 is backcrossed with unpigmented fish, 25 percent of the progeny develops malignant tumors. The result can be explained by an independent segregation of an activated oncogene and a tumor suppressor gene. The following speculative model might translate these results to melanoma in humans (Fig. 6-3). One parental population has an oncogene activated in both alleles, balanced by two active suppressor alleles (B). In the other parental population, the oncogene alleles are not activated but the two tumor suppressor alleles are inactivated (A). In both populations the tumor incidence is low. When the two populations are interbred, the suppressive activity of one suppressor gene in the F1 would still be high enough to counterbalance the activated oncogene, and the individual does not

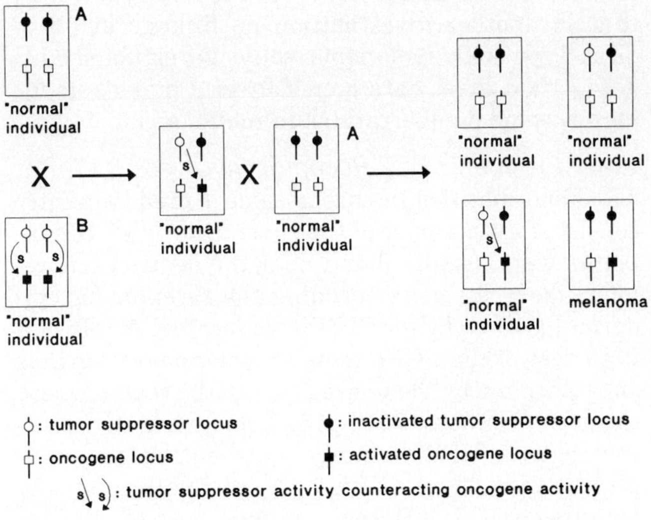

FIG. 6-3. *Elevated incidence of melanoma in the offspring of two different populations with a low incidence.* A hypothetical genetic model. Circles: tumor suppressor locus. Squares: oncogene locus. The open symbols represent normal loci, the closed symbols affected loci. S→ : Activity of the tumor suppressor gene repressing the activity of the activated oncogene. See text for further details.

develop melanoma. However, when the F1 is backcrossed with individual A, Mendelian inheritance predicts that 25 percent of the progeny would develop the tumor because of the lack of tumor suppressor activity (Fig. 6-3).

In conclusion, a number of genes are involved in the origin and development of melanoma. In the case of the FAMMM syndrome autosomal dominant inheritance has been documented. Although the precise mechanism of the inheritance remains obscure, accumulative evidence exists that suppressor oncogenes and/or dominantly activated oncogenes are involved (compare Fig. 6-2). For the expression of the FAMMM phenotype, presumably a somatic mutation is required, although direct experimental evidence for this view is lacking. Most likely, additional genetic alterations are required for the progression from dysplastic nevus to highly malignant melanoma.

CHROMOSOMAL ALTERATIONS IN MELANOMA

In the previous sections, possible mechanisms of inheritance and possible genes involved in familial melanoma were discussed. We will now focus on genetic alterations in melanoma that might provide a clue as to which genes are prevalently altered in melanoma and what might be the biological effect of these alterations. A possible way to trace these genes is to investigate chromosomal alterations and ask what genes are affected by these alterations.

Chromosome 1: A Tumor Suppressor Gene Involved?

Over the past ten years, a vast amount of literature on cytogenetic alterations in melanoma appeared.[58] The most frequent alterations in melanoma are found in chromosomes #1, #6, and #7. Because #1 is the largest, alterations in this chromosome are typical for many forms of human cancer, like carcinomas of the testis, cervix, ovary, and breast.[58] Nevertheless, the specific alterations in melanoma (usually involving 1p12-1p22 and 1p36) might be of significance. This region of chromosome 1 harbors a tumor suppressor gene and has been implicated in other neuroectodermal tumors occurring in multiple endocrine neoplasia and neuroblastoma. It has been shown that loss of heterozygosity in this region correlates with late melanoma progression.[59] Furthermore, a translocation involving 1p36 has been found in normal cells of individuals from a FAMMM family,[60] suggesting that in this family heterozygosity at this locus might be present. The gene encoding Nerve Growth Factor as well as the oncogene N-*ras* are also located at 1p12-1p22. In particular the N-*ras* gene is of interest because this oncogene is frequently activated in melanoma (see the following). However, the activation consists of point mutations augmenting the signal transducing properties of the gene, and neither rearrangements nor partial deletions in ras genes have been reported to be involved in their activation. Therefore, it is disputable whether the cytogenetic changes do affect N-*ras* in a significant way, unless they might cause *in*activation of a wild type *ras* allele thereby allowing the dominant expression of a mutated *ras* gene present in the other allele.

Chromosome 6: HLA Involved?

The alterations in chromosome 6 are interesting for two reasons. First, a functional tumor suppressor gene is located on this chromosome.[55] Second, a linkage between melanoma and the Major Histocompatibility Complex (MHC) located on 6p21-23 has been suggested. Chromosomal aberrations in chromosome 6 are most frequent in 6q.[58,61] Deletions do occur mainly distal of band q23, while translocations (often to chromosome 1) affect 6q11-13.[61] Therefore, the suppressor gene can be tentatively mapped in one of these regions. Various oncogenes have been assigned to 6q, including *mas, ros,* and *myb*. The latter gene encodes a nuclear protein involved in proliferation. A translocation of *myb* to chromosome 12, resulting in deletion of a part of 3′-terminal sequences of the locus, has occurred in one particular melanoma cell line.[62] Such an event may result in the deletion of sequences important for the regulation of transcription of the gene and may lead to an inappropriate expression. Although it has been shown that the gene is expressed in the cell line, it is not known whether this actually contributes to its tumor phenotype. Structural alterations involving *myb* have not been found in other than this particular melanoma cell line.[61] Alterations in the short arm of #6 have also been reported.[63] Often multiple copies of 6p are found, but also deletions in this arm have been detected. This is of interest because MHC genes (HLA in humans) have shown to be involved in progression of melanoma: the HLA Class I (HLA-A,B,C) and Class II (HLA-DP,DQ,DR) proteins do play a pivotal role in presentation of foreign or tumor-associated peptides to the immune system. Alterations in the expression of these proteins may influence the recognition of tumor cells by immune effector cells and impair a proper immune reactivity of the patient against the tumor, leading to progression. HLA Class I expression is often down-modulated in melanomas[44,64] and low HLA Class I expression is associated with progression.[65,66] Monosomy at the MHC locus[67] and restriction fragment length polymorphisms (RFLPs) have been documented,[68,69] but no frequent and gross genomic rearrangements in the HLA region have ever been reported to our knowledge; therefore, it seems unlikely that rearrangements or gene losses at 6p are responsible for the HLA down-modulation. In fact, down-modulation of HLA Class I at the mRNA level is brought about by elevated expression of the c-*myc* oncogene,[44] indicating that subtle regulation at the transcriptional level is responsible for loss of HLA expression, rather than gene loss.

Another issue related to aberrations of 6p is the genetic linkage of melanoma to the expression of certain HLA alleles or haplotypes. The HLA genes are highly polymorphic through the population and HLA-disease association is conceivable if (1) an HLA-mediated immune response to the tumor is occurring in the patient and (2) melanoma-associated peptides are presented only by a restricted number of HLA types. In that case, individuals with certain HLA alleles will not be able to reject the tumor. Altered frequencies of particular HLA Class I[70–73] and Class II[74,75] alleles have been found in patients. In one linkage study,[76] a particular haplotype (HLA-A9, -B35,-Cw4) appeared more frequently in healthy relatives of patients with the FAMMM syndrome and sporadic melanoma, suggesting that this haplotype protects against the occurrence of melanoma. In addition, a higher frequency of this haplotype was observed in healthy relatives of patients with FAMMM syndrome than healthy relatives of patients with sporadic melanoma, suggesting that the latter are at risk. In all cases, a lower frequency of HLA-B35 was found in patients, implying an association of B35 with a protective factor. It should be noted, however, that in another investigation no linkage at all of HLA type with melanoma could be established.[77] Altogether, these data do not favor a major role for chromosome 6p aberrations in melanoma.

Chromosome 7: EGF Receptor Involved?

The abnormalities in chromosome 7 predominantly consist of extra copies of the short arm.[63,78,79] Breakpoints were usually found near the centromeric region where the gene encoding the receptor for epidermal growth factor (EGFR) is located. A role of a high dose of the EGFR gene in melanoma is further substantiated by the finding that in the region where the gene is located (7p12-p13), homogeneously staining regions (HSR), usually representing gene amplifications, were found.[80] A correlation of the expression of EGFR and copy numbers of chromosome 7[81] indicate that increased expression of EGFR is related to an augmentation of malignancy by conferring a growth advantage to the already malignant cells. Very suggestive in this context is the finding that #7 aberrations are correlated with shorter survival of melanoma patients.[82]

Other Chromosomes: Which Genes are Involved?

A number of other chromosomal alterations, although found less frequently than those previously discussed, may be interesting because their locations are connected with the presence of oncogenes, tumor suppressor genes, or other genes contributing to cancer progression. These include HSR or trisomy of #8[67,83] on which the c-*myc* oncogene is located. Multiple copies of #8q comprising c-*myc* were found in uveal melanoma.[84] Expression of c-*myc* has been found to be elevated in cell lines derived from cutaneous melanoma.[44] However, in the lines investigated[44,45] no chromosomal alterations in the c-*myc* gene have been detected by Southern blot analysis, suggesting that the elevated expression is caused by a mechanism other than amplification.

Consistent deletions of chromosome 9 have been described.[85,86] A specific region of 9p (9pter-p22), harboring the interferon genes, is often missing in dysplastic nevi as well as in melanomas,[87] suggesting that the aberrations in #9 are occurring early in progression. A role for interferon is unclear, but one can speculate that decrease in an eventual autocrine production of interferon by tumor cells may lead to progression because interferons have been shown to have growth inhibitory effects on melanoma cells.[88]

Chromosome 11 has drawn attention because a disproportionate distribution of rare H-*ras* alleles localized at 11p15 has been found in cancer patients,[89] in particular in melanoma patients.[89–91] The polymorphism is generated by variable tandem repeat (VTR) sequences upstream of the coding sequences of the gene. Studies in FAMMM families, however, could not establish as yet a linkage between FAMMM and the segregation of these rare alleles.[92,93] The biological consequences of the polymorphism are not clear, although the VTR has a weak enhancer activity. Recently, a rare allele of a FAMMM patient has been cloned, but when compared with the common allele, the sequence alteration did not appear to have consequences for the normal biological activity of the H-*ras* gene.[93] It cannot be excluded, however, that the alterations have remote effects *in cis* on neighboring regions of chromosome 11. In this respect it is noteworthy that a tumor suppressor locus, involved in hereditary renal cancer (Wilm's tumor), is situated at 11p13. Remarkably, one case report describes a Wilm's patient with an interstitial deletion of the short arm of #11, who developed dysplastic nevi at an early age.[94] In another report, the only consistent abnormalities found in melanoma materials from three patients were structural abnormalities in 11p.[95] Combined with the recent finding that chromosomal alterations in chromosome 11 are correlated with shorter survival in melanoma,[82] we conclude that a further investigation of the relevant regions of chromosome 11 in melanoma may be worthwhile and may shed new light on the involvement of alterations in this chromosome in familial and sporadic melanoma.

An interesting translocation involving chromosomes 19 and 1 in three independent melanomas has been found.[96] The breakpoint at #19 resides at band p13, where at least four interesting genes are located[97]: the gene encoding insulin receptor which has an important function in proliferation, the *mel* oncogene, and the oncogenes *junB* and *junD*. The latter genes encode proteins that form heterodimers with the *fos* oncogene, resulting in a complex (AP-1) involved in transcriptional regulation of a wide range of cellular genes.[98] Interestingly, a tumor promoter, the phorbol ester TPA, is capable of enhancing the function of AP-1 via protein kinase C. The latter protein plays an important role in the signaling between growth factor receptors and nuclear transcription processes with modulation of AP-1 activity as a possible end point.[99] It is conceivable that aberrations of 19p13 affect the regulation of jun proteins, thereby modulating AP-1 activity and disturbing the normal transcription regulation of other cellular proteins in such a way that uncontrolled proliferation is induced. Finally, the *mel* gene is located at 19p13.2.[100] This gene has been picked up from DNA from a human melanoma with an assay detecting transforming activity of chromosomal DNA.[101] This gene has homology with *ras,* and in fact belongs to family of genes encoding *ras*-related GTP/GDP binding proteins, Rab/Y pt.[102] Strikingly, in one melanoma, sequences were rearranged and amplified, suggesting a role for *mel* in this particular tumor. (R.A. Padua, personal communication.)

In conclusion, melanoma can be characterized by a complex and often heterogeneous combination of chromosomal alterations, most frequently involving chromosomes 1, 6, and 7. Tumor suppressor genes and oncogenes are likely to be involved, but hitherto no definitive proof is available for this, and no definitive assignment can be made as to which loci are consistently affected. As far as cytogenetic alterations in FAMMM patients and relatives are concerned, only sparse data are available, the main reason probably being that melanocytes from atypical nevi are hard to culture. Recurrent chromosomal alterations in normal fibroblasts and cells from atypical nevi of two FAMMM patients have been described.[60] Earlier, numerical abnormalities were found in normal lymphocytes from members of FAMMM families with melanoma or dysplastic nevi.[103] In addition, random chromosomal rearrangements, including translocations and inversions, were found in normal fibroblast or lymphocytes of FAMMM patients, in contrast to normal relatives and spouses, who showed no alterations.[104] On the basis of these observations, it has been suggested to classify the FAMMM syndrome as a "chromosome instability disorder."[103] The continuously occurring random chromosomal alterations in the patients do reinforce that the effect of the dominantly inherited FAMMM gene by itself is not sufficient to bring the syndrome to full phenotypic expression.

ONCOGENES

As seen from the previous sections, the genetic analysis of familial melanoma together with the current knowledge of chromosomal alterations have provided insight into the patterns of inheritance in the familial cases and have yielded a vast amount of information about which chromosomes or chromosomal regions are involved. However, a definite answer to the question, "What causes melanoma?" cannot as yet be given on the basis of this information. A solution should probably be found in an understanding of the precise molecular events underlying the disease. So far, no clear histological, cytogenetical, and molecular genetic differences between the sporadic and familial forms have been found, and therefore, we assume that, in principle, similar molecular alterations are involved in both types.

Several Classes of Oncogenes

It is now generally accepted that molecular alterations in oncogenes are responsible for the conversion of a normal cell into a tumor cell.[1,2] Usually, these genes exert normal functions in cell proliferation and differentiation (Table 6-1). Roughly, three classes

TABLE 6-1
CELLULAR ONCOGENES INVOLVED IN MELANOMA

GENE	FUNCTION	ACTIVATION[1]	REFERENCES
c-*erbB1*	EGF[2]-receptor	↑ gene copy number	81
		↑ expression	81
c-*erbB2*	EGF-receptor-like	↑ expression	143
c-*fos*	Transcription factor	expressed	113
hst/int2	FGF[3]-like	amplification	144
mel	GTP binding	? (3T3 assay)	101
	(belongs to family of rab proteins)	amplification	148
		rearrangement	148
		expressed	143
c-*myc*	DNA binding factor	↑ expression	44, 113, 115, 143
N-*myc*	Transcription	amplification	43
c-*myb*	Transcription	translocation	62, 145
p53	Transcription ?	expressed	143
H-*ras*	Signal transduction	point mutation	116, 117, 121, 122
	(GTPase)	amplification	146
K-*ras*	Signal transduction	point mutation	122
N-*ras*	Signal transduction	point mutation	117–122, 140
c-*sis*	PDGF-B[4]	↑ expression	113
c-*src*	Tyrosine-kinase	↑ expression	143
		↑ kinase activity	147

[1] ↑ : increase
[2]Epidermal Growth Factor
[3]Fibroblast Growth Factor
[4]Platelet Derived Growth Factor-β

of oncogene proteins can be defined according to their cellular localization. A first class is localized in the cell nucleus and is involved in DNA replication, transcriptional regulation, and proliferation. Well-known examples of this category are c-*myc* (a DNA binding protein),[42,105,106] c-*fos*,[107] and c-*jun*.[108] The latter two form the aforementioned transcription factor AP-1. A second class consists of secreted proteins, usually representing growth factors.[99] An example is c-*sis* encoding PDGF-B (platelet derived growth factor-B). A third class of oncogene proteins is localized in the membrane or in the cytoplasm and is somehow involved in signal transduction, that is it confers a proliferative signal induced by a receptor-ligand interaction from the membrane to the nucleus. Several subclasses can be discerned: (1) integral membrane receptors, usually with tyrosine kinase activity, involved in the actual onset of proliferation, such as the EGF receptor (encoded by c-*erbB1* at chromosome 7); (2) nonreceptor tyrosine kinases localized at the inner side of the membrane, like c-*src*; (3) serine kinases present in the cytoplasm. In addition, the well-known family of *ras* genes (including K-, H-, and N-*ras*) can be classified in this group of signal transducers, although they do not possess kinase activity. The *ras* genes encode membrane proteins of 21 kDa (p21*ras*) with GTPase activity.[109,110] Recently, alteration of the GTP/GDP ratio in these proteins was found upon a receptor-ligand interaction in T-cells[111] and in insulin receptor overexpressing cells,[112] indicating that the protein indeed may play an important role in signal transduction.

Inappropriate expression or structural alteration of oncogenes may disturb their regular action. In such a state, the oncogene is called activated and this may lead to the formation of a cancerous cell.[1,2] Frequently found types of oncogene activation are elevated expression of the gene, structural alterations in the gene, or both.

Oncogenes Activated in Melanoma

Oncogenes found to be activated in melanoma are summarized in Table 6-1. A number of cases involve elevated expression: c-*erbB-2*, c-*src*, c-*sis*, c-*fos*, and c-*myc*. The *hst/int-2* locus encoding secreted proteins with homology to FGF (fibroblast growth factor)[99] has been found to be amplified in a single case. Structural alterations have been found in the c-*myb* and c-*erbB1* genes, encoding proteins involved in transcription and signal transduction, respectively. The most frequent structural alterations in melanoma have been found in the family of *ras* genes. In the remaining part of this section we will focus on *myc* and *ras*, because these oncogenes are predominantly activated in melanoma.

Myc

High c-*myc* expression was found in a panel of melanoma cell lines.[44,45] Activation of c-*myc* and/or

N-*myc* has been reported in two independent other studies.[43,113] The c-*myc* oncogene has an important function in the regulation of cell proliferation and differentiation of normal cells.[42] Deregulation may lead to immortalization of cells, and this may contribute to the transformed state of tumor cells.[105] Apart from being involved in the genetic origin of melanoma tumors, there is another reason why high c-*myc* expression in melanoma is of particular interest: it is capable of switching off expression of the Major Histocompatibility Complex Class I genes, which have an important function in the interaction of tumor cells with the immune system. In human melanoma tumors, frequently low expression of HLA Class I genes has been found.[64,65] Interestingly, HLA-B alleles rather than HLA-A or HLA-C are affected,[45] and therefore it seems that the downregulation is locus-specific. An important function of HLA-B downmodulation by c-*myc* may be to provide an immunosurveillance system whereby cells with high *myc* expression are eliminated by natural killer cells.[114,115]

Ras

Point mutations in all members of the family of *ras* genes (H-*ras,* K-*ras* and N-*ras*) have been found,[116–122] although mutations in N-*ras* are preponderant (Table 6-2). The almost exclusive activation of N-*ras* might be associated with the fact that melanocytes are of neuroendocrine origin.[123] Expression of the N-*ras* gene was found in the neural crest[124,125] and therefore in melanocytes, the N-*ras* gene might be more prone to mutations than H- and K-*ras* due to an altered higher order structure of the DNA at the transcriptionally active site where the N-*ras* gene is located.

The mutations in the *ras* genes were found at amino acid positions 12, 13 or 61. Mutations at these positions do abolish the GTPase activity of the protein, resulting in an activation, which is responsible for its transforming properties. The mutations were found in primary melanomas as well as in metastases, and incidentally even in atypical nevi (K-*ras*).[122] The fraction of melanomas with an activated *ras* gene, as measured in the transformation assay or by determining the mutation directly, was not high: for primary melanomas 4/30,[116] 1/13,[119] 7/37,[120] 1/16,[121] and 4/22[122] and for metastatic melanomas 1/19[121] and 4/14.[122] This means that either (1) in tumors where *ras* is not activated, other events must have contributed to tumor formation or (2) *ras* has no role in melanoma development or progression at all. The latter conclusion is not very likely because of the following argument. In several primary melanomas, two different N-*ras* mutations are found. These different mutations are situated in different cells present in roughly equal amounts in the primary tumor.[120] This can only be explained if the mutation had been induced at about the same time due to one single event (probably a lesion by UV exposure), and from that time on the cells started to proliferate. This is only possible if the N-*ras* activation plays an active role in the progression of the particular melanocyte from which the two populations with different ras mutations originated (see also the following).

In five cases, primary tumor, metastases, or cell lines from the same patient were available and tested for *ras* activation (Table 6-2[120]). In each individual patient the same mutation pattern was found: primary tumor, metastases, and cell lines of two patients contained the same mutation, whereas these materials of the other three patients had no mutation. This indicates that the mutations are not induced during the establishment of the cell lines or during subsequent passaging, and that with respect to the *ras* mutation pattern, the cell lines are representative for the original tumor.

In several studies, more than one mutation has been found in a particular lesion (Table 6-2). In two patients (number 4 and number 10), several metastases of such a lesion were available. One patient had an N-*ras* mutation at different amino acid positions, N13val and N12asp (mutations leading to a valine and asparagine at position 13 and 12 of the N-*ras* protein). Two separate metastases had only a single N-*ras* mutation (one metastasis with N12asp and one with N13val). In the other patient, N13val and N13asp were present in the primary tumor, but in this case, only the cells with N12asp were present in three independent metastases, suggesting a preference of cells with N12asp to metastasize. All lesions, including those with two mutations, harbored in addition a wild type allele. The combined data permit the following conclusions: (1) the original tumors are biclonal, (2) the *ras* mutations are localized on different alleles in different cells, and (3) the mutations are a relatively early event in tumor formation, at least they do occur before the transformed melanocyte starts to proliferate progressively.

More Than One Oncogene Activated

Two cell lines with an N-*ras* mutation (from patient 4 and patient 11, Table 6-2) have, in addition, elevated expression of the c-*myc* oncogene.[115] The concurrence of these activations might be crucial in the etiology of these particular tumors.[126] This is in conjunction with the view that oncogenic transformation is a multistep process, involving activation of at least two genes.[2,6] Moreover, c-*myc* and N-*ras* together have been shown to be capable of transforming primary rodent fibroblasts. On the other hand, considering a larger panel of 12 melanoma cell lines,[115]

TABLE 6-2
RAS MUTATIONS IN MELANOMA

NUMBER OR NAME	PRIMARY TUMOR[1]	METASTASIS[1]	CELL LINE[1]	BASE CHANGE[2]	REFERENCE
Mel-Swift			N61lys	CAA → AAA	118
4	N13val	Met.B: N13val	N13val	GGT → GTT	120
	N13asp	Met.A: N13asp		GGT → GAT	
10	N12asp	Met.A-C: N12asp		GGT → GAT	120
	N13val	(3 metastases)		GGT → GGT	
11			N61arg	CAA → CGA	120
16		Met.A-N: N61lys (14 metastases)		CAA → AAA	120
20	N61lys	N61lys	N61lys	CAA → AAA	120
31	N61lys	N61lys		CAA → AAA	120
32	N61lys			CAA → AAA	120
4 × SK-Mel			N61arg		121
3 × SK-Mel			N61lys		121
SK-Mel-127			N61leu		121
SK-Mel-65			N13arg		121
DW	N61lys				122
PAW-N1	N61arg			CAA → CGA	119
XP44RO(mel)		N61his		CAA → CAT	140
MW		N61his			
		K12val			122
SK-Mel-146			H61lys		121
SK-2			H61leu	CAG → CTG	116
JC	H12val				122
	K12val				
JB	K12asp				122
HB	K12val				122
2 × GE,DP		K12val			122
JD		K12val			122
		K12asp			

[1]The mutations in N-*ras*, H-*ras* or K-*ras* are listed for materials available. For example: N13val, mutation gly → val at amino acid position 13 in the N-*ras* gene. The wild type amino acids are: N12gly, N13gly, N61gln, H61gln, H12gly, K12gly.
[2]No base change listed not known.

these two were the only ones with the double activation of c-*myc* and N-*ras,* and one cell line had neither of the two genes activated. This indicates that in the panel of melanoma cell lines no consistent pattern of oncogene activation can be assigned, stressing that, apart from *myc* and *ras,* other oncogenes are probably involved in the genetic origin of melanoma (Table 6-1).

Ras Activation: A Role for UV?

Epidemiological studies revealed a role for exposure to sunlight and the occurrence of melanoma, in particular lentigo maligna melanoma, but also cutaneous melanoma.[127–131] Also, in patients with the FAMMM syndrome, such a correlation has been found.[10,132,133] This can be explained by the finding that in these patients a direct relationship between sun exposure and the number of nevi was found[134]: an increasing number of nevi may account for an increasing chance to develop a melanoma. There are more indications that UV exposure may be involved in the origin of melanoma. First, in vitro assays have shown an enhanced susceptibility of normal fibroblasts or lymphocytes to UV exposure or to UV mimetic drugs in melanoma patients as compared to normal individuals.[135] Second, the number of micronuclei (a measure of genotoxic damage) in fibroblasts of FAMMM or melanoma patients was increased after UV irradiation as compared to fibroblasts of control individuals.[136] Third, thymidine dimers caused by UV exposure are less efficiently removed in fibroblasts from FAMMM and melanoma patients.[36,137] Finally, patients with DNA repair insufficiencies like xeroderma pigmentosum (XP), who are extremely sensitive to sun exposure, have a more than 2000-fold increased risk to develop a melanoma.[35,138] In two studies analyzing oncogene activation in skin tumors of patients with XP, N-*ras* genes were found to be mutated. In the first,[139] two squamous cell carcinomas of one patient contained an N61his mutation (CAA → CAT). In another study,[140] an N61his mutation was found in a mela-

TABLE 6-3
SOLAR EXPOSURE OF BODY SITES AND RAS MUTATIONS IN MELANOMA

SUN-EXPOSURE	*NUMBER OF PRIMARY MELANOMAS*	*NUMBER OF PRIMARY MELANOMAS WITH A RAS MUTATION*
continuous	10	7
intermittent	16	0
rare	5	0

A Chi-square test for continuous sun exposure and *ras* mutation for patients with known localization of the primary tumor reveals a highly significant correlation: $p < 0.001$ ($\chi^2 = 18.99$, $df = 2$). Even if the patients with occult ($n = 5$) or unknown ($n = 1$) primary tumor localization are included in the category of continuously UV-exposed body sites, the statistical analysis shows a significant correlation between continuous UV exposure and *ras* mutation: $p < 0.05$ ($\chi^2 = 11.35$, $df = 2$).

noma tumor as well as a melanoma cell line from an XP patient. These data suggest that due to impaired DNA repair of a UV-induced thymidine dimer in the strand opposing the coding strand (sequence GTT) an A.T to T.A transversion has occurred at position 61 of the N-*ras* gene. A similar mutation has been found to be responsible for transforming activity of the N-*ras* gene after in vitro irradiation of the isolated gene with UV light of 254 nm.[141] Strikingly, the primary tumors with an N-*ras* mutation (found in 7 out of 37 patients) were invariably localized on continuously sun-exposed body sites and never on intermittently or rarely sun-exposed sites (Table 6-3[120]). This suggests that in all seven patients with a *ras* mutation, sun exposure might be the etiologic agent involved in the origin of these melanomas. Two melanomas were found to be heterogeneous with respect to the *ras* mutations (Table 6-2). The mechanism involving pyrimidine dimer formation at the dipyrimidine site by UV irradiation may explain this finding (Fig. 6-4). One should assume that the lesions in the noncoding strand are not immediately excised and repaired but are still present in two next rounds of replication, thereby causing random incorporation of different nucleotides opposite of the CC dimer in each round. All mutations found in either codon harbor a TT or CC dimer opposite to the coding sequence which further supports the model (Fig. 6-4). It should be noted that the spectrum of transversions and transitions (involving conversion of T or C) is different from the predominant UV-induced G → A transitions found in other systems.[11,142] However, in most systems, the effect of UV irradiations was monitored by detecting gene inactivation, while in the case of the *ras* studies a strong selection has taken place for particular mutations that induce the transforming capacity of the

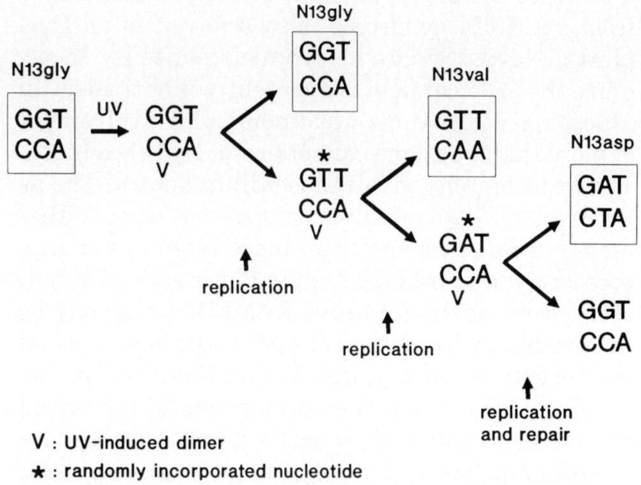

*FIG. 6-4. Mechanism of UV-induced N-*ras *mutation in biclonal melanomas.* Schematic hypothetical model of the generation of two tumor cells with different mutations in the N-*ras* gene (codon 13) by a single UV-induced CC-dimerization event in one cell. v: dimer *: randomly incorporated nucleotide. See text for further details.

gene, and therefore, the spectrum of mutations found in the N-*ras* gene in melanomas is not at all representative for mutations induced in the DNA by UV.

CONCLUSION

In this chapter we have reviewed a number of genetic aspects of the FAMMM syndrome and melanoma. By far the most cases of melanoma occur in a sporadic form. The etiology is not known, but there are indications that sun exposure does play a role and may cause mutations that do contribute to malignant progression, in particular point mutations in the N-*ras* oncogene. Furthermore, consistent chromosomal aberrations have been detected in melanoma, chromosomes 1, 6, and 7 being the most frequently involved. There is evidence for a putative tumor suppressor gene on chromosome 6 that is capable of reverting the transformed properties of melanoma cell lines. Amplification and/or elevated expression of epidermal growth factor receptor (the oncogene c-*erbB1*) sequences on chromosome 7 may play a role in the development of melanoma. This is corroborated by the finding that aberrations involving chromosomes 7 and 11 are correlated with poor survival of melanoma patients. In addition to N-*ras* and c-*erbB1*, other oncogenes have been implied in the oncogenesis of melanoma. One of these is c-*myc*, capable of downmodulating the expression of MHC Class I genes, thus influencing the interaction of the melanoma cells with the immune system of the patient. In around 10 percent of the cases of melanoma a familial history is present. These patients suffer from FAMMM syndrome, also referred to as Dysplastic Nevus Syndrome. The susceptibility to acquire the atypical nevi is apparently inherited as an autosomal dominant trait, although the involvement of more than one gene cannot presently be excluded. The locus or gene involved is still unknown. The as yet available data permit genetic models where either an activated oncogene or an inactivated tumor suppressor gene is inherited. In one model, loss of heterozygosity at the tentative FAMMM locus may be involved in the transition of a phenotypically normal melanocyte to an atypical one proliferating in the dysplastic nevus. For the development of the actual melanoma, additional somatic alterations are involved, most likely involving oncogene activation (for instance the N-*ras* gene by UV exposure) or inactivation of additional tumor suppressor loci.

REFERENCES

1. Weinberg RA. Oncogenes, antioncogenes, and the molecular bases of multistep carcinogenesis. *Cancer Res* 49:3713–3721, 1989.
2. Bishop JM. Molecular themes in oncogenesis. *Cell* 64:235–248, 1991.
3. Ponder BA. Familial cancer: opportunities for clinical practice and research. *Eur J Surg Oncol* 13:463–473, 1987.
4. Ponder BA. Inherited predisposition to cancer. *Trends Genet* 6:213–218, 1990.
5. Marshall CJ. Tumor suppressor genes. *Cell* 64:313–326, 1991.
6. Hunter T. Cooperation between oncogenes. *Cell* 64:249–270, 1991.
7. Greene MH and Fraumeni JF. The hereditary variant of malignant melanoma. In: Clark WH, Goldman LI, and Mastrangelo MJ (eds.), *Human Malignant Melanoma.* Philadelphia: Grune and Stratton, 1979, 139–166.
8. Lynch HT and Fusaro RM. Genetic epidemiology and the familial atypical multiple mole melanoma syndrome. In: Lynch HT, and Tautu P (eds.), *Genetic Epidemiology of Cancer.* Berlin: Springer-Verlag, 1991, 114–131.
9. Clark WH Jr, Elder DE, Guerry D, Epstein MN, Greene MH, and Van Horn M. A study of tumor progression: The precursor lesions of superficial spreading and nodular melanoma. *Hum Pathol* 15:1147–1165, 1984.
10. Greene MH, Clark WH Jr, Tucker MA, Elder DE, Kraemer KH, Guerry D, Witmer WK, Thompson J, Matozzo I, and Fraser MC. Acquired precursors of cutaneous malignant melanoma. The familial dysplastic nevus syndrome. *N Eng J Med* 312:91–97, 1985.
11. Ananthaswamy HN, and Pierceall WE. Molecular mechanisms of ultraviolet radiation carcinogenesis. *Photochem Photobiol* 52:1119–1136, 1990.
12. Kraemer KH, and Greene MH. Dysplastic nevus syndrome. Familial and sporadic precursors of cutaneous melanoma. *Dermatol Clin* 3:225–237, 1985.
13. Tucker MA. Individuals at high risk of melanoma. In: Elwood JM. (ed.), *Melanoma and Nevi. Incidence, Interrelationships, and Implications.* Pigment Cell, vol. 9. Basel, Switzerland: Karger, 1988, 95–109.
14. Crutcher WA and Sagebiel RW. Prevalence of dysplastic naevi in a community practice letter. *Lancet* 1:729–739, 1984.
15. Nordlund JJ, Kirkwood J, Forget BM, Scheibner A, Albert DM, Lerner E, and Milton GW. Demographic study of clinically atypical (dysplastic) nevi in patients with melanoma and comparison subjects. *Cancer Res* 45:1855–1861, 1985.
16. Tucker MA, and Bale SJ. Clinical aspects of familial cutaneous malignant melanoma. *Semin Oncol* 15:524–528, 1988.
17. Norris W. A case of fungoid disease. *Edinb Med Surg J* 16:562–565, 1820.
18. Dracopoli NC and Bale SJ. Genetic aspects of cutaneous malignant melanoma. *Semin Oncol* 15:541–548, 1988.
19. Bergman W, Palan A, and Went LN. Clinical and genetic studies in six Dutch kindreds with the dysplastic naevus syndrome. *Ann Hum Genet* 50:249–258, 1986.
20. Lynch HT, Fusaro RM, Kimberling WJ, Lynch JF, and Danes BS. Familial atypical multiple mole-melanoma (FAMMM) syndrome: Segregation analysis. *J Med Genet* 20:342–344, 1983.
21. Bergman W, van Haeringen A, and Went LN. The FAMMM syndrome in The Netherlands. In: Lynch HT and Fusaro RM. (eds.), *Hereditary Malignant Melanoma.* Boca Raton, FL: CRC Press, 1991.
22. Lynch HT, Fusaro RM, Kimberling WJ, and Lynch JF. The cutaneous evolution of nevi with familial atypical multiple mole melanoma syndrome. *Pediatr Dermatol* 2:289–293, 1985.
23. Greene MH, Clark WH Jr, Tucker MA, Kraemer KH, Elder DE, and Fraser MC. High risk of malignant melanoma in melanoma-prone families with dysplastic nevi. *Ann Intern Med* 102:458–465, 1985.
24. Kopf AW, Hellman LJ, Rogers GS, Gross DF, Rigel DS, Friedman RJ, Levenstein M, Brown J, Golomb FM, Roses DF, et al. Familial malignant melanoma. *JAMA* 256:1915–1919, 1986.
25. Bergman W, Watson P, de Jong J, Lynch HT, and Fusaro RM. Systemic cancer and the FAMMM syndrome. *Br J Cancer* 61:932–936, 1990.
26. Greene MH, Tucker MA, Clark WH Jr, Kraemer KH, Elder DE, and Fraser MC. Hereditary melanoma and the dysplastic nevus syndrome: The risk of cancers other than melanoma. *J Am Acad Dermatol* 16:792–797, 1987.
27. Holly EA, Kelly JW, Shpall SN, and Chiu SH. Number of melanocytic nevi as a major risk factor for malignant melanoma. *J Am Acad Dermatol* 17:459–468, 1987.
28. Swerdlow AJ, English J, Mackie RM, O'Doherty CJ, Hunter JA, Clark J, and Hole DJ. Benign melanocytic naevi as a risk factor for malignant melanoma. *BMJ* 292:1555–1559, 1986.
29. Cannon-Albright LA, Bishop DT, Goldgar DE, and Skolnick MH. Genetic epidemiology of cancer and predisposing lesions. In: Lynch HT and Tautu P. (eds.), Genetic epidemiology of cancer. Berlin: Springer-Verlag, 1991, 58–65.
30. Beitner H, Norell SE, Ringborg U, Wennersten G, and Mattson B. Malignant melanoma: Aetiological importance of individual pigmentation and sun exposure. *Br J Dermatol* 122:43–51, 1990.
31. Crombie IK. Racial differences in melanoma incidence. *Br J Cancer* 40:185–193, 1979.
32. Beral V, Evans S, Shaw H, et al. Cutaneous factors related to the risk of malignant melanoma. *Br J Dermatol* 109:165–172, 1983.
33. Osterlind A, Tucker MA, Hou-Jensen K, Stone BJ, Engholm G, and Jensen OM. The Danish case-control study of cutaneous malignant melanoma. I. Importance of host factors. *Int J Cancer* 42:200–206, 1988.
34. Garbe C, Kruger S, Stadler R, Guggenmoos-Holzmann I, and Orfanos CE. Markers and relative risk in a German

population for developing malignant melanoma. *Int J Dermatol* 28:517–523, 1989.
35. Kraemer KH, Lee MM, and Scotto J. DNA repair protects against cutaneous and internal neoplasia: Evidence from xeroderma pigmentosum. *Carcinogenesis* 5:511–514, 1984.
36. Roth M, Boyle JM, and Muller H. Thymine dimer repair in fibroblasts of patients with dysplastic naevus syndrome (DNS). *Experientia* 44:169–171, 1988.
37. Traupe H. Polygenic vs monogenic inheritance of dysplastic nevi and malignant melanoma: Yesterday's debate or the answer of tomorrow? In: Lynch HT and Tautu P. (eds.), *Genetic Epidemiology of Cancer*. Berlin: Springer-Verlag, 1991, 102–113.
38. Greene MH, Goldin LR, Clark WH Jr, Lovrien E, Kraemer KH, Tucker MA, Elder DE, Fraser MC, and Rowe S. Familial cutaneous malignant melanoma: Autosomal dominant trait possibly linked to the Rh locus. *Proc Natl Acad Sci U S A* 80:6071–6075, 1983.
39. Bale SJ, Dracopoli NC, Tucker MA, Clark WH Jr, Fraser MC, Stanger BZ, Green P, Donis-Keller H, Housman DE, and Greene MH. Mapping the gene for hereditary cutaneous malignant melanoma-dysplastic nevus to chromosome 1p. *N Eng J Med* 320:1367–1372, 1989.
40. Kugoh HM, Hashiba H, Shimizu M, and Oshimura M. Suggestive evidence for functionally distinct, tumor-suppressor genes on chromosome-1 and chromosome-11 for a human fibrosarcoma cell line, HT1080. *Oncogene* 5:1637–1644, 1990.
41. Fong CT, Dracopoli NC, White PS, Merrill PT, Griffith RC, Housman DE, and Brodeur GM. Loss of heterozygosity for the short arm of chromosome 1 in human neuroblastomas: Correlation with N-*myc* amplification. *Proc Natl Acad Sci U S A* 86:3753–3757, 1989.
42. Luscher B and Eisenman RN. New light on *myc* and *myb*. 1. *Myc*. *Genes Dev* 4:2025–2035, 1990.
43. Bauer J, Sokol L, Stribrna J, Kremen M, Krajsova I, Hausner P, and Hejnar P. Amplification of N-*myc* oncogene in human melanoma cells. *Neoplasma* 37:233–238, 1990.
44. Versteeg R, Noordermeer IA, Krüse-Wolters KM, Ruiter DJ, and Schrier PI. c-*Myc* down-regulates class I HLA expression in human melanomas. *EMBO J* 7:1023–1029, 1988.
45. Versteeg R, Krüse-Wolters KM, Plomp AC, van Leeuwen A, Stam NJ, Ploegh HL, Ruiter DJ, and Schrier PI. Suppression of class I human histocompatibility leukocyte antigen by c-*myc* is locus specific. *J Exp Med* 170:621–635, 1989.
46. van Haeringen A, Bergman W, Nelen MR, van der Kooij-Meijs E, Hendrikse I, Wijnen JT, Khan PM, Klasen EC, and Frants RR. Exclusion of the dysplastic nevus syndrome (DNS) locus from the short arm of chromosome 1 by linkage studies in Dutch families. *Genomics* 5:61–64, 1989.
47. Cannon-Albright LA, Goldgar DE, Wright EC, Turco A, Jost M, Meyer LJ, Piepkorn M, Zone JJ, and Skolnick MH. Evidence against the reported linkage of the cutaneous melanoma-dysplastic nevus syndrome locus to chromosome 1p36. *Am J Hum Genet* 46:912–918, 1990.
48. Gruis NA, Bergman W, and Frants RR. Locus for susceptibility to melanoma on chromosome-1p. *N Eng J Med* 322:853–854, 1990.
49. Dracopoli NC, Houghton AN, and Old LJ. Loss of polymorphic restriction fragments in malignant melanoma: Implications for tumor heterogeneity. *Proc Natl Acad Sci U S A* 82:1470–1474, 1985.
50. Orita M, Murakami Y, Ishihara K, and Sekiya T. Loss of heterozygosity at polymorphic chromosomal loci in patients with malignant melanoma. *J Invest Dermatol* 92:280S–283S, 1989.
51. Dracopoli NC, Alhadeff B, Houghton AN, and Old LJ. Loss of heterozygosity at autosomal and X-linked loci during tumor progression in a patient with melanoma. *Cancer Res* 47:3995–4000, 1987.
52. Sanders BM, Jay M, Draper GJ, and Roberts EM. Non-ocular cancer in relatives of retinoblastoma patients. *Br J Cancer* 60:358–365, 1989.
53. Silverman JF, Blahove M, Collins JL, and Norris HT. Cutaneous malignant melanoma in a black patient with neurofibromatosis (von Recklinghausen's disease). *Am J Dermatopathol* 10:536–540, 1988.
54. Xu GF, Oconnell P, Viskochil D, Cawthon R, Robertson M, Culver M, Dunn D, Stevens J, Gesteland R, White R, and Weiss R. The neurofibromatosis type-1 gene encodes a protein related to Gap. *Cell* 62:599–608, 1990.
55. Trent JM, Stanbridge EJ, Mcbride HL, Meese EU, Casey G, Araujo DE, Witkowski CM, and Nagle RB. Tumorigenicity in human melanoma cell lines controlled by introduction of human chromosome 6. *Science* 247:568–571, 1990.
56. Zechel C, Schleenbecker U, Anders A, and Anders F. v-*erbB* related sequences in Xiphophorus that map to melanoma determining Mendelian loci and overexpress in a melanoma cell line. *Oncogene* 3:605–617, 1988.
57. Wittbrodt J, Adam D, Malitschek B, Maueler W, Raulf F, Telling A, Robertson SM, and Schartl M. Novel putative receptor tyrosine kinase encoded by the melanoma-inducing Tu locus in Xiphophorus. *Nature* 341:415–421, 1989.
58. Trent JM, Leong SPL, and Meyskens FL. Chromosome alterations in human malignant melanoma. In: Conti CJ, Slaga TJ, and Klein-Szanto AJP. (eds.), *Skin Tumors: Experimental and Clinical Aspects*. New York: Raven Press, 1989, 165–186.
59. Dracopoli NC, Harnett P, Bale SJ, Stanger BZ, Tucker MA, Housman DE, and Kefford RF. Loss of alleles from the distal short arm of chromosome 1 occurs late in melanoma tumor progression. *Proc Natl Acad Sci U S A* 86:4614–4618, 1989.
60. Hecht F, and Hecht BK. Chromosome rearrangements in dysplastic nevus syndrome predisposing to malignant melanoma. *Cancer Genet Cytogenet* 35:73–78, 1988.
61. Trent JM, Thompson FH, and Meyskens FL Jr. Identification of a recurring translocation site involving chromosome 6 in human malignant melanoma. *Cancer Res* 49:420–423, 1989.
62. Dasgupta P, Linnenbach AJ, Giaccia AJ, Stamato TD, and Reddy EP: Molecular cloning of the breakpoint on chromosome 6 in cutaneous malignant melanoma: Evidence for deletion in the c-*myb* locus and translocation of a segment of chromosome 12. *Oncogene* 4:1201–1205, 1989.
63. Balaban GB, Herlyn M, Clark WH Jr, and Nowell PC. Karyotypic evolution in human malignant melanoma. *Cancer Genet Cytogenet* 19:113–122, 1986.
64. Ruiter DJ, Bergman W, Welvaart K, Scheffer E, van Vloten WA, Russo C, and Ferrone S. Immunohistochemical analysis of malignant melanomas and nevocellular nevi with monoclonal antibodies to distinct monomorphic determinants of HLA antigens. *Cancer Res* 44:3930–3935, 1984.
65. Bröcker EB, Suter L, Bruggen J, Ruiter DJ, Macher E, and Sorg C. Phenotypic dynamics of tumor progression in human malignant melanoma. *Int J Cancer* 36:29–35, 1985.
66. van Duinen SG, Ruiter DJ, Bröcker EB, van der Velde EA, Sorg C, Welvaart K, and Ferrone S. Level of HLA antigens in locoregional metastases and clinical course of the disease in patients with melanoma. *Cancer Res* 48:1019–1025, 1988.

67. Cowan JM, Halaban R, Lane AT, and Francke U. The involvement of 6p in melanoma. *Cancer Genet Cytogenet* 20:255–261, 1986.
68. Angelini G, Fossati G, Radice P, Longo A, Piccioli P, Pierotti MA, Ferrara GB, and Parmiani G. Loss of polymorphic restriction fragments of class I and class I MHC genes in a malignant melanoma. *J Immunogenet.* 13:241–246, 1986.
69. Castelli C, Mazzucchelli F, Sensi M, Fossati G, and Parmiani G. Loss of heterozygosity of DQ *alpha* gene in human malignant melanoma. *Tumori* 75:378–382, 1989.
70. Demenais F, Cesarini JP, Daveau M, Cavelier B, Gony J, Feingold N, and Hors J. A linkage study between HLA and cutaneous malignant melanoma or precursor lesions or both. *J Med Genet* 21:429–435, 1984.
71. Hawkins BR, Dawkins RL, Hockey A, Houliston JB, and Kirk RL. Evidence for linkage between HLA and malignant melanoma. *Tissue Antigens* 17:540–541, 1981.
72. Pellegris G, Illeni MT, Rovini D, Vaglini M, Cascinelli N, and Ghidoni A. HLA complex and familial malignant melanoma. *Int J Cancer* 29:621–623, 1982.
73. Bergholtz B, Brennhovd I, Klepp O, Kaakinen A, and Thorsby E. HLA antigens in malignant melanoma. *Prog Clin Biol Res* 16:175–180, 1977.
74. Pollack MS and Livingston PO. HLA and DR antigen frequencies in melanoma patients: Possible relation to disease prognosis. *Tissue Antigens* 26:262–265, 1985.
75. Mueller-Eckhardt G, Schendel DJ, Hundeiker M, Riedel T, O'Neill GJ, Riethmuller G, and Mueller-Eckhardt C. Possible association between HLA-DR5 and superficial spreading melanoma (SSM). *Int J Cancer* 34:751–755, 1984.
76. Rovini D, Pellegris G, Cascinelli N, Cantoni L, Vaglini M, Placucci M, Santinami M, Belli F, and Illeni MT. HLA antigens in familial and sporadic cutaneous melanoma. *Tumori* 74:657–664, 1988.
77. Bale SJ, Greene MH, Murray C, Goldin LR, Johnson AH, and Mann D. Hereditary malignant melanoma is not linked to the HLA complex on chromosome 6. *Int J Cancer* 36:439–443, 1985.
78. Limon J, Dal Cin P, Sait SN, Karakousis C, and Sandberg AA. Chromosome changes in metastatic human melanoma. *Cancer Genet Cytogenet* 30:201–211, 1988.
79. Sozzi G, Miozzo M, Calderone C, Fossati G, Pierotti MA, Cascinelli N, and Della Porta G. Chromosome abnormalities and fragile sites in human melanoma. *Cancer Genet Cytogenet* 44:61–67, 1990.
80. Trent JM, Thompson FH, and Ludwig C. Evidence for selection of homogeneously staining regions in a human melanoma cell line. *Cancer Res* 44:233–237, 1984.
81. Koprowski H, Herlyn M, Balaban GB, Parmiter AH, Ross AH, and Nowell P. Expression of the receptor for epidermal growth factor correlates with increased dosage of chromosome 7 in malignant melanoma. *Somat Cell Mol Genet* 11:297–302, 1985.
82. Trent JM, Meyskens FL, Salmon SE, Ryschon K, Leong SP, Davis JR, and McGee DL. Relation of cytogenetic abnormalities and clinical outcome in metastatic melanoma. *N Eng J Med* 322:1508–1511, 1990.
83. Brieux de Salum S, Slavutsky I, Besuschio S, and Pavlovsky AA. Homogeneously staining regions (HSR) in a human malignant melanoma. *Cancer Genet Cytogenet* 11:53–60, 1984.
84. Horsman DE, Sroka H, Rootman J, and White VA. Monosomy 3 and isochromosome 8q in a uveal melanoma. *Cancer Genet Cytogenet* 45:249–253, 1990.
85. Pedersen MI, and Wang N. Chromosomal evolution in the progression and metastasis of human malignant melanoma. A multiple lesion study. *Cancer Genet Cytogenet* 41:185–201, 1989.
86. Kacker RK, Giovanella BC, and Pathak S. Consistent karyotypic abnormalities in human malignant melanomas. *Anticancer Res* 10:859–871, 1990.
87. Cowan JM, Halaban R, and Francke U. Cytogenetic analysis of melanocytes from premalignant nevi and melanomas. *J Nat Cancer Inst* 80:1159–1164, 1988.
88. Osanto S, Jansen R, Naipal AM, Gratama JW, van Leeuwen A, and Cleton FJ. In vivo effects of combination treatment with recombinant interferon-gamma and -alpha in metastatic melanoma. *Int J Cancer* 43:1001–1006, 1989.
89. Krontiris TG, DiMartino NA, Colb M, and Parkinson DR. Unique allelic restriction fragments of the human Ha-*ras* locus in leukocyte and tumour DNAs of cancer patients. *Nature* 313:369–374, 1985.
90. Radice P, Pierotti MA, Borrello MG, Illeni MT, Rovini D, and Della Porta G. HRAS1 proto-oncogene polymorphisms in human malignant melanoma: TaqI defined alleles significantly associated with the disease. *Oncogene* 2:91–95, 1987.
91. Hayward NK, Nancarrow DJ, Parsons PG, Kidson C, and Ellem KA. TaqI polymorphism within the c-*Ha-ras-1* VTR is associated with melanoma. *Hum Genet* 83:395–396, 1989.
92. Harnett P, and Kefford RF. Molecular models of tumorigenesis: Application to familial and sporadic melanoma. *Semin Oncol* 15:549–557, 1988.
93. Kasperczyk A, Mermer BA, Parkinson DR, Lonergan JA, and Krontiris TG. Allele-specific deletion in exon I of the *Hras1* gene. *Am J Hum Genet* 45:689–696, 1989.
94. McDonagh AJ, Wright AL, and Messenger AG. Dysplastic naevi in association with partial deletion of chromosome 11. *Clin Exp Dermatol* 15:44–45, 1990.
95. Heim S, Mandahl N, Arheden K, Giovanella BC, Yim SO, Stehlin JS Jr, and Mitelman F. Multiple karyotypic abnormalities, including structural rearrangements of 11p, in cell lines from malignant melanomas. *Cancer Genet Cytogenet* 35:5–20, 1988.
96. Parmiter AH, Balaban G, Herlyn M, Clark WH Jr, and Nowell PG. A t(1;19) chromosome translocation in three cases of human malignant melanoma. *Cancer Res* 46:1526–1529, 1986.
97. Mattei MG, Simon-Chazottes D, Hirai S, Ryseck RP, Galcheva-Gargova Z, Guenet JL, Mattei JF, Bravo R, and Yaniv M. Chromosomal localization of the three members of the *jun* proto-oncogene family in mouse and man. *Oncogene* 5:151–156, 1990.
98. Lewis B. Oncogenic conversion by regulatory changes in transcription factors. *Cell* 64:303–312, 1991.
99. Cross M and Dexter TM. Growth factors in development, transformation, and tumorigenesis. *Cell* 64:271–280, 1991.
100. Nimmo E, Padua RA, Hughes D, Brook JD, Williamson R, and Johnson KJ. Confirmation and refinement of the localisation of the c-*mel* locus on chromosome 19 by physical and genetic mapping. *Hum Genet* 81:382–384, 1989.
101. Padua RA, Barrass N, and Currie GA. A novel transforming gene in a human malignant melanoma cell line. *Nature* 311:671–673, 1984.
102. Nimmo ER, Sanders PG, Padua RA, Hughes D, Williamson R, and Johnson KJ. The MEL gene—A new member of the RAB/Y pt class of Ras-related genes. *Oncogen* 6:1347–1351, 1991.
103. Caporaso N, Greene MH, Tsai S, Pickle LW, and Mulvihill JJ. Cytogenetics in hereditary malignant melanoma and dysplastic nevus syndrome: Is dysplastic nevus syndrome a chromosome instability disorder? *Cancer Genet Cytogenet* 24:299–314, 1987.

104. Jaspers NG, Roza-de Jongh EJ, Donselaar IG, Van Velzen-Tillemans JT, van Hemel JO, Rümke P, and van der Kamp AW. Sister chromatid exchanges, hyperdiploidy, and chromosomal rearrangements studied in cells from melanoma-prone individuals belonging to families with the dysplastic nevus syndrome. *Cancer Genet Cytogenet* 24:33–43, 1987.
105. Cole MD. The *myc* oncogene: Its role in transformation and differentiation. *Annu Rev Genet* 20:361–384, 1986.
106. Alitalo K, Koskinen P, Makela TP, Saksela K, Sistonen L, and Winqvist R. *Myc* oncogenes: Activation and amplification. *Biochim Biophys Acta* 907:1–32, 1987.
107. Curran T and Franza BR Jr. *Fos* and *jun:* The AP-1 connection. *Cell* 55:395–397, 1988.
108. Ransone LJ and Verma IM. Nuclear proto-oncogenes *fos* and *jun*. *Annu Rev Cell Biol* 6:539–557, 1990.
109. Bos JL. *Ras* oncogenes in human cancer: A review. *Cancer Res* 49:4682–4689, 1989.
110. Kumar R, Sukumar S, and Barbacid M. Activation of *ras* oncogenes preceding the onset of neoplasia. *Science* 248:1101–1104, 1990.
111. Downward J, Graves JD, Warne PH, Rayter S, and Cantrell DA. Stimulation of p21 *ras* upon T-cell activation. *Nature* 346:719–723, 1990.
112. Burgering BMTh, Medema R, Maassen JA, Van de Wetering ML, van der Eb AJ, McCormick F, and Bos JL. Insulin stimulation of gene expression mediated by p21 *ras* activation. *EMBO J* 1991.
113. Shin DM, Gupta V, Donner L, Chawla S, Benjamin R, Gutterman J, and Blick M. Aberrant oncogene expression in uncultured human sarcoma and melanoma. *Anticancer Res* 7:1117–1123, 1987.
114. Versteeg R, Peltenburg LTC, Plomp AC, and Schrier PI. High expression of the c-*myc* oncogene renders melanoma cells prone to lysis by natural killer cells. *J Immunol* 143:4331–4337, 1989.
115. Schrier PI, Versteeg R, Peltenburg LTC, Plomp AC, Van't Veer LJ, and Krüse-Wolters KM. Sensitivity of melanoma cell lines to natural killer cells: A role for oncogene-modulated HLA expression? *Semin Cancer Biol* 1991.
116. Sekiya T, Fushimi M, Hori H, Hirohashi S, Nishimura S, and Sugimura T. Molecular cloning and the total nucleotide sequence of the human c-*Ha-ras-1* gene activated in a melanoma from a Japanese patient. *Proc Natl Acad Sci U S A* 81:4771–4775, 1984.
117. Albino AP, Le Strange R, Oliff AI, Furth ME, and Old LJ. Transforming *ras* genes from human melanoma: A manifestation of tumour heterogeneity? *Nature* 308:69–72, 1984.
118. Padua RA, Barrass NC, and Currie GA. Activation of N-*ras* in a human melanoma cell line. *Mol Cell Biol* 5:582–585, 1985.
119. Raybaud F, Noguchi T, Marics I, Adelaide J, Planche J, Batoz M, Aubert C, de Lapeyriere O, and Birnbaum D. Detection of a low frequency of activated *ras* genes in human melanomas using a tumorigenicity assay. *Cancer Res* 48:950–953, 1988.
120. Van't Veer LJ, Burgering BMTh, Versteeg R, Boot AJM, Ruiter DJ, Osanto S, Schrier PI, and Bos JL. N-*ras* mutations in human cutaneous melanoma on sun-exposed body sites. *Mol Cell Biol* 9:3114–3116, 1989.
121. Albino AP, Nanus DM, Mentle IR, Cordon-Cardo C, McNutt NS, Bressler J, and Andreeff M. Analysis of *ras* oncogenes in malignant melanoma and precursor lesions: Correlation of point mutations with differentiation phenotype. *Oncogene* 4:1363–1374, 1989.
122. Shukla VK, Hughes DC, Hughes LE, McCormick F, and Padua RA. *Ras* mutations in human melanotic lesions—K-*Ras* activation is a frequent and early event in melanoma development. *Oncogene Res* 5:121–127, 1989.
123. Le Douarin N. Migration and differentiation of neural crest cells. *Curr Top Dev Biol* 16:31–85, 1980.
124. Ireland CM. Activated N-*ras* oncogenes in human neuroblastoma. *Cancer Res* 49:5530–5533, 1989.
125. Gerosa MA, Talarico D, Fognani C, Raimondi E, Colombatti M, Tridente G, De Carli L, and Della Valle G. Overexpression of N-*ras* oncogene and epidermal growth factor receptor gene in human glioblastomas. *J Natl Cancer Inst* 81:63–67, 1989.
126. Land H, Parada LF, and Weinberg RA. Cellular oncogenes and multistep carcinogenesis. *Science* 222:771–778, 1983.
127. Green A, Siskind V, Bain C, and Alexander J. Sunburn and malignant melanoma. *Br J Cancer* 51:393–397, 1985.
128. Holman CD, Armstrong BK, and Heenan PJ. Relationship of cutaneous malignant melanoma to individual sunlight-exposure habits. *J Natl Cancer Inst* 76:403–414.
129. Rhodes AR, Weinstock MA, Fitzpatrick TB, Mihm MC Jr, and Sober AJ. Risk factors for cutaneous melanoma. A practical method of recognizing predisposed individuals. *JAMA* 258:3146–3154, 1987.
130. Osterlind A, Tucker MA, Stone BJ, and Jensen OM. The Danish case-control study of cutaneous malignant melanoma. II. Importance of UV-light exposure. *Int J Cancer* 42:319–324, 1988.
131. Lee JAH. The melanoma epidemic thus far. *Mayo Clin Proc* 65:1368–1371, 1990.
132. Ramsay RG, Chen P, Imray FP, Kidson C, Lavin MF, and Hockey A. Familial melanoma associated with dominant ultraviolet radiation sensitivity. *Cancer Res* 42:2909–2912, 1982.
133. Perera MI, Um KI, Greene MH, Waters HL, Bredberg A, and Kraemer KH. Hereditary dysplastic nevus syndrome: Lymphoid cell ultraviolet hypermutability in association with increased melanoma susceptibility. *Cancer Res* 46:1005–1009, 1986.
134. Kopf AW, Lindsay AC, Rogers GS, Friedman RJ, Rigel DS, and Levenstein M. Relationship of nevocytic nevi to sun exposure in dysplastic nevus syndrome. *J Am Acad Dermatol* 12:656–662, 1985.
135. Howell JN, Greene MH, Corner RC, Maher VM, and McCormick JJ. Fibroblasts from patients with hereditary cutaneous malignant melanoma are abnormally sensitive to the mutagenic effect of simulated sunlight and 4-nitroquinoline 1-oxide. *Proc Natl Acad Sci U S A* 81:1179–1183, 1984.
136. Roser M, Bohm A, Oldigs M, Weichenthal M, Reimers U, Schmidt-Preuss U, Breitbart EW, and Rudiger HW. Ultraviolet-induced formation of micronuclei and sister chromatid exchange in cultured fibroblasts of patients with cutaneous malignant melanoma. *Cancer Genet Cytogenet* 41:129–137, 1989.
137. Roth M, Sigg Ch, and Emmons LR. Reduced ultraviolet-induced repair in patients with malignant melanoma or dysplastic nevus syndrome. In: Weber W, Laffer UT, and Durig M. (eds.), *Hereditary Cancer and Preventive Surgery*. Basel, Switzerland: Karger, 1990, 58–65.
138. Kraemer KH and Slor H. Xeroderma pigmentosum. *Clin Dermatol* 3:33–69, 1985.
139. Suarez HG, Daya-Grosjean L, Schlaifer D, Nardeux P, Renault G, Bos JL, and Sarasin A. Activated oncogenes in human skin tumors from a repair-deficient syndrome, xeroderma pigmentosum. *Cancer Res* 49:1223–1228, 1989.
140. Keijzer W, Mulder MP, Langeveld JC, Smit EM, Bos JL, Bootsma D, and Hoeijmakers JH. Establishment and char-

acterization of a melanoma cell line from a xeroderma pigmentosum patient: Activation of N-*ras* at a potential pyrimidine dimer site. *Cancer Res* 49:1229–1235, 1989.

141. Van der Lubbe JL, Rosdorff HJ, Bos JL, and van der Eb AJ. Activation of N-*ras* induced by ultraviolet irradiation in vitro. *Oncogene Res* 3:9–20, 1988.

142. Dobetsky EA, Grosovsky AJ, and Glickman BW. The specificity of UV-induced mutations at an endogenous locus in mammalian cells. *Proc Natl Acad Sci U S A* 84:9103–9107, 1987.

143. Chenevix-Trench G, Martin NG, and Ellem KA. Gene expression in melanoma cell lines and cultured melanocytes: Correlation between levels of c-*src*-1, c-*myc* and p53. *Oncogene* 5:1187–1193, 1990.

144. Adelaide J, Mattei MG, Marics I, Raybaud F, Planche J, de Lapeyriere O, and Birnbaum D. Chromosomal localization of the *hst* oncogene and its coamplification with the *int2* oncogene in a human melanoma. *Oncogene* 2:413–416, 1988.

145. Meese E, Meltzer PS, Witkowski CM, and Trent JM. Molecular mapping of the oncogene *myb* and rearrangements in malignant melanoma. *Genes Chromos Cancer* 1:88–94, 1989.

146. Sekiya T, Fushimi M, Hirohashi S, and Tokunaga A. Amplification of activated c-*ha-ras-1* in human melanoma. *Jpn J Cancer Res* 76:555–558, 1985.

147. Barnekow A, Paul E, and Schartl M. Expression of the c-*src* proto-oncogene in human skin tumors. *Cancer Res* 47:235–240, 1987.

148. Padua RA, personal communication.

Chapter 7

BIOLOGY AND PHOTOBIOLOGY OF THE MELANIN PIGMENTARY SYSTEM

Jean-Paul Ortonne

Pigmentation of the skin and hair is brought about by the synthesis of melanins and melanosomes within the neural crest-derived melanocytes and their transport and modification within epidermal and follicular keratinocytes.[1] According to a classic view, the most important biologic role of melanin pigmentation in humans would be that of protection against ultraviolet (UV) radiation.[2,3] This statement is mostly based on the clinical observation that, among humans, heavily pigmented individuals are much less prone to develop sun-induced cancer than are less pigmented ones.

Constitutive skin color in humans corresponds to the genetically determined levels of melanin pigmentation developed in the absence of exposure to solar irradiations or other environmental influences.[1] Facultative skin color or "tan" induced by ultraviolet light is characterized by the increase in melanin pigmentation above the constitutive level.[4] Indeed, ultraviolet radiations are the most common and the most well known agent inducing hypermelanosis of the skin. Thus, photobiology of melanin pigmentation has been extensively studied.[5]

In this chapter, the biology of melanocytes and the biochemical aspects of melanins and melanogenesis will be briefly reviewed. The biochemical recorders of malignant melanomas will be analyzed, as well as the cellular and molecular events following UV irradiation of normal human skin. Finally, phototypes will be described and the photoprotective role of melanins will be discussed.

MECHANISMS OF MELANIN PIGMENT PRODUCTION

Classification of Melanins

Melanins are usually classified on the basis of their color and solubility properties into two major groups, eumelanins and phaeomelanins.[6] The black and brown eumelanins are nitrogenous pigments, insoluble in all solvents that arise by oxidative polymerization of 5,6-dihydroxyindoles derived biogenetically from tyrosine via dopa. The alkali/soluble phaeomelanins, ranging from yellow to reddish brown, contain sulfur in addition to nitrogen and arise by oxidative polymerization of cystein-S-yl-dopas via 1,4-benzothiazines intermediates.[6,7] Trichochromes are sulfur containing pigments with a well-defined structure characterized by a $\Delta 2.2'$-bi(1,4-benzothiazine) chromophore.[6,7]

However, both criteria used in this classification may be misleading.[7] It is possible that some phaeomelanin-like pigments may, in fact, be structural variants of eumelanins resulting from partial photochemical or chemical oxidation of the material.[7] Moreover, there is some suggestion that the size of the pigment granule is at least as important in determining the melanin color as the chemical structure of the pigment.

Thus, the biological situation in mammalian melanocytes is probably more complex than what this clear-cut biochemical classification of melanin pigments suggests. Analysis by chemical degradation of natural pigments whose chemical and physical properties were intermediate between these of pure eumelanin and phaeomelanin polymers provided evidence that they arise by a copolymerization process involving both eumelanin and phaeomelanin precursors by a mechanism which is still little understood.[6] This led to the concept of intermeshing of the eumelanin and phaeomelanin pathways, which appears to be a common feature of melanogenesis in mammals.[6,7]

Metabolic Pathway Leading to Melanins (Figure 7-1)

The overall view of tyrosine metabolism in melanocytes has recently been summarized.[4,7] The amount and types of the product formed from tyrosine in the pigment cells depend on the overall balance of a number of factors under genetic and hormonal control:

- The activity of tyrosinase,
- The availability of molecular oxygen and the primary substrate tyrosine,
- The nature and concentration of heavy metals,
- The redox potential of the pigment cell environment, which is in relation to the oxidation state of the glutathione system.

Enzymatic Control of Melanogenesis

The bifunctional enzyme tyrosinase catalyzes the initial events of the melanogenesis, namely the hydroxylation of tyrosine to dopa and its subsequent oxidation to dopaquinone. This is a most chemically reactive orthoquinone which may give rise to a series of spontaneous reactions including redox exchange, intramolecular cyclization, covalent binding with sulfhydryl components, and oxidative polymerization of the resultant products.[4]

The current state of knowledge about the molecular mechanisms governing the metabolic fate of dopaquinone in melanocytes is the sulfhydryls content of pigment cells, including compounds such as glutathione and cysteine. The primary requirement for eumelanins to be produced is a low sulfhydryl content of melanocytes favoring the conversion of dopaquinone to dopachrome. According to the classic Raper-Mason schema, all the subsequent steps proceed more or less spontaneously without any specific enzymic assistance, dopachrome undergoes some rearrangement and to some extent decarboxylation to give 5,6 dihydroxyindole-2 carboxylic acid.[4]

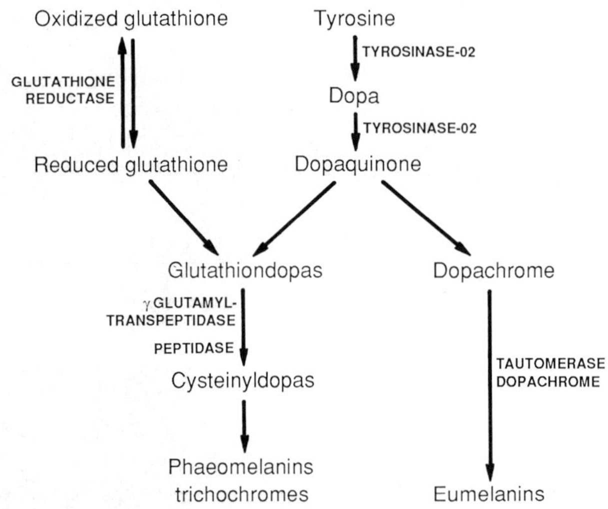

FIG. 7-1. Simplified schema of metabolic pathways leading to melanins.

Recently, a mouse cDNA corresponding to a new member of a family of melanocyte-specific mRNAs, which encodes tyrosinase and related proteins has been cloned and sequenced. It encodes a protein, TRP 2, more recently renamed DOPAchrome tautomerase (DT) which catalyses the conversion of DOPA-chrome to 5,6, dihydroxyindole-2-carboxylic acid. This gene maps to mouse chromosome 14 in the region of the coat color mutation slaty.[7bis] Other investigators suggest that metal ions could play a crucial role in the rearrangement of dopachrome, as well as the subsequent conversion of the resulting 5,6-dihydroxyindoles to melanochromes.[4] The subsequent conversion of these oligomers to eumelanins is still little understood.

In phaeomelanin-forming melanocytes, a switch mechanism leads to the production of sulfur-containing pigments through intervention of SH compounds. Biochemically, the in vivo formation of cysteinyldopas may proceed either by direct addition of cysteine to dopaquinone or by reaction of the latter with reduced glutathion, followed by enzymatic hydrolysis of the resultant glutathionedopas, by the action of gamma-glutamyltranspeptidase and a peptidase known to be present in melanocytes. Several lines of evidence suggest that the first possibility is the more likely to occur within pigment cells. Cysteinyldopas and glutathionedopas may be either metabolized to give sulfur-containing phaeomelanins and trichochromese by way of 1,4-benzothiazine intermediates and/or be released from melanocytes to be eventually excreted in the urine.[4]

Mammalian tyrosinase has been characterized

as a copper containing enzyme.[6] A tyrosinase cDNA from mouse and human have been obtained and the exon-intron structure of the tyrosinase gene is known in both mouse and human.[8] The tyrosinase encoding cDNA has been mapped at or very near the c-*locus*. Mutations involving the tyrosinase gene leading to oculo-cutaneous albinism have been characterized. In addition, another pigment gene (b-*locus*) share homologous nucleotide sequences with the tyrosinase gene. The product of this gene (b-*locus* protein) is present in very high quantities in pigment cell. It has been suggested that this protein is a catalase. A recent study demonstrates that this b-protein has the catalytic function ascribed to tyrosinase.[8]

Thus, it appears that melanogenesis in mammalian melanocytes is regulated by a family of tyrosinase-related genes. In the light of these recent studies, a reassessment of the enzymatic controls involved in the regulation of mammalian pigmentation is required.[8]

Melanocytes, and the "Melanocyte Organ" in Humans

Melanins in the skin are produced by exocrine unicellular glands, melanocytes, that are located on the epidermal basal lamina and project their dendrites into the epidermis.[1,9] Melanocytes are also found in hair follicles, and in mucous membranes. Other melanocytes are present in the eyes, inner ear cochlea, leptomeninges, mesentery and other internal organs. The epidermal melanocytes, however, constitute the dominant part of the melanocyte organ. In the adult human, not recently exposed to sunlight, the functionally active melanocytes form a tissue of 1 to 1.5 cm^3.[10]

In this chapter, the discussion will be mostly restricted to the epidermal melanocyte system. Epidermal melanocytes are derived from the neural crest. Their number varies from region to region of the integument. There are about 2000 or more epidermal melanocytes per square millimeter on the skin of the head and forearms and usually 1000 on the rest of the body.[9] Racial differences in pigmentation are not due to a difference in the number of melanocytes. Melanocytes synthetize specialized cytoplasmic organelles, called melanosomes, which are the sole site of melanin synthesis in the melanocyte. Based largely on the degree of melanin deposition, several stages in the development of the melanosomes have been described.[1,9]

Eumelanosomes, that is melanosomes in which predominant eumelanogenesis occurs, differ in their fine structure from phaeomelanosomes, that is melanosomes associated with phaeomelanins production.[1] There are racial differences in the size of melanosomes and their arrangement within keratinocytes. In caucasoids and mongoloids, melanosomes are small and packaged in complexes in the keratinocytes, whereas in negroids they are large and found as single bodies.[9]

Melanocytes transfer their melanosomes into the keratinocytes and these pigment granules are thereby distributed throughout in the epidermis by the outward movement of keratinocytes. Melanin granules are latter degraded within epidermal keratinocytes. This partnership of melanocytes and keratinocytes has led to the concept of the epidermal melanin unit. This functional unit associates one melanocyte with about 36 viable keratinocytes.[9]

BIOCHEMICAL RECORDERS OF MALIGNANT MELANOMAS

CysteinylDopas

Cysteinyldopas and related substances are excretion products of normal and pathological melanocytes.[11] Free cysteinyldopas can be demonstrated in the melanocytes, but as they are also excreted from these cells, they can be detected in the serum and in the urine. Cysteinyldopas have become of the greatest interest as biochemical recorders of malignant melanoma. Among the cysteinyldopas, 5-S-cysteinyldopa has attracted most attention since it is quantitatively most important. It has been suggested that 5-S-cysteinyldopa is the substance that better than any other small-molecular melanocytic compound provides information on the functional state of the melanocyte system.[11]

The excretion of 5-S-cysteinyldopas in the urine has been determined in several healthy populations. There seem to be no great differences between people of different race or complexion. The normal values are slightly higher in men than in women. Exposure to ultraviolet light increases serum levels and the urinary excretion of 5-S-cysteinyldopas. This probably explains that the quantity of 5-S-cysteinyldopas excreted in the urine varies with the season of the year being greatest in summer and least in winter.[11]

The urinary excretion of 5-S-cysteinyldopa is increased in most patients with disseminated melanoma. However, in some patients, especially those with amelanotic melanoma metastases, the excretion values may be normal in spite of disseminated disease. The age and sex, the body surface area and the effects on cysteinyldopa excretion of even modest sun exposures should all be taken into consideration when evaluating the results.[11]

The determination of 5-S-cysteinyldopa in plasma and urine is of strictly limited value in many primary melanomas, probably because the tumor is so small that it adds relatively little to the volume of the normal melanocyte population. On the other hand, the determination of 5-S-cysteinyldopa may be of great value in the diagnosis of a metastasis in an organ in which a single or multiple metastases give few or no symptoms or are not clinically evident. Several examples of variations of 5-S-cysteinyldopas have been found to decrease after surgical removal of a primary tumor or regression of metastases following chemotherapy.

It has been proposed to increase the diagnostic value of 5-S-cysteinyldopa determination by dopa loading.[11] There is no possibility to improve its diagnostic sensitivity by compensating for differences in basal melanocyte mass or UV-induced melanocyte proliferation.[12]

Several observations suggest that basal 5-S-cysteinyldopa in urine is also derived from sources other than skin melanocytes. The basal 5-S-cysteinyldopa is independent of skin color and of the size of the melanocyte organ.[12] There is a normal 5-S-cysteinyldopa excretion in both tyrosinase-positive, and negative albinos and 5-S-cysteinyldopa has been found in several organs in mice, rats, and guinea pigs.

Other Biochemical Markers

The Thormählen test[11] has been traditionally used for screening the urine in cases of suspected melanoma metastasis. This test detects indol derivatives in the urines of affected patients. The diagnostic value of this test is variously appreciated.[11]

Attempts to measure other precursors of melanins or their metabolites (Tyrosine, dopa) or tyrosinase have been performed in patients with metastatic melanomas but are not a diagnostic value.[11]

Melanogenesis in Malignant Melanomas

Malignant melanomas are composed of subpopulations of cells with a wide range of phenotypic variations especially in terms of pigment synthesis. These tumors can be hypomelanotic or frankly amelanotic. The reason for this decreased ability to produce melanin pigment varies from one tumor to the other. The occurrence of melanogenic inhibitors, including inhibitors of tyrosinase, has been suggested.[13] Electron microscopy study of amelanotic melanomas demonstrate the presence of melanosomes, although these organelles are few, small, and poorly or not melanized, showing that the tumor cells have retained the ability to synthetize melanosomal components.[14] Many cell lines of human and murine melanomas are available, sometimes with melanotic and amelanotic variants.

Biochemical analysis of unpigmented malignant melanomas suggests that these tumors can show significant concentrations of 5-S-cysteinyldopa, and this finding may support the diagnosis of melanoma.[15]

EFFECTS OF UV PHOTO-EXPOSURE ON MELANOCYTES

Acute UV Photo-Exposure

IMMEDIATE PIGMENT DARKENING REACTION (IPD)

This reaction, which involves a grey-brown discoloration of the skin, is induced mainly by long-wave UV radiation (UVA). It is apparent within a few minutes of exposure to UVA, peaks after 1 hour, and gradually fades over a few minutes to several hours.[16] Monitoring cutaneous pigmentation by measuring chromaticity coordinates has shown that IPD does not totally disappear and that a residual tanning response remains unchanged for at least 10 days, which was the observation period in the study.[17] After exposure to large doses of UVA ($\geq$ 18 J/cm^2), the darkening may persist for several days without fading.

From the results of a large-scale study in which the reaction was studied in over 1300 volunteers, it has been suggested that the peak effectiveness is between 320 and 340 nm,[18] with the average irradiation doses needed to produce minimal IPD increasing from phototype I to phototype IV; a lack of the reaction seemed to correlate well with "non-brown" eye color, but did not appear to be related to blonde hair.

At the ultrastructural level, Beitner and Wennersten[19] reported that neither transfer of preformed melanosomes from the melanocytes to the keratinocytes nor a redistribution of the melanosomes within the keratinocytes were observed 24 hours or later after UVA irradiation of skin type III.[19] This is in contrast to previous electron microscopy studies which demonstrated significant changes in the distribution pattern of melanosomes, thick filaments and microtubules, without significant changes in the melanogenic organelles necessary for the synthesis of new melanosomes. It is known, however, that IPD may occur in cadaverous skin, suggesting that the cytoskeleton of melanocytes is very unlikely[20] involved in this process.

Biochemical studies have suggested that the reaction represents an oxidation of the preformed melanin monomeric units via the formation of unstable semiquinone-like free radicals.[21] Another study concluded that the darkening of melanins associated with this immediate reaction is due to a photo-oxidation of semiquinone to quinone, resulting in an increase of carbon-oxygen double bonds that have hyperchromic effects.[22]

The physiological function of the immediate darkening reaction remains unknown and it apparently has no photoprotective properties.[16]

DELAYED TANNING (DT)

DT, which is maximally stimulated by exposure to the "sunburn spectrum," that is UVB radiation (290–

320 nm), and, to a lesser extent, to long-wave UV and visible radiation (320–700 nm) is a gradual process in which skin begins to darken 48 to 72 hours after irradiation.

Light microscopy studies of irradiated skin have shown that multiple exposures to UVA or UVB induce a marked increase in the number of functional melanocytes. Ultrastructural changes include an increase in the number of melanosome synthetized, an increase in the degree of pigmentation of the melanosomes, and an increase in the number of melanosomes transferred to keratinocytes.[23–27] In addition, there are distinct changes to the distribution pattern of melanosomes in keratinocytes, probably as a result of a variation in the size of the melanosomes. It is concluded, therefore, that DT involves synthesis of the new melanosomes, as well as changes in the functional state of melanocytes and keratinocytes. It has also been demonstrated that repeated UVB irradiation induces an increase in the melanocyte population in the protected skin in humans by an, as yet, unidentified mechanism, although this observation suggests release into the circulation of a mitogenic factor for melanocytes.[28,57]

Biochemical studies have shown that exposure to UV radiation is related to changes in specific intermediate metabolites of the melanin biosynthesic pathway in the plasma and in the urine, for example, 5-S-cysteinyldopa, and 6-hydroxy-5-methoxyindole-2-carboxylic acid.[29] Melanogenesis induced by UVA depends on the presence of oxygen or oxygenated molecules, whereas UVB induce pigmentation whether or not oxygen is present.[29]

The signal pathways that mediate UV-induced pigmentation in human melanocytes are unknown. After UV irradiation, a marked decrease in glutathione reductase activity, a decrease in reduced glutathione, and an increase in oxidized glutathione have been observed in the skin.[30] A change in the ratio of reduced to oxidized glutathione starts on about the third day after irradiation and continues for about two weeks and may reflect one of the biochemical mechanisms for post-UV hypermelanosis. Other investigators have suggested that the mechanism of human skin pigmentation after UVB irradiation may be partly explained by a stimulatory effect of Vitamin D3 on the melanocytes. This is based on data showing an increased amount of immunoreactive tyrosinase in human melanocytes after culturing with vitamin D3, with the pigment cells showing morphological changes similar to those observed in melanocytes after UV irradiation.[12] Although attractive, this interpretation is still speculative. It has also been hypothetized that UVR increases the secretion of MSH-like peptides and enhance the availability of MSH receptors on the melanocyte leading to an activation of melanin synthesis. It has also been reported that circulating levels of α-MSH are increased in human following UVR. These results, however, have not been confirmed by recent studies, and it is unlikely that MSH has any direct role in mediating UVR induced melanogenesis.

The intracellular signal pathways mediating UV-induced melanogenesis are also unknown. It has been demonstrated that UV radiation stimulates melanogenesis directly in cultured human melanocytes[31] but no changes in cyclic AMP concentrations were observed following UV exposure, suggesting that cyclic AMP dependent mechanisms do not mediate the UVR signal. More recent datas suggest that the UV-induced signal-activating melanogenesis could be mediated by diacylglycerol[32] and imply that the signal is transduced via an alternative pathway that might be independent of protein kinase C.[33]

It is likely that keratinocyte-derived factors play a role in the induction of melanogenesis after UV irradiation. Several experiments indicate that basic fibroblast growth factor from human keratinocytes is a natural mitogen toward melanocytes in highly proliferative keratinocytes.[34] This has lead to the hypothesis that in vivo UVB stimulates melanocytes indirectly through neighboring irradiated keratinocytes via increased basic fibroblast growth factor production; this hypothesis has not yet been demonstrated. Other experiments suggest that the human melanocyte UV response is not influenced by soluble factors in keratinocyte-conditioned medium. Keratinocytes seem to be able to stimulate melanocytes after UV exposure at least as much as without irradiation, but the physiological mechanism probably requires the simultaneous irradiation of the two cell populations and/or a close cellular contact.[35] In addition, UV radiation acts as an independent mitogen for normal human melanocytes in culture, suggesting that the in vivo UV-induced melanocyte proliferation may be due to a direct effect of pigment cells, perhaps by substituting for the cyclic AMP requirement.[36]

Although pigmentation induced by different spectral regions appears similar to the eye, there are qualitative differences in the protection afforded against subsequent exposure.[37,38] UVB induced tans protect moderately well against all wavelengths. On the other hand, even though a UVA-induced pigmentation is visually impressive as a deep rich brown, it protects poorly against all wavebands.[5] In one study it has been demonstrated that UV tans conferred significant induced protection against UVB induced erythema, while UVA tans were not associated with a similar reduction in the number of pyrimidine dimers in epidermal DNA. It is possible that this difference in the biological effectiveness of these tans is due to the difference in the proliferative response in keratinocytes that UVB produces. It is easily understandable that when increased melanin synthesis occurs in an epidermis undergoing proliferation, melanosomes transferred to keratinocytes will be moved more effectively into the stratum corneum increasing its optical barrier function.

Chronic UV Photo-Exposure of Melanocytes

Although the number of dopa-positive melanocytes in human skin decreases with age,[39,40] melanocyte density is approximately twofold higher in chronically sun-exposed skin than in protected skin at all ages.[41] This suggests that the principal effect of chronic exposure to the sun on human epidermal melanocytes is not premature aging but activation and/or proliferation of the exposed melanocytes. The higher numbers of epidermal melanocytes in sun-exposed human skin may be explained by repeated UV exposure irreversibly increasing the number of dopa-positive melanocytes. On unexposed areas of skin of old subjects, epidermal melanocytes keep their proliferative capacity induced by repeated UV exposure.[41] Preliminary studies suggest, however, that melanocytes derived from adult skin have a considerably shorter life span in vitro, with decreased response to specific mitogens.[42] Various pigmentary changes of the skin are associated with chronic exposure including hyper- and hypomelanoses.[43]

OTHER EFFECTS OF UV ON MELANOCYTES

It is increasingly clear that melanocytes are not only producing melanins. Recent studies have demonstrated that these pigment cells are able to produce many biologically active substances including hormones and cytokines. The production of these factors is sometimes modulated by UVB irradiation. As an example, normal human melanocytes spontaneously release in culture IL-1, IL-6, IL-3 TNFα, GM-CSF, and I-CAM, and this production is strongly upregulated by UVB irradiation.[44] Although the biological significance of these observations is unknown, they open quite a new field for the photobiology of melanocytes.

PHOTOTYPES

Several phototypes have been defined[45] according to the burning and/or tanning reaction of the skin following ultraviolet irradiation (Table 7-1). In another study,[2] six different photogenotypes were identified among the caucasoid population after investigating several different parameters including hair color, winter skin color, freckles, tanning capacity, color of tanning, and erythema after vacational repeated sun exposures (Table 7-2). Excellent correlation were found between melanogenotypes, the shape of melanosomes, reflectometry measurement of unexposed skin, and UVB sensitivity.[2]

TABLE 7-1
DEFINITION OF PHOTOTYPES*

Type I	Always burn without tan[a]
Type II	Always burn and light tan
Type III	Slight burn and good tan
Type IV	No burn and dark tan

*Melski et al. 1977[45]
[a]The volunteers received 3 MED (1 h of midday sun, in June under 40° N latitude). The tanning achieved after a single irradiation was estimated on day 7 following irradiation.

A systematic study of the relationship between the 5-S-cysteinyldopa excretion in the urine and the UV induced melanocyte proliferation, skin type and the erythema reaction has been performed.[28] It was concluded that the skin type had no influence on the basal excretion of 5-S-cysteinyldopa, and no correlation was found between 5-S-cysteinyldopa excretion and UV-induced melanocyte population. During the irradiation, however, skin type II individual developed a more pronounced erythema and had a higher 5-S-cysteinyldopa excretion than those with skin type III. These results further suggest that the basal 5-S-cysteinyldopa in urine is mainly of extra-melanocytic origin. In addition they favor the view that the increase in 5-S-cysteinyldopa is due to damage to the melanocytes.[28]

SKIN AND HAIR COLOR AND CHEMICAL TYPES OF MELANINS

Indirect evidence indicates that the melanins present in black hair and dark-colored skin are mainly eumelanins, whereas the melanins present in red hair and light-colored skin are predominantly phaeomelanins. In order to obtain direct evidence, many attempts have been made to analyze quantitatively the content and the class of melanin pigments in melanogenic tissues.[46,47] Techniques that make unnecessary the isolation of melanins from the melanogenic tissues in order to perform such a characterization are now available. However, there are very few data about possible correlation between the chemical structure of pigments present in human skin and its color. It has been demonstrated that the visual differentiation of hair color does not always reflect the melanogenesis type in human red hair. One study also establishes that the chemical analysis of melanogenesis type corresponds well to the fine structural differentiation of eumelanosomes and phaeomelanosomes.

There is even less information about the chemical structure of melanins in the interfollicular epidermis of human skin. A study performed on normal Japanese individuals suggests that, although eumelanin is dominant in the epidermis, phaeomelanin

TABLE 7-2

MELANOGENOTYPES IN THE WHITE POPULATION: IDENTIFICATION, SUN REACTIONS, CONSTITUTIVE, AND DELAYED PROTECTION FACTORS

MELANOTYPE GENE	HAIR COLOR	WINTER SKIN COLOR	FRECKLES	MED mJ.cm-2	ERYTHEMA BURNING	TANNING	PROTECTION FACTOR DAY 1[a]	PROTECTION FACTOR DAY 21[b]
Rd-Rd	Red	Milky	+ + +	17	easily	never	1	2
Rd-B1	Blonde-Red	Milky	+ +	18	easily	never	1	3
Rd-Br	Chestnut	Pale	+	25	easily	minimal	2	4
B1-B1	Blonde	Pale	0	30	moderate	gradual	2	6
B1-Br	Light brown	Mat	0	40	moderate	good	2.5	8
Br-Br	Dark brown	Mat	0	65	rarely	dark	4	12

[a]The MED of the most sensitive class was taken as a unit value. It corresponds to 15 min of sun exposure at midday under 42 ° N latitude in June.
[b]Protection factor achieved after three weeks of mild, non-sunburning exposures.
From Cesarini JP. 1988[2]

is also synthetized in normal human epidermal melanocytes. A good correlation between the ratio of eu/phaeomelanin and fine structure of melanosomes was also obtained.[48] In another study, the concentration of eumelanin and phaeomelanin in different skin types of caucasoid individuals was determined before and after PUVA.[49] The results also suggest that both types of melanins are present in epidermis. Furthermore, the concentrations of these two pigments appeared to be related to skin type.

THE PHOTOPROTECTIVE ROLE OF MELANINS

Not all individuals share an equal risk for the development of dermatoheliosis and skin cancer. Individuals with black skin rarely get cutaneous cancer. On the other hand, cutaneous cancer and aging of the skin are more common and more severe in people with red hair and light-colored skin. Although the natural defenses of skin against sunlight are complex, involving several different basic mechanisms, a large body of evidence suggest that melanin plays a key role in this process. This may be related partly to the differences in the melanogenesis type in the skin of a given individual. Thus, it has been suggested that differences in the photochemical properties of the different types of melanins may contribute to the harmful effect of the radiation. According to the classic view, it is suggested that eumelanins act as inert sunscreens in cells. They may act as a filter to screen out harmful UV, absorb UV radiation, and dissipate the absorbed energy into heat and scatter and attenuate UV radiation. However, it is also suggested that eumelanins may exert photoprotection in human skin through their ability to act as free radical scavengers for minimizing the harmful effects of other free radicals generated by UV radiations. It is also suggested that melanin acts as a pseudo-dismutase and a scavenger of superoxide anions generated by UVA radiation.[50]

However, irradiation of eumelanins and phaeomelanins has been reported to produce superoxide. UV-visible irradiation of human red hair melanin (RHM) produces considerable amounts of superoxide, whereas the irradiation of black hair melanin (BHM) does not produce detectable amounts of superoxide, suggesting that phaeomelanins may emit toxic radicals able to induce cellular damage. Furthermore, the oxidation of NADH (reduced nicotinamide adenine dinucleotide) by human RHM is enhanced to a larger extent than the NADH oxidation by BHM.[51] This hypothesis is further supported by the demonstration that when subjected to UVA radiation, human RHM produced considerably more cellular damages in Ehrlich ascite cells than human BHM.[52] Several other experiments lead to similar results and also suggest that phaeomelanins degradation products following UV irradiations may have proinflammatory properties, which may account for the increased photosensitivity of light-skinned individuals.[53] It has also been demonstrated that phaeomelanins may become mutagenic after exposure to long-wave length UV-light.[54]

The mechanisms by which phaeomelanin may induce cellular alterations is unknown. It has been suggested that peroxidation of membrane lipids could be involved.[51] Other experiments suggest that phaeomelanin related molecules bind to DNA after activation by UV light with resulting induction of single strand breaks in the DNA.

Recent results also suggest that eumelanin is not simply an inert radioprotective substance. Experimental results demonstrate that eumelanins (synthetic eumelanin prepared by autooxidation of DL DOPA) may be potentially genotoxic[55] and DNA damaging in the absence of radiations. Several melanogenic indole intermediates and metabolites have been shown to be photolabile and initiate DNA damage in vitro in the presence of biologically relevant ultraviolet radiation (that is above 300 km).[56] Thus, the biological functions of melanins and their role in photoprotection and "photoaggression" are more complex than it was though before (for review see ref. 58).

REFERENCES

1. Quevedo WCM, Fitzpatrick TB, Szabo G, and Jimbow K. Biology of melanocytes. In: Fitzpatrick TB, Eisen AZ, Wolff K, Freedberg IM, Austen KF, (eds.), *Dermatology in General Medicine* (3rd ed.) New York: McGraw-Hill, 1987, 224–258.
2. Cesarini JP. Photo-induced events in the human melanocytic system: Photoaggression and photoprotection. *Pigment Cell Res* 1:223–233, 1988.
3. Kollias N and Baqer AH. The role of human melanin in providing photoprotection from solar mid-ultraviolet radiation (280–320 nm). *J Soc Cosmet Chem* 39:347–354, 1988.
4. Prota G. Mechanisms in melanin pigmentation: An up-to-date view. In: Fitzpatrick TB, Forlot P, Pathak MA, and Urback F (eds.), *Psoralens: Past, Present and Future of Photochemoprotection and other biological activities.* Paris: John Libbeyt Eurotext, 1989, 13–23.
5. Gange W and Parrish JA. Photobiology of melanin pigmentation. Fitzpatrick TB, Wick MM, Toda K (eds.), In: *Brown Melanoderma.* Tokyo: University of Tokyo Press, 1986, 75–85.
6. Prota G. Recent advances in the chemistry of melanogenesis in mammals. *J Invest Dermatol* 75:122–127, 1980.
7. Prota G. Chemistry of melanins. *Med Res Rev* 8:525–556, 1988.

7bis. Tsukamoto K, Jackson I, Urabe K, Montague P, and Hearing V. A second tyrosinase-related protein, TRP-2, is a melanogenic enzyme termed DOPAchrome tautomerase. *EMBO J* 11:519–526, 1992.

8. Jimenez M, Tsukamoto T, and Hearing VJ. Tyrosinases from two different loci are expressed by normal and by transformed melanocytes. *J Biol Chem* 266:1147–1156, 1991.
9. Jimbow K. Biology of melanocytes: Cellular and subcellular control of melanocyte differentiation. In: Fitzpatrick TB, Wick MM, and Toda K (eds.), *Brown Melanoderma.* Tokyo: University of Tokyo Press, 1986, 45–62.
10. Rosdahl I and Rorsman H. The size of the "melanocyte organ" in man. In: Bagnara J, Klaus SN, Paul E, and Schartl M (eds.), *Biological, Molecular and Clinical Aspects of Pigmentation.* Tokyo: University of Tokyo Press, 1985, 555–561.
11. Rorsman H, Agrup C, Hansson C, and Rosengren E. Biochemical recorders of malignant melanomas. *Pigment Cell Res* 6:93–115, 1983.
12. Tomita Y, Torinuk W, and Tagami H. Stimulation of human melanocytes by vitamin D3 possibly mediates skin pigmentation after sun exposure. *J Invest Dermatol* 90:882–884, 1988.
13. Mishima Y, Hatta S, Ohyama Y, and Inazu M. Induction of melanogenesis suppression cellularpharmacology and mode of differential action. *Pigment Cell Res* 1:367–374, 1988.
14. Ghadially FN. Is it a melanoma? In: *Diagnosis Electron Microscopy of Tumours.* 2nd Edition. London: Butterworths, 1985, 106–122.
15. Aubert C, Rosengren E, Rorsman H, Rouge F, Foa C, and Lipcey C. 5-S-cysteinyldopa in diagnosis and treatment of human malignant melanomas and ultrastructural observations. *Eur J Cancer* 13:1299–1308, 1977.
16. Beitner H. Immediate pigment-darkening reaction. *Photodermatol Photoimmunol Photomed* 5:96–100, 1988.
17. Porges SB, Kaidbey KH, and Grove GL. Quantification of visible light-induced melanogenesis in human skin. *Photodermatol Photoimmunnol Photomed* 5:197–200, 1988.
18. Poh Agin P, Desrochers D, and Sayre RM. The relationship of immediate pigment darkening to minimal erythemal dose, skin type, and eye color. *Photodermatol Photoimmunol Photomed* 2:288–294, 1985.
19. Beitner H and Wennerstein G. A qualitative and quantitative transmission electronmicroscopic study of the immediate pigment darkening reaction. *Photodermatol Photoimmunol Photomed* 2:273–278, 1985.
20. Meirowski E. Uber pigmentbildung in wom Körper losgelöster Haut. *Frankfurt Z Pathol* 2:439–448, 1909.
21. Pathak MA and Stratton K. Free radicals in human skin before and after exposure to light. *Arch Biochem Biophys* 123:468–476, 1968.
22. Sawamura D, Sato S, Kiuchi H, Hashimoto I, and Katabira Y. UVA induced darkening of lower epidermal cells as an in vitro system of immediate pigment darkening (IPD) and mechanisms of IPD. *J Dermatol* 13:101–107, 1986.
23. Beitner H. The effect of high dose long-wave ultraviolet radiation (UVA) on epidermal melanocytes in human skin: A transmission electron microscopic study. *Photodermatol Photoimmunol Photomed* 3:133–139, 1986.
24. Fitzpatrick TB. Ultraviolet induced pigmentary changes: Benefits and hazards. *Curr Probl Dermatol* 15:25–38, 1986.
25. Jimbow K, Pathak MA, and Fitzpatrick TB. Effect of ultraviolet on the distribution pattern of microfilaments and microtubules and on the nucleus in human melanocytes. *Yale J Biol Med* 46:411–426, 1973.
26. Jimbow K, Pathak MA, Szabo G, and Fitzpatrick TB. Ultrastructural changes in human melanocytes after ultraviolet radiation. In: Fitzpatrick TB (ed.), *Sunlight and Man.* Tokyo: University of Tokyo Press, 1974, 195–215.
27. Jimbow K and Fitzpatrick TB. Changes in distribution pattern of cytofilaments in human melanocytes during ultraviolet mediated melanin pigmentation. *J Cell Biol* 65:481–488, 1975.
28. Stierner U, Rosdahl I, Augustsson A, and Kagedal B. Urinary excretion of 5-S-cysteinyldopa in relation to skin-type, UV. B-induced erythema and melanocyte proliferation in human skin. *J Invest Dermatol* 91:506–510, 1988.
29. Rorsman H and Tegner E. Biochemical observations in UV-induced pigmentation. *Photodermatology* 5:30–38, 1988.
30. Halprin KM and Ohkawara A. Human pigmentation: The role of glutathione. In: Montagna W and Hu F (eds.), *Advances in Biology of Skin,* vol 8, *The pigmentary system.* New York: Pergamon Press, 1967, 241–251.
31. Friedmann PS and Gilchrest BA. Ultraviolet radiation directly induces pigment production by cultured human melanocytes. *J Cell Physiol* 133:88–94, 1987.
32. Gordon PR and Gilchrest BA. Human melanogenesis is stimulated by diacylglycerol. *J Invest Dermatol* 93:700–702, 1989.
33. Friedmann PS, Wren FE, and Matthews JNS. Ultraviolet stimulated melanogenesis by human melanocytes is augmented by Di-Acyl Glycerol but not TPA. *J Cell Physiol* 142:334–341, 1990.
34. Halaban R, Langdon R, Birchall N, Cuono C, Baird A, Scott G, Moellmann G, and McGuire J. Basic fibroblast growth from human keratinocytes is a natural mitogen for melanocytes. *J Cell Biol* 107:1611–1618, 1988.
35. Lacour JP, Gordon PR, Ortonne JP, and Gilchrest BA. Human melanocyte UV response is not influenced by soluble

factors in keratinocyte conditioned medium. *J Invest Dermatol* (abstract) 94:398, 1990.

36. Libow LF, Scheide S, and DeLeo A. Ultraviolet radiation acts as an independent mitogen for normal human melanocytes in culture. *Pig Cell Res* 1:397–401, 1988.
37. Gange RW. Comparison of pigment responses in human skin to UVB and UVA radiation. In: *Advances in Pigment Cell Research.* New York: Alan R. Liss, 1988, 475–485.
38. Kagetsu N, Gange W, and Parrish JA. UVA-induced erythema, pigmentation, and skin surface temperature changes are irradiance dependent. *J Invest Dermatol* 85:445–447, 1985.
39. Quevedo WC, Szabo G, and Virks J. Influence of age and UV on the populations of dopa-positive melanocytes in human skin. *J Invest Dermatol* 52:287–290, 1969.
40. Snell RS and Bischitz PG. The melanocytes and melanin in human abdominal wall skin: A survey made at different ages in both sexes and during pregnancy. *J Anat* 97:361–376, 1963.
41. Gilchrest BA, Blog FB, and Szabo G. Effects of ageing and chronic sun exposure on melanocytes in human skin. *J Invest Dermatol* 73:141–143, 1979.
42. Gilchrest BA. The Skin and Aging Process. Boca Raton, Florida: CRC Press, 1984.
43. Ortonne JP. The effects of ultraviolet exposure on skin melanin pigmentation. *J Intern Med Res* 18:10 pages 1990.
44. Köch A, Schauer E, and Lüger TA. The human melanocyte is an immunocompetent epidermal cell: Production of immunomodulating cytokines. *Arch Dermatol Res* (Abstract) 283:56, 1991.
45. Melski JW, Tanenbaum L, Parrish JA, Fitzpatrick TB, Bleich HL and 28 participant investigators. Oral methoxypsoralen photochemotherapy for the treatment of psoriasis: A cooperative clinical trial. *J Invest Dermatol* 68:328–335, 1977.
46. Ito S, Fujita K, Takahashi H, and Jimbow K. Characterization of melanogenesis in mouse and guinea pig hair by chemical analysis of melanins and of free and bound Dopa and 5-S-Cysteinyldopa. *J Invest Dermatol* 83:12–14, 1984.
47. Jimbow K, Ishida O, Ito S, Hori Y, Witkop CJ, and King RA. Combined chemical and electron microscopic studies of pheomelanosomes in human red hair. *J Invest Dermatol* 81:506–511, 1983.
48. Nayagawa AH, Imokawa G, Etoh T, and Ishibashy Y. Melanogenesis in normal human epidermal melanocytes. *J Invest Dermatol* (Abstract) 92:488, 1989.
49. Thody AJ, Higgins EM, Burchill SA, Marks JM, and Ito S. Epidermal eumelanin and phaeomelanin concentrations in different skin types and in response to PUVA. *Br J Dermatol* 122:288–289, 1990.
50. Pathak MA. Photoprotective role of melanin (eumelanin) in human skin. In: Fitzpatrick TB, Forlot P, Pathak MA, and Urback F (eds.), *Psoralens: Past, Present and Future of Photochemoprotection and other biological activities.* Paris: John Libbeyt Eurotext, 1989, 25–33.
51. Menon IA, Persad S, Ranadive NS, and Heberman HF. Photobiological effects of eumelanin and pheomelanin. In: Bagnara J, Klaus SN, Paul E, and Schartl M (eds.), *Biological, Molecular and Clinical Aspects of Pigmentation.* Tokyo: University of Tokyo Press, 1985, 77–85.
52. Ranadive NS, Shirwadkar S, Persad S, Menon IA. Effects of melanin-induced free radicals on the isolated rat peritoneal mas cells. *J Invest Dermatol* 86:303–307, 1986.
53. Lea PJ, Pawlowski A, Persad SD, Menon A, and Haberman HF. Ultrastructural changes produced in Ehrlich ascites carcinoma cells by ultraviolet-visible radiations in the presence of melanins. *Pigment Cell Res* 1:402–409, 1988.
54. Harsanyi ZP, Post PW, Brinkmann JP, Chedekel MR, and Deibel RM. Mutagenicity of melanin from human red hair. *Experientia* 36:291–292, 1980.
55. Hill HZ and Hill GJ. Eumelanin causes DNA strand breaks and kills cells. *Pigment Cell Res* 1:163–170, 1987.
56. Köch WH and Chedekel MR. Photogeneration of free radicals from eumelanogenic intermediates and metabolites. *Biochim Biophys Acta* 924:458–466, 1987.
57. Stierner U, Rosdahl I, Augustsson A. Indirect effect of UVB-irradiation on the melanocyte system in covered skin. *J Invest Dermatol* 87:447, 1986.
58. Hill HZ. The function of melanin as six blind people examine an elephant. *Bioessays* 14:49–56, 1992.

Chapter 8

ULTRAVIOLET PROTECTION

Rex M. Tyrrell

SOLAR RADIATION

The spectrum of solar radiation at the surface of the earth ranges from approximately 290 nm through the ultraviolet (UV) and visible ranges and into the infrared. The ultraviolet region (see Fig. 8-1) is further subdivided into the UVB (290–320 nm) and UVA (320–380 nm). It should be noted however, that by current international definition, the transition from UVA to UVB is considered to be at 315 nm. The lower limit of UVB reflects the absorption of stratospheric ozone, however, the precise limit varies with time of the day, year, geographical location, climatic conditions, and so on. The intensity of solar radiation also varies throughout the day and is a function of solar zenith angle. From a practical point of view, it is also important to note that the ratio of UVA/UVB varies relatively little throughout the day except at low zenith angles (close to sunrise and sunset). Clouds attenuate UV intensity merely by scattering in a wavelength independent fashion, but significant levels of UV still reach the earth's surface on cloudy and even rainy days.

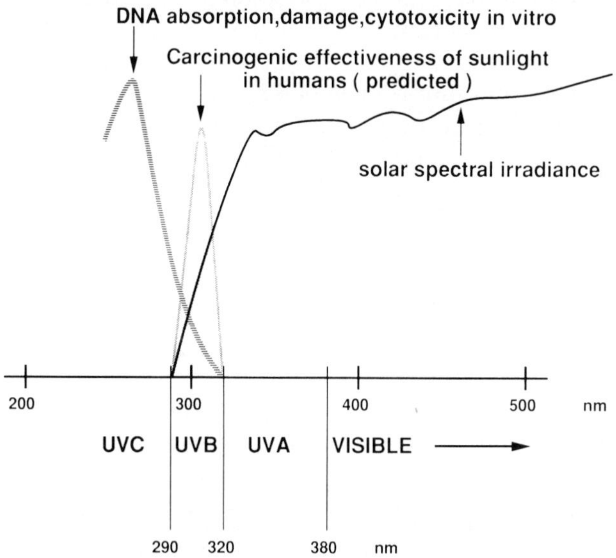

FIG. 8-1 Diagramatic representation of the spectrum of solar radiation reaching the earth's surface that shows the division of UV into A, B, and C.

SOLAR RADIATION AND NONMELANOMA SKIN CANCER

Of the nonmelanoma skin cancers, basal cell carcinoma is by far the most common, accounting for 80 percent of the total cases reported. However, squamous cell carcinomas account for the majority of the mortality. The epidemiological data provides a totally convincing correlation between sunlight exposure and squamous cell carcinoma[1] and the probability of occurrence is strongly correlated with the accumulated solar UV exposure. Since experimental animals (including the mouse) develop squamous cell carcinoma as a result of UV exposure,[2] there has been a considerable effort to determine an "action spectrum" for UV carcinogenesis, that is, to determine the carcinogenic effectiveness of the radiation as a function of wavelength. Initial reports, which have subsequently been confirmed by more recent detailed studies, indicate that the wavelengths which are primarily responsible for carcinogenesis are in the UVB range.[3–6] Nevertheless, these studies have demonstrated that UVA radiation is also carcinogenic in animals although the total accumulated doses required are several orders of magnitude higher than for UVB. Thus, an excellent action spectrum of UV induced squamous cell cancer in an experimental animal model now exists and can be used for calculations providing that the user is aware that there is no direct evidence that such an action spectrum also applies to humans.

Basal cell carcinomas are also related to the solar exposure. However, although they appear more frequently on sun-exposed sites, this is not always the case and the correlation of the total exposure as estimated from the latitude, although significant, is weaker than for squamous cell carcinoma. Experimental UV does not cause basal cell carcinoma in mice so that an action spectrum has not yet been determined.

SOLAR RADIATION AND MELANOMA

Until recently, no animal models existed for UV-induced cutaneous melanoma. However, UVB has now been shown to induce melanomas in the small opossum *Monodelphis domestica*[7] so that our information in this area is likely to increase. The fish hybrid that involves a cross between platy fish and swordtails also develops UVB-induced melanoma[8] and this may prove a particularly simple model for determining action spectra since the fishes are small enough to be irradiated in cuvettes. Indeed, in a recent update of the original preliminary report, Setlow and Grist[9] described an action spectrum showing that UVA radiation is approximately 2 orders of magnitude more effective in inducing melanoma than inducing either DNA damage in mammalian cells or squamous cell carcinoma in mice. If this finding holds for the mammalian melanoma model systems currently under development (marsupials, p53 suppressor gene knock-out mice), the implications for protection of human populations against melanoma would be substantial.

The relationship between solar exposure and cutaneous melanoma has been controversial but it is now generally agreed[10,11] that the correlation between the fairly common lentigo malignant melanoma (LMM) and solar exposure is similar to that seen for the nonmelanoma carcinomas. Furthermore, there is now data available consistent with the possibility that cutaneous melanoma in general, especially the common superficial spreading form, is related to sunlight exposure. This is largely based on the higher melanoma incidence rates that occur in white populations with decreasing latitude. However, there is also a correlation between risk factors for cutaneous melanoma (freckling and nevus formation) and solar exposure. Cutaneous melanoma is also high in *Xeroderma pigmentosum* patients whose cells exhibit a defect in repair of UV-induced DNA damage.[12] There are indications from case-control studies that a history of acute sunburn at an early age increased the risk of cutaneous melanoma. There is also substantial evidence[13] in support of the claim that strong intermittent exposure to UV rather than long-term chronic exposure may be important in determining overall melanoma risk. Except for lentigo maligna melanoma there is no apparent relationship between outdoor occupations and melanoma risk and the site on the body at which the other types of melanoma appear is not correlated with the highest levels of sunlight exposure. Nevertheless, an increasing volume of important epidemiological data should help to settle remaining doubts concerning the correlation between solar exposure and the incidence of the different types of human melanoma.

MOLECULAR GENETICS OF SKIN CANCER

The link between DNA damage, cancer and the causative agents such as sunlight has been strengthened by the analysis of mutations in DNA isolated from tumors (although it must be noted that such mutations may have occurred at a late stage in tumor formation). Several studies now exist in which mutations have been analyzed in oncogenes. In one such study,[14] materials from 37 cutaneous melanomas were analyzed. Seven of these were found to have N-*ras* mutations and all of these were detected in biopsies of melanomas that developed at body sites receiving the most frequent exposures to solar radiation. All the mutations were at bipyrimidine sites where mutagenic UV photoproducts could arise, thereby implicating solar exposure in the etiology. Other studies have indicated that K-*ras* activation is a frequent and early event in melanoma development.[15]

The analysis of p53 tumor suppressor gene mutations has provided even more convincing evidence of the role of sunlight in skin cancer.[16] The majority (14 out of 24) of invasive squamous cell carcinomas from sun-exposed skin had p53 mutations at various sites. In an update of this work, Brash and co-workers[17] have reported that over 90 percent of the invasive squamous cell carcinomas and basal cell carcinomas contain aberrations in the p53 gene and protein. Again, the types of mutations observed clearly indicate that mutation of p53 by solar UV is the first step in the cancer process. Based on the immunohistochemical detection of mutant p53 protein, Stretch et al.[18] have concluded that 45 out of 53 samples from a range of primary and metastatic melanomas had evidence of p53 gene mutations and that such mutations were more prevalent in the metastatic tissue. However, the molecular genetic approach undertaken by Brash and co-workers is really essential in order to obtain clues as to the role of specific mutagens, and UV in particular, in the carcinogenic process that leads to the melanomas.

ACTION SPECTRA AND THE ESTIMATION OF THE CARCINOGENIC EFFECTIVENESS OF SUNLIGHT

On the assumption that damage to the DNA is the initiating event in the carcinogenic process, it has been considered informative to derive action spectra for photoproduct formation in DNA and to use such information to determine the wavelengths in sunlight that are effective in producing skin cancer.[19] In order to predict carcinogenic effectiveness of sunlight as a function of wavelength, it is necessary to know the action spectrum of the biological end-point chosen (e.g., photoproduct formation) as well as to have available the transmission of solar radiation to the target cells of interest as a function of wavelength and spectroradiometric data for selected solar exposure conditions. Careful human skin transmission measurements have been available for some time[20] and there is substantial literature on DNA photoproduct formation as a function of wavelength.[21] Analysis of such data has led to the inference[19] that the UVB region of the spectrum is the most effective in causing human skin cancers. However, the picture may not be so simple for melanomas.

Although the correlation between sunlight and DNA damage is crucial in the analysis of the carcinogenic pathways leading to skin cancer, other wavelength dependent parameters merit consideration. For example, the apparent correlation between acute sunburn and melanoma may indicate that extensive tissue destruction and subsequent repopulation may play a role early in the development of the disease. Action spectra for inactivation of cultured human skin cells (fibroblasts and keratinocytes) follow the DNA absorption spectra out to 320 nm but cells become more sensitive than predicted simply from DNA damage measurements at longer wavelengths.[22] This is undoubtedly related to a series of observations that show that UVA radiation constitutes a severe oxidative stress to cells[23] so that non-DNA targets susceptible to oxidation (e.g., membranes) are increasingly damaged at longer wavelengths. Based on convolution of action spectra, skin transmission and solar irradiance data (as mentioned), it was calculated that even at noon on a summer day (Albuquerque, NM) 50 percent of the cytotoxic effectiveness of solar UV at the basal layer of the epidermis would be contributed by the UVA region. Early and late in the day, the contribution would be as much as 80 percent. The destructive power of the UVA component of the sunlight should therefore not be underestimated, particularly in view of the provocative melanoma action spectrum results recently reported by Setlow (as mentioned).

Other wavelength dependent phenomena may play a role in the development of skin cancer. For example, it is now well established that UVB radiation causes both local and systemic alterations of the immune system.[24] It is clear that sunlight-induced changes in the immune system in people could influence various stages in the development of cutaneous malignancies (see Chapter 3).

PROTECTION AGAINST SOLAR RADIATION

From the foregoing it is evident that for nonmelanoma skin cancer, the UVB radiation component of sunlight is of critical importance. However, UVA clearly contributes significantly to the total carcinogenic effectiveness of sunlight. Although some animal data and the human DNA damage spectra are consistent with the assumption that the UVB region is important for sunlight-induced melanoma, recent data underlines how dangerous it would be to ignore the possibility that UVA plays a significant or even major role. For better delineation of the role of UVA, considerable work is still necessary in the animal model systems relevant to humans. A clear definition of the contribution of the longer wavelengths is also important because the use of primarily UVB absorbing sunscreens (as is the current practice) will allow more time for solar exposure and thereby increase the total exposure to the UVA radiation component. It is important that for proper protection against cutaneous malignancies, and melanoma in particular, the use of sunscreens that absorb both UVA and UVB radiations as uniformly as possible should be encouraged.

Most clothing materials absorb the whole spectrum of UV fairly uniformly and provide important protection. The level of protection is mainly correlated with the tightness of the weave and with the material employed. For high protection on uncovered areas of the body, sunscreens such as zinc oxide and titanium oxide may be used. These function primarily by reflection and scattering and, therefore, protect against the entire UV spectrum. For routine use on exposed areas, chemical sunscreens are most commonly employed. These change the quantity and spectral distribution of the radiation passing into the skin. Until recently, most sunscreens absorbed primarily UVB radiation and included *para*-aminobenzoic (PABA) derivatives, salicylate, cinnamates, and camphor derivatives. To increase the UVA absorption properties, dibenzoyl methanes, anthranilates, and benzophenones have been introduced. However, ideal chemical sunscreens which absorb equally throughout the ultraviolet spectrum and essentially act as neutral density filters have not yet been developed.

Sunscreen packaging now generally indicates whether the preparation absorbs both UVA and UVB radiations. In addition, the most useful parameter which should appear on a sunscreen is the sun protection factor (SPF) which is defined as the ratio of the least amount of ultraviolet radiation required to produce minimal erythema after application of a standard quantity of the sunscreen product film to the skin to that required to produce the same erythema without sunscreen application. Under ideal conditions, this means that solar exposure can be increased by a factor equivalent to the SPF but in practice, because of variation in application, and so on, exposure should be kept to well within the calculated limits. An associated problem is that there is considerable variation between laboratories in SPF evaluation[25] but this problem should gradually be eliminated as international standards for light sources and measurement protocols are introduced. Because of the predominant effectiveness of UVB in the test light source (as in sunlight), the SPF is a poor indication of UVA protection. Several in vivo and in vitro methods have been proposed for defining protection against UVA but opinions differ sharply as to the best one. In practice such a factor would probably do more to confuse than help users in their selection of a suitable product since exposure is normally to total solar radiation not either UVA or UVB. In view of this, Diffey[26] recommends that a ratio calculated from the mean of the UVA absorbance of the product divided by the mean of the UVB absorbance would be the most reproducible method for a manufacturer to employ since it obviates the need for clinical endpoints. In this case, the SPF value will remain the primary guide to the choice of product but would be accompanied by a description of the range of wavelengths against which the product protects (e.g., UVB or UVB + UVA as is often provided now) together with the quantitative description of the UVA/UVB absorbance ratios for comparative purposes.

Sunscreens are evaluated on their efficiency in protecting against erythema. Although protection against skin cancer is not examined routinely during sunscreen testing, certain sunscreens have been shown to protect against UV-induced skin tumor formation in mice[27–30] and the assumption that they are protective against chronic effects in humans would appear reasonable. Although there are many acute toxic side effects of various sunscreen agents, such formulations are rapidly being eliminated from the market as safer sunscreens become available.

SUMMARY

The data currently available clearly indicates solar radiation as an important factor in the causation of melanoma. The relationship is likely to strengthen as more epidemiological data is gathered, especially since the profile of information required to validate analysis is now known. Molecular genetics may also be used to implicate UV as a causative factor.

In general, protection against melanoma should follow the approach taken to protect against skin cancer in general. This includes the use of adequate protective clothing (including the use of a hat) and the avoidance of direct sunlight exposure between 10 AM and 3 PM, if necessary by seeking shade. As an adjunct to this natural protective behavior, sunscreens with high SPF factors should be employed. In view of a total lack of knowledge concerning the action spectrum for melanoma induction in mammals, it would appear prudent to use broadband (e.g., UVA + UVB) protection. Particular care should be taken to protect and eventually educate small children with the goal of avoiding any single incidence of acute sunburn.

ACKNOWLEDGMENTS

The work of the author is supported by grants from the Swiss League Against Cancer and the Swiss National Science Foundation (31.30880.91).

REFERENCES

1. Scotto J, Fears TR, and Fraumeni JF. Incidence of non-melanoma skin cancer in the United States. *US Dept Health and Human Services, NIH* 82:2433, 1981.
2. Blum HF. Carcinogenesis by ultraviolet light. Princeton, NJ: Princeton University Press, 1959.
3. Freeman RG. Data on the action spectrum for ultraviolet carcinogenesis. *J Nat Cancer Int* 55:1119–1121, 1975.
4. Slaper H. Skin cancer and UV exposure: Investigation on the estimation of risks, PhD thesis, University of Utrecht, 1987.
5. Sterenborg HJCM, and van der Leun JC. Action spectra for tumorigenesis by ultraviolet radiation. In: Pauschier WF, and Bosnjakovic BFN (eds.) *Human Exposure to Ultraviolet Radiation: Risk and Regulation*. Amsterdam: Elsevier Science Publishing, 1987, 137–140.
6. deGruijl FR, and van der Leun JC. Action spectra for carcinogenesis. In: Urbach F (ed.) *Biological Responses to Ultraviolet A Radiation*. Overland Park, KS: Valdenmar Publishing, 1992, 91–97.
7. Ley RD, Applegate LA, Padilla RS, and Stuart TD. Ultraviolet radiation-induced malignant melanoma in Monodelphis domestica *Photochem Photobiol* 50:1–5, 1989.
8. Woodhead AD, Grist E, Schultz R, and Setlow RB. A fish model for estimating the wavelengths effective in melanoma induction. Tenth International Congress on Photobiology, Jerusalem, Program and Abstracts, 1988, 32.
9. Setlow RB, and Grist E. Action spectrum for melanoma induction. Eleventh International Congress on Photobiology, Kyoto, Program and Abstracts, 1992, 184.
10. USEPA. Assessing the risk of trace gases that can modify the stratosphere, Vol. III Chapters 6 to 18, EPA 400/1-87/001C, 1987.
11. UNEP-report on Environmental effects of ozone depletion. Van der Leun, JC, and M Tevini (eds.), 1989.
12. Kraemer K, Lee MM, and Scotto J. Xeroderma pigmentosum cutaneous ocular and neurobiological abnormalities in 830 published cases. *Arch Dermatol* 23:241–250, 1987.
13. Gallagher RP. Solar UV radiation and human skin cancer: Is timing and character of exposure important? Eleventh International Congress on Photobiology, Kyoto, Program and Abstracts, 1992, 183.

14. Van't Veer LJ, Burgering, BMTh, Versteeg R, Boot AJM, Ruiter DJ, Osanto S, Schrier PI, and Bos JL. N-ras mutations in human cutaneous melanoma on sun-exposed body sites. *Mol Cell Biol* 9:3114–3116, 1989.
15. Shukla VK, Hughes DC, Hughes LE, McCormick F, and Padua RA. *Ras* mutations in human lesions: K-*ras* activation is a frequent and early event in melanoma development *Oncogene Res* 5:121–127, 1989.
16. Brash DE, Rudolph JA, Simon JA, Lin A, McKenna GJ, Baden HP, Halperin AJ, and Pontén J. A role for sunlight in skin cancer: UV induced p53 mutations in squamous cell carcinoma. *Proc Natl Acad Sci USA* 88:10124–10128, 1991.
17. Brash DE, Ziegler A, Simon J, and Kunala S. UV-mutations of the p53 gene in human skin cancers. Eleventh International Congress on Photobiology, Kyoto, Program and Abstracts, 1992, 184.
18. Stretch JR, Gatter K, Ralfkraer E, Lane DP, and Harris AL. Expression of mutant p53 in melanoma. *Cancer Res* 51:5976–5979, 1991.
19. Setlow RB. The wavelengths in sunlight effective in producing skin cancer. *Proc Natl Acad Sci USA* 71:3363–3366, 1974.
20. Bruls WA, Sloper H, van der Leun JC, and Berrens C. Transmission of human epidermis and stratum corneum as a function of thickness in the ultraviolet and visible wavelengths. *Photochem Photobiol* 40:415–494, 1984.
21. Tyrrell RM. Damage and repair from non-ionizing radiations. In: Hurst A, and Nasim A (eds.) *Repairable Lesions in Microorganism.* Academic Press, 1984, 85–124.
22. Tyrrell RM, and Pidoux M. Action spectra for human skin cells: Estimation of the relative cytotoxicity of the middle ultraviolet, near ultraviolet and violet regions of sunlight on epidermal keratinocytes. *Cancer Res* 47:1825–1829, 1987.
23. Tyrrell RM. UVA as an oxidative stress. In: Sies H (ed.) *Oxidative Stress-Oxidants and Antioxidants.* London: Academic Press, 1991, 57–84.
24. Kripke ML. Immunological unresponsiveness induced by ultraviolet radiation. *Immunol Rev* 80:87–102, 1984.
25. Urbach F. Testing the efficacy of sunscreen: Effect of choice of source and spectral power distribution of ultraviolet radiation, and choice of end-point. *Photodermatology* 6:177–181, 1989.
26. Diffey BL. The need for sunscreens with broadspectrum protection. In: Urbach F (ed.) *Biological Responses to Ultraviolet A Radiation.* Overland Park, KS: Valdenmar Publishing, 1992, 321–328.
27. Knox JM, Griffin AC, and Hakin RE. Protection from ultraviolet carcinogenesis. *J Am Acad Dermatol* 3:30–35, 1980.
28. Kligman LH, Akin FJ, and Kligman AM. Sunscreens prevent ultraviolet photocarcinogenesis. *J Am Acad Dermatol* 3:30–35, 1980.
29. Wulf HC, Pouslen T, Brodthagen H, and Hou-Jensen K. Sunscreens for delay of ultraviolet induction of skin tumors. *J Am Acad Dermatol* 7:194–202, 1982.
30. Gallagher CH, Greenoak GE, Reeve VE, Carfield PJ, Baker RSU, and Bonin AM. Ultraviolet carcinogenesis in the hairless mouse skin—influence of the sunscreen 2-ethylhexyl-p-methoxycinnamate. *Aust J Expt Biol Med Sci* 62:577–588, 1984.

APPENDIX: GUIDELINES FOR PROTECTION AGAINST SUNLIGHT DAMAGE

1. Sun damage has a cumulative effect over a lifetime. Avoid sunburns especially at an early age. Educate children about danger of sunburns and teach them about proper use of sunscreens.
2. Avoid unnecessary exposure to sun especially between the hours of 10 AM and 3 PM. Do not schedule outdoor activities at this time. Use tightly woven clothing and apply sunscreens on exposed skin. Use a widebrimmed hat to avoid sunburn over the scalp, neck, and ears.
3. Most sunscreen lotions offer protection against UVB. To avoid possible significant harmful effects of UVA, use a sunscreen that offers protection against both UVA and UVB.
4. When choosing the sun protection factors (SPF) of sunscreen lotions, use a minimum SPF of 15. People with very light skin, easy tendency to burn and blonds and redheads should use a higher SPF.
5. It is important to learn how to apply sunscreen lotion properly. Apply the lotion at least 15 to 30 minutes ahead of exposure. Following heavy perspiration, or swimming, reapply sunscreen lotion. Unless a longer lasting sunscreen lotion is used, reapply lotion every 2 hours. Do not forget to apply sunscreen over ears, scalp, forehead, nose, and neck.
6. Avoid cosmetic tanning. UVA may significantly damage the skin and may be a contributing factor for melanoma and other skin cancer.
7. Some drugs may increase photosensitivity and increase the skin damage with less sun exposure than normally encountered. During the use of these medications, sun exposure should be minimized.

Chapter 9

POTENTIAL PRECURSORS OF CUTANEOUS MELANOMA

Arthur R. Rhodes

INTRODUCTION

Early diagnosis is the key to preventing death from melanoma, and easy access to the skin for examination makes this goal feasible. In 18 to 85 percent of cases, melanoma develops in a pre-existing nevus.[1] The historic "in-contiguity" relationship between nevi and melanoma may be corroborated by family photographs[2] and substantiated histopathologically by the presence of a nevomelanocytic nevus in contiguity with melanoma in 18 to 72 percent of cases.[1] This observation poses a dilemma, because 73 to 92 percent of adults have one or more nevi.[3–5] While it would seem that there is insufficient knowledge among the lay public to differentiate typical nevi from melanoma, and other pigmented non-melanocytic lesions from melanocytic and nevomelanocytic benign neoplasms, most affected people are aware of their melanomas and that something is abnormal. Among 69 melanoma patients who were aware of a "stable" pre-existing nevus at the tumor site for at least 3 years,[6] the median duration of "change" of the nevus before seeking consultation was 6 months (Arthur R. Rhodes, unpublished data). Among 125 melanoma patients in Scotland,[7] 105 (84 percent) noted a changing nevus or a new nevus at least 3 months prior to excision, and in 42 cases (34 percent), the interval was more than 1 year. Delay in diagnosis and treatment usually relates to patient denial or ignorance about the consequences of a new or changing nevus rather than physician delay in diagnosis and treatment.[7]

The task of reducing death from melanoma may be more readily accomplished by selectively screening people who have significant melanoma risk factors. The purpose of screening people at high risk for developing melanoma is to diagnose tumors in an early stage of development, before metastasis has occurred, and perhaps even to prevent melanoma in some cases if a potential precursor of melanoma can be identified and surgically removed. Selective screening tends to increase the prevalence of problems being sought, and therefore, improves the predictive value of any diagnostic screening test, including the use of gross morphologic features of nevi in guessing at histopathologic features. The most important risk factors for melanoma identified to date, plus estimates of their relative risks, are shown in Table 9-1. Most of the relative risks listed are selected estimates from case-control studies, while some relative risks are derived from prospective studies.[8] It should be noted that prominent nevi and potential melanoma precursors are the most important risk factors identified to date. Prominent nevi (i.e., relatively large size and number) indicate an increased melanoma risk, even in the absence of recognizable melanoma precursors. For instance, melanoma risk is increased 10-fold for the presence of 5 nevomelanocytic nevi at least 5 mm in diameter,[9] 16-fold for 5 nevi at least 7 mm in diameter,[10] 20-fold for the presence of more than 120 nevi at least 1 mm in diameter,[9] 41-fold for 12 nevi at least 5 mm in diameter,[11] and 64-fold for 50 nevi at least 2 mm

TABLE 9-1
RISK FACTORS FOR DEVELOPMENT OF CUTANEOUS MELANOMA[a]

RISK FACTOR	*ESTIMATED RELATIVE RISK[b]*
1. New mole, or mole that has changed or is changing	Very high[c]
2. Adulthood (≥15 years versus <15 years)	88
3. Unique nevus and/or prominent nevus pattern	
a. Dysplastic nevus, prior melanoma, and familial melanoma	500
b. Dysplastic nevus and familial melanoma	148
c. Dysplastic nevus but no familial melanoma	27
d. Congenital nevus	21
e. Lentigo maligna	10
f. 50 nevomelanocytic nevi ≥2 mm diameter	64
g. 12 nevomelanocytic nevi ≥5 mm diameter	41
h. 5 nevomelanocytic nevi ≥7 mm diameter	16
i. 5 nevomelanocytic nevi ≥5 mm diameter	10
4. Caucasian race (versus Black)	12
5. Prior cutaneous melanoma	9
6. Cutaneous melanoma in a first degree blood relative	8
7. Immunosuppression	4
8. Sun-induced freckles	4
9. Sun sensitivity	3
10. Excessive sun exposure	3

[a]Table modified from Table 2, p. 3147, Ref. 8.
[b]Degree of increased risk for people with the risk factor compared to people without the risk factor. Relative risk of 1.0 implies no increased risk.
[c]Risk estimated roughly to be increased 10-fold to 400-fold.

in diameter.[10] Pigmentary traits other than nevi (including freckling) may be additive in risk to the nevus trait.

The modern classification of cutaneous melanoma[12–14] cites unique patterns of intraepidermal spread (i.e., Pagetoid appearance in superficial spreading melanoma and absence of intraepidermal spread in nodular melanoma) and potential precursors of melanoma (i.e., lentigo maligna, dysplastic nevus, and congenital nevus). While melanoma may develop in any melanocyte in any location, a significantly higher proportion of melanomas develop in contiguity with unique varieties of "benign" melanocytic neoplasms. The potential melanoma precursors that will be covered herein are listed in Table 9-2. While the exact degree of risk associated with each of the melanocytic neoplasms discussed may be controversial or unknown, the purpose of describing the various tumors as potential melanoma precursors is to emphasize the heterogeneity of origin of melanoma. Recognition and management of individuals who are at high risk for melanoma by virtue of having one or more of these recognizable melanocytic neoplasms provide a unique intervention strategy that is difficult or not possible for the vast majority of noncutaneous cancers.

TABLE 9-2
POTENTIAL PRECURSORS OF CUTANEOUS MELANOMA

Acquired dysplastic melanocytic nevus
Congenital nevomelanocytic nevus
Lentigo maligna
Cellular blue nevus
Nevus of Ota, nevus of Ito
Nevus spilus, dysplastic and/or congenital
Melanocytic dysplasia on acral or mucosal surface
Spindle cell and/or epithelioid cell nevus

ACQUIRED DYSPLASTIC MELANOCYTIC NEVUS

DEFINITION

Melanocytic dysplasia is a histopathologic term and implies a disordered proliferation of melanocytes associated with discontinuous and variable cellular atypia. The acquired dysplastic melanocytic nevus (DMN) is suspected clinically based on the presence of one or more relatively large and irregular-appearing nevi (see Plates 2 and 3) and defined histopathologically by the presence of intraepidermal melanocytic dysplasia in a lentiginous epidermal pattern on nonacral and nonmucosal sites (see Plate 4). (There are varieties of intraepidermal melanocytic dysplasia on acral and mucosal sites, and other terms are used to describe such lesions. See section on Acral and Mucosal Melanocytic Dysplasias later in this chapter.) DMN may be suspected clinically based on gross morphologic features. DMN are important because they are potential histogenic precursors of melanoma and markers of increased melanoma risk.

While the concept of DMN as a precursor to melanoma has been popularized only recently, this lesion has been evident for many years and probably used synonomously for intraepidermal melanoma and "atypical" or "active junctional nevi." In 1820, Norris[15] described a family in which two members developed cutaneous melanoma, and other family members were striking for the presence of "many moles on various parts of their bodies." Very likely, the moles described by Norris were DMN. Published reports delineating DMN as histogenic precursors and markers of increased risk in the setting of familial melanoma were described in 1978[16–20] and called atypical moles, B-K moles, and atypical multiple mole-melanoma syndrome (FAMMM). The terminology for DMN is still in flux, and there is an ongoing discussion of the precursor and risk marker role for DMN in the histogenesis of melanoma.

EPIDEMIOLOGY

In the United States, DMN may be suspected in 1.8 to 4.9 percent of white adults.[21,22] The marked variation in prevalence, including very high rates in some populations,[23–28] may relate to true population heterogeneity or inconsistent gross and/or histopathologic definitions used for diagnosis.

Familial aggregation occurs in approximately 10 percent of cutaneous melanomas (i.e., two or more members with melanoma), and DMN are markers of increased melanoma risk as well as potential histogenic precursors in this setting. There may be more than 30,000 people with familial melanoma and DMN in the United States.[29] Such kindreds have been recognized in the United States, Germany, France, Great Britain, the Netherlands, and Japan. To this author's knowledge, the syndrome of familial melanoma and DMN has not been described in darkly pigmented races. DMN may aggregate in families in which melanoma has not (yet) been detected.[30–33] In one sample of 18 patients with DMN but without a family or personal history of melanoma, DMN were detected in 24 of 95 sibs and 3 of 36 parents.[30] DMN also have been detected in patients with "sporadic" melanoma[1,21,34,35] and their first-degree relatives.[36–39] (The term "sporadic" or spontaneous mutation when applied to the absence of familial aggregation of DMN assumes that at least three generations in a given kindred have been examined for the trait of DMN and/or melanoma, and such information is rarely available to the responsible physician.) Compared with the relatively low prevalence rate of DMN in white adults without melanoma, DMN may be detected in approximately 50 percent of blood relatives in the familial melanoma setting[16–20] and at least 17 percent of white adults with melanoma outside of the familial melanoma setting.[21–23,35,39,40–43]

PATHOGENESIS

Intraepidermal melanocytes in DMN occupy an intermediate position between typical and malignant, and intraepidermal melanocytic dysplasia in DMN may be interpreted as a block in normal differentiation. These notions are based on nuclear and cytoplasmic features,[1,34,35,44–47] DNA distribution pattern in Feulgen-stained imprints,[46,48,49] patterns of staining for major histocompatibility antigens in tissue sections,[48,50–52] deranged melanogenesis associated with increased pheomelanin content and abnormal melanosomes, enlarged cell bodies, increased dopa-positivity, and a disordered proliferation of melanocytes associated with an inflammatory host response and unique mesenchymal features.[1,34,44,45,53–56] The faulty differentiation in DMN may be due to a combination of genetic, hormonal, and environmental factors.

Genetic analysis of melanoma-prone families has shown that the DMN-melanoma trait segregates as an autosomal dominant disorder,[1,16–19,57–62] that DMN and melanoma may represent pleiotropic effects of a highly penetrant single gene,[60] and that the susceptibility gene in familial melanoma may be located on chromosome band 1p36.[60,63] Other workers exclude the DMN-familial melanoma trait from the short arm of chromosome 1,[64] and still other workers favor polygenetic or multifactoral inheritance for DMN.[65,66] Delayed appearance of the DMN trait (i.e., DMN may not become manifest until the end of the first decade of life), incomplete expression, heterogeneity of populations studied, and disagreement about minimum features required for gross and microscopic diagnosis confound ascertainment of familial patterns of DMN. In one study of familial melanoma,[59] 15 clinically unaffected individuals were documented to be gene carriers.

There are numerous associated biologic features in people with DMN and familial melanoma. Abnormalities include marked sensitivity of fibroblasts to cell killing by ultraviolet radiation (UVR) and the UVR-mimetic carcinogen 4-nitroquinoline-1-oxide,[67–69] enhanced UVR sensitivity of lymphoblastoid cell lines,[70] hypermutability of lymphoblastoid cell lines to UVR,[71] and increased hyperdiploidy and density-independent growth regulation in fibroblast cultures.[20] In response to ionizing irradiation, skin fibroblasts from patients with DMN in the familial melanoma setting show significantly more chromatid breaks and gaps.[72] There appears to be general chromosomal instability in subjects with DMN in the presence or absence of a personal history of melanoma.[73] Lymphoblastoid cell lines show normal DNA repair, normal recovery of DNA synthesis, and normal cell survival to UVR.[71] Growth and survival of cultured nevomelanocytes and epidermal melanocytes from DMN do not appear to be more sensitive to UVR than normal epidermal melanocytes cultured from neonatal foreskin and other controls.[74] No consistent association with HLA antigens or ABO blood groups has been detected for familial melanoma.[75]

CLINICAL MANIFESTATIONS

Atypical histologic features should be suspected in relatively large melanocytic lesions that have one or more of the following: very dark pigmentation and/or haphazard disposition of multiple hues (shades of brown and red), coloration pink to red with minimal or no pigmentation, a target appearance, a macular component periperally and a raised component centrally, and irregular and/or poorly demarcated outlines (see Plate 3). While size alone cannot be used to exclude melanocytic dysplasia, DMN are commonly 5 mm or larger in greatest diameter. There are varieties of melanocytic tumors smaller than 5 mm in greatest diameter that have histopathologic features similar to DMN.[76–78] Individuals who have DMN may have one, several, scores, or even hundreds of DMN (see Plate 2). In one study, patients who had DMN outside the familial melanoma setting had an average of 10 DMN per person.[29]

DMN first appear as rather large moles in the middle or end of the first decade of life, but gross and microscopic features may not be sufficiently evolved to establish a diagnosis until puberty. (There may be varieties of congenital nevomelanocytic nevi associated with intraepidermal melanocytic dysplasia. See section on Congenital Nevomelanocytic Nevus later in this chapter.) DMN usually appear by age 20 years, and affected individuals may continue to develop additional DMN over time.[58]

Establishing a diagnosis of DMN requires a high index of suspicion and experience correlating gross characteristics with histopathologic patterns of intraepidermal melanocyte architecture and cellular morphologic features. Degree and quantity of cellular atypia in DMN usually parallel degree of clinical atypia,[34,49] and clinical diagnosis agrees with histopathologic diagnosis in 69 to 92 percent of cases,[25,78–80] depending on the experience of the clinician and familiarity with the histopathologic features by the examining pathologist. Examination of the pigment pattern using high magnification of the brightly illuminated mineral oil-covered lesion surface (the procedure is being called *epiluminescent microscopy, dermatoscopy,* and other names)[81] may be useful in predicting melanocytic dysplasia and degree of cellular atypia, as well as differentiating melanoma from dysplastic nevi and nevomelanocytic nevi and melanocytic hyperplasias from nonmelanocytic lesions.[82–85]

Historically stable melanocytic tumors that are selected for typical appearance can be expected not to manifest intraepidermal melanocytic dysplasia.[34,49] There are varieties of nonpigmented or lightly pigmented tumors associated with intraepidermal melanocytic dysplasia, particularly among people who are unable to make melanin, that is, individuals with type I skin or albinism.[86,87] Nonpigmented varieties of DMN may be difficult to diagnose without a high index of suspicion, that is, relatively large size, minimal surface distortion relative to breadth, and sometimes the presence of a peripheral rim of pale pigmentation or central pigmentation.

PATHOLOGY

Diagnostic histopathologic features of DMN may be defined as absolute (necessary for diagnosis) and relative (frequently associated). *Absolute criteria* include (1) a proliferation of intraepidermal melanocytes disposed singly and/or in irregular nests in the epidermal basal unit or slightly above, in a lentiginous epidermal pattern (elongated, club-shaped, and/or fused rete ridges); and (2) variable and discontinuous cellular atypia of melanocytes (see Plate 4). *Relative histologic criteria* include (1) lymphohistiocytic infiltrates in the dermis, with or without melanin-laden macrophages; (2) dermal mesenchymal features consisting of concentric eosinophilic fibrosis (condensed papillary dermal collagen along epidermal rete ridges), lamellar fibroplasia (delicate collagen fibrils and elongated fibroblasts parallel to the epidermal surface and situated at the tips of epidermal rete ridges), and/or neovascularization; (3) a proliferation of ellipsoidal and irregularly nested melanocytes disposed at the epidermal basal unit, frequently bridging epidermal rete ridges; (4) nevomelanocytes in the dermis, often associated with impairment of maturation and synthesis of pigment; and (5) extension of melanocytic hyperplasia beyond the dermal nevomelanocytic component if a dermal nevomelanocytic component is present.

In contrast to DMN, intraepidermal (in situ) melanoma may be arbitrarily defined as intraepidermal melanocytic proliferation showing fully evolved cellular atypia that is side-to-side and continuous for a sufficient breadth.[44] There is a spectrum of cellular atypia from slight to marked in DMN.[14,34,44,88] Inadequate sampling and heterogeneity of pathologic features may result in a false negative diagnosis.

DIFFERENTIAL DIAGNOSIS

Lesions that may be mistaken for DMN include intraepidermal (in situ) melanoma, seborrheic keratosis, pigmented actinic keratosis, benign pigmented keratosis, pigmented basal cell carcinoma, pigmented Bowen's disease, traumatic hematoma, pyogenic granuloma, sclerosing hemangioma, pigmented spindle cell and/or epithelioid cell nevus, dermatofibroma, common and cellular varieties of blue nevus, combined melanocytic nevus-blue nevus, cocardiform nevus, darkly pigmented solar lentigo, and darkly pigmented varieties of lentiginous nevomelanocytic nevus without significant cellular atypia. Without a high index of suspicion, it may be difficult to suspect nonpigmented varieties of DMN among individuals who are relatively deficient in their ability to make melanin.[86,87]

TREATMENT

For people who have only one or two lesions suspicious for being DMN, excision is reasonable, but periodic examination at least yearly should be offered for a lifetime. Affected people may be expected to develop new DMN over time,[89] and there is a general impression that melanoma may develop from normal-appearing skin or in innocuous-appearing pigmented lesions in individuals who have DMN (or melanoma). Prophylactic removal of each and every nevus in patients who have DMN (or melanoma) is impractical, mutilating, and will not obviate the need for lifetime periodic examination. Lesions that are difficult to monitor (i,e., hairy scalp, umbilicus, perianal or genital areas) should be considered for prophylactic excision. Other lesions to be considered for prophylactic excision include those that are extremely atypical in gross appearance, those that are documented to have changed significantly, those in patients for whom adequate medical follow-up is deemed unlikely, and those in patients who have altered immunologic function. For people who have numerous DMN, clinical photographs are invaluable for detecting new or changing lesions over time during periodic complete cutaneous examinations.

A histopathologic diagnosis provides a more solid basis for making management recommendations. However, it is reasonable to defer routine histopathologic confirmation and to offer periodic follow-up for people who have minimally irregular DMN and/or prominent nevi in which the degree of cellular atypia is not likely to be sufficient to confirm a histopathologic diagnosis of DMN.

Surgical excision using 2 to 3 mm lateral margins is currently the recommended method of removing DMN. Recurrence is unlikely unless excision is incomplete.[90,91] Wood's lamp examination may be useful in delineating borders for lesions with poorly demarcated outlines. Incompletely excised DMN should be re-excised or examined periodically for recurrence, depending on the degree and quantity of cellular atypia. Deep excision margins of DMN should extend to below the deepest component of the lesion. Usually, the dermal nevus component (if present) of most acquired DMN extends no deeper than the papillary dermis or upper reticular dermis. Topical chemotherapy using 5 percent 5-fluorouracil[92] or tretinoin,[93] and methods of destructive therapy, should be regarded as experimental for treatment of DMN in the usual case.

People who have DMN and a personal and/or family history of melanoma are probably at greater risk for developing melanoma than people who have DMN and no personal or family history of melanoma. However, overall management of affected individuals is similar. People who have DMN should practice self-examination at least once every 4 to 6 weeks. People who have DMN (and/or melanoma) may develop new DMN (and melanoma) over time, so periodic physician examination for atypical nevi and melanoma is indicated indefinitely. Particular attention should be paid to hidden areas such as the scalp, anus, umbilicus, and genitalia. The hairy scalp may be the source of lethal melanoma even in children.[94] Relatives or spouses should be enlisted to assist in monthly home examinations, particularly the posterior torso and hairy scalp. Affected people should be made aware of the signs and symptoms of early melanoma. Patients who have DMN should be examined every 3 to 6 months, depending on "activity" and gross abnormalities of nevi and demonstrated melanoma risk in the individual or kindred, by a physician experienced in the clinical-pathological correlation of nevi. It is reasonable to recommend that patients who have had DMN (or melanoma) and who have no pigmented lesions remaining still be examined indefinitely at yearly intervals.

The relation between hormonal factors and the progression of DMN to melanoma is unknown. Therefore, puberty and pregnancy, and administration of oral contraceptives or estrogen replacement therapy, may require more frequent follow-up.

All bloodline relatives in melanoma-prone families should be examined for DMN and/or melanoma, and, if unaffected, at least yearly until 20 years of age.[58] Children who have a prominent mole pattern but without obvious DMN should be re-examined periodically until at least 20 years of age. If DMN are not apparent by age 20, and prominent moles are not evident, it is considered unlikely that an individual will express the DMN trait.[58]

Although there are no definitive data, it may be presumed that excessive exposure to ultraviolet radiation may promote cellular alterations and perhaps neoplastic progression in genetically "initiated" melanocytes in DMN (or even normal skin in such individuals). Until conclusive information becomes available, it is suggested that people who have DMN should avoid sunbathing or getting red in the sun, including nonmedical use of artificial ultraviolet radiation (i.e., tanning beds). Cover-up with tightly woven clothing, and maximum sunscreen protection to body sites that cannot be covered easily, should be used during unavoidable ultraviolet radiation exposure.

Eye care given to patients who have DMN has been controversial because of the occasional association of cutaneous melanoma and ocular melanoma. Both types of melanoma may show familial aggregation. Until there is more conclusive information, people who have DMN, whether or not there is a personal or family history of melanoma, are recommended to receive the same level of eye care as the general population.

There are anecdotal examples of other malignancies developing in patients who have DMN and familial melanoma. A detailed analysis of 14 melanoma kindreds in one study failed to document a significant association with other tumor types.[95] An extensive investigation for other malignancies appears not to be warranted for asymptomatic patients who have DMN, even in the familial melanoma setting.

COURSE AND PROGNOSIS

DMN may remain stable, progress to melanoma, or possibly regress over time. The most important study to date linking DMN to the development of melanoma is the investigation and follow-up of 14 melanoma-prone kindreds.[58] In this study, comprised of 401 individuals in 14 melanoma-prone families, 128 primary cutaneous melanomas were documented in 69 family members, including 40 new melanomas diagnosed during the period of initial examination to an average follow-up of 4 years. The 40 new melanomas developed only among family members who had one or more DMN. Results of this prospective study, combined with photographic documentation of invasive melanoma developing in contiguity with DMN[16,96] and the in contiguity of DMN in association with cutaneous melanoma (see Plate 5) in one-fifth to one-third of cases[14,45,58,97–101] (Table 9-3), help to demonstrate that DMN are formal histogenic precursors of melanoma.

The estimated risk of melanoma developing in people who have DMN in the familial melanoma setting may be as high as 56 percent from age 20 to 59 years, and 100 percent by age 76 years.[58] In contrast, bloodline relatives without DMN or melanoma in the familial melanoma setting have a cumulative melanoma risk that appears to be no greater than that of the general population.[58] Familial melanoma patients are striking for a tendency to develop multiple primary melanomas and at a younger age compared to nonfamilial melanoma. Close surveillance of this high-risk group has resulted in detection of melanoma in a curable phase of development in the vast majority of people followed prospectively.[58] Prepuberal metastatic melanoma developing in association with DMN has been reported in the familial melanoma setting.[94]

People who have DMN outside the familial melanoma setting (i.e., with or without a personal or family history of melanoma) have a 7-fold to 70-fold increased risk of developing melanoma,[10,21,23,29,102–104] and a lifetime melanoma risk of at least 18 percent.[29] According to a prospective study of DMN patients followed with repetitive examinations, the melanoma risk was increased 57-fold for people with DMN in the absence of a personal or family history of melanoma, to more than 400-fold for people with a personal and family history of melanoma.[105–107]

Even a single DMN appears to be a significant risk factor for developing melanoma. In the familial melanoma setting, melanoma has been observed in histologic contiguity with a DMN in the absence of DMN elsewhere.[58] The presence of any DMN in patients with melanoma increases the risk for another primary melanoma 6-fold, and the presence of two or more DMN increases the risk for another primary melanoma 9-fold.[108] DMN patients who are followed

TABLE 9-3
IN CONTIGUITY HISTOPATHOLOGIC ASSOCIATION BETWEEN MELANOMA AND DYSPLASTIC MELANOCYTIC NEVUS

AUTHOR(S)	*MELANOMA CASES (TOTAL NUMBER)*	*CASES IN CONTIGUITY WITH MELANOCYTIC DYSPLASIA (%)*	*REFERENCE*
Rhodes et al.	225[a]	49 (21.8)	14
Clark et al.	219[a]	73 (33.3)	45
Cook and Robertson	226[b]	62 (27.4)	97
McGovern et al.	723[c]	282 (39.0)	99
Black	500[c]	162 (32.4)	100
Greene et al.	111[d]	78 (70.3)	58
Duray and Ernstoff	13	6 (46.0)	98
Gruber et al.	188	32 (17.0)	101

[a]Excludes lentigo maligna melanoma.
[b]Includes intraepidermal (in situ) as well as invasive melanoma.
[c]Includes only cases of superficial spreading melanoma.
[d]Includes only cases of familial melanoma.

closely and who develop melanoma are likely to have their tumors discovered in a curable phase of development.[58,105,106,109]

People who have DMN and who are also immunosuppressed may have an increased risk of developing melanoma.[110,111]

CONGENITAL NEVOMELANOCYTIC NEVUS

DEFINITION

The congenital nevomelanocytic nevus (CNN) is a nevomelanocytic nevus apparent at birth (see Plates 6, 7, and 8), consisting of nevomelanocytes in the epidermis and/or dermis. There are rare varieties of relatively large nevomelanocytic nevi that appear for the first time between 3 months and 2 years according to parental photographs but which are likely congenital based on large size (≥ 1.5 cm diameter) and are, therefore, called "tardive" CNN, presumably related to delayed epidermal pigmentation overlying the nevus. Nevomelanocytic nevi ≥ 1.5 cm in diameter appearing after birth but within the first year of life constitute a small proportion of all nevomelanocytic nevi that are excised.[112] Nevi that are at least 1.5 cm in diameter in adults and are not DMN or melanoma may be regarded as CNN for management purposes.

CNN have been separated as small or large based on ease of removal, relative size, and absolute size. A lesion may be defined as small if it can be excised easily and the wound defect closed primarily without using skin flaps or grafts. A lesion may be defined as large if it does not fulfill the definition of small, and giant if it occupies, a significant portion of a major anatomic site.[113,114] Based on these practical definitions, otherwise "small" CNN on the torso or buttocks might be regarded as "large" on more critical sites such as the face, hands and feet, and perineum. Other definitions for CNN abound. CNN have been defined as giant if occupying the area of the patient's palm for the face or neck, and twice that area for other anatomic sites[115,116] (the palmar surface occupies 1.25 percent of total body surface area throughout life); 30 percent of the body surface area[114]; and 930 cm^2.[117] Some authors arbitrarily divide CNN according to largest diameter as small (< 1.5 cm), medium (1.5 to 19.9 cm), and large (≥ 20 cm),[118] regardless of anatomic location or age of the affected individual.

Absolute size or area definitions are confusing when differential changes in lesion area and body surface area during natural growth are considered. For instance, lesions that are called "small" or "medium" in the newborn period may be designated medium or large, respectively, by late childhood or adulthood if CNN grow in proportion to body growth. Definitions of small and large based on ease of excision are not restricted by anatomic location or body size. Another important consideration in classifying CNN by size is malignant potential. Melanoma is more likely to destroy or obscure a small CNN than a large CNN. Parents and physicians are more likely to take note of a large CNN than a small one. Classification by absolute or relative size may obscure a causal association between small varieties of CNN and melanoma.

EPIDEMIOLOGY

While at least 2.5 percent of newborns have some sort of pigmented lesion,[119] only 1 percent of newborns have biopsy-confirmed nevomelanocytic nevi, with no sexual predilection.[119–122] Most CNN are small and singular. In two combined series of cases,[119,120] only 1 of 61 infants with a total of 62 CNN had more than one lesion; 57 of the 62 CNN were 30 mm in diameter or less, 44 were 10 mm in diameter or less, and 4 lesions were considered large, the largest lesion being 26 cm by 18 cm (Joseph Alper, MD and Lewis Holmes, MD, personal communication). CNN at least 41 mm in diameter occur in 1 of every 6900 newborns, lesions at least 99 mm in diameter occur in 1 of every 20,000 newborns, and lesions that may be regarded as giant occur in 1 of 500,000 newborns.[123]

PATHOGENESIS

The congenital divided nevus of the eyelid (see Plate 6) is an important experiment in nature, for it demonstrates the probable time of appearance of CNN in utero. The eyelids form between 5 and 6 weeks in utero, begin to fuse at about 8 to 9 weeks, and then reopen during the sixth uterine month.[124] Since melanocytes begin to appear in fetal skin before 40 days estimated gestational age,[125] it is likely that CNN form after that time but before the sixth uterine month.[124,126]

Nevomelanocytic nevi in general are probably derived from neural crest melanoblasts or their progeny, and number and size of nevi are probably determined by genetic and environmental factors. Familial aggregation has been demonstrated for large and small varieties of CNN.[127]

CLINICAL MANIFESTATIONS

In general, small CNN are round or oval plaques with skin markings that distort the skin surface at least slightly when assessed by oblique lighting (see Plate 7). Pigmented CNN have diffuse fine brown speckles on a lighter background when viewed by high magnification of the mineral oil-coated surface,[120] similar to acquired nevi.[81–85] At birth, some CNN have coarse and long hair, but others are relatively hairless or develop hair after 6 to 12 months. Lesions may have a smooth, pebbly, rugose, verrucous, cerebriform, or grossly lobular surface (see Plate 8b). Outlines are usually smooth and regular, but some varieties of CNN may have an atypical appearance characterized by haphazard pigmentation and irregular and/or indistinct outlines.

Large CNN have been associated with multiple smaller CNN[121,123] (see Plate 8), ocular malformation and glaucoma,[121,128] choroidal lesions,[129] club foot, underlying bony atrophy, deafness,[121] spina bifida occulta,[130] neurofibromatosis,[130,131] neuroblastoma of the adrenal gland,[130] Wilm's tumor,[132] leptomeningeal melanocytosis,[130,133–137] and in one patient a myriad of hamartomas and brain malformation.[138]

Leptomeningeal melanocytosis, associated with CNN of the head, neck, or posterior midline, may be asymptomatic or result in communicating or noncommunicating hydrocephalus, seizures, focal neurologic deficits, mental retardation, or even melanoma. The frequency of asymptomatic leptomeningeal melanocytosis associated with head, neck, and posterior midline CNN is unknown. Leptomeningeal melanocytosis is not usually detectable by standard imaging techniques in the absence of mass lesions. Symptomatic leptomeningeal melanocytosis carries a poor prognosis, even in the absence of malignancy.

PATHOLOGY

CNN are characterized by the presence of nevomelanocytes in the epidermis and/or dermis. Histopathologic features are cited as being useful in distinguishing nevi as congenital or acquired,[112,139,180] but currently, there are no known features that are 100 percent specific and 100 percent sensitive for establishing age of first appearance of a given nevomelanocytic nevus.

The differentiation of nevi as acquired or congenital based on histopathologic features is central to defining a histogenic relation between small varieties of CNN and melanoma. CNN are significantly more likely than acquired nevi to have nevomelanocytes in the lower two-thirds of the reticular dermis or deeper as sheets of cells and/or single cells, and involve appendageal and neurovascular structures in the lower two-thirds of the reticular dermis[112,139] (see Plate 9). However, there are CNN with histopathologic features similar to acquired nevi,[140] and acquired nevi with histopathologic features similar to CNN.[112,121,122,139] The sensitivity of deep reticular dermal involvement with nevomelanocytes is low for small CNN. In series of mostly small CNN, nevomelanocytes extended to the deep reticular dermis in only 37 to 79 percent of cases. While CNN selected for excision in children and adults had nevomelanocytes in the deep reticular dermis in up to 98 percent of cases,[112,139,141] only 2 of 11 unselected relatively small CNN biopsied in the newborn period had nevomelanocytes in the deep reticular dermis, and in 3 cases, nevomelanocytes were confined to the epidermis[119]; when the same cases were studied using more sensitive techniques, however, nevomelanocytes were demonstrated in deeper anatomic zones.[140] Most giant CNN have pan-dermal involvement with nevomelanocytes.[130,142] Deep dermal and/or appendageal and neurovascular involvement by nevomelanocytes strongly suggests the diagnosis of CNN; absence of these features does not preclude the diagnosis of CNN. In a study of 112 nevomelanocytic nevi excised from 85 patients, 107 (96 percent) were assigned correctly as historically congenital or acquired based on histopathologic features alone.[143]

A neuroid type of CNN, consisting of nevomelanocytic elements taking on the appearance of Wagner-Meissner corpuscles and neuroidal tissue, may be responsible for lobulation and redundancy of tissue in some cases (pachydermatous or cerebelliform appearance). There are spindle cell and/or epithelioid cell varieties of giant CNN, often with atypical cellular and architectural features, making differentiation from melanoma difficult. There are giant congenital varieties of blue nevi, and giant CNN with blue nevus elements. Nevomelanocytes in giant CNN may be present in underlying muscle, bone, placenta, umbilical cord, cranium, and dura mater. Very extensive CNN may be intermixed with elements of vascular malformation, hemangiomas, increased numbers of mast cells, cartilage, calcification, and bone.

There are small and large varieties of CNN that manifest intraepidermal melanocytic dysplasia.[14,144,145] A similar proportion of CNN and acquired nevi excised in a pediatric hospital over a 30-month period revealed melanocytic dysplasia (i.e., 7 percent and 9 percent, respectively).[112] The presence of melanocytic dysplasia in CNN is not dependent on patient age. In 11 small CNN biopsied within the first 72 hours of life,[119] none showed intraepidermal or dermal nevomelanocytic dysplasia (A. J. Cox, personal communication), and when the same lesions were excised more than a decade later, there was still no evidence of atypical cellular features, mitotic activity, or dysplasia.[140] Histopathologic features of CNN do not appear to change over time.[140,142]

Leptomeningeal melanocytosis consists of dense perivascular proliferations of often anaplastic, nonpigmented, or pigmented nevomelanocytes and melanin-laden macrophages as nests or nodules at the basal subarachnoid cisterns, often penetrating neural tissues and frequently causing obstruction of cerebrospinal fluid flow and interference of reabsorption in the arachnoid villi, or causing acqueductal stenosis or obstruction of outflow foramina.[130]

DIFFERENTIAL DIAGNOSIS

Lesions that may be mistaken for CNN include Mongolian spots, café au lait macules, lentigo simplex, epidermal nevus, nevus sebaceous, arrector pili (smooth muscle) hamartoma, and Becker's nevus. While congenital nonmelanocytic pigmented lesions can usually be distinguished grossly from CNN, a small biopsy may be required for diagnosis, particularly in lightly pigmented and "flat" varieties of CNN for which the differential diagnosis is café au lait macule or uncharacterized pigmentation.

TREATMENT

Management of patients who have CNN is dependent on the perceived melanoma risk plus cosmetic and functional considerations. Strongly stated positions on both sides of the issue are reflected in clinical practice. In a survey of military and civilian dermatologists in 1979,[146] 57 percent of 187 respondents said that they always excise CNN. In a questionnaire survey of academic and nonacademic dermatologists in 1984,[147] a consensus of opinion included the following: (1) a majority of physicians refer their patients with very large CNN for surgical evaluation, (2) infants with very large CNN were usually treated by 12 months of age, (3) an incidence of conversion to melanoma of 0.1 percent or greater warrant prophylactic removal of small CNN, (4) half the respondents excise small CNN in children and adults, and (5) fewer than 40 percent of respondents "follow" small CNN rather than excise.

While there is disagreement about the exact frequency of the in contiguity association between CNN and melanoma, most students of the controversy agree that at least some melanomas develop in CNN, both large and small. Melanoma may develop in giant CNN even in the first several years of life. Therefore, excision should be considered as early as possible, but it is probably prudent to wait until after 6 months of age to reduce surgical and anesthesia risks. Management will depend on a lesion's appearance (typical versus atypical), size, location, and difficulty of removal, plus perceived risks of surgery and general anesthesia, cosmetic improvement or deficit that may be anticipated, and general health considerations. It may not be possible to remove each and every nevomelanocyte in very large lesions, particularly when there is deep involvement and/or involvement of vital structures. Extensive involvement, with precious little normal skin available for graft donar sites, may necessitate abandoning prophylactic removal and accepting life-long periodic examination to detect the earliest signs of melanoma. Artificial skin replacement and tissue expansion may be used to resurface very large wound defects. The goal of surgery for very large CNN is to remove as much of the nevus as possible while preserving function and improving cosmetic appearance. Other indications for surgical excision of very large CNN include chronic pruritus, ulceration, and infection. Dermabrasion and other modes of destructive therapy do not address the malignant potential of CNN—nevus cells may remain in the dermis (if present initially),[142,148] and cosmetic results are unpredictable. At least two cases of melanoma have been reported following dermabrasion of large CNN,[149] and one case of "pseudomelanoma" after laser treatment of a CNN.[150]

The malignant potential associated with small CNN is more controversial than that associated with large CNN. Thus, management of patients who have small CNN is also controversial. Most students of the controversy agree that at least some melanomas develop in small CNN. Given the uncertainties, the following recommendations should be considered guidelines for managing patients who have small CNN.

1. All CNN should be documented at birth, preferably in the form of high-quality photographs which can be used to aid follow-up by parents and physicians. During follow-up, suspicious changes require urgent evaluation. Follow-up will be complicated by the natural evolutionary changes in surface, size, color, and hair that take place in a nevus during body growth.[151]
2. Atypical-appearing CNN should be considered for immediate excision, because even small CNN may occasionally develop melanoma during infancy and childhood.
3. All small CNN should be evaluated for prophylactic removal before 12 years of age, after which time the risk of melanoma rises sharply. Management of patients who have small CNN will depend on a patient's general health; gross appearance, size, and location of the CNN; and cosmetic and functional deficits (or improvement) resulting from excision. Life-long photographic follow-up may be preferable to excision for small CNN in some patients.
4. There is usually no need to excise benign-appearing small CNN during infancy and early childhood if general anesthesia is required and lesions can be followed and examined easily.

Morbidity and mortality risks of general anesthesia probably outweigh malignant potential of benign-appearing small CNN during the first decade of life.
5. Given the familial occurrence of CNN (large and small),[127,152] an inquiry should be made about CNN in family members.
6. Currently, there is no obvious way of adjusting recommendations for prophylactic excision of CNN based solely on race.

COURSE AND PROGNOSIS

While CNN in adults should maintain a stable appearance, CNN have a dynamic development during body growth.[140,151] In a 12-year follow-up of 7 CNN biopsied in the newborn period, Nickoloff et al.[140] confirmed a 2-fold to 8-fold increase in size in 5 cases, and no increase in size in 2. In a follow-up study of 32 CNN, Zina et al.[151] noted that during the first 13 to 18 months of life, most nevi increased in size by 2-fold or 3-fold. The great variation in CNN growth may be related to the fact that different anatomic sites of the human body grow at different rates. These issues are relevant to optimal timing of prophylactic surgery for the smallest possible scar.

CNN may become more elevated over time or remain the same.[151] Varieties of giant CNN may develop lobular masses caused by proliferation of nevomelanocytes. CNN have been associated with fading or complete loss of pigmentation, halo depigmentation, and even regression.[115,130,153,154] Tumors developing in CNN other than melanoma include melanoma simulants, schwannoma, neuroid tumor, lipoma, rabdomyosarcoma, neurofibroma, sebaceous nevus, blue nevus, hemangioma, lymphangioma, and mastocytoma.

Causal Association Between Congenital Nevus and Melanoma

LARGE CONGENITAL NEVUS

The histogenic relation between melanoma and large CNN is well documented.[118] The risk of developing melanoma by age 10 years in the general population is 1 in 100,000.[8] The chance that someone with melanoma will also have a very large CNN $\geqslant$ 99 mm in greatest diameter is 1 in 2000 to 1 in 20,000.[120,123] The chance that someone with a very large CNN will develop melanoma by age 10 years is the product of the two individual probabilities, or less than 1 in 200 million. The large number of reported cases of melanoma developing in patients who have very large CNN suggests a causal association.[114–118,130,155–159] In a review of 68 patients who had prepuberal metastatic melanoma, 20 cases (29 percent) were associated with very large CNN,[160] a frequency more than 500 times greater than expected. The lifetime melanoma risk for patients with very large CNN has been estimated to be at least 6.3 percent,[155] based on a questionnaire follow-up study of 151 persons with very large CNN examined between 1915 and 1973 in Denmark.[115,116] In a study of 39 individuals with giant CNN born between 1960 and 1980 in England, 2 cases were documented to have died with metastatic melanoma, and the melanoma risk was estimated to be 8.5 percent during the first 15 years of life.[161] While melanoma may develop in very large CNN at any time of life, diagnosis was established in the first 3 to 5 years of life in about half of affected patients who ultimately developed melanoma in association with giant CNN.[114,117,130,149,160] Lethal melanoma has been reported in newborns with giant CNN.[129,162] The prognosis of patients who develop melanoma in association with giant CNN is usually grave.[130] There are cases of lethal melanoma developing in giant CNN in black children.[163–165]

Malignant degeneration in large CNN may be associated with relatively sudden appearance of a dermal or subcutaneous nodule, a focal darkening of superficial pigmentation (or occasionally a pink or red color), itching, pain, bleeding, or ulceration. A nonepidermal origin of melanoma in very large CNN occurs in perhaps two-thirds of cases,[130,155] and thus, the usual gross morphologic features generally used for suspecting malignant change in pre-existing pigmented lesions may not apply.

SMALL CONGENITAL NEVUS

Parental history, medical records, and/or family photographs are required to document small CNN as a precursor of melanoma, or a remnant of the small CNN must remain intact for histopathologic confirmation. A valid histogenic relation between small CNN and melanoma is more difficult to establish than for large CNN.

It has been estimated that only one of every 170,000 melanomas should develop in contiguity with small CNN based on surface area considerations and chance alone.[166] Based on historical data from published series, a pigmented mole at the tumor site from birth was alleged for 9 to 58 percent of melanoma cases (Table 9-4). In one series of 134 melanomas, 15 percent of patients reported the existence of a birth mole at the tumor site, corroborated by parental statements and family photographs in some cases.[177] Melanoma was documented to occur at age 35 years in a CNN about 7 cm in diameter in a 35-year-old white woman; the CNN was documented photographically at age 5 months.[179] Among 19 cases of melanoma on volar and subungual skin, 6 cases (32 percent) were alleged to have developed in CNN.[178]

Available histopathologic studies corroborate historic observations of melanoma developing in small

TABLE 9-4
HISTORICAL ASSOCIATION OF CUTANEOUS MELANOMA DEVELOPING IN A SMALL-PIGMENTED MOLE PRESENT AT BIRTH

AUTHOR(S) (YEAR)	AGE AT DIAGNOSIS, IN YEARS	TOTAL NUMBER OF MELANOMA CASES	NUMBER WITH SMALL BIRTH MOLE AT TUMOR SITE (%)[a]	REFERENCE
Williams and Martin (1937)	19–81	25	5 (20)	167
Daland and Holmes (1939)	7–88	128	24 (19)	168
Driver and MacVicar (1943)	Not stated	60	25 (42)	169
Ackerman (1948)	10–90	75	15 (20)	170
Wright (1949)	8–84	94	20 (21)	171
Booher and Pack (1957)	12–77	122	11 (9)	172
Helwig (1963)	10–89	392	92 (24)	173
Bader et al. (1979)	<20	70[b]	13 (19)	174
Pratt et al. (1981)	0.2–21	31	11 (35)	175
Mole et al. (1982)	2–15	12	7 (58)	176
Rhodes and Melski (1982)	16–75	134	20 (15)	177
Vázquez et al. (1984)	36–113	19	6 (32)	178
Fong and Sagebiel (1989)	<15	11[c]	3 (27)	157

[a]Cases reporting birth mole at tumor site, based on patient history.
[b]One case associated with a giant congenital nevus.
[c]Two cases associated with a giant congenital nevus.

CNN. When histopathologic features were used to differentiate dermal nevi as congenital or acquired, dermal nevi having one or more microscopic features regarded as characteristic of CNN were detected in contiguity with 1 percent to 8.1 percent of primary melanomas.[45,118,166,180] The histogenic relation between melanoma and small CNN is dependent on the *specificity* of methods used for histopathologic ascertainment of a nevus as congenital or acquired.[112,166,177,180,181] Additional issues impact on the problem: (1) unselected CNN may have histopathologic features indistinguishable from acquired nevi[119]; (2) small CNN cannot always be adequately documented; and (3) histogenic precursors (including small CNN) may be obscured or obliterated by biologically aggressive melanomas.[180] These uncontrollable biases in ascertainment may account for observed discrepancies in the historic and histologic associations reported for melanomas developing in contiguity with small CNN.

Another approach to documenting age onset of a given nevus in contiguity with melanoma is nevus size. Any nevus that is 1.5 cm in diameter or larger and is not a dysplastic nevus or melanoma is likely to be congenital. Illig et al.[180] documented an in contiguity association between such "relatively large" nevomelanocytic nevi (between 1.5 cm and < 10 cm in diameter) and melanoma (see Plate 10). Individual case reports of melanoma developing in contiguity with relatively small varieties of CNN[98,182–190] (including multiple small CNN)[121] support the hypothesis that some small CNN may develop melanoma. The observed association between small CNN and melanoma (based on historic, histopathologic, and size criteria) is several orders of magnitude greater than expected based on body surface area considerations and chance alone.[166,181]

Very large CNN, present in only 1 in 2000 to 1 in 20,000 newborns, constitute a significant threat for individuals who have them, but are responsible for less than 1 percent of all cutaneous melanomas (3 of 1173 melanomas reviewed in Table 9-4). In contrast, small CNN are present in 1 percent of newborns,[119,120,123] carry a lifetime melanoma risk of perhaps 5 percent,[177] and may be responsible for 3 to 15 percent of melanomas in general[166,177] and a higher proportion of melanomas diagnosed during childhood (Table 9-4).

LENTIGO MALIGNA

DEFINITION

Lentigo maligna (LM) may be defined as a relatively large, haphazardly pigmented macule on sun-damaged skin (see Plate 11), usually in the elderly, consisting of a nonnested proliferation of variably atypical melanocytes in an atrophic epidermis (see Plate 12). LM may be stable or progress to intraepidermal (in situ) and invasive melanoma (see Plate 13). While some authors characterize LM as synonomous with melanoma in situ, this author regards LM a variety of intraepidermal melanocytic dysplasia in sun-damaged skin.

Additional terms that have been used to describe LM include Hutchinson's freckle, senile freckle, circumscribed precancerous melanosis, lentigo malin des Viellards, melanosis premaligna, melanose de Dubreuilh, melanosis circumscripta preblastomatosa, and precancerous nonnevoid melanocytoma.

EPIDEMIOLOGY

The age-specific prevalence of LM at least 1 cm in diameter has been estimated to be 0.7/1000 at ages 1 to 44 years, 3.8/1000 at ages 45 to 64 years, and 11.7/1000 at ages 65 to 74 years.[191] Of 85 cases of LM and lentigo maligna melanoma (LMM) in one series,[192] age at biopsy ranged from 20 to 85 years for men (average 58 years) and 31 to 73 years for women (average 55 years); 11 percent of those affected were younger than 40 years. According to one study, median age at diagnosis of LMM was 70 years, while the average age of onset of the original lesion (presumably LM) was reported to be 47 years.[193] In another study, 33 of 119 cases of LMM in three registries were diagnosed at or above the age of 75 years.[191] Onset of LM often precedes diagnosis of LMM by decades. LM does not have a consistent sex predilection. Almost all cases of LM occur in whites.[192]

PATHOGENESIS

LM is postulated to develop from an abnormal clone of intraepidermal melanocytes on sun-damaged skin. Ultraviolet radiation (UVR) is believed to have a causative role. While LM has been argued by some to be synonymous with in situ (intraepidermal) melanoma, the concept of intraepidermal melanocytic dysplasia (as distinct from intraepidermal melanoma) may be changing this view. LM may be regarded as a variety of intraepidermal melanocytic dysplasia induced by UVR in susceptible individuals.

Nevomelanocytic nevi do not seem to play a causative role in the histogenesis of LM.[192–194] LMM was the predominant melanoma type in one case series of xeroderma pigmentosum (XP) patients from Japan.[195] Patients with XP have numerous solar lentigines, first appearing early in life, characterized by atypical melanocytic proliferations.[196–198] It is likely that at least some melanomas in XP patients develop in atypical solar lentigines. It is highly likely that LM in non-XP patients also develop in atypical solar lentigines.[199]

Compared with other varieties of melanoma in one case-control study,[200] LMM is most strongly linked to a relative or absolute inability to tan in response to UVR. Genetic factors also may be playing a role. The significant association between frequency of use of nonpermanent hair dyes and LM (3.4-fold increased risk) in one case-control study[201] may be related to the confounding factor of an increased tendency to use hair dyes among persons who tan little or not at all and are most likely to have very lightly pigmented hair.

CLINICAL MANIFESTATIONS

LM first appears as a small, well-circumscribed tan or light brown macule which usually enlarges and becomes darker and more variegated over time, producing a markedly haphazard array of lighter and darker pigmentation, hypopigmentation, and occasionally depigmentation (see Plate 11). Some areas expand peripherally while other areas remain stationary or regress. Examination of the brightly illuminated mineral oil-coated surface with high magnification reveals a widened reticular pattern of pigmentation, with pseudopod extensions at the periphery.[82] Lesions may be as small as 3 to 5 mm in diameter or several centimeters in diameter and larger.[193]

Fully evolved melanoma associated with LM may be a darkly pigmented plaque or nodule superimposed on a circumscribed macule composed of various shades of brown pigmentation and areas of regression (see Plate 13), or a pink nodule of melanoma in the case of amelanotic LM.

PATHOLOGY

Several phases of evolution may be apparent within the same lesion. LM in its earliest phase of development is usually a tan macule, or a pink patch in the case of amelanotic LM, composed of a disordered proliferation of variably atypical melanocytes admixed with typical melanocytes in the basal layer of a thinned epidermis usually overlying solar degeneration of dermal collagen (see Plate 12). In younger patients, solar degeneration of dermal collagen may not be evident, and some epidermal areas may be almost identical to solar lentigo.[202] The variably atypical melanocytes in LM may be almost normal in size but with hyperchromatic nuclei, pleomorphism, and an enlarged retraction artifact, or variably large with abundant vacuolated cytoplasm and irregular and hyperchromatic nuclei. Melanocytes in LM are individually disposed and nonnested, some having prominent dendrites and an expanded retraction artifact, or spindle-shaped with elongated perikarya and hyperchromatic nuclei. Variably atypical melanocytes may extend down hair follicle epithelium. Macular areas of LM with these histopathologic features are unlikely to show intraepidermal (in situ) or invasive melanoma. Early forms of LM are usually associated with a perivascular or bandlike infiltrate of lymphocytes and melanin-laden macrophages in the papillary dermis. In the usual case, there is no associated nevomelanocytic nevus in LM.

Darker brown areas of LM may show greater numbers of more atypical melanocytes, but nest formation is still not usually seen. Black areas of lentigo maligna commonly show continuous proliferations of markedly atypical melanocytes disposed in cords, irregular nests, and strips above the basement membrane, with spindle forms predominating. This latter phase, showing a side-to-side and continuous proliferation of markedly atypical melanocytes at or above the epidermal basement membrane as single cells or irregular nests, may be called intraepidermal (in situ) melanoma. When intraepidermal nesting of markedly atypical melanocytes is present, invasive melanoma in the same specimen is highly likely.[13,203] Special stains, including S-100, may be necessary to detect microinvasive melanoma in lesions of LMM apparently confined to the epidermis. In one study, 14 of 91 cases diagnosed as LM were determined to have microinvasive melanoma based on stains for S-100 protein.[204] There is considerable confusion in the terminology of LM versus intraepidermal (in situ) melanoma associated with LM. Invasive melanoma must be carefully sought in lesions fulfilling the definition of intraepidermal melanoma associated with LM.

Areas associated with LM that have a distorted skin surface as a plaque or nodule usually indicate invasive melanoma and show a dermal accumulation of usually pure collections of spindle-shaped malignant melanocytes, inflammatory cells, and melanin-laden macrophages amidst solar degeneration of dermal collagen.[192] Blue-gray areas of LMM usually correspond to histopathologic features of regression, namely, areas of dermal fibrosis and melanin-laden macrophages but without malignant melanocytes.

DIFFERENTIAL DIAGNOSIS

Lesions that may be mistaken for LM include irregular varieties of solar lentigo, junctional nevus, seborrheic keratosis, pigmented superficial basal cell epithelioma, pigmented actinic keratosis, and benign pigmented keratosis. Diagnosis should be suspected in any patch of irregular macular pigmentation on sun-damaged skin. Amelanotic varieties of LM will appear as a red patch and are commonly misdiagnosed by experienced clinicians as actinic keratosis, squamous cell carcinoma, psoriasis, or eczematous dermatitis.

TREATMENT

Surgical excision with adequate margins of normal appearing skin is probably the most reliable method of adequately removing LM. Wood's lamp examination may be required to define lesion outlines. Advanced patient age and complicating illness, and cosmetic or functional aspects of treatment, may require other therapeutic options such as cryotherapy, grenz-irradiation, topical 5-fluorouracil, dermabrasion, ionizing radiation, electrodesiccation and curettage, and laser. For relatively stable lesions of LM in frail individuals, it may be appropriate to offer frequent periodic photographic observation to detect the earliest signs of malignant change. Plaque-like or nodular elevations, as well as darkly pigmented "macular" areas, should be sampled for histopathologic examination. Superficial destructive therapy, including cryotherapy[205] and laser,[206] may be associated with high-recurrence rates, often related to deep residual involvement of LM in epithelial appendages and neurovascular structures, or alternatively, incomplete delineation of lesion borders. Topical treatment of LM using tretinoin creme[207] and azelaic acid[208] have a significant failure rate and should be considered experimental.

COURSE AND PROGNOSIS

LM may remain stable or progress to intraepidermal (in situ) and invasive melanoma (see Plate 13). It is not uncommon to have a duration of 10 to 15 years or more before LM progresses to intraepidermal and invasive melanoma. While lesion size greater than 4 cm in diameter is associated with a high likelihood of detecting melanoma, size alone may not be reliable for predicting the presence of associated melanoma in LM. Of 59 cases of LM with and without associated melanoma, of cases smaller than 3 cm in diameter, 27 (47 percent) were associated with invasive melanoma.[192]

Patients usually seek medical evaluation for lesions of LM when a nodule develops, when the lesion enlarges, when a localized area darkens, and/or when an evaluation is urged by family and friends because of unusual appearance. Of 45 patients with LMM, only 15 (33 percent) were noted clinically to have a discrete nodule.[192] When melanoma develops in nonpigmented varieties of LM (usually a red or pink patch), there is often a delay in diagnosis by the unsuspecting clinician and usually an associated poorer prognosis.[209,210]

The risk of invasive melanoma attributable to LM is a controversial issue. Of 85 cases of LM reported by Wayte and Helwig,[192] 45 cases (53 percent) were associated with invasive melanoma at the time of diagnosis. In a series of 48 cases reported by Clark and Mihm,[193] 35 cases (73 percent) were associated with invasive melanoma at the time of diagnosis. These risk figures reflect highly selected tumors, that is, atypical-appearing or changing lesions are more likely to be biopsied than innocuous-looking lesions. Reported histologic series of LM/LMM consisting of changing or highly suspicious lesions examined in consultation tend to inflate the frequency of associated melanoma at the time of diagnosis. Another method of assessing melanoma risk attributable to LM is based on prevalence of LM in the general population, and melanoma case fraction in which LM is the precursor. LM is the precursor in 4 percent of cutaneous melanomas when strict definitions are applied,[14] but the range may vary from 2.5 to 5.0 percent.[191] Based on available figures for the age-adjusted prevalence rate of LM at least 1 cm in diameter and diagnosed clinically in the general population, and the proportion of melanomas attributable to LM, the following estimates have been derived: (1) risk of melanoma developing in LM may be estimated to be approximately 1 in 750 affected people per year over the age of 45 years; (2) risk appears to increase with age; and (3) risk to age 75 years may be as high as 1.2 to 3.3 percent, and lifetime risk as high as 2.2 to 4.7 percent, depending on age at presentation.[191]

Deeply invasive melanoma, metastatic melanoma, and death may be associated with LMM.[192,193,211]

NEVUS SPILUS

DEFINITION

Nevus spilus is defined as circumscribed tan pigmentation consisting of lentigo simplex (melanocytic hyperplasia in a lentiginous epidermal pattern), in which more darkly pigmented raised and/or flat speckled nevomelanocytic or melanocytic hyperplasias are present[212] (see Plate 14). Cases fitting the gross and microscopic description of nevus spilus have been called speckled lentiginous nevus and zosteriform lentiginous nevus. More than 30 years ago, café-au-lait pigmentation without speckling also was called nevus spilus.

EPIDEMIOLOGY

Nevus spilus is usually acquired. Rare cases are present at birth. There were no cases of nevus spilus described among 4641 newborn infants examined in Boston, Massachusetts,[120] or among 1058 newborn infants examined in Stanford, California.[119] In contrast to the rarity of nevus spilus in newborns, this lesion was detected in 14 (2.3 percent) of 601 predominantly white adults in a private dermatology practice in New York City[213] and 20 (2.1 percent) of 939 predominantly white school children aged 8 to 16 years in Switzerland.[214] Nevus spilus appears to have no sexual predilection.

PATHOGENESIS

Nevus spilus likely represents a localized genetic defect in neural crest melanoblasts. Environmental factors also may be playing a role.

CLINICAL MANIFESTATIONS

Nevus spilus usually becomes evident during late infancy or early childhood. Lesions may be localized and small (see Plate 14), have a segmental distribution, or occupy a major portion of the body surface. Nevus spilus rarely has been associated with skeletal and muscle abnormalities, cerebral hemisphere atrophy, nevus flammeus, verrucous epidermal nevus, seizure disorder, and peripheral vascular abnormalities.

PATHOLOGY

Flat, dark speckles of nevus spilus usually consist of lentiginous melanocytic hyperplasia. Raised elements usually contain collections of nevomelanocytes in the epidermis and/or dermis. The tan background pigmentation usually consists of increased numbers of melanocytes in a lentiginous epidermal pattern.[212,215–220] Speckled elements of nevus spilus may consist of epithelioid cell and/or spindle cell nevi, melanocytic dysplasia,[221] or blue nevi.[222]

DIFFERENTIAL DIAGNOSIS

Nevus spilus must be differentiated from café-au-lait macules and lentigo simplex, relatively flat and hairless varieties of large congenital nevus, and Becker's nevus. Irregular or very darkly pigmented speckles of nevus spilus may require biopsy to determine the presence of epithelioid cell and/or spindle cell elements, blue nevus, melanocytic dysplasia, or melanoma.

TREATMENT

Clinical appearance, history of stability or instability, congenital or noncongenital onset, and perceived melanoma risk will determine treatment. Atypical-appearing lesions and new and/or unstable elements in nevus spilus should be evaluated for histopathologic examination or close photographic follow-up for malignant change. The speckled melanocytic and/or nevomelanocytic elements of congenital nevus spilus should be considered for prophylactic excision (if lesions are small enough) or periodic lifetime photographic follow for suspicious change.

COURSE AND PROGNOSIS

There are well-documented cases of melanoma developing in contiguity with nevus spilus[221,223–230] (see Plate 15). While the exact biologic events leading to melanoma in nevus spilus are unknown, this occurrence may be related to a multistep process in genetically initiated atypical melanocytes (i.e., melanocytic dysplasia or congenital nevi), an environmentally induced change in typical or atypical melanocytes (i.e., UVR, toxic exposure, or viral infection), or a combination of factors.

When viewed as a risk marker for the development of melanoma, nevus spilus may have a trend for being more common in melanoma cases compared to controls. Kopf et al.[227] detected nevus spilus in 5 of 105 (4.8 percent) white adults with melanoma, compared to 14 of 601 (2.3 percent) dermatology outpatients. Kelly et al.[40] detected nevus spilus in 12 of 121 (10 percent) melanoma patients, compared to 9 of 139 (6 percent) outpatient controls. Overmatching of cases and controls, which would tend to reduce the estimated melanoma risk, cannot be excluded in these case-control studies.

CELLULAR BLUE NEVUS

DEFINITION

The cutaneous blue nevus consists of an acquired or congenital blue, blue-gray, or blue-black papule, nodule, or plaque-like aggregate of aberrant dermal melanocytes actively producing melanin. Three types of cutaneous blue nevus are recognized: (1) common blue nevus, (2) cellular blue nevus, and (3) combined blue nevus-nevomelanocytic nevus. The cellular blue nevus (see Plate 16) differs from the common and combined blue nevus in that the cellular blue nevus is usually larger, more elevated, and potentially more aggressive biologically. The importance of the cellular blue nevus is its association with development of melanoma.

EPIDEMIOLOGY

Cellular blue nevus is rare. In two major studies of pigmented lesions in 5699 newborns,[119,120] cellular blue nevus was notably absent. The prevalence rate of blue nevus was 3.2 percent among 9996 healthy Japanese males 18 to 26 years of age, the vast majority of lesions being 1 to 2 mm deep blue macules or papules (likely common blue nevi),[231] while only 0.12 percent (12 people) had large blue-black nodules (likely cellular blue nevus) (A. Hidano, personal communication). Among 139 white adult outpatients in San Francisco, California, 6 (4 percent) were noted to have (common) blue nevi.[40]

PATHOGENESIS

Although a schwannian or endoneural origin is postulated for blue nevus based on ultrastructural features and isolation of cholinesterase activity,[232] a melanocytic origin is suggested by the presence of obvious melanin synthesis in common varieties of blue nevi and ultrastructural evidence of melanin synthesis in cells of cellular blue nevi.[233] Blue nevi, together with Mongolian spots and the nevus fuscoceruleus ophthalmomaxillaris of Ota and nevus acromiodeltoideus of Ito (see following section), are believed to represent ectopic accumulations of melanin-producing melanocytes in the dermis, arrested during their migration from the neural crest to sites in the skin. The rare occurrence of blue nevi in oral mucosa, uterine cervix, vagina, spermatic cord, prostate gland, and lymph node supports this notion. An alternative hypothesis is that the neural crest derived melanoblasts from which common and cellular varieties of blue nevus develop are abnormal from the outset.

CLINICAL MANIFESTATIONS

Cellular blue nevus is a blue-gray or blue-brown nodule or plaque, 1 to 3 cm in diameter (see Plate 16), occasionally larger, usually apparent at birth. The lesion surface is usually smooth, but may be irregular. About half the cases of cellular blue nevus are located on buttocks or sacrum.[234] Very large congenital blue nevi, often with multiple satellite lesions, have been reported.[130,235–240] Cellular blue nevus may occasionally develop in association with congenital nevomelanocytic nevus.[130,241] In contrast to the cellular blue nevus, the common blue nevus is usually an acquired, solitary, asymptomatic blue, blue-gray, or blue-black minimally elevated papule, usually smaller than 5 mm in diameter.

PATHOLOGY

In the common blue nevus, dermal melanocytes appear as melanin-containing fibroblast-like cells grouped in irregular bundles admixed with melanin-containing macrophages, intimately associated with excessive production of fibrous tissue in the mid or upper reticular dermis, occasionally extending downward to the subcutaneous fat or upward to the papillary dermis (see Plate 17). In the cellular blue nevus, there are usually components of common blue nevus associated with fascicles of spindle-shaped cells with ovoid nuclei and abundant pale cytoplasm with little or no melanin, and often epithelioid cells, in the dermis and often subcutaneous fat, in nests, bundles, and neuroid forms, with little or no intervening stroma (see Plate 17). Histopathologic diagnosis may be difficult when the common blue nevus component and melanin production are sparse or inapparent. Atypical melanosomes may be seen in cellular blue nevus. Histopathologic differentiation among cellular blue nevus, melanoma, and melanoma developing in cellular blue nevus may be difficult.[242,243]

Occasionally, small groups of well-differentiated nevomelanocytes are present in the marginal sinuses or parenchyma of lymph nodes draining the anatomic site of cellular blue nevus, making it difficult to distinguish true metastasis from pseudometastasis. These "inert" deposits in the capsules and peripheral sinuses of lymph nodes may be passively transported from the primary tumor site to lymph nodes, or alternatively, cellular deposits in lymph nodes may represent ectopic embryologic "rests."[234,242]

Like melanoma and typical acquired nevomelanocytic nevus, cellular blue nevus shows positive cytoplasmic staining with antivimentin antibody and negative staining with antineurofilament antibodies. Staining for S-100 protein has been determined to be positive in some cases of blue nevus and negative in others, while HMB-45 immunoreactivity (generally thought of as melanoma-specific) has been noted to be strongly positive in cellular blue nevus and variable in common blue nevus.[244]

DIFFERENTIAL DIAGNOSIS

Cellular blue nevus may be confused clinically for sclerosing hemangioma, dermatofibroma, histiocytoma, glomus tumor, primary or metastatic melanoma, pyogenic granuloma, pigmented spindle cell nevus, and traumatic tattoo with excessive scarring. There are acquired variants of macular dermal melanocytosis that may cause confusion for blue nevus. Mongolian spots, nevus of Ota, and nevus of Ito also are accumulations of melanin-producing melanocytes in the dermis, but unlike cellular blue nevus, these forms of dermal melanocytosis are usually broad in extent and macular.

TREATMENT

Cellular blue nevus should be evaluated for excision because of its malignant potential. Sudden appearance of a blue nodule, expansion of a pre-existing blue plaque, a congenital blue nodule, or a relatively large blue nodule or plaque (10 mm in diameter or larger) demand consideration for histopathologic examination. Excision of cellular blue nevus should include deep cutaneous fat to ensure complete removal.

COURSE AND PROGNOSIS

The natural evolution of cellular blue nevus has not been studied adequately because lesions are usually excised. Melanoma developing in cellular blue nevus usually presents as an expanding dermal nodule, with or without ulceration. Melanoma developing in cellular blue nevus may spread to lymph nodes and cause death due to local invasion and visceral metastasis.[233,235,236,242,243,245–247]

Melanoma developing in cellular blue nevus, often called *malignant blue nevus,* is distinguished from cellular blue nevus by invasiveness, significant cellular atypia, pleomorphism, atypical mitoses, and areas of necrosis. In a series of 12 cases of strictly defined "malignant blue nevus," an origin in cellular blue nevus was demonstrated in 11 cases.[245] The cellular blue nevus may be regarded as a potential precursor of melanoma, and the malignant blue nevus may be regarded as melanoma developing in cellular blue nevus. In contrast to cellular blue nevus, common blue nevus has not been associated with development of melanoma.

NEVUS OF OTA AND NEVUS OF ITO

DEFINITION

Nevus of Ota, also called *nevus fuscoceruleus ophthalmomaxillaris,* consists of unilateral (occasionally bilateral) slate gray and blue-brown speckled macular pigmentation usually occurring in the distribution of the first and second divisions of the trigeminal nerve, involving periorbital, temporal, malar, and/or frontal areas of the facial skin, as well as underlying anatomic structures (see Plate 18). Nevus of Ito, also called *nevus fuscoceruleus acromiodeltoideus,* has the same clinical features as nevus of Ota, except that lesions are located on the scapula and/or deltoid area (see Plate 19).

EPIDEMIOLOGY

Approximately 50 percent of cases of nevus of Ota and nevus of Ito are congenital or appear very early in childhood, with the remainder developing by the second decade of life, occasionally after pregnancy.[248] Lesions occur mostly in Asians and blacks, rarely in whites. The prevalence has been reported to be 0.2 to 1.0 percent of Japanese outpatients.[249,250] The prevalence in whites and other races is unknown but thought to be rare (less than 1 in 10,000 outpatients). Familial aggregation has been noted occasionally for nevus of Ota.[248] There appears to be a strong female to male predominance in Asians and whites, up to 4:1.[249,251]

PATHOGENESIS

Nevus of Ota and nevus of Ito are believed to represent ectopic accumulations of melanin-producing melanocytes in the dermis, "arrested" during their migration from the neural crest to sites in the skin. The reasons for their relative permanence and racial and sex predilection are unknown, but the neural crest melanoblasts responsible for these lesions are believed to be abnormal from the outset. A genetic basis, influenced by hormonal and possibly environmental factors, is possible.

CLINICAL MANIFESTATIONS

Skin pigmentation in nevus of Ota and nevus of Ito may be black, black-purple, blue-black, deep blue, slate-blue, purple-brown, or faint brown (see Plates 18 and 19). Pigmentation is usually macular, but papular elements may occur. Pigmentation intensity is said to vary from day to day, particularly in females.[249] Lesions are unilateral in most cases, and bilateral in up to 10 percent in Japanese cases.[251] Pigmentation also may be noted in the ipsilateral scleral connective tissue in 49 to 61 percent of cases.[251] Other eye involvement may include palpebral conjunctiva, iris, choroid, retrobulbar fat, periosteum and orbital bone, and optic nerve. Vision is not usually affected, but associated glaucoma has been reported.[252] Lips, oral palate, and nasal mucosa also may be involved. Rare cases are associated with sensorineural deafness.[253,254] Nevus of Ota has been associated with leptomeningeal melanocytosis.[255–257]

PATHOLOGY

Pathology of nevus of Ota and nevus of Ito is similar, with melanin-producing bipolar, dendritic, or stellate melanocytes and melanin-laden macrophages usually in the upper and mid-reticular dermis. Leptomeninges may be affected with melanocytosis and melanosis in nevus of Ota.[255–257] The dopa reaction is strongly positive in weakly pigmented melanocytes in nevus of Ota; melanocytes are negative to tyrosine incubation.[250]

DIFFERENTIAL DIAGNOSIS

Nevus of Ota and nevus of Ito may be mistaken for traumatic bruising, congenital dermal melanocytosis (Mongolian spot) (see Plate 20), and nevomelanocytic nevi. Nevomelanocytic nevi are usually brown or flesh-colored plaques or papules. Congenital dermal melanocytosis is defined by the presence of blue-gray macular pigmentation occurring at birth and is noted in 90 percent of darkly pigmented races, 70 percent of native hispanic and American Indian populations, and 10 percent of whites. Congenital dermal melanocytosis may occur at any site in the newborn period, but is most common on the buttocks and sacrum (see Plate 20). While congenital dermal melanocytosis usually disappears by puberty, lesions are persistent in about 4 percent of cases. The more superficial location of melanin in nevus of Ota and nevus of Ito is responsible for the brownish cast to these lesions, compared to the blue-gray color of congenital dermal melanocytosis, notable for more deeply situated melanin-containing melanocytes.

TREATMENT

Excision, dermabrasion, or laser surgery may be considered for skin pigmentation on an individual basis. Repeated cryotherapy combined with argon laser has been reported to fade pigmentation in some cases,[258] but repigmentation may occur with time. Cosmetic cover-up may be helpful.

COURSE AND PROGNOSIS

Pigmentation may fade with time, and some benign cutaneous elevations may occur. Melanoma developing in the skin of nevus of Ota and nevus of Ito is rare but has been reported in at least 5 cases.[259–262] Nevus of Ota has been associated with melanoma developing in the leptomeninges,[255–257] pineal gland,[263] iris, choroid, orbit, and uveal tract.[254,264–266] A case of dermal melanocytosis similar to nevus of Ota and nevus of Ito, except for its generalized distribution of lesions, has been reported in association with disseminated melanoma.[267] Most of the reported cases of melanoma associated with nevus of Ota and nevus of Ito, from skin or noncutaneous sites, have occurred in whites, although cases have been reported in a Japanese man[254] and a black woman.[265]

ACRAL AND MUCOSAL MELANOCYTIC DYSPLASIA

DEFINITION

There are atypical varieties of pigmented macules on acral sites[268–272] (see Plates 21, 22, and 23), penis,[273–277] vulva[274,278–280] conjunctiva,[281–283] and oral mucosa[284,285] that are characterized by a disordered proliferation of intraepidermal melanocytes with variable cellular atypia (see Plate 22) and that may be relevant to melanoma progression, both in whites and nonwhites.[5,178,271,272,279,286–301] Acral and mucosal melanocytic dysplasia should probably be separated nosologically from dysplastic melanocytic nevus (see Acquired Dysplastic Melanocytic Nevus in the beginning of the chapter). Melanoma occurring in the setting of dysplastic nevus and familial melanoma are only rarely associated with an acral or mucosal location.[301] Terms such as atypical lentigo simplex or melanocytic dysplasia on acral or mucosal sites distinguish this variety of lesion from lentigo maligna (LM) and dysplastic nevus. Separating acral and mucosal melanocytic dysplasia from dysplastic melanocytic nevus and LM is useful for melanoma intervention purposes. It is important to consider acral and mucosal sites during examination for the presence of melanocytic dysplasia and melanoma.

PATHOGENESIS

Intraepidermal melanocytic dysplasia on palms, soles, and mucous membranes may be regarded as a genetically and/or environmentally initiated trait that has a histogenic relationship to melanoma occurring in these sites.[5,178,268,281,286–289,302] Factors responsible for melanocytic dysplasia on acral and mucosal sites require further study.

EPIDEMIOLOGY

The prevalence of pigmented melanocytic nevi on acral sites and mucosal sites appears to be race related. Pigmented nevi were detected on the palms in 6 percent of 632 whites and 19 percent of 114 blacks, and on the plantar surface in 8 percent of 632 whites and 18 percent of 114 blacks.[303] In a study of 251 blacks, pigmented lesions were detected on the soles in 22.3 percent and on the palms in 24.7 percent.[268] The darker the skin color in blacks, the higher the prevalence of acral pigmented lesions.[268] In a survey of 23,165 Japanese outpatients, 770 (3.3 percent) had pigmented nevi of the plantar surface.[304] Conjunctival nevi were noted in 0.9 percent of 632 whites and 4 percent of 114 blacks.[303] Pigmented lesions on the external genitalia are relatively common, present in 14.2 percent of 10,000 males ages 17 to 25 years[305] and in 10.3 percent of 301 predominantly white adult females.[306]

The prevalence of pigmented nevi of the nail bed, manifested as a longitudinal band of pigmentation (see Plate 23), also is race-related. Among 800 Japanese, 20 percent of males and 23 percent of females had pigmented bands of the fingernails.[307] Nail bands in blacks show an age-related increase in prevalence, from 2.5 percent among individuals aged 0 to 3 years, to 96 percent among individuals older than 50 years.[308] In contrast, pigmented nail bands are extremely rare in whites. In one survey,[303] no nail bands were detected on fingernails or toe nails in 632 whites. Given the low prevalence of nail bands in whites, their presence in whites must raise suspicion for melanoma or potential melanoma precursor.[309]

CLINICAL MANIFESTATIONS

Acral and mucosal melanocytic dysplasias appear as irregularly pigmented, relatively large macules on palms, soles, or mucous membranes (see Plate 21). Lesions may be a few millimeters in diameter to a very large size. Lesions may be acquired or congenital, stable or unstable. Melanocytic tumors in darkly pigmented races are less amenable to diagnosis based on gross morphologic features than in whites. On nonacral and nonmucosal surfaces, melanocytic tumors in darkly pigmented races are often darkly pigmented, and other criteria, such as irregular borders, irregular topography and/or ulceration, eccentric pigmentation, appearance of a spot or papule, or unstable growth history are required to suspect melanocytic dysplasia (or melanoma).

In nonwhites, suspicion about melanocytic dysplasia or early malignant change of pigmented nevus of the nail bed (see Plate 23) must be based on clinical appearance (very dark, very wide, and/or spill-over to periungual skin) and instability. In whites, a nail nevus should be considered for histopathologic examination whether or not the lesion is acquired or congenital, stable or unstable.

PATHOLOGY

Pigmented lesions on palms, soles, and mucous membrances may be nevomelanocytic nevi, lentiginous proliferations of typical or atypical melanocytes, or pigmentation without melanocytic proliferation.[268,304] Vulvar- and penile-pigmented lesions may consist of lentiginous melanocytic hyperplasia,[273,278,279,306] and varieties of such lesions have been called genital lentiginosis.[274] There are histologically atypical varieties of lentiginous melanocytic hyperplasia on acral sites (see Plate 22),[268–272] penis,[273–277] vulva,[274,279,280] conjunctiva,[281–283] and oral mucosa.[284,285] Although it has been stated (based on observation of selected cases) that pigmented lesions of the genitalia frequently show atypical histology, this was not the case when pigmented lesions were studied consecutively in women presenting for routine gynecologic examination.[306]

Pigmented bands of the fingernails in Japanese are due to a focal increase in number, dopa positivity, and dendricity of melanocytes in the nail matrix.[310]

DIFFERENTIAL DIAGNOSIS

Melanocytic dysplasias on acral sites must be distinguished from typical nevomelanocytic nevus, lentigo simplex without atypia, benign melanosis without melanocytosis, verruca vulgaris, foreign body reaction, pigmented bowenoid papulosis (on mucosal site), pigmented squamous cell carcinoma, callus, clavus, and traumatic hematoma. Melanocytic dysplasia of the oral, genital, or anal mucosa must be distinguished from benign melanosis without melanocytic hyperplasia, lentigo simplex without atypia, typical nevomelanocytic nevus, pigmented bowenoid papulosis, pigmented squamous cell carcinoma, traumatic hematoma, condyloma accuminatum, and amalgum tattoo (oral mucosa). Melanocytic dysplasia of the nail bed must be distinguished from typical nevomelanocytic nevus, lentigo simplex without atypia, pigmented squamous cell carcinoma, verruca vulgaris, foreign body reaction, traumatic hematoma, and chronic bacterial or fungal infection.

TREATMENT

Pigmented lesions on acral and mucosal surfaces must be evaluated individually based on clinical appearance, stability or instability, and the perceived risk of melanoma. Very darkly pigmented nevi on acral surfaces should be viewed with suspicion, regardless of skin pigmentation. Melanocytic and nevomelanocytic hyperplasias may be precursors of melanoma in these sites. Pigmented nevi of the oral mucosa (apart from the gums),[286] vaginal mucosa, and anal mucosa are very uncommon and ought to be viewed with suspicion.

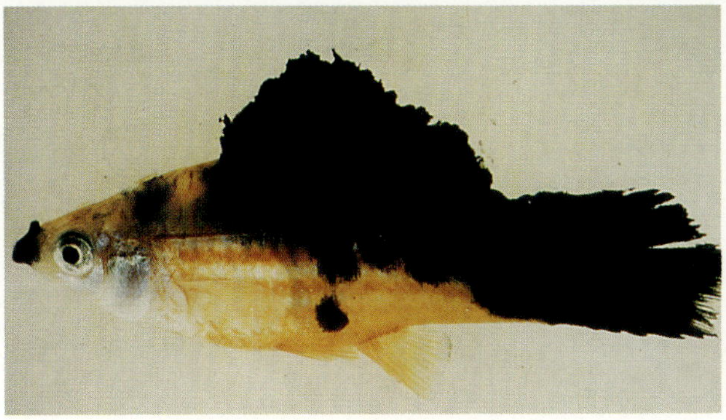

PLATE 1. *Platyfish-swordtail hybrid developing melanoma "spontaneously."*

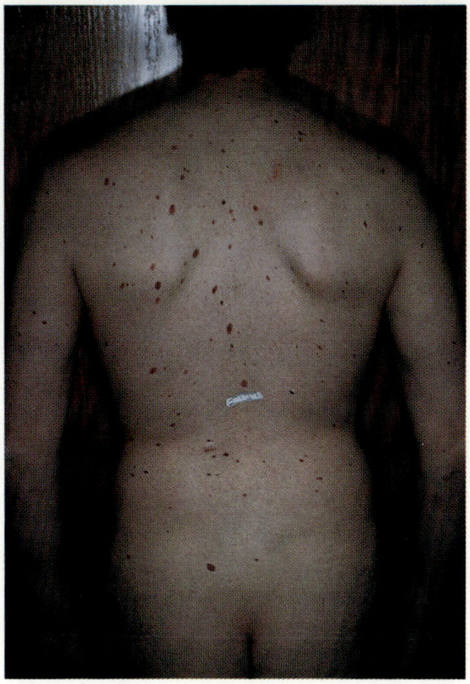

PLATE 2. *Dysplastic melanocytic nevi. Numerous prominent pigmented nevi are noted on the back of a 21-year-old white male who had more than 50 nevi at least 5 mm in diameter, atypical appearing nevi, histopathologically documented dysplastic nevi, a personal history of melanoma, dysplastic nevi in two brothers, and autopsy-documented melanoma in his father.*

PLATE 3. *Dysplastic melanocytic nevi, close-up view. (a) Dysplastic compound nevus with focally severe cellular atypia, on the midback of a 27-year-old white male for an indeterminate duration. (b) Dysplastic compound nevus with slight cellular atypia, on the midback of a 33-year-old white male since early childhood, becoming more irregular in coloration for several years. (c) Junctional dysplastic nevus with slight cellular atypia, on the upper back of a 57-year-old white male for an indeterminate duration. (d) Dysplastic compound nevus with moderate cellular atypia, on the upper back of an 18-year-old white female, reportedly stable in appearance since early childhood. (e) Dysplastic compound nevus with slight cellular atypia, on the parietal scalp of a 7-year-old white male, reportedly stable for several years. (f) Junctional dysplastic nevus with moderate cellular atypia, on the shoulder of a 69-year-old white male, present for at least 4 years and reportedly stable. Note the variability in appearance of the nevi, some with irregular and dark pigmentation and/or a target appearance, irregular or fuzzy outlines, relatively large size, and "flattish" surface relative to breadth. Scale in mm.*

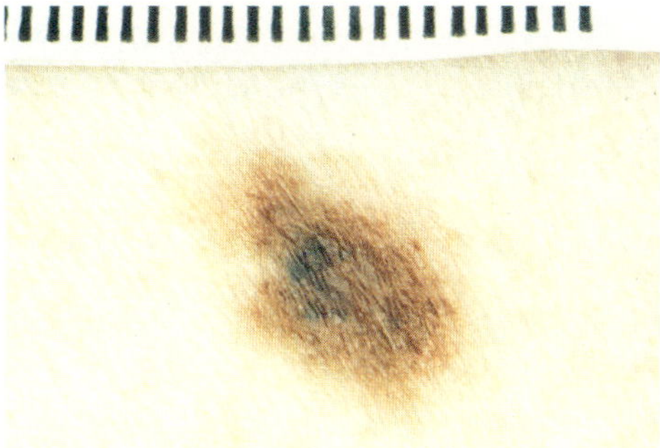

(a)

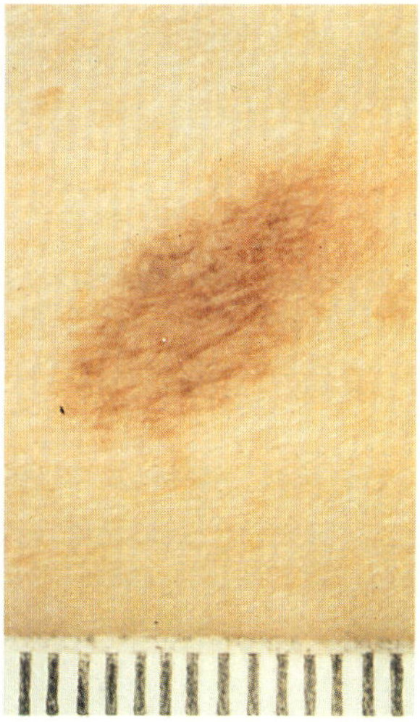

(b)

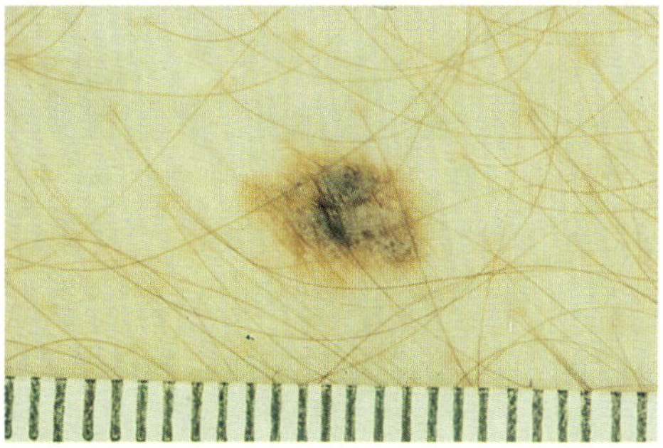

(c)

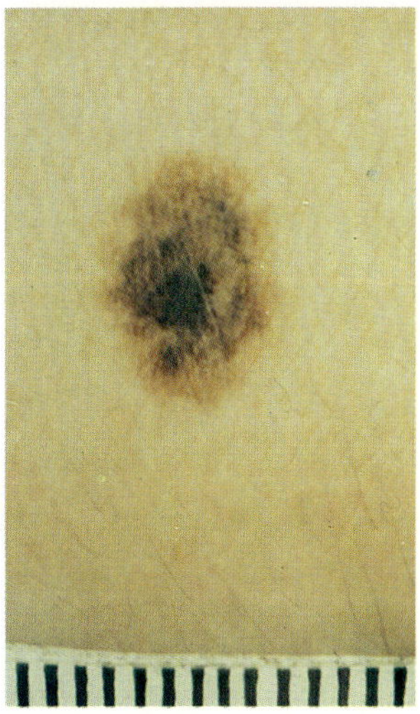

(d)

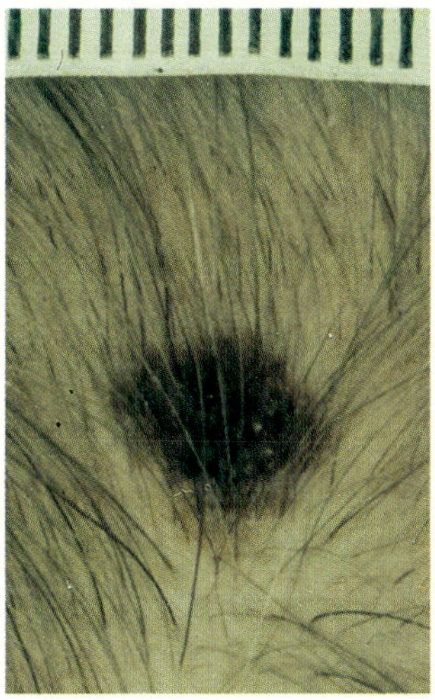

(e)

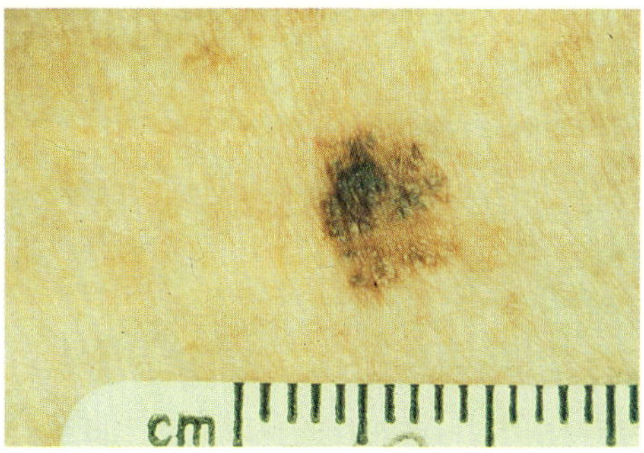

(f)

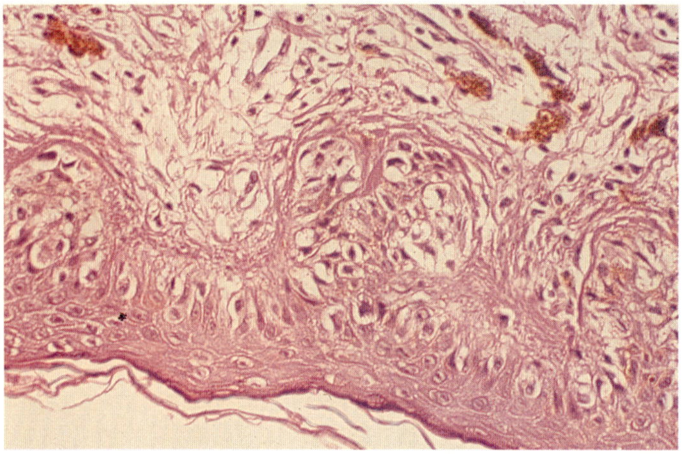

(a)

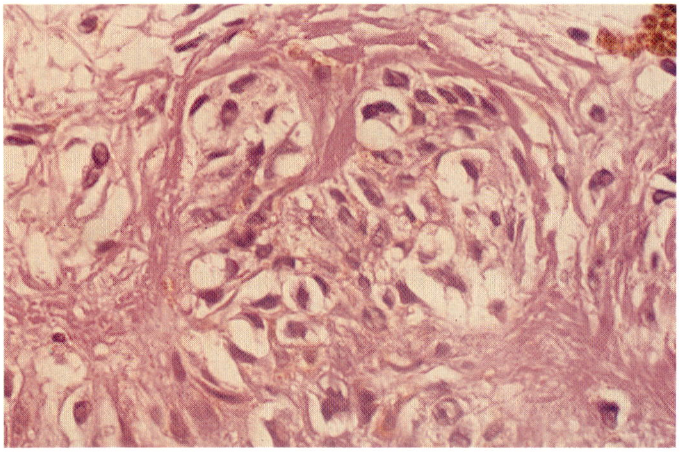

(b)

PLATE 4. *Histopathologic features of dysplastic melanocytic nevus shown in Plate 3(f). (a) Low magnification, showing lentiginous epidermal hypertrophy with elongated epidermal rete ridges, proliferation of intraepidermal melanocytes, cellular atypia of melanocytes, eosinophilic fibrosis surrounding rete ridges, and increased melanin in macrophages. Original magnification × 550. (b) Higher magnification of (a), showing disordered intraepidermal melanocytic proliferation with variable and discontinuous cellular atypia. Original magnification × 1100. Hematoxylin and eosin stain.*

PLATE 5. *Melanoma developing in contiguity with dysplastic melanocytic nevus. (a) Intraepidermal (in situ) superficial spreading melanoma developing in contiguity with a dysplastic nevus, the pre-existing lesion present for at least 20 years and darkening for 3 years, on the upper back of a 72-year-old white male. Note the dark and irregular pigmentation on the lower pole (in situ melanoma) of an irregular brown plaque (dysplastic nevus). (b) Superficial spreading melanoma, invasive to level IV/2.0 mm thickness, developing in contiguity with a dysplastic nevus, the pre-existing lesion present for at least 20 years and darkening with nodular elevation for an indeterminate duration, on the posterior thigh of a 41-year-old white female. Note the black nodule of melanoma on the inferior pole of a variegated brown plaque (dysplastic nevus). (c) Superficial spreading melanoma, invasive to level IV/1.32 mm thickness, developing in contiguity with a dysplastic nevus, present for an indeterminate duration, on the back of a 51-year-old white male. Note the central black nodule (melanoma) and the surrounding "macular" pigmentation (dysplastic nevus). Scale in mm.*

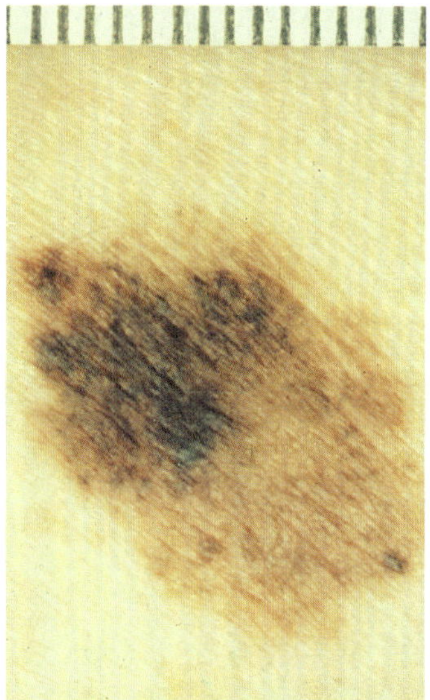

(a)

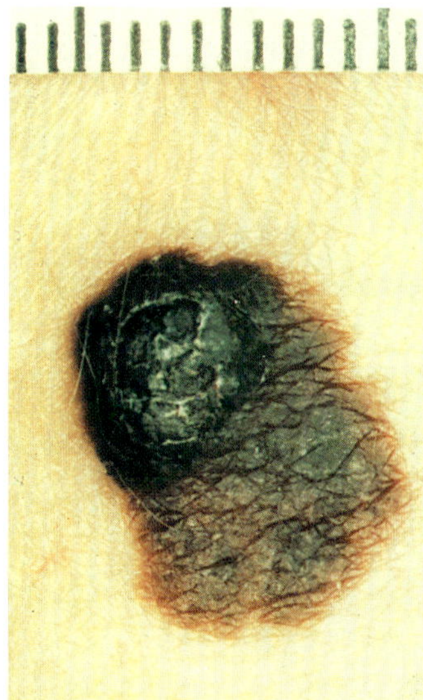

(b)

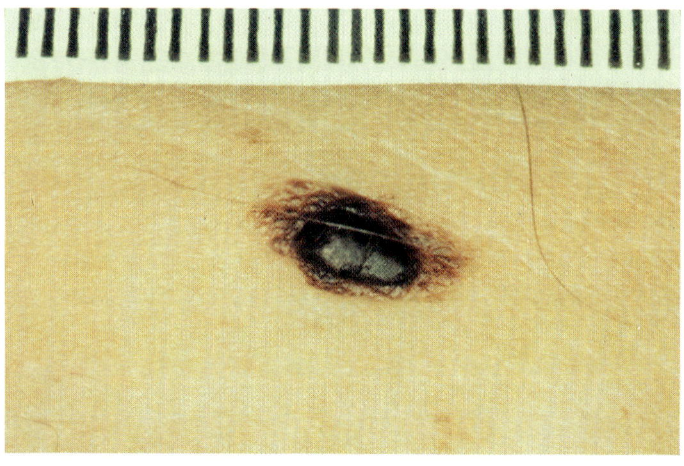

(c)

PLATE 6. *Congenital split nevomelanocytic nevus of the medial upper and lower eyelids of a 9-year-old white male.*

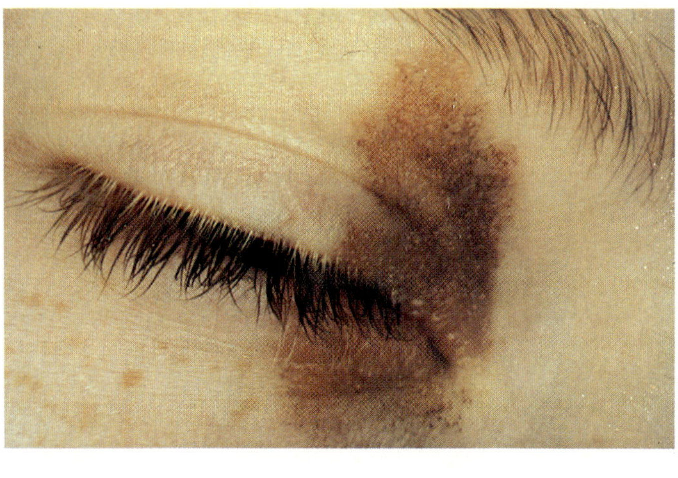

PLATE 7. *Small congenital nevomelanocytic nevi, benign in appearance, on the buttock of a 4-year-old white female (a), the nose of a 2-month-old white female (b), the leg of a 12-year-old white male (c), and the low back of a 1-day-old Japanese male (d). Scale in mm.*

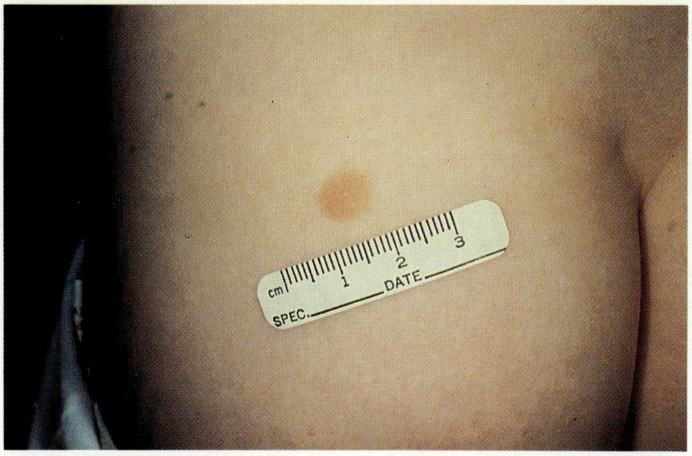

(a)

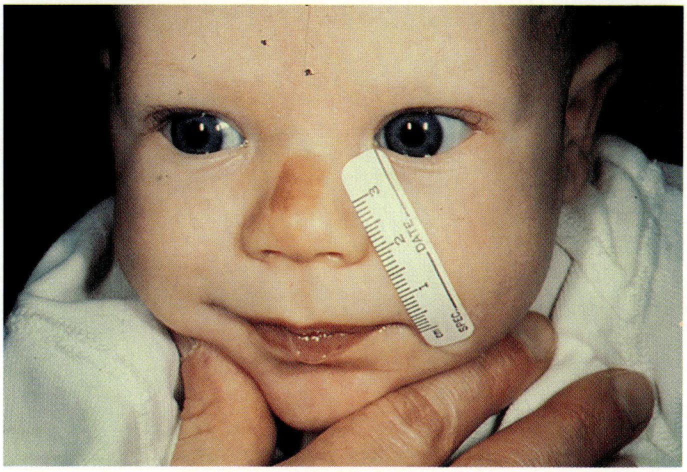

(b)

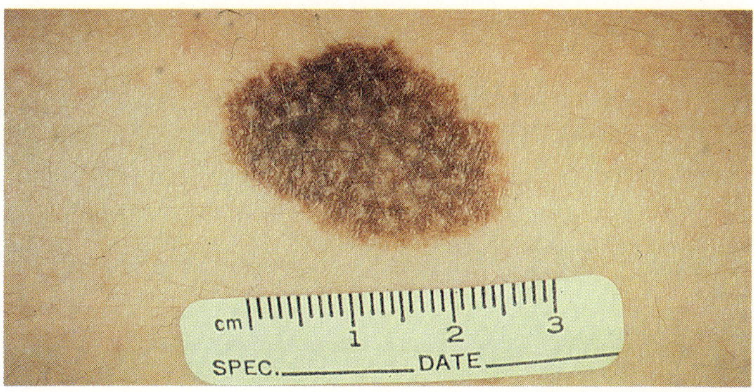

(c)

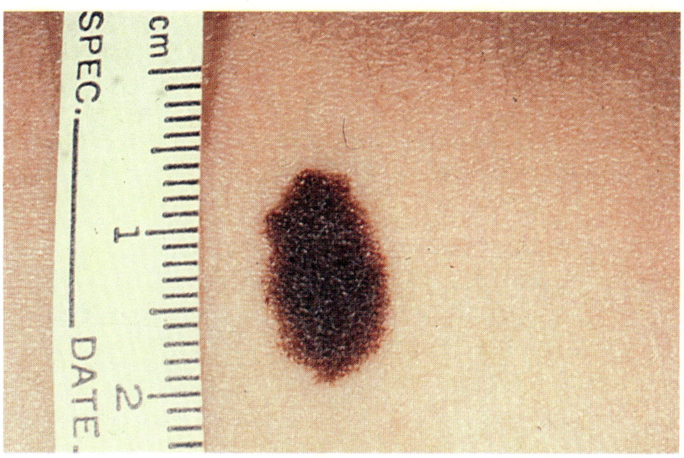

(d)

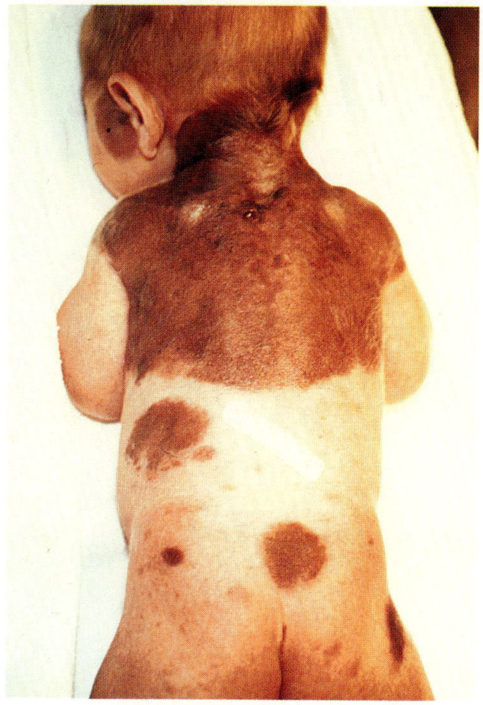

(a)

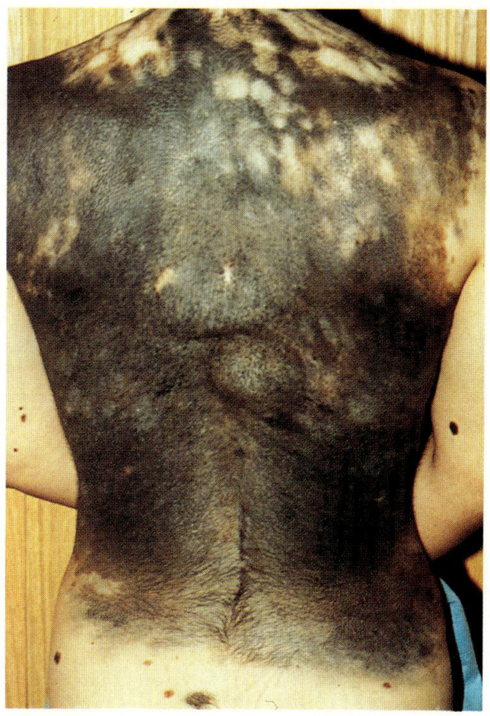

(b)

PLATE 8. *Giant congenital nevomelanocytic nevi. (a) Giant "cape" nevus on the neck and torso of a 2-day-old white male. (b) Giant nevus on the posterior torso and buttocks of a 47-year-old Japanese female. Note the soft tumorous masses and areas of pigment loss in (b) and the numerous satellite congenital nevi in both cases.*

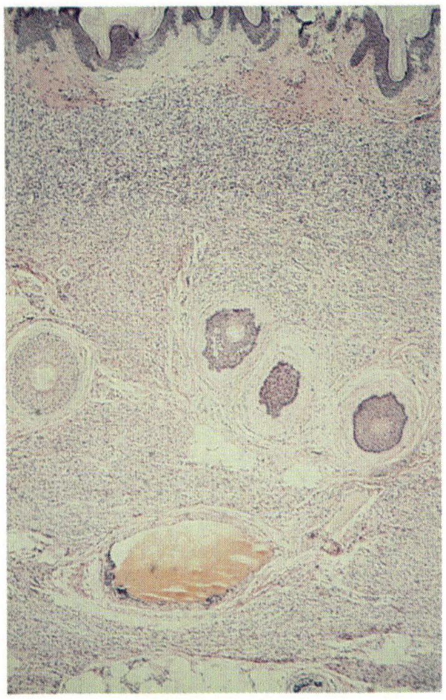

(a)

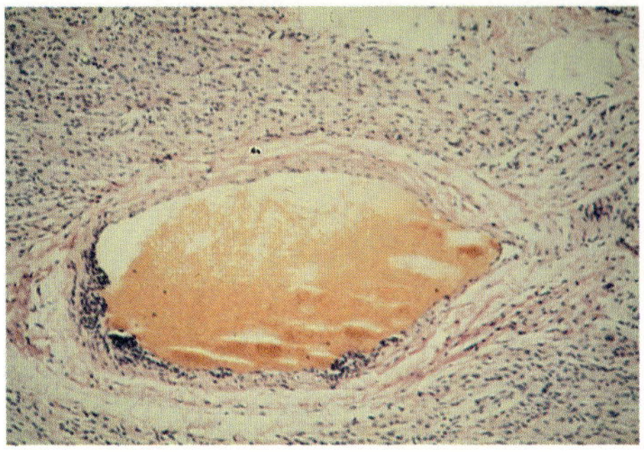

(b)

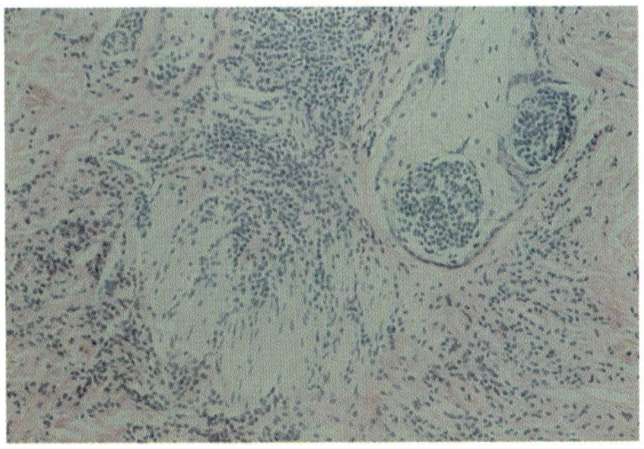

(c)

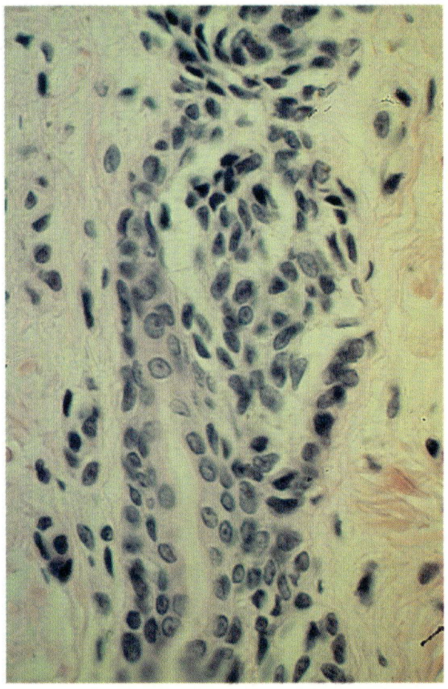

(d)

PLATE 9. *Histopathologic features characteristic of congenital nevomelanocytic nevus. (a) Sheets of nevomelanocytes in the lower two-thirds of the reticular dermis and involving the panniculus. Original magnification × 92. (b) Higher magnification of (a), showing nevomelanocytes within the wall of a small vein in the deep reticular dermis. Original magnification × 230. (c) Nevomelanocytes within the capsule of a sebaceous gland and within a malformed arrectores pilorum, plus nevomelanocytes in single array and sheets, in the deep reticular dermis. Original magnification × 800. (d) Nevomelanocytes within the epithelium of an eccrine duct in the mid reticular dermis. Original magnification × 800. Hematoxylin and eosin stain.*

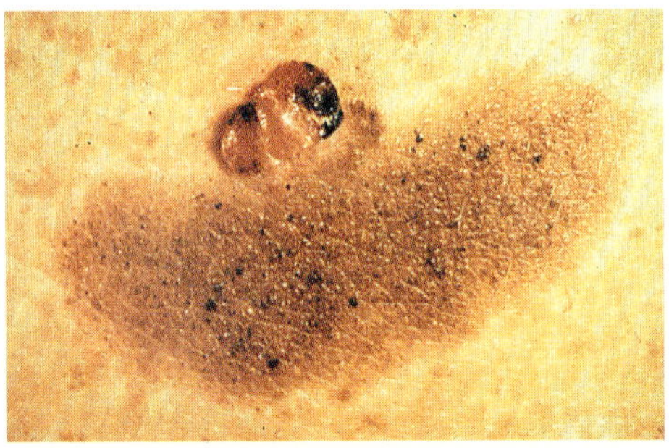

(a)

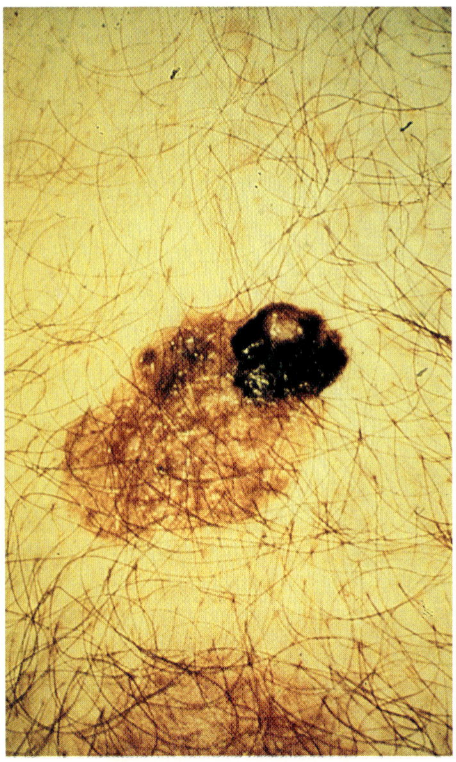

(b)

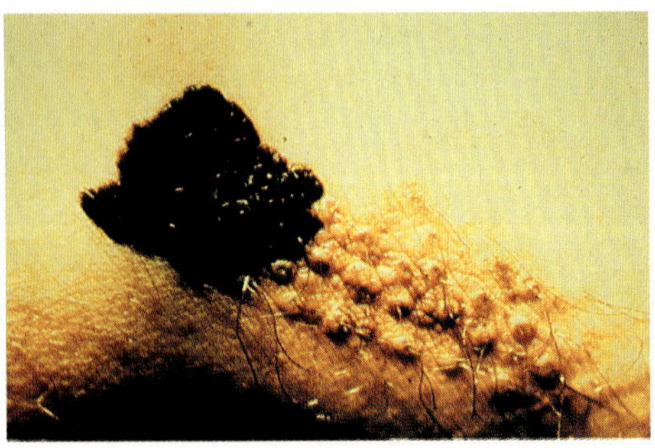

(c)

PLATE 10. *Melanoma developing in contiguity with relatively small varieties of "presumed" congenital nevomelanocytic nevi based on nevus size. (a) Melanoma developing in nevus measuring 7 × 4 cm on the back of a 52-year-old white female. (b) Melanoma developing in nevus measuring 3 × 2 cm on the breast of a 56-year-old white male. (c) Melanoma developing in nevus measuring 2 × 1.5 cm on the thigh of a 29-year-old white male. (Courtesy of Drs. L Illig, F Weidner, M Hundeiker, H Gartmann, B Biess, F Leyh, and E Paul, with permission from the publisher, Archives of Dermatology, October 1985, volume 121, pp 1274–1281, Copyright 1985, American Medical Association.)*

PLATE 11. *Lentigo maligna present for "many years" on the cheek of an 80-year-old white male. Note the haphazardly distributed shades of light brown, medium brown, and dark brown macular pigmentation and irregularity of borders. Scale in mm.*

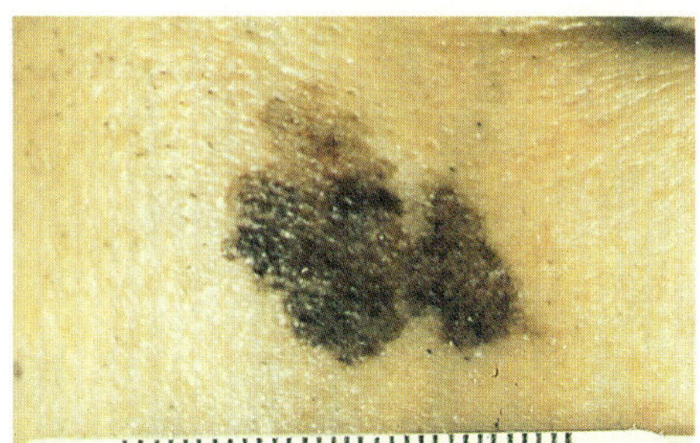

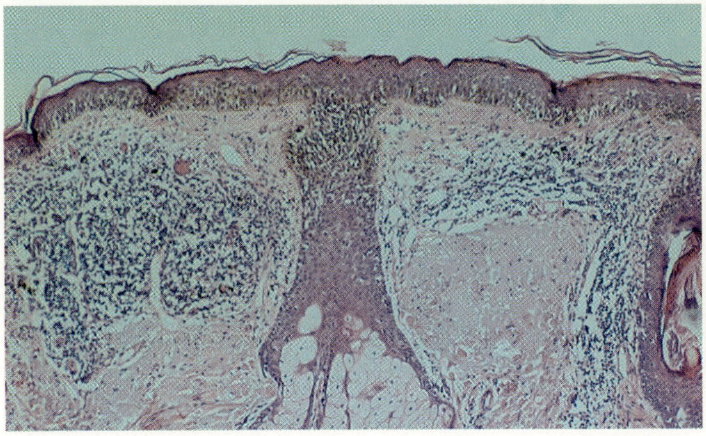

(a)

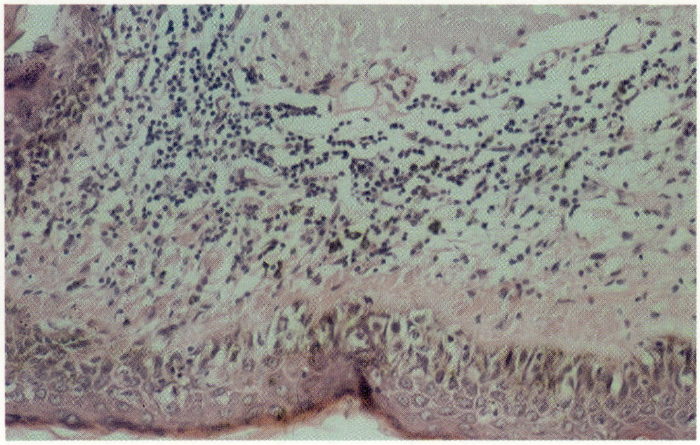

(b)

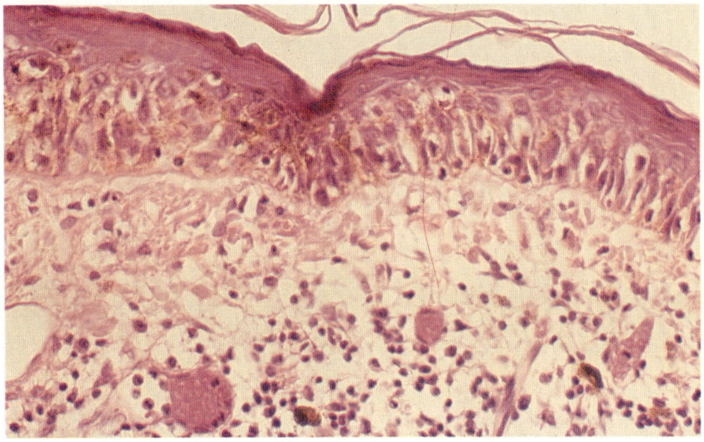

(c)

PLATE 12. *Histopathologic features of lentigo maligna shown in Plate 11. (a) Low magnification, showing an atrophic epidermis, intraepidermal melanocytic hyperplasia with variable cellular atypia, dense lymphohistiocytic infiltrates, and degeneration of collagen in the papillary dermis. Note involvement of hair follicle epithelium in the center of the field. Original magnification × 70.56. (b) Higher magnification of (a), showing intraepidermal melanocytic hyperplasia with variable cellular atypia within an effaced epidermis, associated with a dense lymphohistocytic infiltrate and degeneration of collagen in the dermis. Original magnification × 180. (c) Higher magnification, another field of same lesion, showing intraepidermal melanocytic hyperplasia with variable cellular atypia, associated with a dense lymphohistiocytic infiltrate in the dermis. Original magnification × 400. Hematoxylin and eosin stain.*

PLATE 13. *Melanoma (two separate foci, level III and level IV, respectively) developing in contiguity with lentigo maligna on the cheek of a 93-year-old white male. Note the two prominent black nodules within the patch of irregular macular black pigmentation. Scale in mm.*

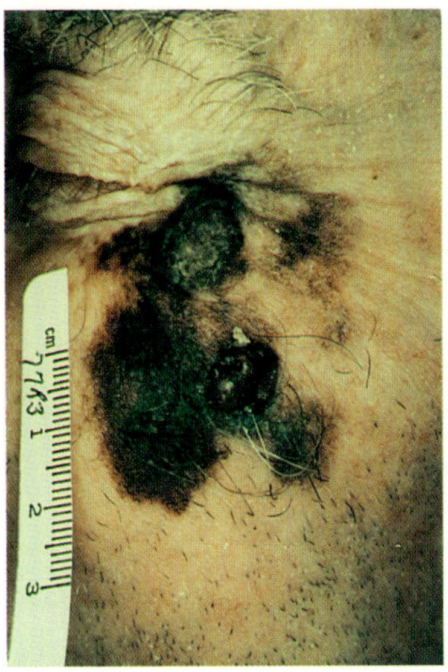

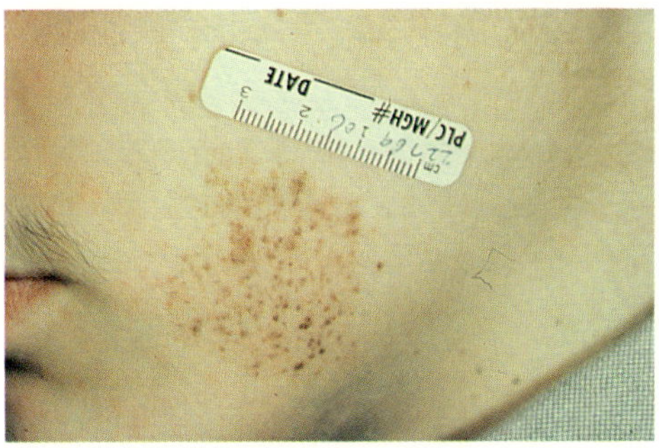

PLATE 14. *Nevus spilus on the cheek of a 13-year-old white male. Note the light brown and medium brown speckles of raised and flat pigmentation on a tan background. Scale in mm.*

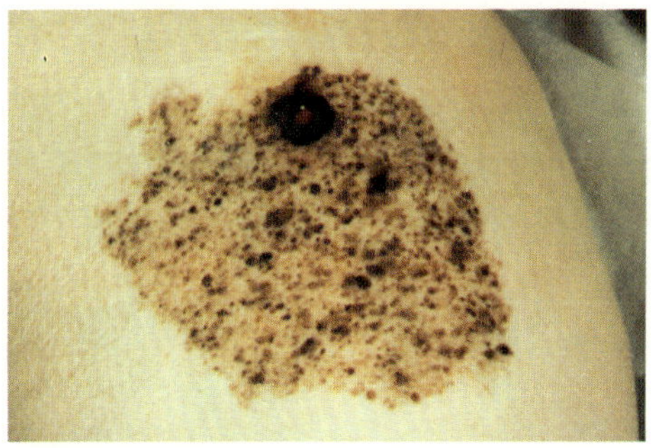

PLATE 15. *Melanoma developing in a congenital "dysplastic" nevus spilus on the leg of a 79-year-old white female. (Courtesy of Rhodes AR and Mihm MC, Archives of Dermatology, April 1990, volume 126, pp 500–505, Copyright 1990, American Medical Association.)*

PLATE 16. *Cellular blue nevus, present since infancy or birth, on the temporal scalp of a 32-year-old white male. Scale in mm.*

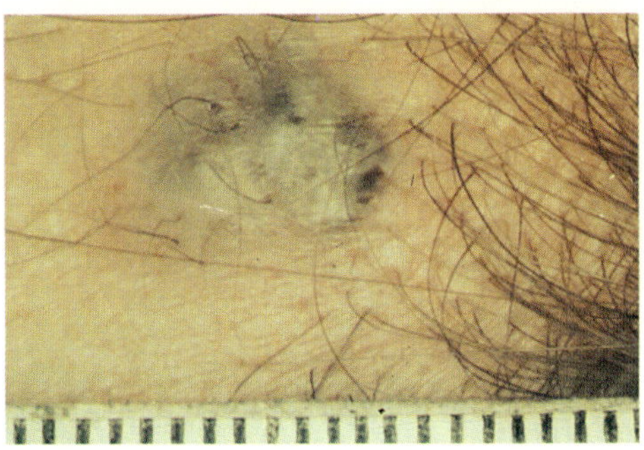

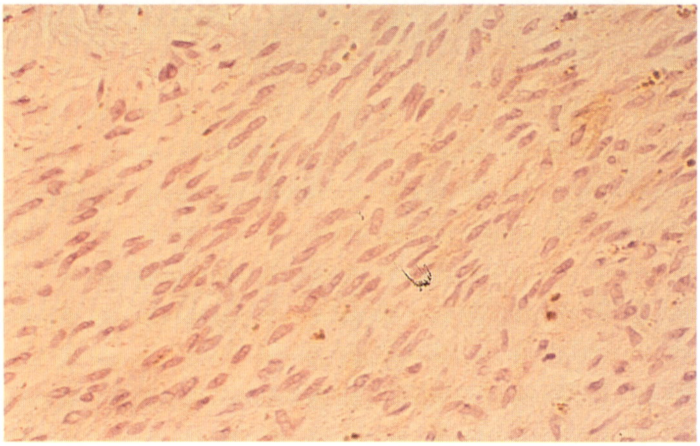

(a)

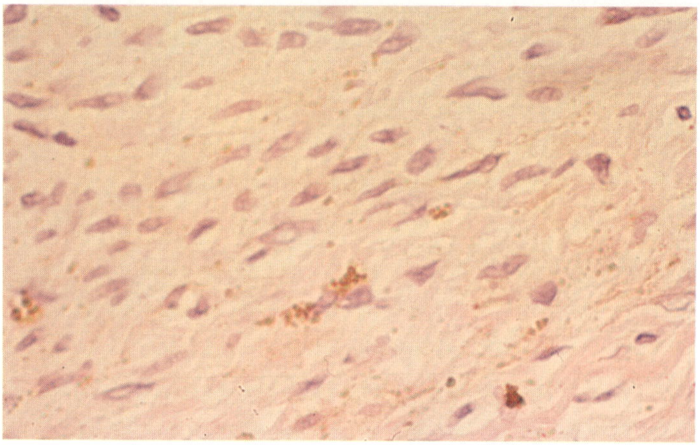

(b)

PLATE 17. *Histopathologic features of cellular blue nevus shown in Plate 16. (a) High magnification, showing nests and fascicles of spindle-shaped cells in the mid and deep reticular dermis. Original magnification × 560. (b) Higher magnification of another field, showing nests and fascicles of spindle-shaped cells with ovoid nuclei and abundant pale cytoplasm with no evident melanin, adjacent to similar cells with scattered melanin granules. Original magnification × 1120. Hematoxylin and eosin stain.*

PLATE 18. *Nevus of Ota. The blue-grey macular pigmentation on the temple and cheek of this 4-year-old Japanese female has been present since early infancy.*

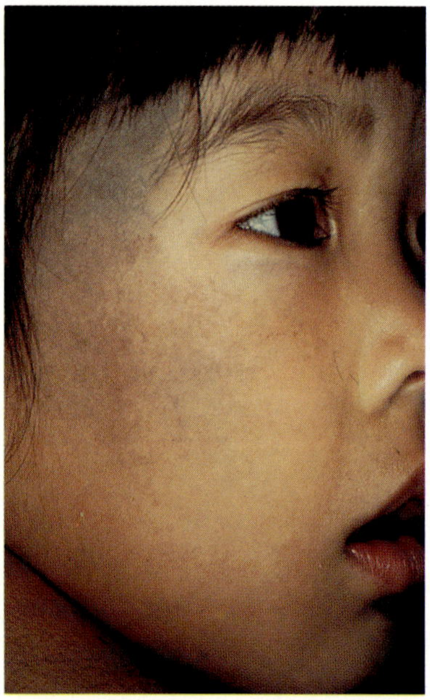

PLATE 19. *Nevus of Ito. The blue-grey macular pigmentation on the upper chest of this 25-year-old Japanese female has been present since early infancy.*

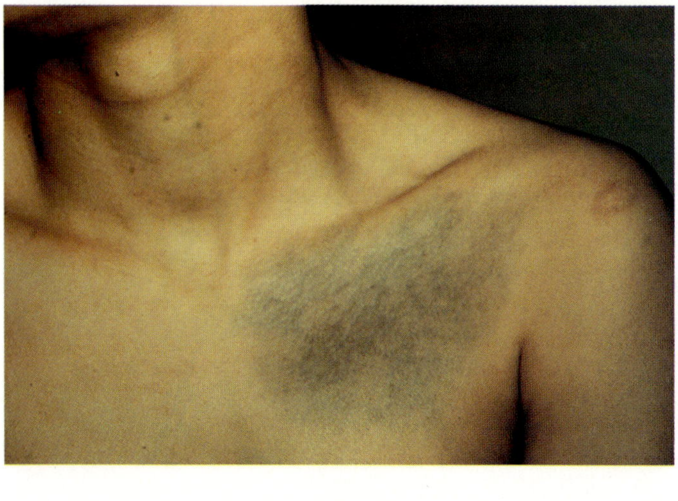

PLATE 20. *Congenital dermal melanocytosis (Mongolian spots), manifested as circumscribed blue-grey macules on the buttocks and sacrum of a 2-day-old Chinese female.*

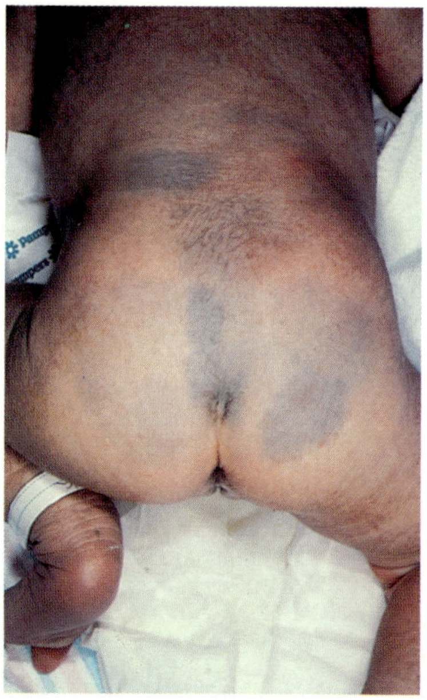

PLATE 21. *Acral melanocytic dysplasia, appearing as a circumscribed 5 × 3 mm macule with slightly variegated pigmentation and fuzzy borders, on the right plantar foot of a 44-year-old white male. Scale in mm.*

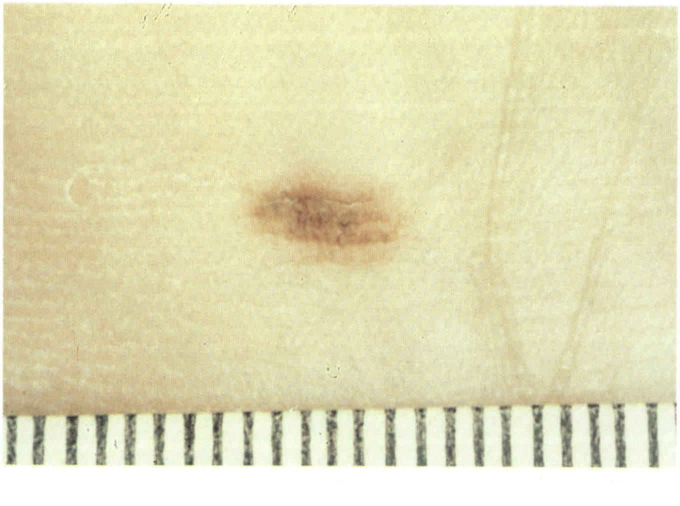

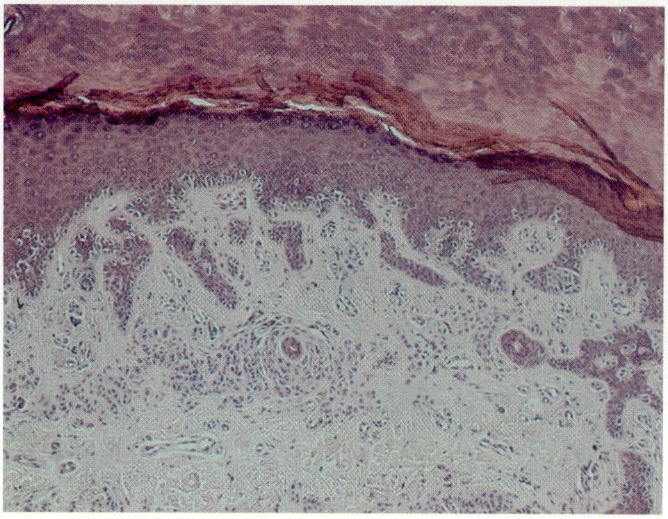

(a)

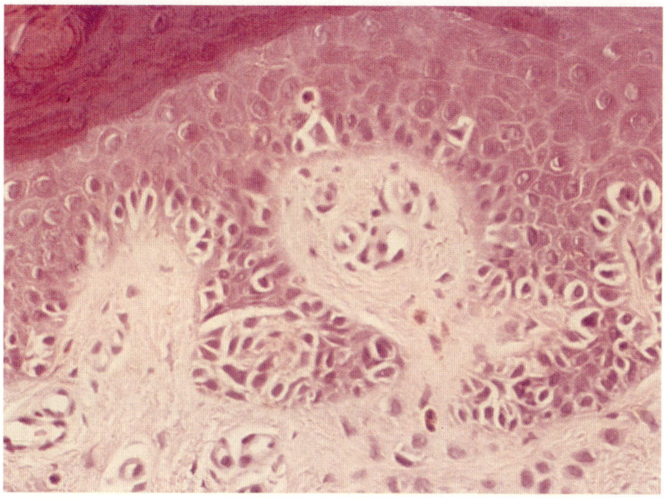

(b)

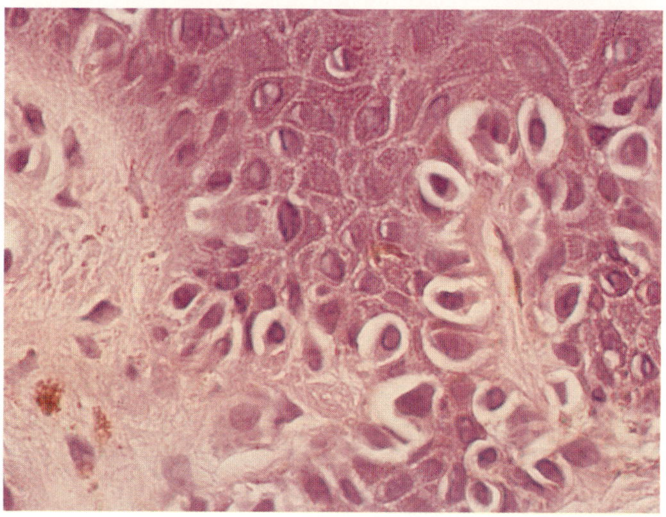

(c)

PLATE 22. *Histopathologic appearance of acral melanocytic dysplasia (lesion shown in Plate 21). (a) Low-power view, showing disordered intraepidermal melanocytic hyperplasia in a lentiginous epidermal pattern, associated with variable cellular atypia of individual melanocytes and a typical nest of nevus cells. Original magnification × 600. (b) Higher magnification of (a), showing intraepidermal melanocytic hyperplasia with mostly slight cellular atypia. Original magnification × 1200. Hematoxylin and eosin stain.*

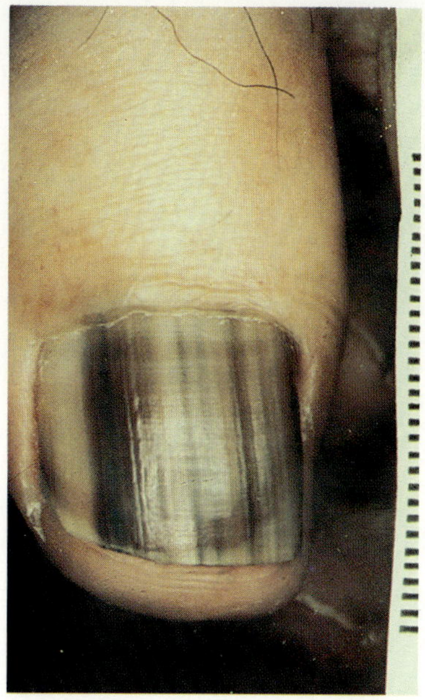

PLATE 23. *Acral melanocytic dysplasia of the nail bed on the first toe of a 65-year-old white male, present for many years and stable historically, histopathologically manifesting intraepidermal melanocytic hyperplasia with slight cellular atypia. Scale in mm.*

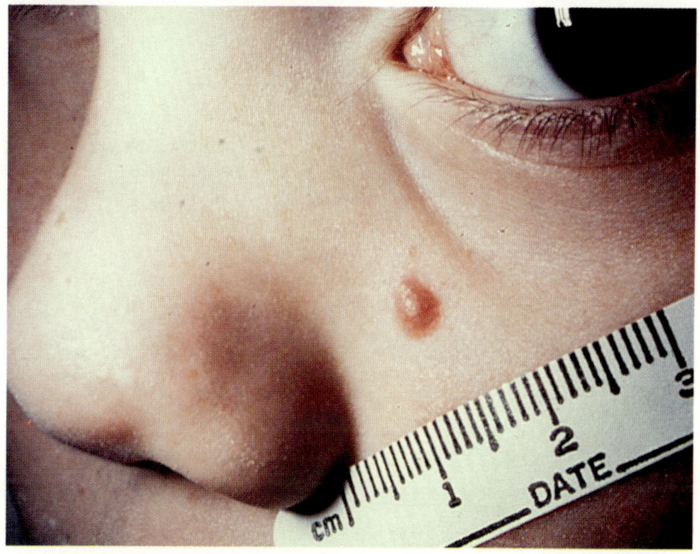

PLATE 24. *Epithelioid cell and/or spindle-cell nevus (Spitz tumor), predominantly epithelioid cell type, appearing as a dome-shaped, pink rubbery nodule on the left cheek of a 3-year-old white male, evolving over the course of 1 month approximately 10 months before. Scale in mm.*

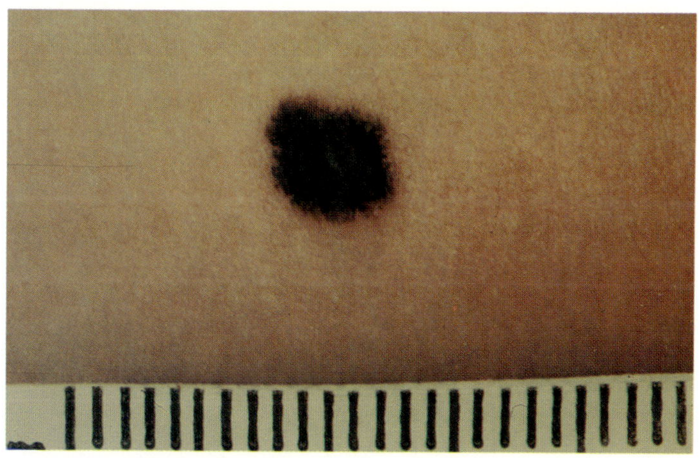

PLATE 25. *Pigmented spindle-cell nevus, appearing as a very dark brown plaque at age 1 year and slowly becoming darker and larger, on the forearm of a 3-year-old white female. Scale in mm.*

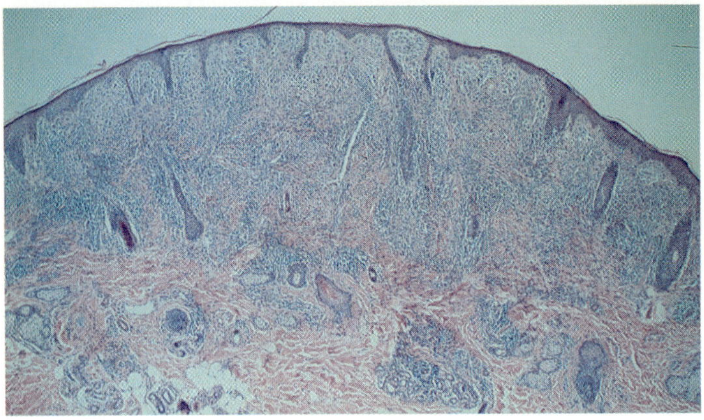

(a)

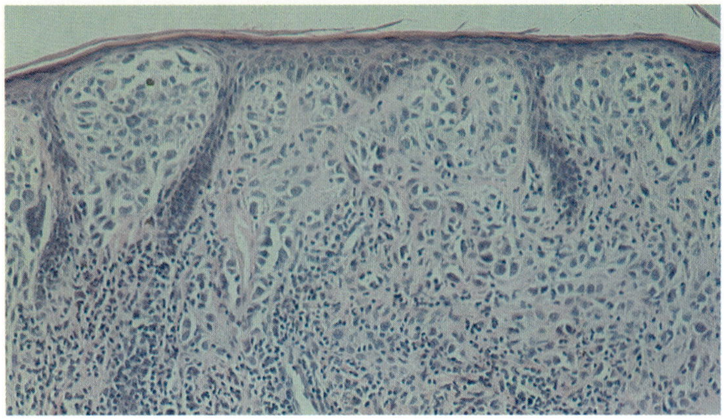

(b)

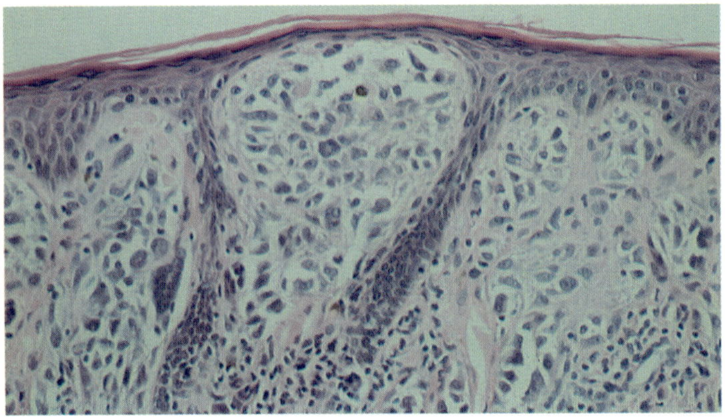

(c)

PLATE 26. *Histopathologic features of epithelioid cell and/or spindle-cell nevus, predominantly epithelioid cell type (Spitz tumor) (lesion shown in Plate 24). (a) Low-power view, showing a symmetrical tumor (side-to-side and top-to-bottom) with a wedge shape, plus a lymphohistiocytic infiltrate in the dermis. Original magnification × 28. (b) Higher magnification, showing polygonal and acidophilic cells with abundant cytoplasm disposed in irregular nests in the papillary dermis, some nests with artifactural clefts, with maturation of cells with increasing depth, associated with a lymphohistiocytic infiltrate. Original magnification × 112. (c) Higher magnification of (b), showing bizarre polygonal and acidophilic cells with abundant cytoplasm disposed in irregular nests in the papillary dermis, associated with multinucleated cells. Original magnification × 180. Hematoxylin and eosin stain.*

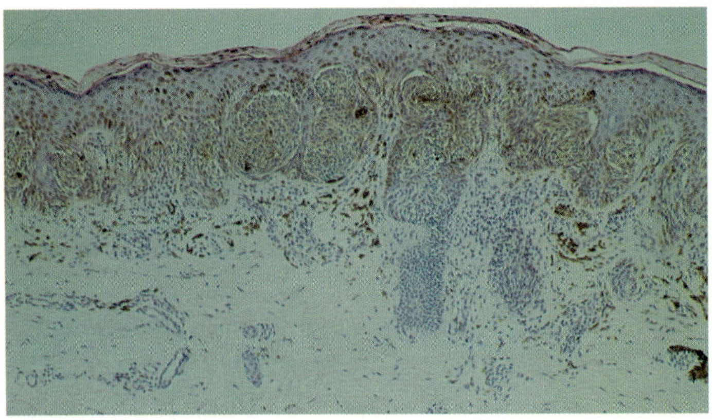

(a)

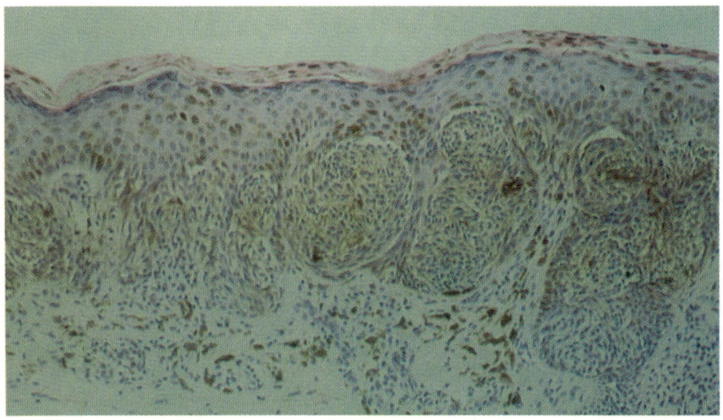

(b)

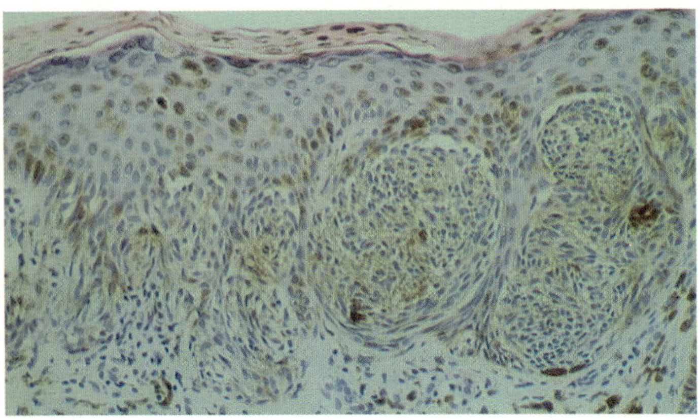

(c)

PLATE 27. *Histopathologic features of pigmented spindle-cell nevus (lesion shown in Plate 25). (a) Low magnification, showing irregular intraepidermal nests of compactly aggregated spindle-shaped, pigment-producing melanocytes, plus lymphohistiocytic infiltrates at the base of the tumor. Original magnification × 70.6 (b) Higher magnification of (a), showing compact intraepidermal nests of spindle-shaped, pigment-producing melanocytes. Original magnification × 112. (c) Higher magnification of (b), showing compact nests of pigment-producing, spindle-shaped melanocytes in the epidermis, plus a lymphohistiocytic infiltrate and melanin-containing macrophages in the papillary dermis. Original magnification × 180. Hematoxylin and eosin stain.*

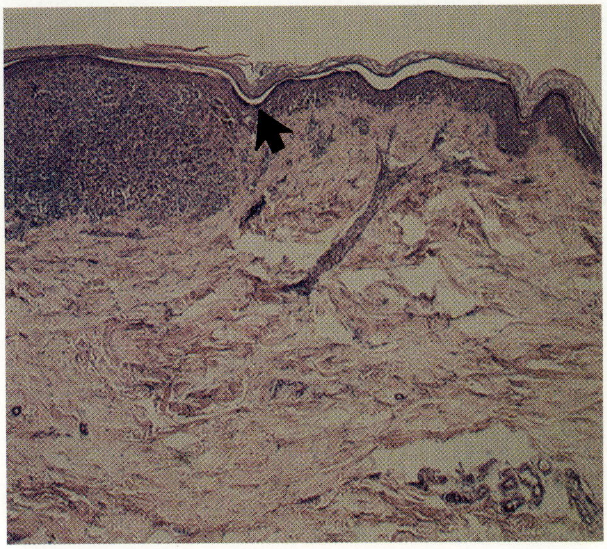

PLATE 28. Superficial spreading melanoma: *A superficial spreading malignant melanoma in its radial (arrow) and vertical growth phases. The latter phase is characterized by an expansile nodule of epithelioid cells filling and expanding the papillary dermis (double arrow) (×32.5). (inset) Close-up view demonstrates both growth phases. Note atypical melanocytes scattered throughout the epidermis, characteristic of the radial growth phase (×130).*

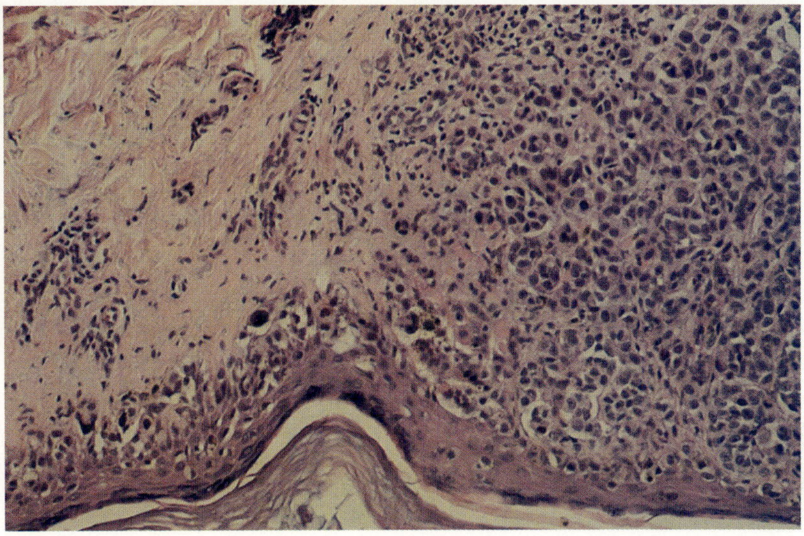

(inset)

PLATE 29. Acral lentiginous melanoma: *Large, heavily pigmented dendritic atypical melanocytes involve the epidermis and are proliferating into the reticular dermis (×28.3) (inset) Highly dendritic, large melanocytes with coarsely granular melanin (×520).*

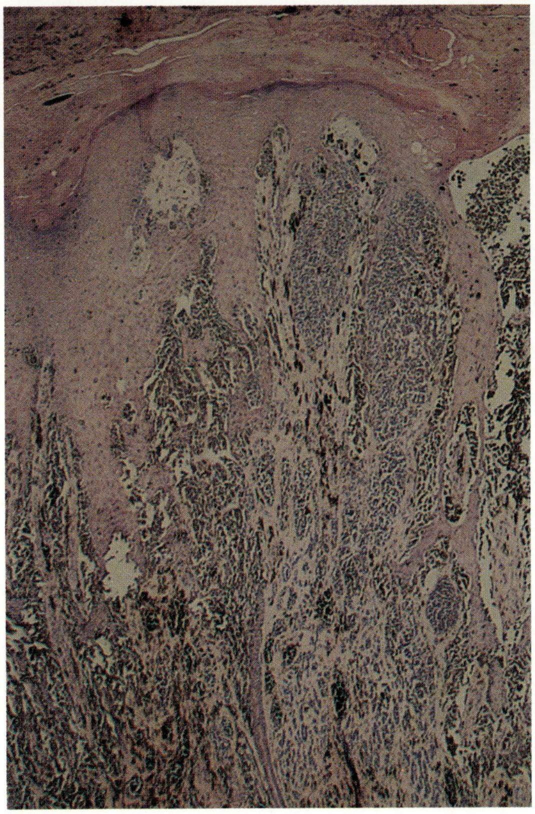

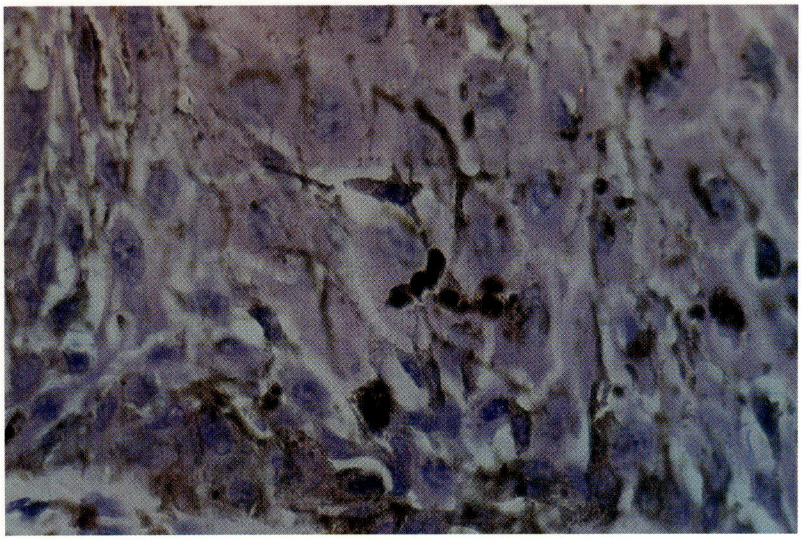

(inset)

(inset)

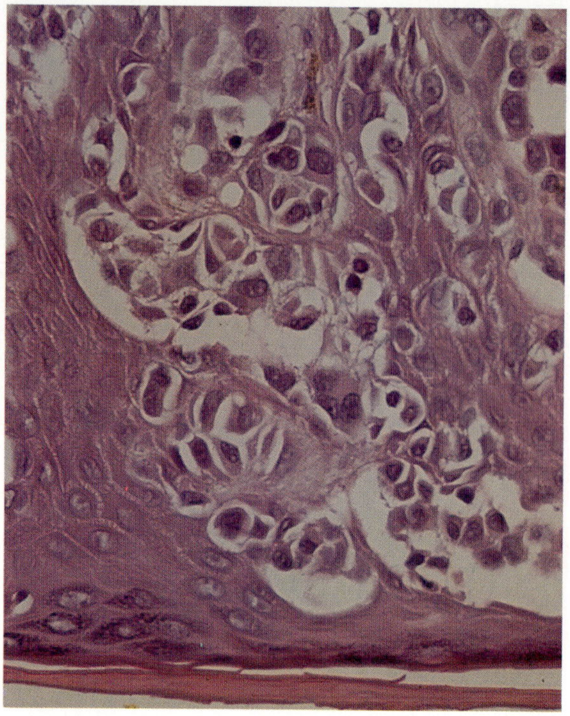

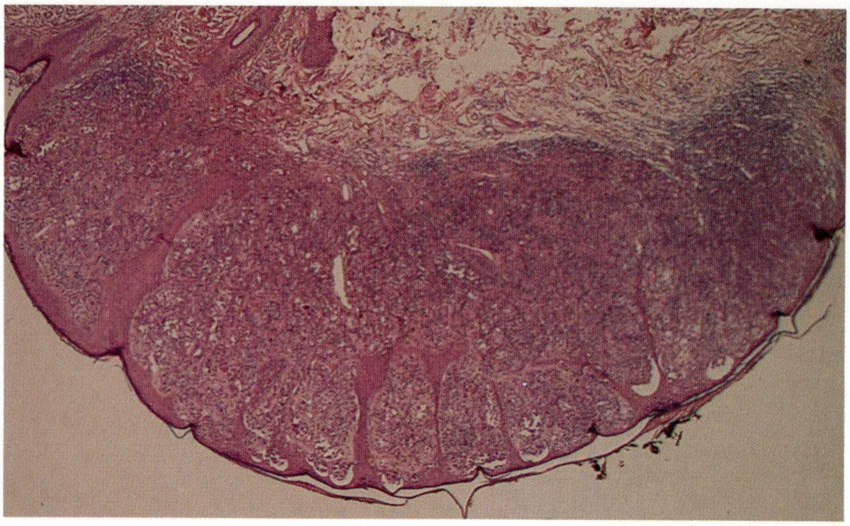

PLATE 30. Nodular melanoma: *An expansile nodule is filling the papillary dermis and invading the reticular dermis. This "pure" vertical growth phase is characteristic of nodular melanomas. (×32.5). (inset) Note anaplastic cells with markedly hyperchromatic nuclei and large nuclear-to-cytoplasmic ratios (×520).*

PLATE 31. Desmoplastic melanoma: *Randomly arrayed spindle cells and melanophages are observed amid a prominently fibrotic stroma (×32.5). (inset) The infiltrative nature of this neoplasm is noted here occurring along the eccrine ducts (arrow) and the neural bundles (double arrow). The hypercellularity of the nerve represents early invasion (×130).*

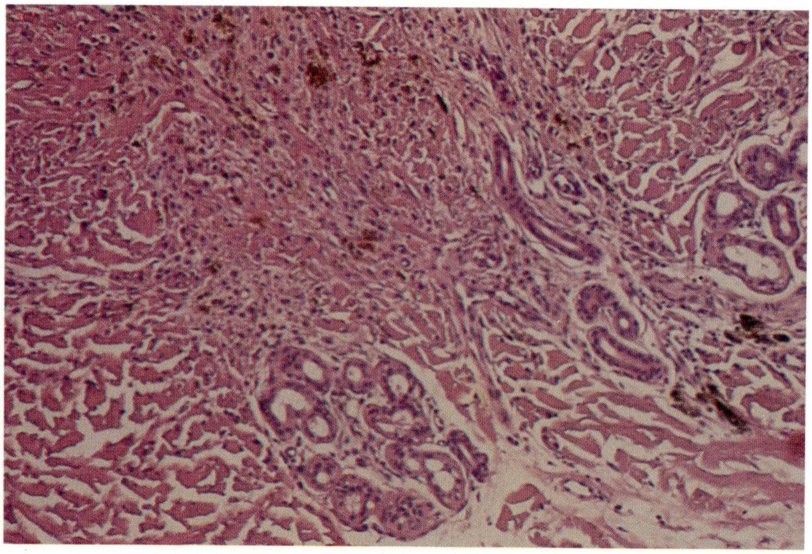

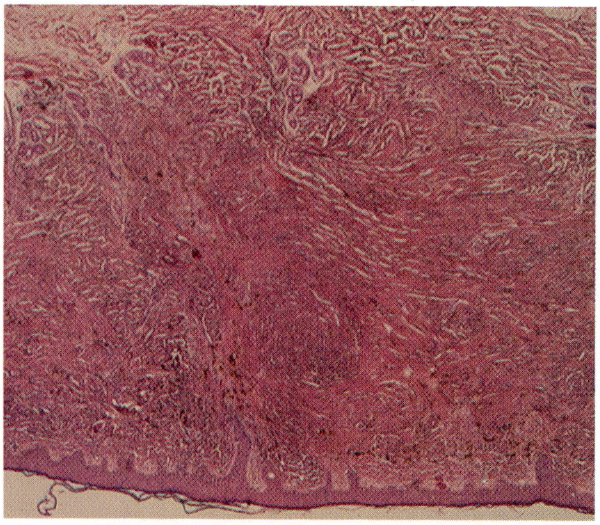

PLATE 32. Regressed melanoma: *Dense fibrosis amid a residual papillary dermal inflammatory infiltrate and aggregates of melanophages characterize this melanoma undergoing regression. Note the prominent fibrosis (arrow), melanophages (arrow-head), and ectatic blood vessels (double arrow) (×67.5).*

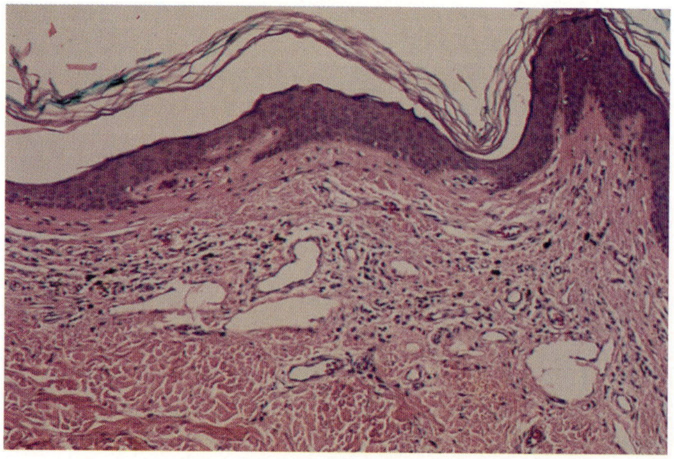

(inset)

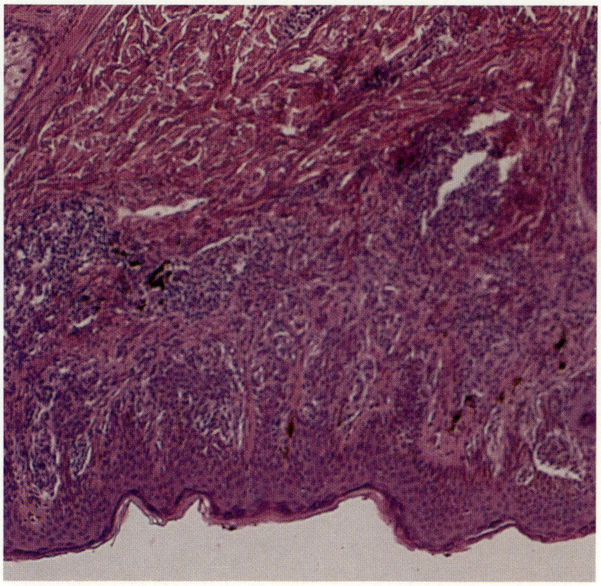

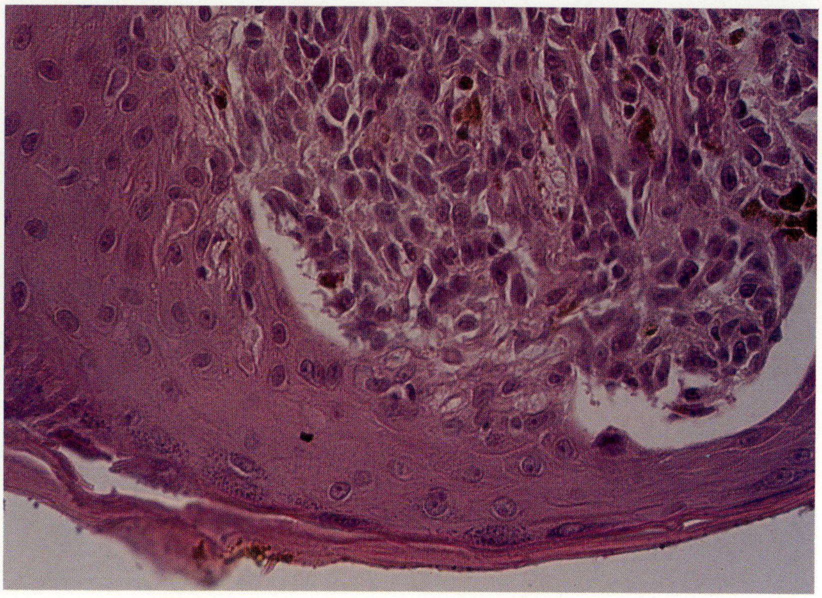

PLATE 33. Spitz nevus: *Spindle and epithelioid cells are arranged in intraepidermal nests and dermal fascicles exhibiting the "maturation" phenomenon amid prominent dermal fibrosis (×35). (inset) "Supra-nest capping" is a commonly observed feature in Spitz nevi (×350).*

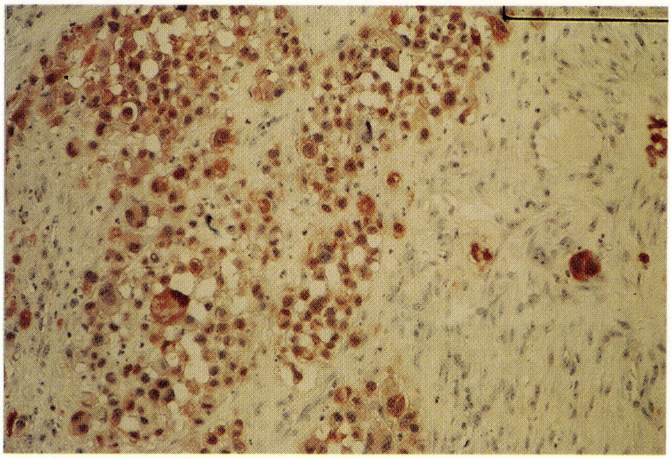

PLATE 34. *Paraffin section of melanoma metastasis stained with anti-S100 polyclonal antibody. The immunostaining is visualized by aminoethylcarbazole (×160, counterstained with hematoxylin).*

PLATE 35. *Frozen section of amelanotic melanoma metastasis stained with NKI/beteb monoclonal antibody. Note the granular intracytoplasmic staining pattern in clusters of positive tumor cells (×400, aminoethylcarbazole, counterstained with hematoxylin).*

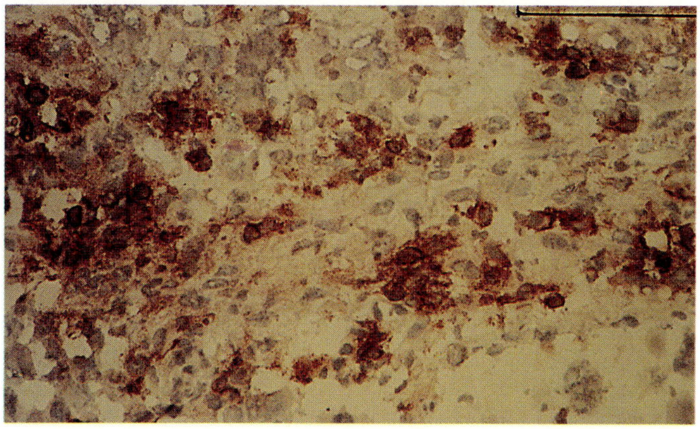

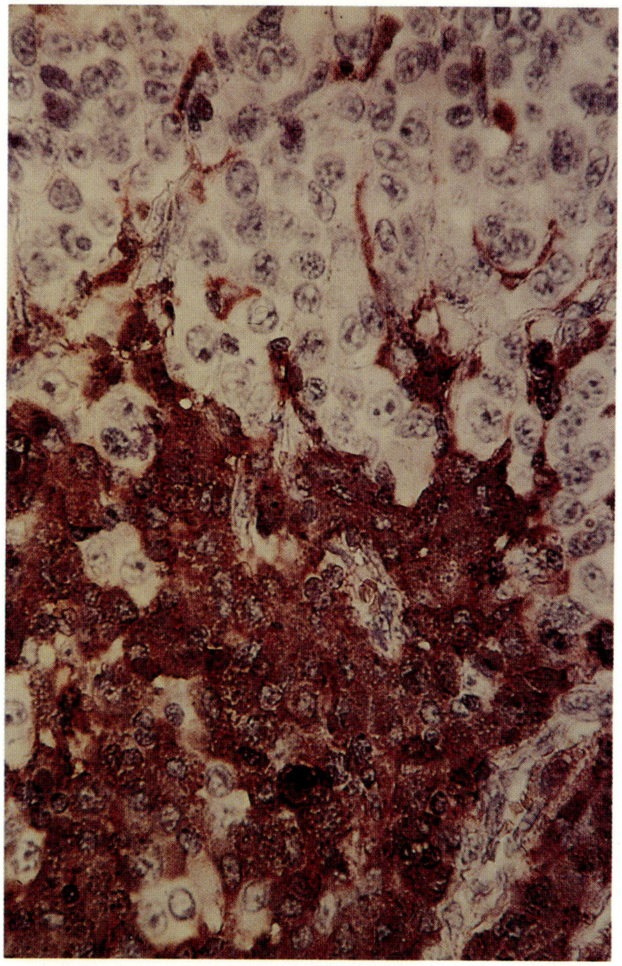

PLATE 36. *Formalin-fixed paraffin section of a melanoma metastasis stained with the anti-HLA-DR-mAB 910 D7.*[65] *Note the intralesional heterogeneity of antigen expression.*

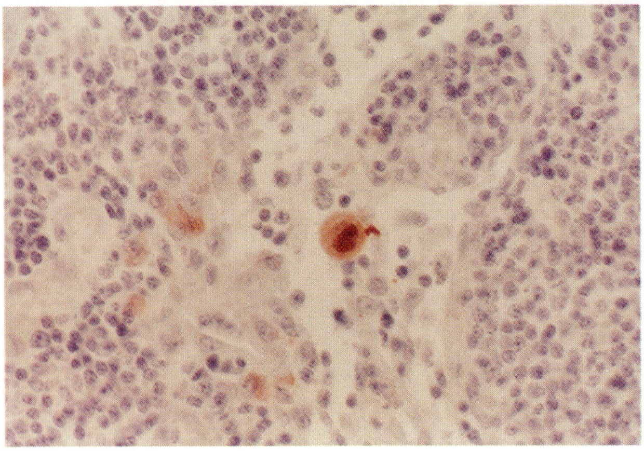

(a)

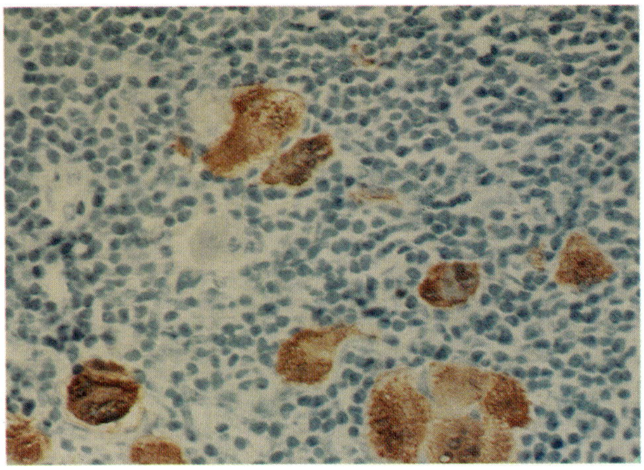

(b)

Plate 37. *"Occult" melanoma cells in blue dyed delineated "sentinel" nodes. (a) In this case tumor cells were not visible in frozen or permanent sections stained with hematoxylin and eosin, but they were readily visible in sections stained intraoperatively by our rapid immunohistochemical technique (× 250) and in sections from the formalin-fixed, paraffin-embedded block prepared from the frozen tissue. (b) In this case, small numbers of tumor cells were detected in the sentinel nodes intraoperatively in H & E and immuno-stained frozen sections and confirmed in the permanent preparations (× 340). (In both cases, the first antibody is anti-S-100 protein, the developer aminoethylcarbazole and the counterstain hematoxylin.)*

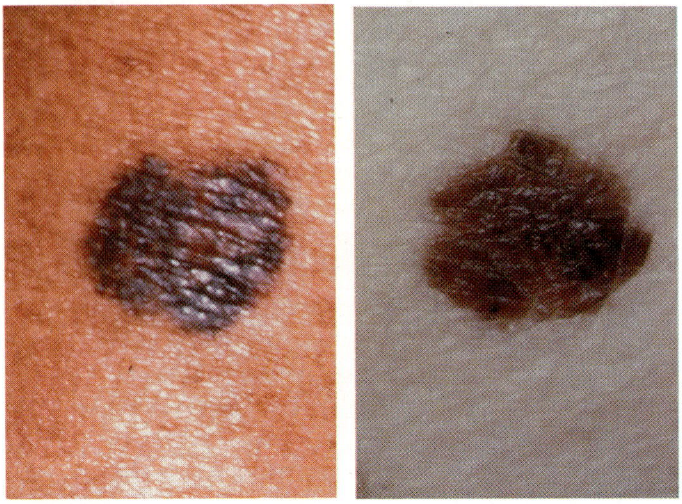

PLATES 38 AND 39. *Nonpalpable melanoma; typical dark lesions with well-defined margins. The shape is slightly asymmetric in both lesions.*

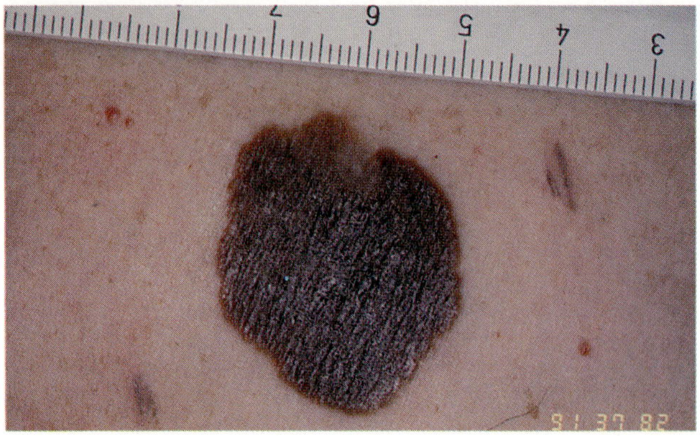

PLATE 40. *Palpable melanoma; raised, dark, pigmented lesion with irregular margins.*

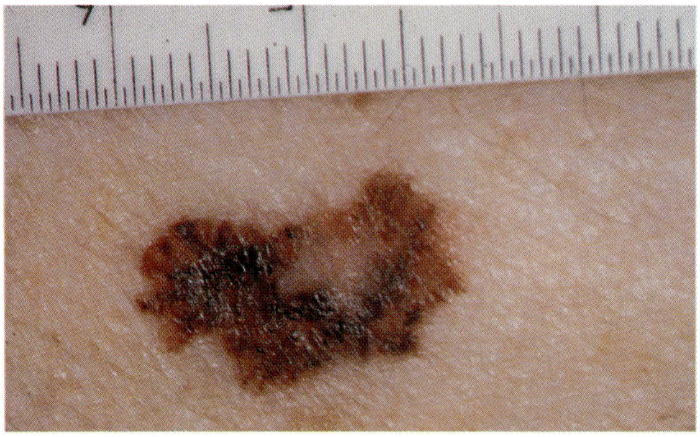

PLATE 41. *Spontaneous regression, in its initial phase, the lesion being lightly pigmented with irregular margins and heterogenous distribution of the color.*

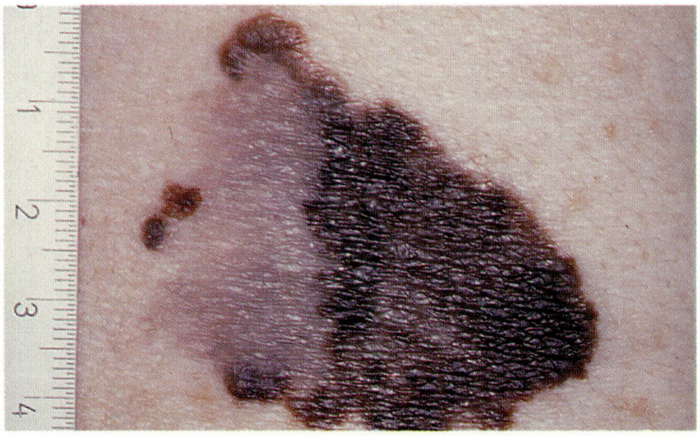

PLATE 42. *Advanced regression of a dark-pigmented lesion.*

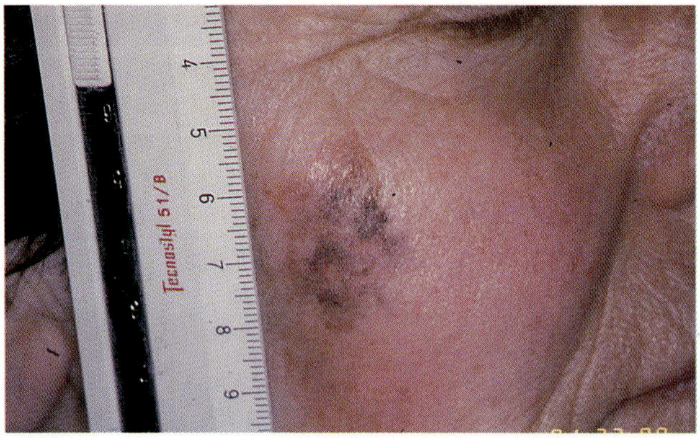

PLATE 43. *Flat facial lesion commonly found in the older patient. Irregularly distributed pigmentation.*

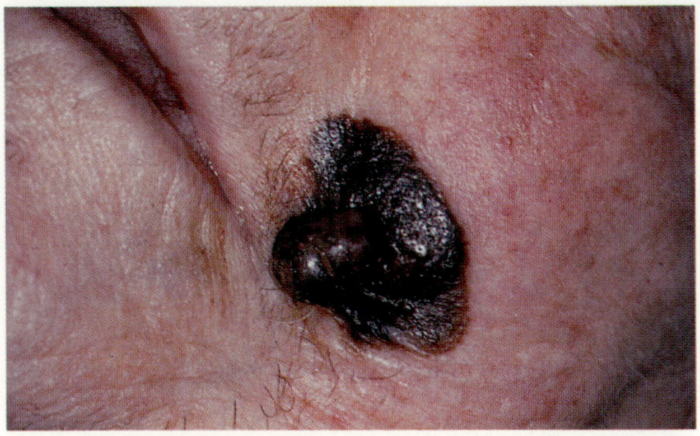

PLATE 44. *Cutaneous melanoma of the face in a more advanced stage than that shown in Plate 43, with increased pigmentation and nodular development.*

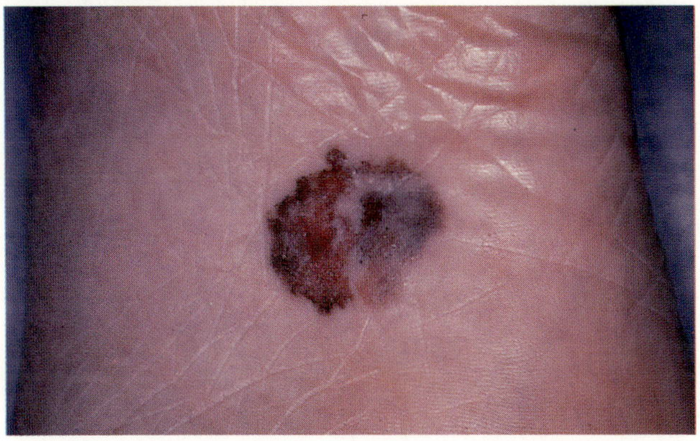

PLATE 45. *Advanced plantar lesion in a caucasian patient. In this lesion, the typical features of primary melanoma are particularly evident.*

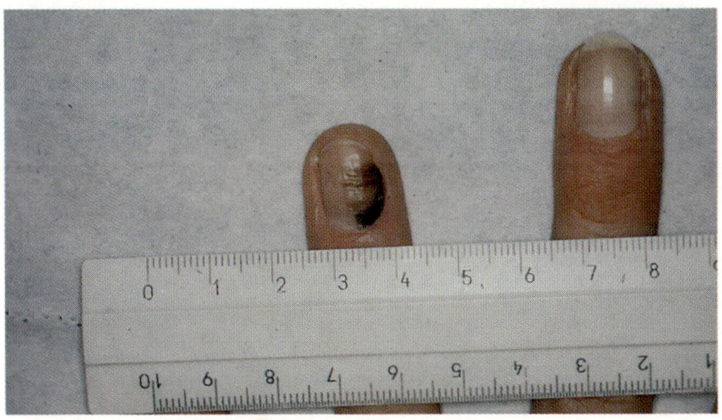

PLATE 46. *Photograph of a subungual melanoma. Final diagnosis is possible only after removal of the nail and biopsy of the nail bed.*

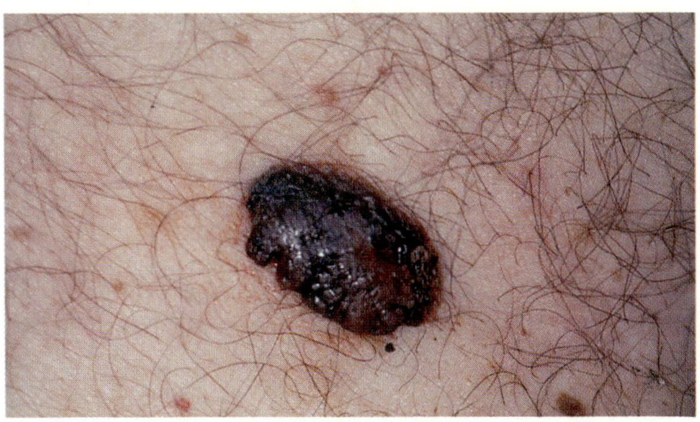

PLATE 47. *A raised nodular melanoma with marginal ulceration.*

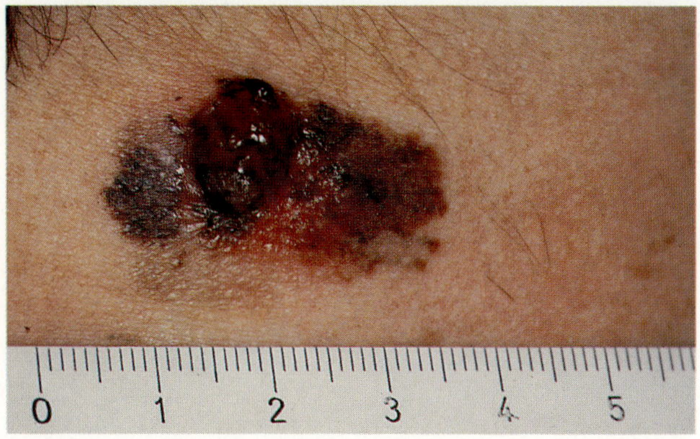

PLATE 48. *A flat melanoma with a large nodule on its surface. The nodule is less pigmented and ulcerated.*

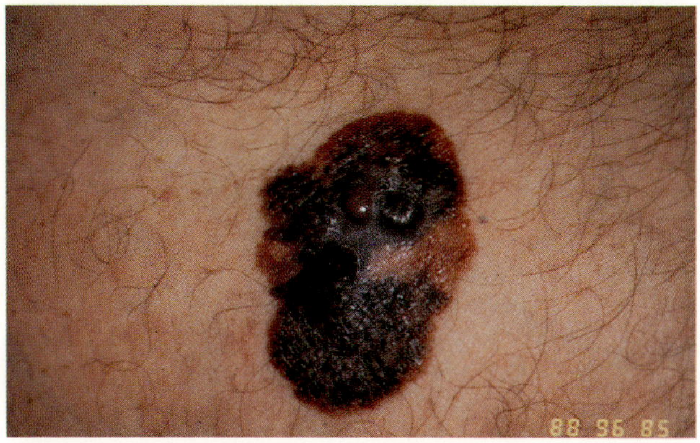

PLATE 49. *Black and brown nodules developing in a palpable melanoma. There is also an area of spontaneous regression.*

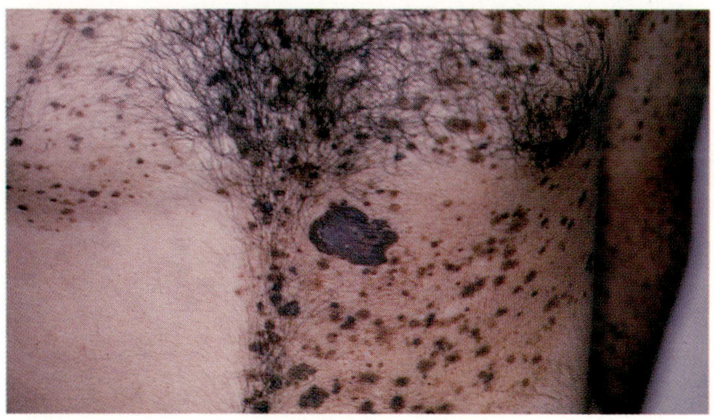

PLATE 50. *Giant nevus in a young male patient in which a palpable melanoma has developed.*

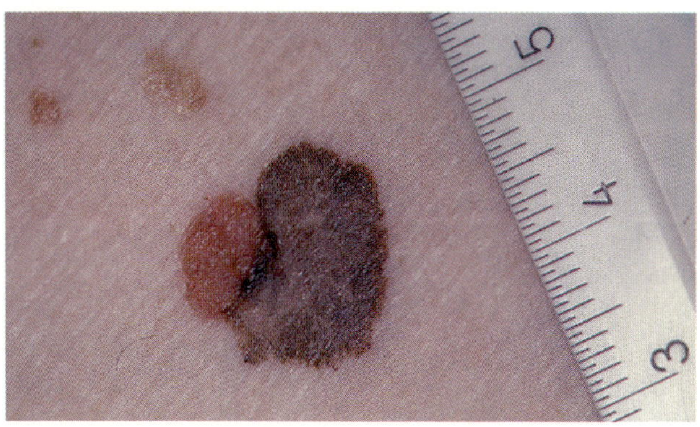

PLATE 51. *A thin melanoma developing near compound navus.*

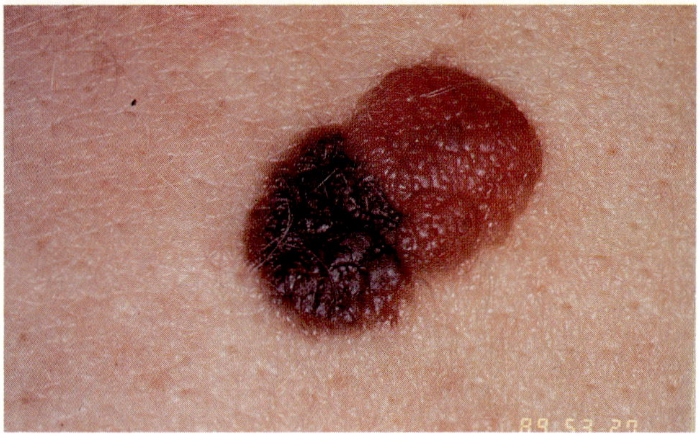

PLATE 52. *A palpable melanoma developing near acquired intradermal nevus.*

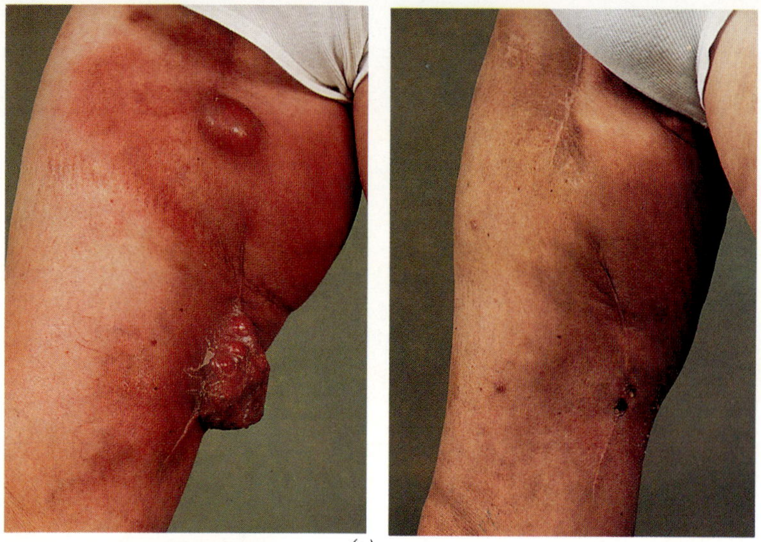

(a) *(b)*

Plate 54. *Inflammatory recurrent melanoma in the inguinal region in a 63-year-old female patient (left photograph). Complete remission is seen 2 months after a "borderline" true hyperthermic perfusion (tissue temperatures between 41–42°C during the whole hour of Melphalan perfusion) (right photograph). The duration of the complete remission was short, namely 4 months; the patient died 13 months after perfusion of hematogenic metastases.*

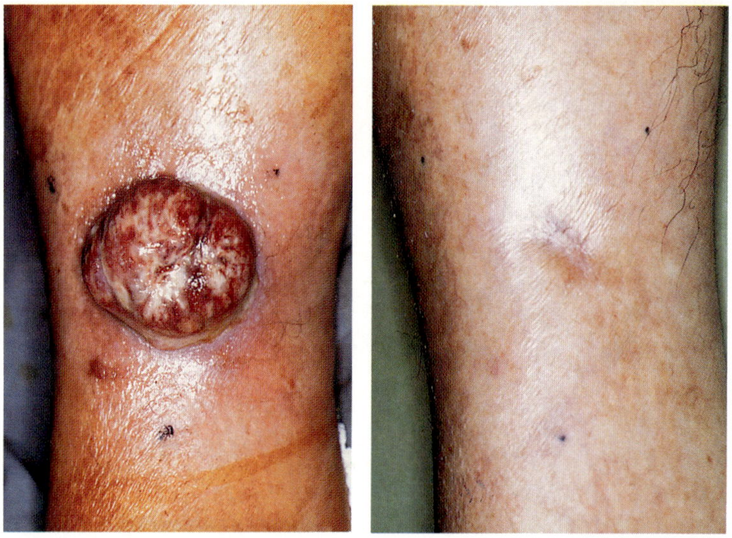

(a) *(b)*

Plate 53. *A local recurrence of the lower leg in an 83-year-old female patient (left photograph). Complete remission is obtained 3 months after a single normothermic (tissue temperatures between 37–38°C) perfusion with Melphalan (right photograph). The patient is alive with no evidence of disease, 5 years after perfusion treatment. (Reprinted with permission of Dreschler J.M. et al, De Kankerpatiënt, Bohn, Stafleu, Van Loghum, The Netherlands, 1988.)*

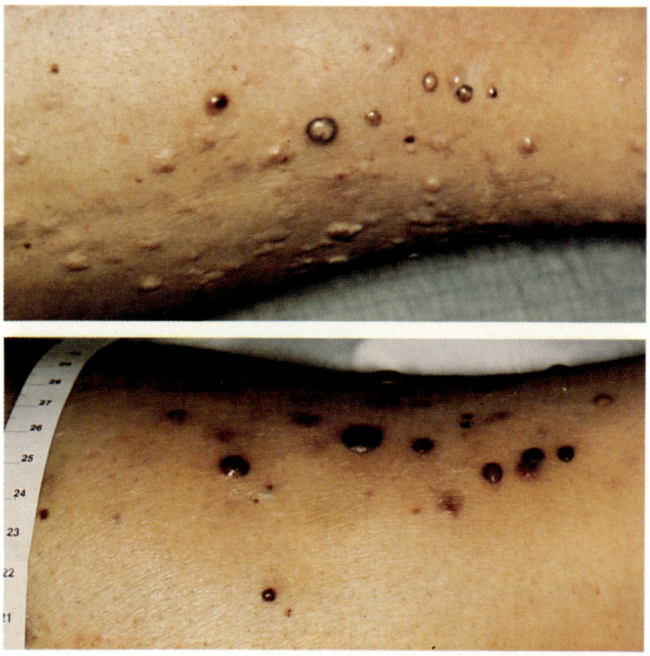

(a)

(b)

Plate 55. *Female, age 56, presenting more than 100 amelanotic in transit melanoma metastasis on right lower limb. No prior therapy. (a) External aspect of the R. thigh before isolation perfusion. (b) Same region 48 hours after isolation perfusion with 3 mg rTNFα alone for 60 minutes at 40°C. Tumor nodules have become hemorragic and necrotic.*

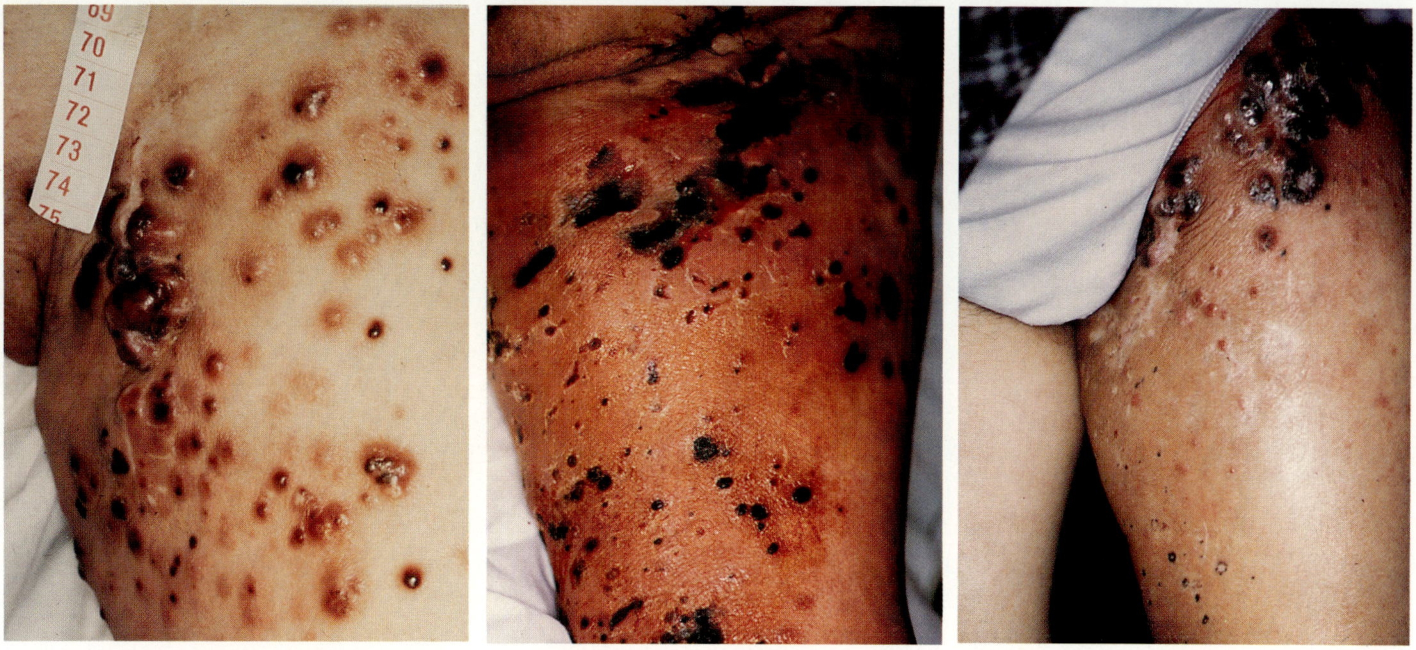

(a) (b) (c)

Plate 56. *Female, age 83, presenting more than 100 in transit melanoma metastasis on left lower limb including proximal inguinal region. No prior therapy. (a) L. thigh antero-internal aspect before isolation perfusion. (b) Same region 11 days after isolation perfusion. Black areas correspond to complete tumor necrosis according to the histological study. (c) Same region 8 months after perfusion. Bulky recurrences in the proximal area while the rest of the thigh remains tumor free. Black dots on distal part are tatoos resulting from tumor regression.*

Plate 57. *Female, age 56, same as Plate 55. Continuing complete remission 23 months after two isolation perfusions with rTNFα, INFγ, and melphalan.*

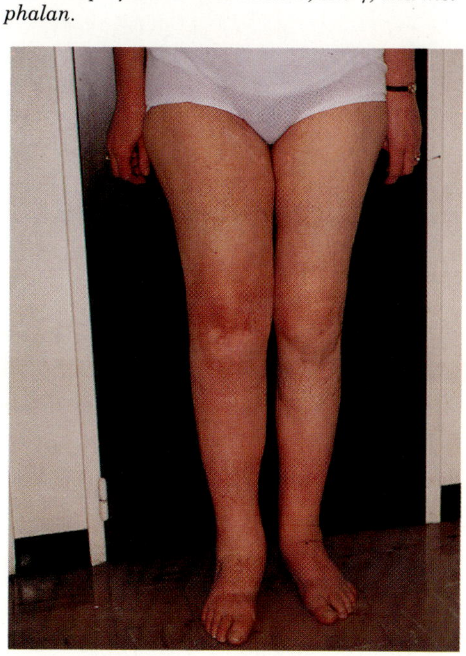

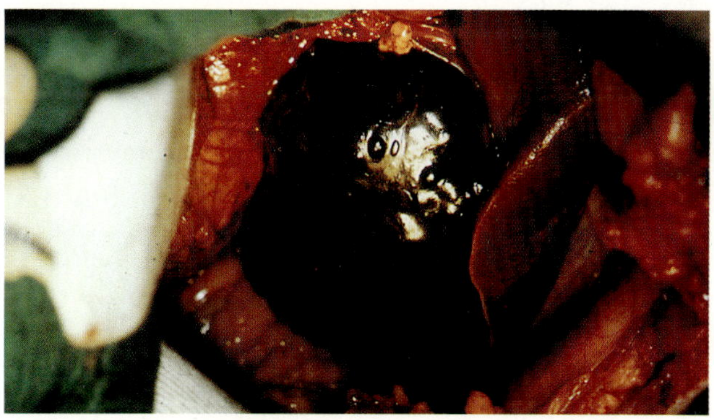

Plate 58. *Melanoma liver metastasis before chemoembolization.*

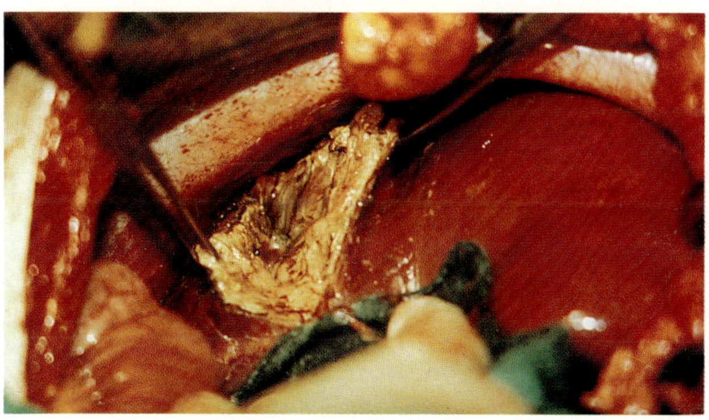

Plate 59. *Necrotic melanoma liver metastasis at second look laparotomy.*

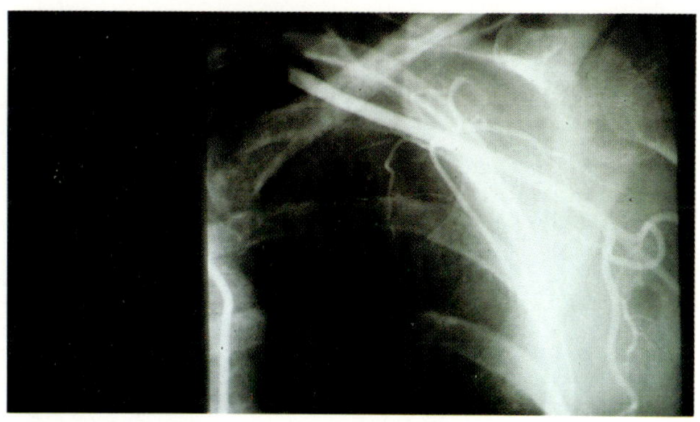

Plate 60. *Subclavian artery blocking with balloon catheter.*

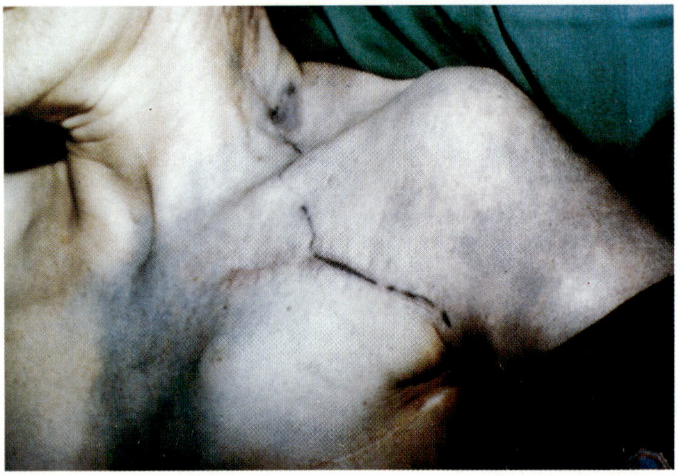

Plate 61. *Blue staining of subclavian infusion area. Upper arm is blocked with pneumatic cuff.*

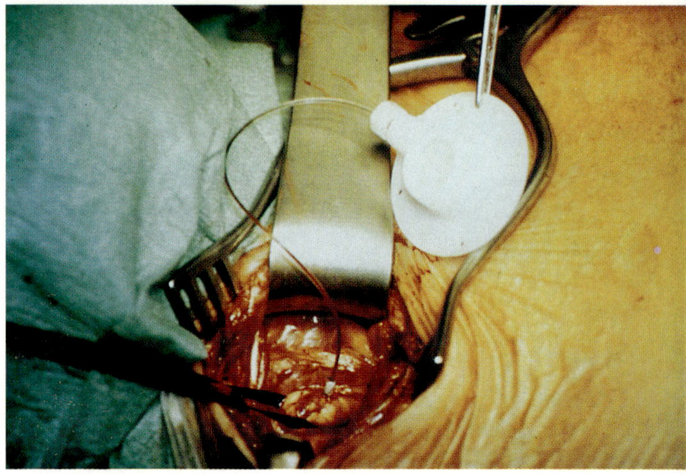

Plate 62. *End-to-side implantation of Jet Port Allround catheter in proximal subclavian artery.*

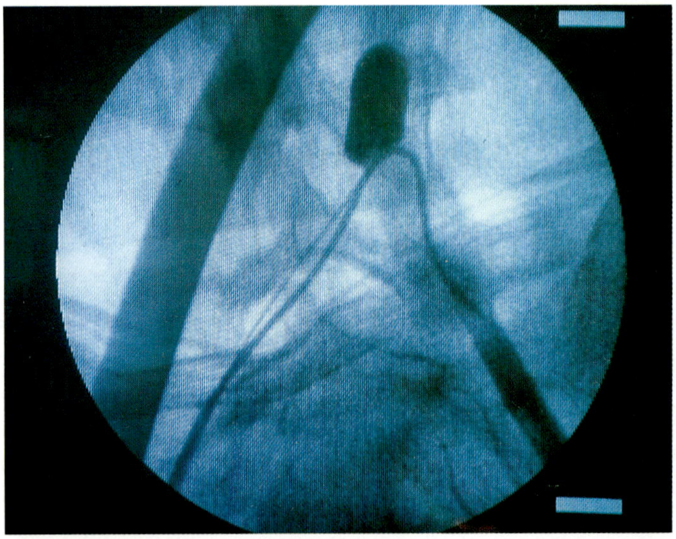

Plate 63. *Balloon blocking of aortic bifurcation. Infusion of left common iliac artery through side winder catheter.*

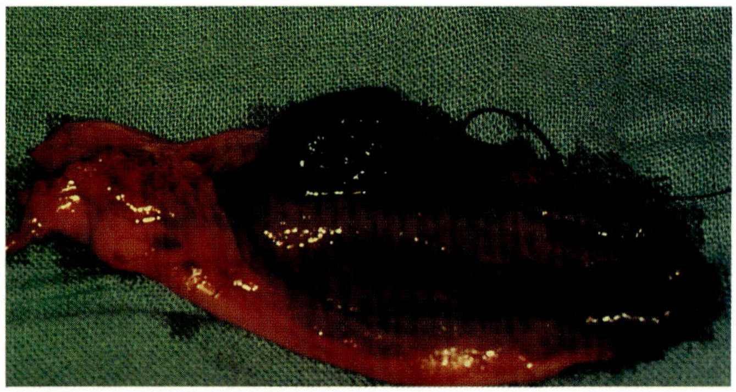

PLATE 64. *Malignant melanoma metastasis into the resected gallbladder of the same patient. She is still alive more than 3 years later with no evidence of disease.*

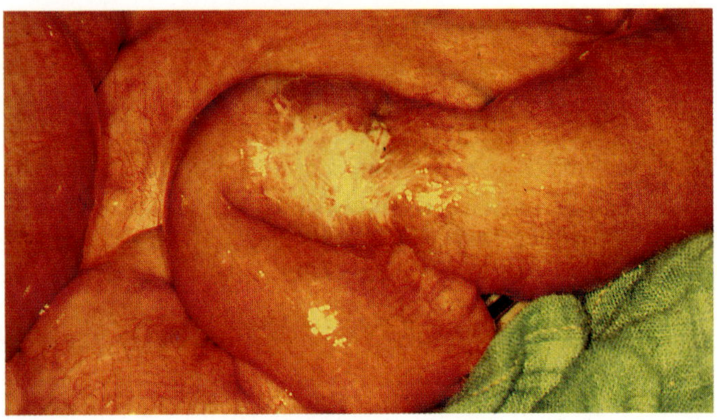

PLATE 65. *Percutaneous cholangiogram showing a tumor occupying the proximal common bile duct in a 58-year-old female patient with a history of malignant melanoma of the left lower limb presenting with an obstructive jaundice, 3 years after excision of the primary lesion. The resection of the extrapancreatic main bile duct with a Y-shaped hepaticojejunostomy was performed. The patient was discharged in an excellent general condition, with normal bilirubin levels. She died from disseminated disease, 2 years and 5 months after the resection of the biliary metastasis.*

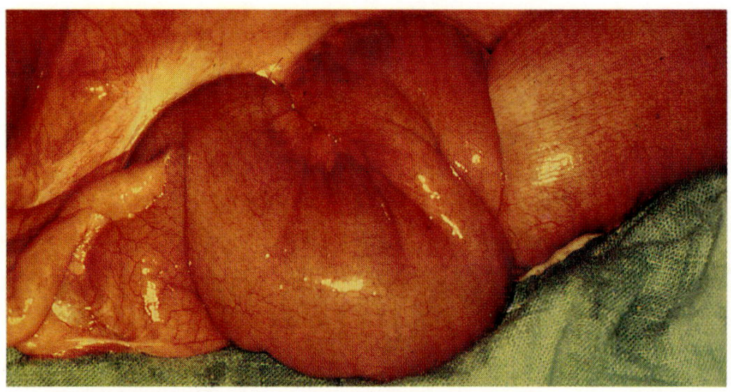

PLATE 66. *Intussusception of the small bowel due to a malignant melanoma metastatic polyp.*

Lesions that are suspected of being melanocytic dysplasia (or melanoma) should be considered for histopathologic examination. If the histopathologic features of a clinically atypical-appearing lesion is interpreted as "typical," sampling of other parts of the lesion and/or periodic lifelong photographic follow-up are strongly suggested.

Any pigmented nevus of the nail bed should be considered for histopathologic examination in whites, and evaluated on an individual basis in darkly pigmented races.

COURSE AND PROGNOSIS

Based on observations of intraepidermal melanocytic dysplasias in contiguity with at least some acral and mucosal melanomas,[178,272,287,289–296,298–300,302] it may be presumed that some varieties of acral and mucosal melanocytic dysplasias may be potential precursors of melanoma. In a report of 60 acral lentiginous melanomas,[287] an associated dermal nevomelanocytic nevus could be identified in continuity with the tumor in 13 percent of cases. Congenital nevomelanocytic nevi have been identified as precursors of acral lentiginous melanoma in some cases.[178,287] The absence of an identifiable dermal nevomelanocytic nevus component in continuity with 69 melanomas in another series of acral melanomas[288] suggests that precursor lesions with dermal nevomelanocytes may have been missed due to inadequate sampling or destruction of the precursor by the melanoma, that the populations studied may have been different, or that the nature of precursor melanocytic lesions on palms and soles may be different from those on other cutaneous sites and/or misinterpreted as the radial growth phase of, or response to, melanoma.

EPITHELIOID CELL AND/OR SPINDLE-CELL NEVUS

DEFINITION

Epithelioid cell and/or spindle-cell nevomelanocytic nevus (EC-SC nevi) is usually an acquired, benign melanocytic tumor so alarming in its clinical presentation and sufficiently bizarre histopathologically to cause diagnostic confusion for melanoma. The tumor was named juvenile melanoma by Sophie Spitz in 1948[311] and benign juvenile melanoma by Kopf and Andrade in 1966.[312] A variant of EC-SC nevus called *pigmented spindle-cell nevus* was reported by Reed et al. in 1975.[313] Other terms for EC-SC nevus include Spitz's juvenile melanoma, benign juvenile melanoma, Spitz tumor, prepuberal melanoma, nevus prominens et pigmentosus, pseudomelanoma, spindle and epithelioid cell nevus, nevus of large spindle and/or epithelioid cells, and compound melanocytoma.

EPIDEMIOLOGY

EC-SC nevus may develop at any age. In one series of 308 patients with EC-SC nevi,[314] 15 percent of the cases appeared during adolescence or later, the oldest patient being 56 years of age. In other case series, 7 percent of tumors appeared at birth,[312] 33 percent before age 10 years,[315] 61 percent older than 14 years,[316] 31 percent older than 20 years,[315] and 8 percent older than 45 years.[316] In Australia, EC-SC nevus was estimated to have an annual incidence rate of 1.4 cases per 100,000 population at a time when the annual incidence rate of melanoma was 25.4 per 100,000.[315]

CLINICAL MANIFESTATIONS

The most common variety of EC-SC nevus is the acquired solitary, asymptomatic, pink or red, hairless, firm, dome-shaped, verrucous, or smooth-surfaced telangiectatic papule or nodule (see Plate 24). Very darkly pigmented lesions are usually pigmented spindle cell nevi and constitute a minority of EC-SC nevus, up to 7 percent of cases,[311,312] The pigmented spindle cell nevus is usually a sharply circumscribed, uniformly darkly pigmented papule or plaque (see Plate 25). EC-SC nevi are usually asymptomatic, but pruritus, tenderness, and/or bleeding may occur occasionally. The duration of solitary EC-SC nevus before diagnosis is usually less than 9 months. A congenital history has been documented for some cases of EC-SC nevus.[311,312] EC-SC nevi may enlarge over time, gradually or rapidly.

PATHOLOGY

Although the bizarre histopathologic features and frequent occurrence of dermal inflammation may cause diagnostic confusion, EC-SC nevus can usually be differentiated from melanoma. EC-SC nevi in children and adults are histopathologically indistinguishable.[317]

Features believed to typify EC-SC nevus (and to distinguish EC-SC nevus from melanoma) include *presence* of bizarre mononuclear and multinucleated giant cells, maturation of tumor cells with increasing depth (as reflected in mean nuclear size and DNA content), prominent coalescent eosinophilic globules, and artifactual clefts of junctional nests, and *absence* of atypical mitoses, nuclear pleomorphism, prominent upward spread of nevomelanocytes as single cells or small nests in the epiderms, or hyperchromasia of tumor cells. Potential for metastasis is favored when there is deep dermal presence, intense melanin production in the dermis, arrangement of epithelioid cells in contiguous aggregates, atypical mitoses, and lack of maturation of nevomelanocytes with increasing tumor depth.

Epithelioid cells predominate in 21 percent of EC-SC nevi (see Plate 26). Spindle cells predominate in 45 to 54 percent of EC-SC nevi, and a relatively equal combination of cell types occurs in 24 to 34 percent of cases. The pigmented spindle-cell nevus consists of compactly aggregated spindle-shaped, pigment-producing melanocytes (see Plate 27), distinguished from melanoma by its uniform nuclei, uniform cellular detail, and distinctive pattern of growth. Almost all cases of the pigmented spindle-cell nevus have a lymphohistiocytic host response. Spindle cells extend down eccrine ducts in 40 percent and involve hair follicles in 22 percent of cases. There are atypical variants of the pigmented spindle-cell nevus, in which there are architectural alterations and striking cellular atypia.

Cellular DNA content measured cytofluorometrically in EC-SC nevus is reported to show a diploid pattern, with only rare polyploid cells, similar to typical acquired nevus.[318–320] Nevomelanocytes in EC-SC nevus show reactivity for S-100 protein, HMB-45, and neuron-specific enolase.[321]

DIFFERENTIAL DIAGNOSIS

Diagnosis of the EC-SC nevus was suggested preoperatively in only 15 of 43 cases in one series.[312] Nonpigmented EC-SC nevus may resemble juvenile xanthogranuloma, hemangioma, pyogenic granuloma, molluscum contagiosum, dermal nevomelanocytic nevus, solitary mastocytoma, granuloma (i.e., sarcoid, foreign body reaction), insect bite reaction, and dermatofibroma. Pigmented EC-SC nevus may resemble nodular melanoma, dysplastic melanocytic nevus, fibrous histiocytoma, sclerosing hemangioma, appendage tumor, and pigmented keloid. Warty variants of the EC-SC nevus may be confused for verrucca vulgaris, seborrheic keratosis, and epidermal nevus.

TREATMENT

Conservative excision with 3 to 5 mm margins of normal skin (depending on location) is this author's treatment of choice for a single "typical" EC-SC nevus. Incompletely excised lesions may recur,[312,322–324] as many as 7 to 16 percent of cases. In another study, there were no recurrences after 1 to 10 years of follow-up among 24 cases of the EC-SC nevus that were incompletely excised.[325] Despite such data, this author still strongly recommends that incompletely excised lesions be re-excised. Recurrence is usually related to inapparent junctional activity extending beyond the visible borders and/or deep dermal involvement extending laterally from the main body of the tumor. Recurrent lesions may have a more worrisome histopathologic appearance and cause even more confusion for melanoma.

COURSE

Tumors believed to have histologic features similar to the EC-SC nevus may occasionally develop metastasis and death.[326,327] In fact, of the 13 cases originally described in children by Spitz,[311] one patient died of metastatic melanoma. There is a concern that some varieties of the EC-SC nevus may progress to melanoma or represent melanoma from the outset. Histopathologic remnants of the EC-SC nevus were reported in contiguity with melanoma in 5.9 percent of 362 cases.[328] Other authors disagree with this observation.[312,329] In one report, melanoma originally diagnosed as spindle-cell nevus eventuated in metastatic melanoma (and death) in a 10-year-old child.[327] The diagnosis of the EC-SC nevus should be made with care and circumspection, regardless of patient age.

NONMALIGNANT CAUSES OF CHANGE IN NEVOMELANOCYTIC NEVI

There may be relatively sudden changes in nevomelanocytic nevi that are unrelated to malignant transformation. These changes may be physiologic in nature. For instance, epidermal melanocytes overlying acquired nevi may be stimulated to produce melanin and thus appear suddenly or become more prominent in response to sun exposure, corticosteroid and corticotropin,[330] blistering disease,[331] chemotherapy,[332] and other factors which are not well-defined.[333] In these physiologic and environmental causes of change, all of the nevi in a given individual in cases of physiologic change, or all of the nevi in a given location in case of environmental or traumatic-induced change, should change together. Any single nevus that is noted to change independently should be cause for alarm.

"Benign" changes in a single nevus that may simulate malignant transformation include cystic dilatation of a hair follicle, epidermal cyst formation, folliculitis, abscess formation, trauma and hemorrhage, and in the case of a pedunculated nevus, strangulation and thrombosis. These benign causes of local change require close observation until resolution occurs over the course of a few weeks in the case of trauma or inflammation. Consideration should be given to histopathologic examination for lesions that do not revert to normal.

Common acquired nevi are believed to enlarge and increase in number during puberty. During pregnancy, nevi are believed to darken and perhaps to increase in number as well. In fact, 58 of 86 pregnant women noted no change of their nevi during pregnancy; most changing and new lesions were skin tags and dermatofibromas.[334] Although sometimes stated otherwise, atypical histopathologic features are not usual in nevi excised during pregnancy.[334,335] In one study, there was no significant atypia detected in 92 percent of 128 nevi removed from 86 pregnant volunteers.[334] While "physiologic" causes of change in nevi may be confused for dysplasia or melanoma and may cause alarm, complacency about "expected" changes during puberty and pregnancy may be responsible for missing malignant tumors.

In darkly pigmented races, dark pigmentation is common for typical acquired nevi on nonacral and nonmucosal surfaces. However, black pigmentation of nevi on acral and mucosal surfaces in any race should be viewed with suspicion and considered for excisional biopsy. Blue, gray, red, and white areas in a nevus are not typical features and also ought to be viewed with suspicion. Pigmented nevi on nonacral and nonmucosal surfaces in darkly pigmented races are more difficult to evaluate than in lightly pigmented races because of heavy background pigmentation and obscuration of overall pigment pattern.

Recurrent melanocytic nevus (pseudomelanoma) is the name given to recurrent lesions following incomplete removal of a nevomelanocytic nevus.[336] A markedly atypical clinical and histological appearance may accompany recurrence. Atypical changes in a recurrent nevus may be related to trauma of prior partial removal per se or unique characteristics of the original pigmented lesion excised. Recurrent junctional activity and repigmentation are not uncommon after dermabrasion and superficial shave biopsy of dermal nevi. Moreover, when the original lesion was reviewed for 99 of 175 recurrent nevi, melanocytic atypia was considered absent or mild in 99 percent of cases.[337] When dermal nevi are partially excised, leaving a rim of dermal nevus cells, re-epithelization is characterized by a hyperplasia of dendritic melanocytes, and lymphocytic infiltrates are common in the superficial dermis.[337] In contrast to these observations, there was no atypical melanocytic hyperplasia on subsequent total excision of 15 benign melanocytic nevi that had undergone incisional biopsy.[338]

The *scar lentigo* is a pigmented macule appearing in an excision scar or skin graft.[339] The pathology of pigmented macules occurring in scars is unsettled. Such lesions have been described as consisting of a normal number of epidermal melanocytes on the one hand (i.e., melanosis) or increased number of epidermal melanocytes on the other (lentigo). This author favors the latter view, and typical varieties of such lesions require only periodic observation.

CONCLUSIONS AND GUIDELINES FOR TREATMENT OF MELANOCYTIC TUMORS

INDICATIONS FOR TREATMENT

The vast majority of typical acquired nevomelanocytic nevi may be left alone. Although the following guidelines may be used in assessing indications for excision, each case must be individualized.

1. *Cosmetic removal.* A patient's desire to have a nevus removed is sufficient indication for excision. It is not surprising that pathologists detect histologic dysplasia or even melanoma in prominent or "ugly" nevi removed for "cosmetic" purposes.
2. *Continual irritation.* While there is no evidence that continual physical trauma of a nevus induces malignant transformation, nevi that demonstrate periodic enlargement and/or discoloration related to continual physical trauma are best excised to avoid confusion for neoplasia. Location alone (i.e., beneath a belt, brassiere strap, or collar) should not be regarded as an absolute indication for excision if the lesion remains stable, benign in appearance, and asymptomatic.
3. *Hidden sites.* As a general public health recommendation, it is reasonable to advise periodic self-examination of nevi for symptomatic or asymptomatic change. Nevi that are difficult or impossible to follow because of hidden location (i.e., hairy scalp or perineum) are candidates for excision, particularly when lesions are atypical in appearance and/or occurring in the setting of a family and/or personal history of melanoma and/or dysplastic nevi. Nevi in hidden sites require individual assessment.
4. *Atypical appearance.* An atypical appearance of a nevus is reason enough to recommend excision. Absolute size, and presence or absence of hair, are usually less specific indicators of dysplasia or malignancy than are pigment pattern, overall architecture, or growth history, although melanocytic tumors that have atypical histopathologic features are usually larger than normal because of clinical selection bias, and melanoma usually lacks hair. Relative to the importance of size, of 1098 cutaneous melanomas invasive to level II or deeper, 98.6 percent (1085 cases) were at least 5 mm in diameter; 2 melanomas were 2 mm in diameter, 1 case was 3 mm in diameter, and 10 cases were 4 mm in diameter (Darrell S. Rigel, MD and Rene S. Rodriguez-Sains, MD, New York University Melanoma Registry, personal communication).
5. *Atypical evolution.* Nevi usually grow in proportion to overall body growth (possibly faster than overall body growth) for a given anatomic

location, and nevi tend to increase in number, during early childhood and puberty. During growth spurts, all nevi in a given individual should be changing together. Any nevus undergoing independent growth, "marching out of step" with the others, may require evaluation for histopathologic examination, or close observation if atypical histopathologic features are not suspected.

6. *Lesions at high risk.* Melanocytic and nevomelanocytic tumors known to have a high risk for developing melanoma (see previous text) require either prophylactic excision or periodic follow-up indefinitely.
7. *Anatomic location.* There can be no rules about wholesale removal of pigmented nevi based on anatomic site alone. Based on their low prevalence, pigmented nevi of nail beds and conjunctivae in whites should be evaluated for histopathologic examination or followed periodically and indefinitely for malignant change. Based on their high prevalence, pigmented nevi of the nail bed in darkly pigmented races should be assessed on an individual basis. Rapid growth, very wide and dark pigmentation, and pigmentation involving the nail fold are indications for the histopathologic examination of nail nevi, regardless of race.

TREATMENT

Removal of nevi is usually accomplished by complete surgical excision. Leaving a partially excised nevus, regardless of the histopathologic features, is fraught with potentially alarming consequences of repigmentation and/or regrowth simulating neoplasia (pseudomelanoma), but this is not always the case, and individual judgement should be exercised about the need for complete excision of a partially excised histopathologically "benign" nevus. Lesions that have atypical histologic features should be excised completely or followed indefinitely for malignant change if complete excision is not feasible without compromising function or causing mutilation. Incisional biopsy, even for melanoma, is necessary at times, particularly for lesions that cannot be excised easily and that require histopathologic diagnosis before recommending further therapy.

Destructive modes of therapy (electrodesiccation, cryotherapy, chemotherapy, and dermabrasion) should not be considered in the usual management of melanocytic and nevomelanocytic hyperplasias and dysplasias. Destructive therapy prevents adequate histopathologic evaluation. Although dermabrasion has been used to eliminate pigmentation of nevomelanocytic nevi, residual nevus cells in the dermis are to be expected, cosmetic outcome is often unpredictable, and recurrence with worrisome gross and histopathologic features may complicate further evaluation.

REFERENCES

1. Elder DE et al. Acquired melanocytic nevi and melanoma: the dysplastic nevus syndrome. In Ackerman AB (ed). *Pathology of Malignant Melanoma.* New York: Masson, 1981, 185–215.
2. Paul E. Growth dynamics of malignant melanomas: A photodocumentary investigation. *Arch Dermatol* 116:182–185, 1980.
3. MacKie RM et al. The number and distribution of benign pigmented moles (melanocytic naevi) in a healthy British population. *Br J Dermatol* 113:167–174, 1985.
4. Swerdlow AJ et al. Benign naevi associated with high risk of melanoma. *Lancet* 2:168, 1984.
5. Lewis MG, and Johnson K. The incidence and distribution of pigmented nevi in Ugandan Africans. *Br J Dermatol* 80:362–366, 1968.
6. Rhodes AR, and Melski JW. Small congenital nevocellular nevi and the risk of cutaneous melanoma. *J Pediatr* 100:219–224, 1982.
7. Doherty VR, and MacKie RM. Reasons for poor prognosis in British patients with cutaneous malignant melanoma. *BMJ* 292:987–989, 1986.
8. Rhodes AR et al. Risk factors for cutaneous melanoma: A practical method of recognizing high-risk individuals. *JAMA* 258:3146–3154, 1987.
9. Grob JJ, Gouvernet J, Aymar D, Mostaque A, Romano MH, Collet AM, Noe MC, Diconstanzo MP, and Bonerandi JJ. Count of benign melanocytic nevi as a major indicator of risk for nonfamilial nodular and superficial spreading melanoma. *Cancer* 66:387–395, 1990.
10. Swerdlow AJ, English J, MacKie RM, O'Doherty CJ, Hunter JAA, Clark J, and Hole DJ. Benign melanocytic nevi as a risk factor for malignant melanoma. *BMJ* 292:1555–1559, 1986.
11. Reynolds P, and Austin DF: Epidemiologic-based screening strategies for malignant melanoma of the skin. In: Engstrom PF, Anderson PN, and Mortenson LE (eds.) *Advances in Cancer Control: Epidemiology and Research.* New York: Alan R. Liss, 1984, 245–254.
12. Clark WH Jr, From L, Bernardino EA, and Mihm MC. The histiogenesis and biologic behavior of primary human malignant melanoma of the skin. *Cancer Res* 29:705–727, 1969.
13. McGovern VJ. The classification of melanoma and its relationship with prognosis. *Pathology* 2:85–98, 1970.
14. Rhodes AR, Harrist TJ, Day CL, Mihm MC Jr, Fitzpatrick TB, and Sober AJ. Dysplastic melanocytic nevi in histologic association with 234 primary cutaneous melanomas. *J Am Acad Dermatol* 4:563–574, 1983.
15. Norris W. Case of fungoid disease. *Edin Med Surg J* 16:562–565, 1820.
16. Clark WH Jr et al. Origin of familial malignant melanomas from heritable melanocytic lesions: The BK mole syndrome. *Arch Dermatol* 114:732–738, 1978.
17. Reimer RR et al. Precursor lesions in familial melanoma: A new genetic preneoplastic syndrome. *JAMA* 239:744–746, 1978.
18. Frichot BC et al. New cutaneous phenotype in familial malignant melanoma. *Lancet* 1:864–865, 1977.
19. Lynch HT et al. Familial atypical multiple mole-melanoma syndrome. *J Med Genet* 15:352–356, 1978.
20. Lynch HT et al. A review of hereditary malignant melanoma including biomarkers in familial atypical multiple

mole-melanoma syndrome. *Cancer Genet Cytogenet* 8:325–358, 1983.
21. Rhodes AR et al. Possible risk factors for primary cutaneous malignant melanoma. *Clin Res* 28:252A, 1980.
22. Crutcher WA, and Sagebiel RW. Prevalence of dysplastic naevi in a community practice. *Lancet* 1:729, 1984.
23. Nordland JJ, Kirkwood J, Forget BM, et al. Demographic study of clinically atypical (dysplastic) nevi in patients with melanoma and comparison subjects. *Cancer Res* 45:1855–1861, 1985.
24. Scheibner A et al. Multiple primary melanoma—A review of 90 cases. *Australas J Dermatol* 23:1–8, 1982.
25. Cooke KR, Spears GFS, Elder DE, and Greene MH. Dysplastic naevi in a population-based survey. *Cancer* 63:1240–1244, 1989.
26. Sander C, Tschochohei H, and Hagedorn M. Zur Epidemiologie des dysplastischen Nävus. *Hautarzt* 40:758–760, 1989.
27. Piepkorn M, Meyer L, Goldgar G, Seuchter SA, Cannon-Albright LA, Skolnick MH, and Zone JJ. The dysplastic melanocytic nevus: A prevalent lesion that correlates poorly with clinical phenotype. *J Am Acad Dermatol* 20:407–415, 1989.
28. Augustsson A, Stierner U, Suurküla M, and Rosdahl I. Prevalence of common and dysplastic naevi in a Swedish population. *Br J Dermatol* 124:152–156, 1991.
29. Kraemer KH et al. Dysplastic naevi and cutaneous melanoma risk. *Lancet* 2:1076–1077, 1983.
30. Crijns B, Vink J, and Bergman W. Does the sporadic dysplastic nevus syndrome really exist? *Clin Res* 37:716A, 1989.
31. Albert LS, Rhodes AR, and Sober AJ. Dysplastic melanocytic nevi and cutaneous melanoma: Markers of increased melanoma risk for affected persons and blood relatives. *J Am Acad Dermatol* 22:69–75, 1990.
32. White IR, and MacDonald DM. Familial multiple melanocytic naevi—The B-K mole syndrome. *Clin Exp Dermatol* 6:549–553, 1981.
33. Tucker MA, Crutcher WA, Hartge P, and Sagebiel RW. Dysplastic nevi patients frequently have family members with dysplastic nevi or cutaneous melanoma. *Proc Am Assoc Cancer Res* 30:320, 1989 (abstract).
34. Rhodes AR et al. Increased intraepidermal melanocyte frequency and size in dysplastic melanocytic nevi and cutaneous melanoma: A comparative quantitative study of dysplastic melanocytic nevi, superficial spreading melanoma, nevocellular nevi, and solar lentigines. *J Invest Dermatol* 80:452–459, 1983.
35. Elder DE et al. The dysplastic nevus syndrome: A phenotypic association of sporadic cutaneous melanoma. *Cancer* 46:1787–1794, 1980.
36. Munro DD. Multiple active junctional nevi with family history of malignant melanoma. *Proc R Soc Med* 67:594–595, 1974.
37. MacKie RM. Multiple melanomas and atypical melanocytic naevi: Evidence of an activated and expanded melanocytic system. *Br J Dermatol* 107:621–629, 1982.
38. Hagstrom WJ et al. Dysplastic nevus syndrome (B-K mole syndrome). *Plast Reconstr Surg* 71:219–224, 1983.
39. English DR, Menz J, Heenan PJ, Elder DE, Watt JD, and Armstrong BK. The dysplastic naevus syndrome in patients with cutaneous malignant melanoma in Western Australia. *Med J Aust* 145:194–198, 1986.
40. Kelly JW, Holly EA, Shpall SN, and Ahn DK. The distribution of melanocytic naevi in melanoma patients and control subjects. *Australas J Dermatol* 30:1–8, 1989.
41. Grob JJ, Andrac L, Romano MH, Dvain D, Collet-Villette AM, Munoz MH, and Bonerandi JJ. Dysplastic naevus in non-familial melanoma. A clinicopathological study of 101 cases. *Br J Dermatol* 118:745–752, 1988.
42. Scheibner A et al. Clinical features, prognosis, and incidence of multiple primary malignant melanomas. *Aust N Z Surg* 51:386, 1981 (abstract).
43. Barnhill RL, and Roush GC. Histopathologic spectrum of clinically atypical melanocytic nevi. II. Studies of nonfamilial melanoma. *Arch Dermatol* 126:1315–1318, 1990.
44. Rhodes AR, Mihm MC Jr, and Weinstock MA. Dysplastic melanocytic nevi: A reproducible histologic definition emphasizing cellular morphology. *Mod Pathol* 2:306–319, 1989.
45. Clark WH Jr et al. A study of tumor progression: The precursor lesions of superficial spreading and nodular melanoma. *Hum Pathol* 15:1147–1165, 1984.
46. Schmiegelow P, Schroiff R, Breitbart E, Bahnsen J, Lindner J, and Jänner M. Malignant melanoma: Its precursors and its topography of proliferation. *Virchows Arch A Pathol Anat Histopathol* 409:47–59, 1986.
47. Elder DE et al. The dysplastic nevus syndrome: Our definition. *Am J Dermatopathol* 4:455–460, 1982.
48. Bergman W, Ruiter DJ, Scheffer E, and Van Vloten WA. Melanocytic atypia in dysplastic nevi: Immunohistochemical and cytophotometrical analysis. *Cancer* 61:1660–1666, 1988.
49. Bergman W et al. Histopathological, immunohistochemical and cytophotometrical characterization of dysplastic nevi. *J Invest Dermatol* 82:542–543, 1984.
50. Ruiter DJ et al. Monoclonal antibodies selected to discriminate between malignant melanoma and nevocellular nevi. *J Invest Dermatol* 85:4–8, 1985.
51. Ruiter DJ et al. Major histocompatibility antigens and mononuclear inflammatory infiltrate in benign nevomelanocytic proliferations and malignant melanoma. *J Immunol* 129:2808–2815, 1982.
52. Elder DE. Distinguishing cancer and noncancer. *J Invest Dermatol* 85:1–3, 1985.
53. Yamada K, Salopek T, Jimbow K, and Ito S. An extremely high content of pheomelanin in dysplastic melanocytic nevi. *Clin Res* 37:723A, 1989.
54. Takahashi H, Horikoshi T, and Jimbow K. Fine structural characterization of melanosomes in dysplastic nevi. *Cancer* 56:111–123, 1985.
55. Rhodes AR, Seki Y, Fitzpatrick TB, and Stern RS. Melanosomal alterations in dysplastic melanocytic nevi: A quantitative ultrastructural investigation. *Cancer* 61:358–369, 1988.
56. Salopek T, Yamada K, and Jimbow K. Morphologic and biochemical features of dysplastic melanocytes in vitro. *J Invest Dermatol* 92:511, 1989.
57. Lynch HT et al. Tumour spectrum in the FAMMM syndrome. *Br J Cancer* 44:553–560, 1981.
58. Greene MH et al. High risk of malignant melanoma-prone families with dysplastic naevi. *Ann Intern Med* 102:458–465, 1985.
59. Bergman W, Palan A, and Went LN: Clinical and genetic studies in six Dutch kindreds with the dysplastic naevus syndrome. *Ann Hum Genet* 50:249–258, 1986.
60. Bale SJ, Chakravarti A, and Greene MH. Cutaneous malignant melanoma and familial dysplastic nevi: Evidence for autosomal dominance and pleiotropy. *Am J Hum Genet* 38:188–196, 1986.
61. Wassilew S et al. Familiäre multiple naevogene Melanome. *Z Hautkr* 56:931–941, 1981.
62. Landthaler M, and Braun-Falco O. Familiares hereditares malignes Melanome. *Med Klin* 74:353–357, 1979.
63. Bale SJ, Dracopoli NC, Tucker MA, Clark WH Jr, Fraser MC, Stanger BZ, Green P, Donis-Keller H, Housman DE,

and Greene MH. Mapping the gene for hereditary cutaneous malignant melanoma-dysplastic nevus to chromosome 1p. *N Engl J Med* 320:1367–1372, 1989.

64. Van Haeringen A, Bergman W, Nelen MR, Van Der Kooij-Meijs E, Hendrikse I, Wijnen JT, Khan PM, Klasen EC, and Frants RR. Exclusion of the dysplastic nevus syndrome (DNS) locus from the short arm of chromosome 1 by linkage studies in Dutch families. *Genomics* 5:61–64, 1989.
65. Traupe H, Macher E, Hamm H, and Happle R. Mutation rate estimates are not compatible with autosomal dominant inheritance of the dysplastic nevus "syndrome." *Am J Med Genet* 32:155–157, 1989.
66. Happle R et al. Arguments in favor of a polygenetic inheritance of precursor nevi. *J Am Acad Dermatol* 6:540–543, 1982.
67. Howell JN et al. Fibroblasts from patients with hereditary cutaneous malignant melanoma are abnormally sensitive to the mutagenic effect of simulated sunlight and 4-nitroquinoline 1-oxide. *Proc Natl Acad Sci U S A* 81:1179–1183, 1984.
68. Smith PJ et al. Abnormal response to the carcinogen 4-nitroquinoline 1-oxide of cultured fibroblasts from patients with dysplastic nevus syndrome and hereditary cutaneous melanoma. *Carcinogenesis* 4:911–916, 1983.
69. Smith PJ et al. Abnormal sensitivity to UV-irradiation in cultured skin fibroblasts from patients with hereditary cutaneous malignant melanoma and dysplastic nevus syndrome. *Int J Cancer* 30:39–45, 1982.
70. Ramsay RG et al. Familial melanoma associated with dominant ultraviolet radiation sensitivity. *Cancer Res* 42:2909–2912, 1982.
71. Perera MIR, Um K, Greene MH, Waters HL, Bredberg A, and Kraemer KH. Hereditary dysplastic nevus syndrome: Lymphoid cell ultraviolet hypermutability in association with increased melanoma susceptibility. *Cancer Res* 46:1005–1009, 1986.
72. Sanford KK, Tarone RE, Parshad R, Tucker MA, Greene MH, and Jones GM. Hypersensitivity to G2 chromatid radiation damage in familial dysplastic naevus syndrome. *Lancet* 2:1111–1116, 1987.
73. Caporaso N, Greene MH, Tsai S, Pickle LW, and Mulvihill JJ. Cytogenetics in hereditary malignant melanoma and dysplastic nevus syndrome: Is dysplastic nevus syndrome a chromosome instability disorder? *Cancer Genet Cytogenet* 24:299–314, 1987.
74. Yohn J, Robinson W, and Norris D. Melanocytes and nevus cells from dysplastic nevus syndrome patients do not have increased sensitivity to ultraviolet B radiation. *Clin Res* 36:706A, 1988 (abstract).
75. Hersey P et al. Low natural killer-cell activity in familial melanoma patients and their relatives. *Br J Cancer* 40:113–122, 1979.
76. Santucci M, Urso C, Giannini A, and Bondi R. Common acquired melanocytic nevi, melanocytic dysplasia and malignant melanoma: A morphometric study. *Appl Pathol* 7:111–115, 1989.
77. Eng AM. Solitary small active junctional nevi in juvenile patients. *Arch Dermatol* 119:35–38, 1983.
78. Black WC, and Hunt WC. Histologic correlations with the clinical diagnosis of dysplastic nevus. *Am J Surg Pathol* 14:44–52, 1990.
79. Roush GC, Kirkwood JM, Ernstoff M, Somma SJ, Duray PH, Klaus SN, Stenn KS, Titus LJ, and Lerner AB. Reproducibility and validity in the clinical diagnosis of the nonfamilial dysplastic nevus: Work in progress. *Recent Results Cancer Res* 102:154–158, 1986.
80. Kelly JW, Crutcher WA, and Sagebiel RW. Clinical diagnosis of dysplastic melanocytic nevi: A clinicopathologic correlation. *J Am Acad Dermatol* 14:1044–1052, 1986.
81. Bahmer FA, Fritsch P, Kreusch J, Pehamberger H, Rohrer C, Schindera I, Smolle J, Soyer HP, and Stolz W. Terminology in surface microscopy. *J Am Acad Dermatol* 23:1159–1162, 1990.
82. Fritsch P, and Pechlaner R. Differentiation of benign from malignant melanocytic lesions using incident light microscopy, In: Ackerman AB (ed.) *Pathology of Malignant Melanoma.* New York: Masson, 1981, 301–312.
83. Pehamberger H, Steiner A, and Wolff K. In vivo epiluminescence microscopy of pigmented skin lesions. I. Pattern analysis of pigmented skin lesions. *J Am Acad Dermatol* 17:571–583, 1987.
84. Steiner A, Pehamberger H, and Wolff K. In vivo epiluminescence microscopy of pigmented skin lesions. II. Diagnosis of small pigmented skin lesions and early detection of malignant melanoma. *J Am Acad Dermatol* 17:584–591, 1987.
85. Soyer HP, Smolle J, Hödl S, Pachernegg H, and Kerl H. Surface microscopy: A new approach to the diagnosis of cutaneous pigmented tumors. *Am J Dermatopathol* 11:1–10, 1989.
86. Pehamberger H et al. Dysplastic nevus syndrome with multiple primary amelanotic melanomas in oculocutaneous albinism. *J Am Acad Dermatol* 11:731–735, 1984.
87. Levin DL, Roth DE, and Muhlbauer JE. Sporadic dysplastic nevus syndrome in a tyrosinase-positive oculocutaneous albino. *J Am Acad Dermatol* 19:393–396, 1988.
88. Sigg C, Pelloni F, and Schnyder UW. Fokale melanocytäre Atypien in dysplastishen Nävuszellnävi. *Hautarzt* 40:701–707, 1989.
89. Barnes LM, and Nordlund JJ. The natural history of dysplastic nevi: A case history illustrating their evolution. *Arch Dermatol* 123:1059–1061, 1987.
90. Sagebiel RW. Histopathology of borderline and early malignant melanomas. *Am J Surg Pathol* 3:543–552, 1979.
91. Ackerman AB, and Mihara I. Dysplasia, dysplastic melanocytes, dysplastic nevi, the dysplastic nevus syndrome, and the relation between dysplastic nevi and malignant melanomas. *Hum Pathol* 16:87–91, 1985.
92. Bondi EE et al. Topical chemotherapy of dysplastic melanocytic nevi with 5% fluorouracil. *Arch Dermatol* 117:89–92, 1981.
93. Meyskens FL, Edwards L, and Levine NS. Role of topical tretinoin in melanoma and dysplastic nevi. *J Am Acad Dermatol* 15:822–825, 1986.
94. Tucker MA et al. Dysplastic nevi on the scalp of prepubertal children from melanoma-prone families. *J Pediatr* 103:65–69, 1983.
95. Greene MH, Tucker MA, Clark WH Jr, Kraemer KH, Elder DE, and Fraser MC. Hereditary melanoma and the dysplastic nevus syndrome: The risk of cancers other than melanoma. *J Am Acad Dermatol* 16:792–797, 1987.
96. Greene MH et al. Acquired precursors of cutaneous malignant melanoma. The familial dysplastic naevus syndrome. *N Engl J Med* 312:91–97, 1985.
97. Cook MG, and Robertson I. Melanocytic dysplasia and melanoma. *Histopathology* 9:647–658, 1985.
98. Duray PH, and Ernstoff MS. Dysplastic nevus in histologic contiguity with acquired nonfamilial melanoma. *Arch Dermatol* 123:80–84, 1987.
99. McGovern VJ, Shaw HM, and Milton GW. Histogenesis of malignant melanoma with an adjacent component of the superficial spreading type. *Pathology* 17:251–254, 1985.

100. Black WC. Residual dysplastic and other nevi in superficial spreading melanoma: Clinical correlations and association with sun damage. *Cancer* 62:163–173, 1988.
101. Gruber SB, Barnhill RL, Stenn KS, and Roush GC. Nevomelanocytic proliferations in association with cutaneous malignant melanoma: A multivariate analysis. *J Am Acad Dermatol* 21:773–780, 1989.
102. Garbe C, Krüger S, Stadler R, Guggenmoos-Holzmann I, and Orfanos CE. Markers and relative risk in a German population for developing malignant melanoma. *Int J Dermatol* 28:517–523, 1989.
103. Kraemer KH, Tucker M, Tarone R, Elder DE, and Clark WH Jr. Risk of cutaneous melanoma in dysplastic nevus syndrome types A and B. *N Engl J Med* 315:1615–1616, 1986.
104. Halpern AC, Guerry D IV, Elder DE, Clark WH Jr, Synnestvedt M, Norman S, and Ayerle R. Dysplastic nevi as risk markers of sporadic (nonfamilial) melanoma: A case-control study. *Arch Dermatol* 127:995–999, 1991.
105. Rigel DS, Rivers JK, Friedman RJ, and Kopf AW. Risk gradient for malignant melanoma in individuals with dysplastic naevi. *Lancet* 1:352–353, 1988.
106. Rigel DS, Rivers JK, Kopf AW, Friedman RJ, Vinokur AF, Heilman ER, and Levenstein M. Dysplastic nevi: Markers for increased risk for melanoma. *Cancer* 63:386–389, 1989.
107. Tiersten AD, Grin CM, Kopf AW, Gottlieb GJ, Bart RS, Rigel DS, Friedman RJ, and Levenstein MJ. Prospective follow-up for malignant melanoma in patients with atypical-mole (dysplastic-nevus) syndrome. *J Dermatol Surg Oncol* 17:44–48, 1991.
108. Titus-Ernstoff L, Duray PH, Ernstoff MS, Barnhill RL, Horn PL, and Kirkwood JM. Dysplastic nevi in association with multiple primary melanoma. *Cancer Res* 48:1016–1018, 1988.
109. Basen HFA, Bergman W, Van Haeringen A, Scheffer E, and Van Slooten EA. The familial dysplastic nevus syndrome: Natural history and the impact of screening on the prognosis. A study of nine families in the Netherlands. *Eur J Cancer Clin Oncol* 25:337–341, 1989.
110. Greene MH et al. Malignant melanoma in renal transplant recipients. *Lancet* 1:1196–1199, 1981.
111. Tucker MA et al. Cutaneous malignant melanoma after Hodgkin's disease. *Ann Intern Med* 102:37–41, 1985.
112. Rhodes AR et al. A histologic comparison of congenital and acquired nevomelanocytic nevi. *Arch Dermatol* 121:1266–1273, 1985.
113. Kaplan EN. The risk of malignancy in large congenital nevi. *Plast Reconstr Surg* 53:421–428, 1974.
114. Lanier V et al. Congenital giant nevi: clinical and pathological considerations. *Plast Reconstr Surg* 58:48–54, 1976.
115. Pers M. Naevus Pigmentosus giganticus: Indikationer for operativ Behandling. *Ugeskr Laeger* 125:613–619, 1963.
116. Lorentzen M et al. The incidence of malignant transformation in giant pigmented nevi. *Scand J Plast Reconstr Surg* 11:163–167, 1977.
117. Greeley PW et al. Incidence of malignancy in giant pigmented nevi. *Plast Reconstr Surg* 36:26–37, 1965.
118. Kopf AW et al. Congenital nevocytic nevi and malignant melanomas. *J Am Acad Dermatol* 1:123–130, 1979.
119. Walton RG et al. Pigmented lesions in newborn infants. *Br J Dermatol* 95:389–396, 1976.
120. Alper J et al. Birthmarks with serious medical significance: nevocellular nevi, sebaceous nevi, and multiple cafe-au-lait spots. *J Pediatr* 95:696–700, 1979.
121. Bonifazi E, Lospalluti M, and Meneghini C. Congenital melanocytic naevus. *Bollettino di Dermatologia Pediatrica* 5:12–44, 1986.
122. Clemmensen OJ, and Kroon S. The histology of "congenital features" in early acquired melanocytic nevi. *J Am Acad Dermatol* 19:742–746, 1988.
123. Castilla EE et al. Epidemiology of congenital pigmented nevi; incidence rates and relative frequencies. *Br J Dermatol* 104:307–315, 1981.
124. Hamming N. Anatomy and embryology of the eyelids: A review with special reference to the development of divided nevi. *Pediatr Dermatol* 1:51–58, 1983.
125. Holbrook KA, Underwood RA, Vogel AM, Gown AM, and Kimball H. The appearance, density and distribution of melanocytes in human embryonic and fetal skin revealed by the anti-melanoma monoclonal antibody, HMB-45. *Anat Embryol* 180:443–455, 1989.
126. Harrison R, and Okun M. Divided nevus: A clue to the intrauterine development of melanocytic nevi. *Arch Dermatol* 82:235–236, 1960.
127. Rhodes AR et al. Familial aggregation of small congential nevomelanocytic nevi. *Am J Med Genet* 22:315–326, 1985.
128. De Anda G et al. Giant pigmented hairy nevus. *Rev Argent Dermatol* 64:208, 1983.
129. Broadway D, Lang S, Harper J, Madanat F, Pritchard J, Taranneh M, and Taylor D. Congenital malignant melanoma of the eye. *Cancer* 67:2642–2652, 1991.
130. Reed WB et al. Giant pigmented nevi, melanoma, and leptomeningeal melanocytosis: A clinical and histopathological study. *Arch Dermatol* 91:100–119, 1965.
131. Conway H. Bathing trunk nevus. *Surgery* 6:585, 1939.
132. Pack GT, and Davis J. Nevus giganticus pigmentosus with malignant transformation. *Surgery* 49:347–354, 1961.
133. Fox H et al. Neuro-cutaneous melanosis. *Arch Dis Child* 39:508–516, 1964.
134. Savitz HM, and Anderson PJ. Primary melanoma of the leptomeninges: a review. *Mt Sinai J Med (NY)* 41:774–791, 1974.
135. Lamas E et al. Neurocutaneous melanosis: Report of a case and review of the literature. *Acta Neurochir* 36:93–105, 1977.
136. Kudel TA et al. Computed tomographic findings of primary malignant leptomeningeal melanoma in neurocutaneous melanosis. *Am J Radiol* 133:950–951, 1979.
137. Kaplan AM et al. Neurocutaneous melanosis with malignant leptomeningeal melanoma. *Arch Neurol* 32:669–671, 1975.
138. Mimouni F, Han BK, Barnes L, Ballard JL, Dignan PS, Kiessling MA, and Lucky AW. Multiple hamartomas associated with intracranial malformation. *Pediatr Dermatol* 3:219–225, 1986.
139. Mark GJ et al. Congenital melanocytic nevi of the small and garment type. *Hum Pathol* 4:395–418, 1973.
140. Nickoloff BJ, Walton R, Pregerson-Rodan K, et al. Immunohistologic patterns of congenital nevocellular nevi. *Arch Dermatol* 122:1263–1268, 1986.
141. Stenn KS et al. Patterns of congenital nevocellular nevi: A histologic study of thirty-eight cases. *J Am Acad Dermatol* 9:388–393, 1983.
142. Zitelli JA, Grant MG, Abell E, and Boyd JB. Histologic patterns of congenital nevocytic nevi and implications for treatment. *J Am Acad Dermatol* 11:402–409, 1984.
143. Walsh MY, and MacKie RM. Histological features of value in differentiating small congenital melanocytic naevi from acquired naevi. *Histopathol* 12:145–154, 1988.
144. Ainsworth AM et al. Melanocytic nevi, melanocytomas, melanocytic dysplasias, and uncommon forms of melanoma. In: Clark WH Jr et al. (ed.) *Human Malignant Melanoma*. New York: Grune & Stratton, 1979, 167–208.

145. Silvers DN, and Helwig EB. Melanocytic nevi in neonates. *J Am Acad Dermatol* 4:166–175, 1981.
146. Aeling JL. Dermatologic therapeutic survey. *J Assoc Mil Dermatol* 5:1, 1979.
147. Sweren RJ. Management of congenital nevocytic nevi: A survey of current practices. *J Am Acad Dermatol* 11:629–634, 1984.
148. Tritsch H. Histologie zur Dermabrasion des Riesen-Naevus. *Z Hautkr* 60:47–54, 1985.
149. Hori Y, Nakayama J, Okamoto M, Nagae S, Taniguchi S, Takayama O, and Oohara K. Giant congenital nevus and malignant melanoma. *J Invest Dermatol* 92:310S–314S, 1989.
150. Trau H, Orenstein A, Schewach-Miller M, and Tsur H. Pseudomelanoma following laser therapy for congenital nevus. *J Dermatol Surg Oncol* 12:984–986, 1986.
151. Zina G, Bundino S, Ubertalli S, and Gavinelli R. Studio clinico-evolutivo dei neicongeniti su di un campione di 3.072 neonati. *Giornale Italiano di Dermatologia e Veneroleogia* 120:5–15, 1985.
152. Groh V, and Schnyder UW. Zuk Klinik und Genetik kongenitaler Pigmentnaevi. *Hautarzt* 35:240–248, 1984.
153. Hogan DJ, Murphy F, and Bremner RM. Spontaneous resolution of a giant congenital melanocytic nevus. *Ped Dermatol* 5:170–172, 1988.
154. Zack LD, Stegmeier O, and Solomon LM. Pigmentary regression in a giant nevocellular nevus: A case report and a review of the subject. *Ped Dermatol* 5:178–183, 1988.
155. Rhodes AR et al. Nonepidermal origin of malignant melanoma associated with a giant congenital nevocellular nevus. *Plast Reconstr Surg* 67:782–790, 1981.
156. Boddie AW et al. Malignant melanoma in children and young adults: Effect of diagnostic criteria on staging and end results. *South Med J* 71:1074–1078, 1978.
157. Fong JC, and Sagebiel RW. Malignant melanoma in childhood and adolescence: UCSF Melanoma Clinic Survey. *J Cutan Pathol* 16:303, 1989.
158. Padilla RS, McConnell TS, Gribble JT, and Smoot C. Malignant melanoma arising in a giant congenital melanocytic nevus: A case report with cytogenetic and histopathologic analyses. *Cancer* 62:2589–2594, 1988.
159. Partoft S, Østerlind A, Hou-Jensen K, and Drzewiecki KT. Malignant melanoma of the skin in children (0 to 14 years of age) in Denmark, 1943–1982. *Scand J Plast Reconstr Surg* 23:55–58, 1989.
160. Trozak DJ et al. Metastatic melanoma in prepubertal children. *Pediatrics* 55:191–204, 1975.
161. Quaba AA, and Wallace AF. The incidence of malignant melanoma (0 to 15 years of age) arising in "large" congenital nevocellular nevi. *Plast Reconstr Surg* 78:174–179, 1986.
162. Schneiderman H, Wu AY-Y, Campbell WA, Forouhar F, Yamase H, Greenstein R, and Grant-Kels JM. Congenital melanoma with multiple prenatal metastases. *Cancer* 60:1371–1377, 1987.
163. Derrick JR, and Thompson JA. Fatal malignant melanoma in a negro child. *Pediatrics* 21:222–225, 1958.
164. Fish J, Smith EB, and Canby JP: Malignant melanoma in childhood. *Surgery* 59:309–315, 1966.
165. Dobson L. Prepubertal malignant melanomas. *Am J Surg* 89:1128–1135, 1955.
166. Rhodes AR et al. The malignant potential of small congenital nevocellular nevi: An estimate of association based on a histologic study of 234 primary cutaneous melanomas. *J Am Acad Dermatol* 6:230–241, 1982.
167. Williams IG, and Martin LC. Naevocarcinoma of the skin and mucous membranes. *Lancet* 232:135, 1937.
168. Daland EM, and Holmes JA. Malignant melanoma: A clinical study. *N Engl J Med* 220:651, 1939.
169. Driver JR, and MacVicar DN. Cutaneous melanoma—A clinical study of sixty cases. *JAMA* 121:413, 1943.
170. Ackerman LV. Malignant melanoma of the skin—A clinical and pathological analysis of 75 cases. *Am J Clin Pathol* 18:602, 1948.
171. Wright CJE. Prognosis in cutaneous and ocular malignant melanoma: A study of 222 cases. *J Pathol Bacteriol* 61:507, 1949.
172. Booher RJ, and Pack TG. Malignant melanoma of the feet and hands. *Surgery* 42:1084, 1957.
173. Helwig EB. Malignant melanoma of the skin in man. *Natl Acad Inst Monogr* 10:287, 1963.
174. Bader JL et al. Malignant melanoma in patients under 20 years of age: An epidemiologic study. *Proc Am Assoc Cancer Res* 20:316, 1979.
175. Pratt CB et al. Malignant melanoma in children and adolescents. *Cancer* 47:392–397, 1981.
176. Mole B et al. Melanomes malins de l'enfant. Revne amatonio-clinique de 12 cas. *Ann Chir Plast* 27:87–90, 1982.
177. Rhodes AR, and Melski JW. Small congenital nevocellular nevi and the risk of cutaneous melanoma. *J Pediatr* 100:219–224, 1982.
178. Vázquez M et al. Melanomas of volar and subungual skin in Puerto Ricans. A clinicopathologic study. *J Am Acad Dermatol* 10:39–45, 1984.
179. Paul E. Growth dynamics of malignant melanoma and their relationship to melanocytic naevi as revealed by photocatamnestical investigations. *Pigment Cell Res* (Karger, Basel) 9:59–76, 1988.
180. Illig L et al. Congenital nevi ≤ 10 cm as precursors to melanoma: 52 cases, a review, and a new conception. *Arch Dermatol* 121:1274–1281, 1985.
181. Rhodes AR. The risk of malignant melanoma arising in congenital melanocytic nevi: An argument against the assignment of risk based on size alone. *Am J Dermatopathol* 6 (Suppl 1):184–188, 1984.
182. Sharpe RJ, Salasche SJ, Barnhill RL, and Sober AJ. Nonepidermal origin of cutaneous melanoma in a small congenital nevus. *Arch Dermatol* 126:1559–1561, 1990.
183. Steijlen PM, Hamm H, Van Erp PEJ, Johnson JP, Ruiter DJ, and Bröcker EB. Immunohistologic evidence for the malignant potential of congenital melanocytic nevi. *J Invest Dermatol* 92:366–370, 1989.
184. Paull WH, Polley D, and Fitzpatrick JE. Malignant melanoma arising intradermally in a small congenital nevus of an adult. *J Dermatol Surg Oncol* 12:1176–1178, 1986.
185. Truaz KF, and Page HG. Prepubertal malignant melanoma. *Ann Surg* 137:255–260, 1953.
186. Dargeon HW, Eversole JW, and DelDuca V. Malignant melanoma in an infant. *Cancer* 3:299–306, 1950.
187. Keall J, McElwain TJ, and Wallace AF. Malignant melanoma in childhood. *Br J Plast Surg* 34:340–341, 1981.
188. Rosin MA, and Braun M. Malignant melanoma and levodopa. *Cutis* 33:572–574, 1984.
189. Lyall D. Malignant melanoma in infancy. *JAMA* 202:93, 1967.
190. Lerner AB, and Kirkwood JM. Vitiligo and melanoma: Can genetically abnormal melanocytes result in both vitiligo and melanoma within a single family? *J Am Acad Dermatol* 11:696–701, 1984.
191. Weinstock MA, and Sober AJ. The risk of progression of lentigo maligna to lentigo maligna melanoma. *Br J Dermatol* 116:303–310, 1987.
192. Wayte DM, and Helwig EB. Melanotic freckle of Hutchinson. *Cancer* 21:893–911, 1968.
193. Clark WH Jr, and Mihm MC Jr. Lentigo maligna and lentigo maligna melanoma. *Am J Pathol* 55:39–67, 1969.

194. Mishima Y. Melanosis circumscripta precancerosa (Dubreuilh): non-nevoid premelanoma distinct from junctional nevus. *J Invest Dermatol* 34:361–375, 1960.
195. Takebe H, Nishigori C, and Tatsumi K. Melanoma and other skin cancers in xeroderma pigmentosum patients and mutation in their cells. *J Invest Dermatol* 92:236S–238S, 1989.
196. Robbins JH, and Moshell AN. DNA repair processes protect human beings from premature solar damage: Evidence from studies on xeroderma pigmentosum. *J Invest Dermatol* 73:102–107, 1979.
197. Kraemer KH, Herlyn M, Yuspa SH, Clark WH Jr, Townsend GK, Neises GR, and Hearing VJ. Reduced DNA repair in cultured melanocytes and nevus cells from a patient with xeroderma pigmentosum. *Arch Dermatol* 125:263–268, 1989.
198. Soyer HP, Elder DE, Smolle J, Tanew A, Hödl H, and Kerl H. Pigmented lesions in xeroderma pigmentosum. *J Cutan Pathol* 14:372, 1987 (abstract).
199. Rhodes AR, Albert LS, Barnhill RL, and Weinstock MA. Sun-induced freckles in children and young adults: A correlation of clinical and histopathologic features. *Cancer* 67:1990–2001, 1991.
200. Holman CDJ, and Armstrong BK. Pigmentary traits, ethnic origin, benign nevi, and familial history as risk factors for cutaneous malignant melanoma. *JNCI* 72:257–266, 1984.
201. Holman CDJ, and Armstrong BK. Hutchinson's melanotic freckle melanoma associated with non-permanent hair dyes. *Br J Cancer* 48:599–601, 1983.
202. Sanchez JL, Ramos-Caro F, and Ackerman AB. Histopathologic findings in supposed solar lentigines of Puerto Ricans. In Ackerman AB (ed.) *Pathology of Malignant Melanoma.* New York: Masson, 1981, 107–118.
203. Cramer SF, and Kiehn CL. Sequential histologic study of evolving lentigo maligna melanoma. *Arch Pathol Lab Med* 106:121–125, 1982.
204. Penneys NS. Microinvasive lentigo maligna melanoma. *J Am Acad Dermatol* 17:675–680, 1987.
205. Zacarian SA. Cryosurgical treatment of lentigo maligna. *Arch Dermatol* 118:89–92, 1982.
206. Arndt KA. New pigmented macule appearing 4 years after argon laser treatment of lentigo maligna. *J Am Acad Dermatol* 14:1092, 1986.
207. Rivers JK, and McCarthy WH. No effect of topical tretinoin on lentigo maligna. *Arch Dermatol* 127:129, 1991.
208. McLean DI, and Peter KK. Apparent progression of lentigo maligna to invasive melanoma during treatment with topical azelaic acid. *Br J Dermatol* 114:685–689, 1986.
209. Borkovic SP, and Schwartz RA. Amelanotic lentigo maligna melanoma manifesting as a dermatitis-like plaque. *Arch Dermatol* 119:423–425, 1983.
210. Stoll DB et al. Lentigo maligna in a woman with oculocutaneous albinism. *Arch Dermatol* 117:360–361, 1981.
211. Michalik EE et al. Rapid progression of lentigo maligna to deeply invasive lentigo maligna melanoma. *Arch Dermatol* 119:831–835, 1983.
212. Cohen HJ et al. Nevus spilus. *Arch Dermatol* 102:433–437, 1970.
213. Kopf AW et al. Prevalence of congenital-nevus-like nevi, nevi spili, and cafe-au-lait spots. *Arch Dermatol* 121:766–769, 1985.
214. Sigg C, Pelloni F, and Schnyder UW. Frequency of congenital nevi, nevi spili and cafe-au-lait spots and their relation to nevus count and skin complexion in 939 children. *Dermtologica* 180:118–123, 1990.
215. Matsuda H et al. Zosteriform lentiginous nevus. *Arch Dermatol* 107:902–905, 1973.
216. Konrad K et al. Nevus spilus—ein Pigmentnaevus mit Riesenmelanosoman. Klinik, Histologie und Ultrastruktur. *Hautarzt* 25:585–593, 1974.
217. Stewart DM et al. Speckled lentiginous nevus. *Arch Dermatol* 114:895–896, 1978.
218. Sato S et al. Divided nevus spilus and divided form of spotted grouped pigmented nevus. *Nippon Hifuga Gakkai Zasshi* 88:909–911, 1978.
219. Nguyen KQ et al. Mosaic speckled lentiginous nevi. *Cutis* 30:65–68, 1982.
220. Pritchett RM, and Pritchett PS. Zosteriform speckled lentiginous nevus with giant melanosomes. *Cutis* 30:329–334, 1982.
221. Rhodes AR, and Mihm MC Jr. Origin of cutaneous melanoma in a congenital dysplastic nevus spilus. *Arch Dermatol* 126:500–505, 1990.
222. Ishibashi A, Kimura A, and Kukita A. Plaque-type blue nevus combined with lentigo (nevus spilus). *J Cutan Pathol* 17:241–245, 1990.
223. Perkinson NG. Melanoma arising in a café-au-lait spot of neurofibromatosis. *Am J Surg* 93:1018, 1957.
224. Rütten A, and Goos M. Nevus spilus with malignant melanoma in a patient with neurofibromatosis. *Arch Dermatol* 126:539–540, 1990.
225. Vion B, Belaich S, Grossin M, and Preaux J. Les aspects evolutifs du naevus sur naevus: Revue de la literature a propos de 7 observations (Developmental aspects of nevus spilus: Review of the literature apropos of seven cases). *Ann Dermatol Venereol* 112:813–819, 1985.
226. Brufau C, Moran M, and Armijo M. Naevus sur naevus. A propos de 7 observations, trois associees a d'antres dysplasies, et une a un melanome malin invasif (Nevus on nevus: Apropos of seven case reports, three of them associated with other dysplasias, and one with an invasive malignant melanoma). *Ann Dermatol Venereol* 13:409–418, 1986.
227. Kopf AW et al. Congenital nevus-like nevi, nevi spili, and cafe-au-lait spots in patients with malignant melanoma. *J Dermatol Surg Oncol* 11:275–280, 1985.
228. Wagner RF, and Cottel WI. In situ malignant melanoma arising in a speckled lentiginous nevus. *J Am Acad Dermatol* 20:125–126, 1989.
229. Guillot B, Bessis D, Barnéon G, Monpoint S, and Guilhou JJ. Malignant melanoma occurring on a "naevus on naevus." *Br J Dermatol* 124:610–611, 1991.
230. Bolognia JL. Fatal melanoma arising in a zosteriform speckled lentiginous nevus. *Arch Dermatol* 127:1240–1241, 1991.
231. Hidano A. Persistent Mongolian spot in the adult. *Arch Dermatol* 103:680–681, 1971.
232. Nakai T, and Rappaport H. A study of the histogenesis of experimental melanotic tumors resembling cellular blue nevi: The evidence in support of their neurogenic origin. *Am J Pathol* 43:175–199, 1963.
233. Mishima Y. Cellular blue nevus: Melanogenic activity and malignant transformation. *Arch Dermatol* 101:104–110, 1970.
234. Rodriguez HA, and Ackerman LV. Cellular blue nevus. Clinicopathologic study of 45 cases. *Cancer* 21:393–405, 1968.
235. Silverberg GD et al. Invasion of the brain by a cellular blue nevus of the scalp. *Cancer* 27:349–355, 1971.
236. Hendrickson MR, and Ross JC. Neoplasms arising in congenital giant nevi. Morphologic study of 7 cases and review of the literature. *Am J Surg Pathol* 5:109–135, 1981.
237. Gooneratne S et al. Multicentric giant pigmented nevi of the scalp with local invasion of the cranium and dura mater. *J Pediatr Surg* 17:55–58, 1982.
238. Ikeda S, Makita A, Tajima M, Kawamura T, Mizutani H.

Clinical and histologic studies of blue nevus. In: Fitzpatrick TB et al. (eds.), *Biology and Diseases of Dermal Pigmentation*. Tokyo: University of Tokyo Press, 1981, 95–106.
239. Marano SR, Brooks RA, Spetzler RF, and Rekate HL. Giant congenital cellular blue nevus of the scalp of a newborn with an underlying skull defect and invasion of the dura mater. *Neurosurg* 18:85–89, 1986.
240. Iemoto Y, Kondo Y. Congenital giant cellular blue nevus resulting in dystocia. *Arch Dermatol* 120:798–799, 1984.
241. Grouls V et al. Combined nevus: Malignant blue nevus and giant pigmented nevus. *Z Hautkr* 56:943–946, 1981.
242. Lambert WC, and Brodkin RH. Nodal and subcutaneous cellular blue nevi: A pseudometastasizing pseudomelanoma. *Arch Dermatol* 120:367–370, 1984.
243. Kwittken J, and Negri L. Malignant blue nevus: Case report of a Negro woman. *Arch Dermatol* 94:64–69, 1966.
244. Wood WS, and Tron VA. Analysis of HMB-45 immunoreactivity in common and cellular blue nevi. *J Cutan Pathol* 18:261–263, 1991.
245. Connelly J, and Smith Jr JL. Malignant blue nevus. *Cancer* 67:2653–2657, 1991.
246. Goldenhersh MA, Savin R, Barnhill RL, and Stenn KS. Malignant blue nevus: Case report and literature review. *J Am Acad Dermatol* 19:712–722, 1988.
247. Hernandez FJ. Malignant blue nevus. *Arch Dermatol* 107:741–744, 1973.
248. Hidano A, Kajima H, Ikeda S, Mizutani, Miyasato H, and Niijura M. Natural history of nevus of Ota. *Arch Dermatol* 95:187–195, 1967.
249. Kukita A, Hori Y, Ohhara K, Kawashima M, and Takehara K. Nevus of Ota. In: Fitzpatrick TB, Kukita A, Morikawa F, Seiji M, Sober AJ, and Toda K (eds.) *Biology and diseases of dermal pigmentation*. Tokyo: University of Tokyo Press, 1981, 67–76.
250. Kopf AW, and Weidman AL. Nevus of Ota. *Arch Dermatol* 85:195–208, 1962.
251. Cowan TH, and Malistocky M. The nevus of Ota or oculodermal melanocytosis. *Arch Ophhalmol* 65:483–492, 1961.
252. Mishima Y, and Mevorah B. Nevus Ota and nevus Ito in American Negroes. *J Invest Dermatol* 36:133–154, 1961.
253. Reed WB, and Sugarman GI. Unilateral nevus of Ota with sensorineural deafness. *Arch Dermatol* 109:881–883, 1974.
254. Yamamoto T. Malignant melanoma of the choroid in the nevus of Ota. *Ophthalmologica* 159:1–10, 1969.
255. Sang DN, Albert DM, Sober AJ, and McMeekin TO. Nevus of Ota with contralateral cerebral melanoma. *Arch Ophthalmol* 95:1820–1824, 1977.
256. Botticelli AR, Villani M, Angiari P, and Peserico L. Meningeal melanocytoma of Meckel's cave associated with ipsilateral Ota's nevus. *Cancer* 51:2304–2310, 1983.
257. Sagar HJ, Ilgren EB, and Adams CBT. Nevus of Ota associated with meningeal melanosis and intracranial melanoma. *J Neurosurg* 58:280–283, 1983.
258. Cosman B, Apfelberg DB, and Druker D. An effective cosmetic treatment for Ota's nevus. *Ann Plast Surg* 22:36–42, 1989.
259. Dorsey CS, and Montgomery H. Blue nevus and its distinction from mongolian spot and the nevus of Ota. *J Invest Dermatol* 22:225–236, 1954.
260. Lerner AB, Nordlund JJ, and Kirkwood JM. Effects of oral contraceptives and pregnancy on melanomas. *N Engl J Med* 301:47, 1979 (letter).
261. Van Krieken JHJM, Boom BW, and Scheffer E. Malignant transformation in a naevus of Ito. A case report. *Histopathology* 12:100–102, 1988.
262. Kopf AW, and Bart RS. Malignant blue (Ota's?) nevus. *J Dermatol Surg Oncol* 8:442–445, 1982.
263. Enriquez R, Egbert B, and Bullock J. Primary malignant melanoma of the central nervous system. Pineal involvement in a patient with nevus of Ota and multiple pigmented skin nevi. *Arch Pathol* 95:392–395, 1973.
264. Hulke JW. A series of cases of carcinoma of the eyeball. *Ophthalmic Hosp Rep* 3:279–286, 1861.
265. Nik NA, Glew WB, and Zimmerman LE. Malignant melanoma of the choroid in the nevus of Ota of a Black patient. *Arch Ophthalmol* 100:1641–1643, 1982.
266. Croxatto JO, Charles DE, and Malbran ES. Neurofibromatosis associated with nevus of Ota and choroidal melanoma. *Am J Ophthalmol* 92:578–580, 1981.
267. Levene A. Disseminated dermal melanocytosis terminating in melanoma. A human condition resembling equine melanotic disease. *Br J Dermatol* 101:197–205, 1979.
268. Coleman WP et al. Nevi, lentigines, and melanomas in Blacks. *Arch Dermatol* 116:548–551, 1980.
269. Kato T, Usuba Y, Takematsu H, Kumasaka N, Tanita Y, Hashimoto K, Tomita Y, and Tagami H. A rapidly growing pigmented nail streak resulting in diffuse melanosis of the nail. *Cancer* 64:2191–2197, 1989.
270. Coleman WP et al. Acral lentiginous melanoma. *Arch Dermatol* 116:773–776, 1980.
271. Freinkel AL, and Rippey JJ. Foot pigmentation in blacks. *S Afr Med J* 50:2160–2161, 1976.
272. Saida T. Malignant melanoma in situ on the sole of the foot: Its clinical and histopathologic characteristics. *Am J Dermatopathol* 11:124–130, 1989.
273. Leicht S, Youngberg G, and Diaz-Miranda C. Atypical pigmented penile macules. *Arch Dermatol* 124:1267–1270, 1988.
274. Barnhill RL, Albert LS, Shama SK, Goldenhersh MA, Rhodes AR, and Sober AJ. Genital lentiginosis: A clinical and histopathologic study. *J Am Acad Dermatol* 22:453–460, 1990.
275. Bhawan J, and Cahn TM. Atypical penile lentigo. Case report. *J Dermatol Surg Oncol* 10:99–100, 1984.
276. Kopf AW, and Bart RS. Tumour conference #43: Penile lentigo. *J Dermatol Surg Oncol* 8:637–639, 1982.
277. Revuz J, and Clerici T. Penile melanosis. *J Am Acad Dermatol* 20:567–570, 1989.
278. Rhodes AR et al. Mucocutaneous lentigines, cardiomucocutaneous myxomas, and multiple blue nevi: The "LAMB" syndrome. *J Am Acad Dermatol* 10:72–82, 1984.
279. Rudolph RI. Vulvar melanosis. *J Am Acad Dermatol* 23:982–984, 1990.
280. Sison-Torre EZ, and Ackerman AB. Melanosis of the vulva: A clinical simulator of malignant melanoma. *Am J Dermatopathol* 7:51–60, 1985.
281. Guillen FJ et al. Pigmented melanocytic lesions of the conjunctiva—a new approach to their classification. *Pathology* 17:275–280, 1985.
282. Folberg R et al. Primary acquired melanosis of the conjunctiva. *Hum Pathol* 16:129–135, 1985.
283. Folberg R et al. Malignant melanoma of the conjunctiva. *Hum Pathol* 16:136–143, 1985.
284. Takagi M et al. Primary malignant melanoma of the oral cavity in Japan. *Cancer* 34:358–370, 1974.
285. Page LR, Corio RL, Crawford BE, Giansanti JS, and Weathers DR. The oral melanotic macule. *Oral Surg* 44:219–226, 1977.
286. Buchner A, Henson LS. Pigmented nevi of the oral mucosa: A clinicopathologic study of 36 new cases and a review of 155 cases from the literature. *Oral Med Oral Pathol* 63:566–572, 1987.
287. Kerl H, Hodl S and Stettner M. Acral lentiginous melanoma. In: Ackerman AB (ed.) *Pathology of Malignant Melanoma*. New York: Masson, 1981, 217–242.

288. Feibleman CE et al. Melanomas of the palm, sole, and nailbed: A clinicopathologic study. *Cancer* 46:2492–2504, 1980.
289. Lee RB, Buttoni L, Dhru K, and Tamimi H. Malignant melanoma of the vagina: A case report of progression from preexisting melanosis. *Gynecol Oncol* 19:238–245, 1984.
290. Bart RS, and Kopf AW. A darkly pigmented lesion of a great toe (acral lentiginous melanoma). *J Dermatol Surg Oncol* 3:158–159, 1977.
291. Braitmen M. Subungual malignant melanoma. *Cutis* 23:617–623, 1979.
292. Collins RJ. Melanoma in the Chinese of Hong Kong: Emphasis on volar and subungual sites. *Cancer* 54:1482–1488, 1984.
293. Lewis MG. Malignant melanoma in Uganda (the relationship between pigmentation and malignant melanoma on the soles of the feet). *Br J Cancer* 21:483–495, 1967.
294. McCaffrey TV et al. Malignant melanoma of the oral cavity: Review of 10 cases. *Laryngoscope* 90:1329–1335, 1980.
295. Chimenti S et al. Malignant melanoma of the oral cavity. *J Dermatol Surg Oncol* 7:220–224, 1981.
296. Rapini RP et al. Primary malignant melanoma of the oral cavity: A review of 177 cases. *Cancer* 55:1543–1551, 1985.
297. Rhodes AR. Acral lentiginous melanoma in situ. *Plast Reconstr Surg* 70:617–619, 1982.
298. Rippey JJ, and Lewin JR. Acral lentiginous melanoma or Hutchinson's melanotic freckle of the extremities. *S Afr Med J* 53:1076–1077, 1978.
299. Rippey JJ, and Rippey E. Malignant melanoma with adjacent Hutchinson's melanotic freckle in black Africans. *Pathology* 9:105–109, 1977.
300. Seiji M, and Takahashi M. Malignant melanoma with adjacent intraepidermal proliferation. *Tohoku J Exp Med* 114:93–107, 1974.
301. Gleicher N et al. Familial malignant melanoma of the female genitalia: A case report and review. *Obstet Gynecol Surg* 34:1–15, 1979.
302. Arrington JH et al. Plantar lentiginous melanoma: A distinctive variant of human cutaneous malignant melanoma. *Am J Surg Pathol* 1:131–143, 1977.
303. Allyn B et al. Incidence of pigmented nevi. *JAMA* 186:890–893, 1963.
304. Kukita A, and Ishihara K. Clinical features and distribution of malignant melanoma and pigmented nevi on the soles of the feet in Japan. *J Invest Dermatol* 92:210S–213S, 1989.
305. Cullen SI. Incidence of nevi: Report of survey of the palms, soles and genitalia of 10,000 young men. *Arch Dermatol* 86:40–43, 1962.
306. Rock B, Hood AF, and Rock JA. Prospective study of vulvar nevi. *J Am Acad Dermatol* 22:104–106, 1990.
307. Tasaki K. On band or linear pigmentation of the nails. *Jpn J Dermatol* 33:568, 1983.
308. Leyden JJ et al. Diffuse and banded melanin pigmentation in nails. *Arch Dermatol* 105:548–550, 1972.
309. Kopf AW, and Waldo E. Melanonychia striata. *Australas J Dermatol* 21:59–70, 1980.
310. Higashi N. Melanocytes of nail matrix and nail pigmentation. *Arch Dermatol* 97:570–574, 1968.
311. Spitz S. Melanomas of childhood. *Am J Pathol* 3:591, 1948.
312. Kopf AW, and Andrade R. Benign juvenile melanoma. In: Kopf AW, Andrade R (eds.) *Yearbook of Dermatology 1965–1966*. Chicago: Year Book Medical Publishers, 1966, 7–52.
313. Reed RJ et al. Common and uncommon melanocytic nevi and borderline melanomas. *Semin Oncol* 2:119–147, 1975.
314. Allen AC. Juvenile melanomas. *Ann N Y Acad Sci* 100:29–48, 1963.
315. Weedon D, and Little JH. Spindle and epithelioid cell nevi in children and adults: A review of 211 cases of Spitz nevus. *Cancer* 40:217–225, 1977.
316. Paniago-Pereira C et al. Nevus of large spindle and/or epithelioid cells (Spitz's nevus). *Arch Dermatol* 114:1811–1823, 1978.
317. Echevarria R, and Ackermann LV. Spindle and epithelioid cell nevi in the adult. *Cancer* 20:175–189, 1967.
318. SeBoit PE, and Van Fletcher H. A comparative study of Spitz nevus and nodular malignant melanoma using image analysis cytometry. *J Invest Dermatol* 88:753–757, 1987.
319. Winokur RS, Palazzo JP, Johnson WC, and Duray PH. Evaluation of DNA ploidy in dysplastic and Spitz nevi by flow cytometry. *J Cutan Pathol* 17:342–347, 1990.
320. Chi H-I, Ishibashi Y, Shima A, Mihara I, and Otsuka F. Use of DAPI cytofluorometric analysis of cellular DNA content to differentiate Spitz nevus from malignant melanoma. *J Invest Dermatol* 95:154–157, 1990.
321. Palazzo JP, and Durray PH. Congenital agminated Spitz nevi: Immunoreactivity with a melanoma-associated monoclonal antibody. *J Cutan Pathol* 15:166–170, 1988.
322. Omura EF, and Kheir SM. Recurrent Spitz's nevus. *Am J Dermatopathol* 6:207–212, 1984.
323. Stern J. Recurrent spindle and epithelial cell nevi. *Arch Dermatol* 119:849, 1983.
324. Paties CT, Borroni G, Rosso R, and Vassallo G. Relapsing eruptive multiple Spitz nevi or metastatic Spitzoid malignant melanoma. *Am J Dermatopathol* 9:520–527, 1987.
325. Kaye VN, and Dehner LP. Spindle and epithelioid cell nevus (Spitz nevus). *Arch Dermatol* 126:1581–1583, 1990.
326. Okun MR. Melanoma resembling spindle and epithelioid cell nevus. *Arch Dermatol* 115:1416–1420, 1979.
327. Goldes J et al. Melanoma masquerading as Spitz nevus following acute lymphoblastic leukemia. *Pediatr Dermatol* 1:295–298, 1984.
328. Allen AC, and Spitz S. Malignant melanoma. A clinicopathological analysis of the criteria for diagnosis and prognosis. *Cancer* 6:1, 1953.
329. Kernan JA, and Ackerman LV. Spindle cell nevi and epithelioid cell nevi (so-called juvenile melanomas) in children and adults. *Cancer* 13:612, 1960.
330. Goldman L, and Richfield DF. Effect of corticotrophin and cortisone on the development and progress of pigmented nevi. *JAMA* 147:941, 1951.
331. Soltani K et al. Eruptive nevocytic nevi following erythema multiforme. *J Am Acad Dermatol* 1:503–505, 1979.
332. de Wit PEJ, de Vaan GAM, de Boo ThM, Lemmens WAJG, and Rampen FHJ. Prevalence of naevocytic naevi after chemotherapy for childhood cancer. *Med Pediatr Oncol* 18:336–338, 1990.
333. Eady RAJ et al. Eruptive nevi: Report of two cases, with enzyme histochemical, light and electron microscopic findings. *Br J Dermatol* 97:267–278, 1977.
334. Foucar E et al. A histopathologic evaluation of nevocellular nevi in pregnancy. *Arch Dermatol* 121:350–354, 1985.
335. Sanchez JL et al. Behavior of melanocytic nevi during pregnancy. *Am J Dermatopathol* 6 (suppl 1):89–91, 1984.
336. Kornberg R, and Ackerman AB. Pseudomelanoma: Recurrent melanocytic nevus following partial surgical removal. *Arch Dermatol* 111:1588–1590, 1975.
337. Park HK, Leonard DD, Arrington JH, and Lund HZ. Recurrent melanocytic nevi: Clinical and histologic review of 175 cases. *J Am Acad Dermatol* 17:285–292, 1987.
338. Curley RK, Fallowfield ME, Cook MG, and Marsden RA. Effect of incisional biopsy on subsequent histology of melanocytic nevi. *Br J Dermatol* 123:503–506, 1990.
339. Jackson R. Pigmented lesion following complex removal of melanoma. *Arch Dermatol* 115:1089–1090, 1979.

Chapter 10

HISTOGENETIC TYPES OF PRIMARY SKIN MELANOMA

Ramsay S. Kurban, Abdul-Ghani Kibbi, and Martin C. Mihm, Jr.

INTRODUCTION

Four major subtypes of cutaneous malignant melanoma are recognized. A proliferation of malignant melanocytes in the epidermis, termed *radial growth phase,* is identifiable in three of the subtypes, namely superficial spreading melanoma, lentigo maligna melanoma, and acral lentiginous melanoma. The presence of an invasive dermal nodule of melanoma cells with competence for metastasis signifies the *vertical growth phase.* This phase may be preceded by a radial growth phase, or it may arise *de novo,* in which case it represents the fourth subtype, nodular melanoma.[1] Besides the aforementioned four major subtypes, several variants of malignant melanoma in its vertical growth phase exist. Some of these include desmoplastic spindle cell melanoma, minimal deviation melanoma, and malignant blue nevus. In addition, the discussion of the histology of cutaneous malignant melanoma would not be complete without mention of histologic simulants such as the spindle and epithelioid cell nevus (Spitz nevus) and its variant, the pigmented spindle cell nevus of Reed.

HISTOLOGICAL SUBTYPES OF MALIGNANT MELANOMA

Although there exists some debate on the validity of subclassifying malignant melanomas,[2,3] the classification as described originally by Clark et al.[4,5] and based on clinicopathological criteria remains useful and is widely accepted. Approximately 90 percent of melanomas examined can be placed in one of these four categories; the remainder are labeled "type unclassified."[6] The distinctive, but in some instances subtle, histologic differences unique to each of the subtypes are best appreciated in lesions of small primary melanomas or in specimens taken from the periphery of the radial growth phase of larger melanomas.[7]

Superficial Spreading Melanoma

In its **radial growth phase,** superficial spreading melanoma usually shows large, round, or epithelioid melanocytes scattered asymmetrically as single cells or in nests at all levels of the epidermis. These melanocytes have abundant cytoplasm that contains finely dispersed granular melanin. The nuclei are large and hyperchromatic; pink-staining and enlarged nucleoli are characteristically noted. Nuclear atypia and mitotic figures are often prominent.[5,8,9] A distinctive feature is that the tumor cells in the epidermis, although strikingly atypical when compared with normal melanocytes, are very uniform in their anaplastic appearance. In some instances, these intraepidermal cells may form an uninterrupted aggregate, two to three layers thick, replacing the basal keratinocytic layer.[7] Single-cell infiltration of the papillary dermis may occur and is characteristically accompanied by a marked superficial dermal lymphocytic infiltrate.

As an expansile nodule forms and fills the papillary dermis, the melanoma is then considered to be in its **vertical growth phase** and has acquired competence for metastasis. Superficial spreading melanoma cells in this phase are usually epithelioid and form one or more nodules that are significantly larger than the small clusters of invasive cells usually associated with the radial growth phase. Only rarely (in about 2 percent of cases) does the vertical growth phase of superficial spreading melanoma exhibit neurotropism and desmoplasia.[7] Maturation of cells as they descend into the dermis is minimal or absent, while intradermal necrosis or degeneration of melanocytes is invariably present.[9] A lymphocytic host response is noted, though often less intense than that seen in the radial growth phase (Plate 28).

Lentigo Maligna Melanoma

The radial growth phase of lentigo maligna melanoma resembles closely the early, preinvasive stages of this process (lentigo maligna).[10] Initially, melanocytes are only slightly increased in number and appear round in shape.[11] Subsequently, the individual melanocytes begin to exhibit variations in size and shape, increase in number along the basal layer of an atrophic epidermis, and extend along the external root sheaths of hair follicles. Atypical melanocytic nests appear and are initially widely separated from each other.[7] The cells within the nests are pleomorphic, may be small or spindle shaped, and may exhibit cellular dehesion. At this stage, single-cell invasion appears, and pagetoid spread of cells through the epidermis may be noted. The melanocytic proliferation along the external root sheath may eventually envelop the entire follicle; at times, eccrine ducts may be involved by the same process. The changes in the dermis include a prominent inflammatory infiltrate amid marked solar elastosis.[5,7,10] The term *lentigo maligna melanoma* is applied once invasion into the papillary dermis ensues.

Superficial invasion by the atypical melanocytes may be difficult to discern because the microinvasive component is often obscured by an inflammatory infiltrate. In addition, it is often hard to determine if the atypical cells amid the inflammatory infiltrate are malignant melanocytes or fibrohistiocytes. However, careful examination of multiple step sections coupled with the appropriate use of certain immunohistochemical techniques (for example, demonstration of S100 protein) in areas of suspicious dermal fibrosis or inflammation may be helpful adjuncts in detecting microinvasive foci.[12]

The vertical growth phase of lentigo maligna melanoma may be composed of either epithelioid or spindle cells. They are often admixed with a large number of melanophages; however, spindle cells are more often encountered. Desmoplasia and often neurotropism are seen in 12 to 15 percent of cases.[7]

Acral Lentiginous Melanoma

In its radial growth phase, acral lentiginous melanoma shows large, highly dendritic cells filled with finely or coarsely granular melanin. These melanocytes have round nuclei containing variably dispersed chromatin and prominent nucleoli. The nuclei appear less anaplastic than those seen in superficial spreading melanoma. In the intraepidermal component, acral lentiginous melanoma cells are uniformly large and are located in the basal layer, exhibiting the characteristic lentiginous pattern. The cells and their complex, heavily pigmented dendritic processes extend between three or four layers of adjacent keratinocytes[13] (Plate 29). Nesting of atypical melanocytes is usually not prominent, but, when present, tends to occur at the tips of rete ridges.[7] The cells within the nests are usually ovoid.[13] A characteristic feature in acral lentiginous melanoma is the presence of a prominent lichenoid lymphocytic infiltrate, associated with melanophages, obscuring the dermal-epidermal junction.[7] Because of the site of involvement, the biopsy specimen frequently shows marked acanthosis and elongation of the rete ridges.[14]

The cells involved in the vertical growth phase of acral lentiginous melanoma are commonly spindle shaped and often appear pigmented. Less frequently, these cells may appear epithelioid; or an admixture of spindle cells, large epithelioid cells, and small round cells may be observed.[13] One very important aspect of the vertical growth phase of acral lentiginous melanoma is its tendency to proliferate into the reticular dermis along eccrine ducts. Regressive changes may be noted in up to 39 percent of cases,[13] while neurotropism is noted in about 14 percent of cases.[7]

Nodular Melanoma

Nodular melanoma is a "pure" vertical growth phase disease in which a small expansile nodule in the papillary dermis progresses to invade the reticular dermis and subcutis. A radial growth phase is absent at all times. Although intraepidermal atypical melanocytes may be seen, these are almost always found overlying the invasive nodule and do *not* extend laterally within the epidermis beyond three rete ridges away from the vertical growth phase (Plate 30).

The cell type morphology may vary from monomorphous epithelioid to spindle shaped, to small nevus-like, to mixed. Desmoplasia and neurotropism are rarely noted.

PROGNOSIS ACCORDING TO HISTOLOGICAL CHARACTERISTICS

In our opinion, the histological reporting of cutaneous malignant melanomas should include the following parameters: malignant melanoma subtype (Clark classification), anatomic level of invasion, measured depth, and margins of resection. If a vertical growth phase is present, the following additional parameters are then included: mitotic rate, vertical growth phase cell type, and the presence or absence of ulceration, microscopic satellites, vascular/lymphatic invasion, inflammatory response, or regression.[6,11]

We hope that reporting of such parameters and analysis of the resulting data will help achieve a better understanding of the etiology, pathogenesis, prognosis, and optimal therapy of malignant melanoma.

The single most important factor in predicting survival for patients with cutaneous malignant melanoma that lacks regional lymph node involvement is tumor thickness.[15,16] This measurement is reported by assessing the depth of tumor penetration into the dermis and is expressed in millimeters (as described by Breslow).[17] The anatomic level (as described by Clark et al.)[5] is identified according to anatomic landmarks in the skin. (For a more detailed description of Clark's and Breslow's methods for measurement of depth of invasion, refer to Chap. 12 Pathologic Staging.)

Anatomic level is intimately linked with the likelihood of lymph node involvement: In a clinicopathologic study of 151 patients with malignant melanoma of the extremities, Wanebo et al. found a 4 percent incidence of lymph node metastasis in level II melanoma, 7 percent in level III, 25 percent in level IV, and 70 percent in level V.[18]

Regarding the prognostic value of melanoma subtypes, no difference in clinical outcome is recognized for the subtypes (if controlled for the variable of depth).[16,19–22] The melanomas do differ, however, in many other ways, including familial and racial incidence, median age of patient when diagnosed, association with dysplastic nevi, fine structure of the cells of the radial growth phase, rate of growth, the location of the primary tumor, and etiology.[7]

When the various histologic parameters are adjusted for maximum tumor thickness, in one series only two variables are found to be still significant: ulceration and the number of mitoses.[16]

The presence of ulceration indicates an adverse prognostic feature. The five-year survival rate is reduced from 80 percent for nonulcerated stage I melanomas to 55 percent in the presence of ulceration.[23] A high mitotic index also affects the prognosis adversely.[24] Cell type, which is not significant by itself, becomes so when adjusted by maximum tumor thickness. Thin spindle-cell melanomas have an excellent prognosis, with a higher survival rate than any other cell type in melanomas of the same thickness category.[16] The presence of a lymphocytic infiltrate around the tumor is regarded by some investigators as a favorable prognostic sign.[25,26]

Recently, Srivastava et al. reported that increased vascularity at the base of intermediate-thickness melanomas has adverse prognostic significance.[27,28] Most recently, Clark et al. identified six independently significant factors: mitotic rate per square millimeter, tumor-infiltrating lymphocytes, tumor thickness, anatomic site of the primary melanoma, sex of the patient, and histologic regression.[29] By reference to various tables, the prognosis of individual patients could be predicted. For example, a female patient with a "thin" melanoma on an extremity showing no evidence of regression, no mitoses, and many tumor-infiltrating lymphocytes would have an excellent prognosis.

In light of the foregoing, it is clear that the measured depth of the tumor thickness according to the method of Breslow remains the most significant predictive factor. Other variables that have been identified arise from different populations of patients and different study designs. These different variables must be taken in the light of each author's approach to diagnosis and management.

MALIGNANT MELANOMA VARIANTS

Desmoplastic and Neurotropic Melanoma

Desmoplasia is not an uncommon feature in the vertical growth phase of acral lentiginous and lentigo maligna melanomas. In 1971, Conley et al.[30] described seven cases of a rare variant of spindle-cell melanoma to which they applied the term *desmoplastic malignant melanoma*. Frequently, this neoplasm arises from a benign-appearing melanotic lesion and evolves into an aggressive and infiltrating tumor.

Histologically, these lesions are characterized by a dermal population of spindle cells amid a prominently fibrotic stroma. Closer to the epidermis, these spindle cells are arrayed in hyperchromatic nests lying randomly with respect to the long axis of the skin's surface. Below these nests, the spindle cells assume an angulated, very hyperchromatic appearance and may be mistaken for fibroblasts. A common variant of desmoplastic melanoma is desmoplastic/neurotropic melanoma,[31–34] in which the neoplasm is noted to infiltrate and expand the nerves, or may show fascicular neural-like differentiation. In addition, the spindle cells may infiltrate the perineurium and endoneurium and are sometimes seen at significant distances away from the main tumor. This infiltrative pattern contributes to the high recurrence rate, aggressive nature, and metastatic potential of this tumor[30,35,36] (Plate 31).

Occasionally, focal areas of mucinosis may be

encountered within the tumor and lead to misdiagnoses such as myxoma or myxoid liposarcoma. The presence of a proliferation of single atypical melanocytes in the overlying epidermis may be the clue to the correct diagnosis.

Amelanotic Melanoma

Amelanotic melanoma refers to a malignant melanoma, almost invariably in its vertical growth phase, in which no pigment is found by routine light microscopy.[1] The differential diagnosis of such lesions would therefore include various types of highly malignant nonmelanocytic tumors. On low power, an expansile gray-appearing mass is noted. On higher power, individual cells of the tumor exhibit round or ovoid nuclei that have prominent nucleoli with vesicular patterns of chromatin, often clumped along the nuclear margin.[1] The tumor mass may be composed of spindle cells, epithelioid cells, nevus-like cells, small cells, or a mixture of these types. These cells are often arrayed in clusters of varying sizes and also in fascicles. Infiltrating tumor cells are accompanied by nuclear debris and some lymphocytic response. Clues to the diagnosis of this variant of malignant melanoma include the presence of atypical melanocytes in various levels of the epidermis (pagetoid spread), a collarette of hyperplastic epidermis around the tumor nodule, and the occasional observation of melanophages throughout the tumor.

The application of an immunohistochemical stain, such as S100 protein, vimentin, or HMB45, is useful as a diagnostic indicator of malignant melanoma, especially the amelanotic variant. The intensity of S100 protein immunostaining appears to be inversely proportional to the amount of melanin pigment present.[37]

Gibson and Goelliner studied 15 cases of amelanotic melanoma and found that the Fontana-Masson stain was positive in only 4 of the cases, while immunostaining with the S100 protein showed a positive reaction in 13 cases.[38] Ultrastructural examination showed melanosomes in 13 cases, including 2 cases which were negative for S100 protein. Thus, electron microscopy is considered by these investigators as the most definitive method of diagnosis for amelanotic melanomas.[38]

Minimal-Deviation Melanoma and Borderline Melanoma

These rare nevomelanocytic tumors have sufficiently well-differentiated features to be classified separately from the common forms of melanoma. Their histopathologic characteristics include the presence of an expansile nodule in the papillary dermis showing either no reticular dermal invasion (borderline type), or infiltration of the reticular dermis by cords of tumor cells (minimal-deviation type).[39]

The cells of minimal-deviation melanoma most commonly resemble the spindle and epithelioid cell nevus line. However, cells looking like type B (and, rarely, type A or type C) nevus cells may also make up the uniform population in the expansile dermal nodule.

Characteristically, the cells appear cytologically **uniform** with only mild to moderate atypia. They have abundant, eosinophilic cytoplasm without prominent melanization, large nuclei with chromatin that is slightly irregular at the nuclear margin, and blue-staining nucleoli. Mitotic figures and a host response are infrequently observed and, when present, speak against the diagnosis. Also, atypical mitoses, tumor necrosis, microscopic satellites, and lymphatic/vascular invasion are absent. Although minimal-deviation melanoma was thought to behave in a less aggressive manner as compared to the common forms of melanomas,[39] the difference has not yet been statistically established in well-controlled studies.[40]

Pedunculated Melanoma (Polypoidal Melanoma)

This variant of melanoma assumes clinically a pedunculated appearance. On histological examination, the protruding core of the lesion is filled with nests and sheets of melanoma cells. With time, these lesions may exhibit infiltration by malignant cells into the pedicle and subjacent dermis. The surface of the nodule may show ulceration. Metastasis to regional lymph nodes is often detected even in those tumors that have remained confined to the areas above the pedicle,[41,42] Nonetheless, the measured depth of invasion according to Breslow is the most significant determining prognostic factor.

Balloon Cell Melanoma

Certain nevi contain large vesicular or foamy cells, known as balloon cells, that are thought to be altered nevus cells.[43] The malignant counterpart of this rare "balloon-cell nevus" is a tumor composed predominantly of such cells. Transitions from pigmented epithelioid cells with nuclear anaplasia to the vesicular balloon cells is usually seen.[44] The diagnosis is best made by examining the epithelioid cells closely and recognizing them as fully evolved melanoma cells.

Regressed Melanoma

In primary cutaneous malignant melanoma, regressive changes commonly occur and are either complete or incomplete. The complete type is characterized by the absence of atypical melanocytes in an area overlying the papillary dermis, which exhibits fibrosis, melanophages, and prominent, usually ectatic, blood vessels.[45,46] These histologic findings are nondiagnostic, because they may be observed in other nonmelanomatous nevomelanocytic lesions, such as regressed halo nevus or nonnevomelanocytic conditions, exemplified by post-inflammatory hyperpigmentation. However, in regressed melanoma, the degree of the changes is more striking, and there are prominent aggregates of melanophages, dense fibrosis, and strikingly increased vasculature (Plate 32).

Partial regression is characterized by the focal presence of the prior findings in a malignant melanoma. The prognostic significance of the presence of partial regression in melanoma remains controversial.[47–49]

Malignant Blue Nevus

This rare form of malignant melanoma arises most commonly in the cellular variant of blue nevi. The histology of the precursor lesion is characterized by an uninvolved epidermis and the presence of bipolar, thin, and wavy melanocytes in the dermis, occasionally extending to the subcutis. In addition, collections of paler melanocytes with oval to spindle-shaped nuclei are noted in large, broad fascicles and bundles. The bipolar melanocytes contain abundant melanosomes within long cytoplasmic dendrites, while the "paler" melanocytes appear clear with sparse amounts of melanin pigment. These latter cells, with their plump nuclei and their densely packed array, make up the larger proportion of cellular blue nevi.[50]

The existence of malignant blue nevi has been questioned.[51] This dilemma is partly attributed to the presence of benign nests of nevic cells in the regional lymph nodes draining the sites of benign cellular blue nevi.[51,52] However, isolated case reports of malignant, widely metastatic blue nevi do exist in the literature and have recently been reviewed.[53]

The histologic recognition of malignant blue nevi involves finding dense fascicular collections of pigmented, pleomorphic spindle cells. Adnexal structures are obliterated, and tremendous regional variation in the appearance of the tumor and the degree of pigmentation is noted. Mitotic figures and foci of necrosis are not uncommon.[53] Ultrastructural examination of the atypical melanocytes shows large nuclei with multiple nucleoli and a cytoplasm containing melanosomes at various stages of development.[54]

Malignant blue nevi differ from primary malignant melanomas, notably by their lack of an intraepidermal junctional component. However, differentiating a malignant blue nevus from a metastatic lesion of malignant melanoma may be quite difficult and rests on identifying the characteristic morphology of cells of the malignant blue nevi.

BENIGN CLINICOPATHOLOGIC SIMULANTS OF MALIGNANT MELANOMA

There are several benign nevomelanocytic tumors that mimic cutaneous malignant melanoma on clinical and histopathologic grounds. The immense global investigation of various pigmented lesions over the past two decades has led to the resolution of several controversial issues, particularly those pertaining to growth pattern, biologic behavior, histopathologic markers, and prognosis. Familiarization with the various histologic types of malignant melanoma and the recognition of the salient clinical and histopathologic attributes of benign melanocytic growths and their variants is indispensable in distinguishing benign from malignant melanocytic tumors.

Of the benign lesions that are frequently confused with cutaneous malignant melanoma, the spindle and epithelioid cell nevus,[55] or Spitz nevus, and the pigmented spindle cell nevus [56] are the most common. Although dysplastic nevi belong to this group of frequently overdiagnosed lesions, their clinical and histopathologic spectral features are relatively well understood and, therefore, pose little difficulty in separating them from malignant melanoma

The Spindle and Epithelioid Cell Nevus (Spitz Nevus)

The spindle and epithelioid cell nevus is a benign, dome-shaped, and rapidly growing tumor of nevomelanocytes.[1] It arises most commonly over the face, the lower extremities, and the buttocks but may be seen elsewhere over the body. Young individuals are more frequently affected than the elderly. These lesions are typically pink and are confused with vascular tumors, especially pyogenic granuloma. A few lesions are pigmented and ulcerated, both features causing the lesion to be misinterpreted clinically as malignant.

A prototype spindle and epithelioid cell nevus possesses a rather characteristic histopathologic appearance. [55] The architecture of the tumor and the cytology of its cells are typical, although these features may occasionally vary. On low power, the spindle and epithelioid cell nevus assumes the shape of an inverted triangle, the base of which is at the dermoepidermal interface and the apex of which is in the reticular dermis. The intraepidermal component is predominantly nested at the basal cell portion of the epithelium; however, a few individual cells may be dispersed within the lower half of the epidermis. These intraepidermal nests are expansile in character and extend into the papillary and reticular dermis, gradually losing their orderly nested pattern. "Supra-nest capping," that is the separation of the intraepidermal nests at their roof from adjacent keratinocytes, is commonly observed. Stromal changes include edema and ectatic vessels, especially in the superficial dermis. A lymphocytic host response, although variable in intensity, is frequent throughout the superficial and deep portions of the tumor.

Melanophages may be present, albeit in varying quantities. Dermal fibrosis or sclerosis may be seen, particularly when there is no epidermal component. In these lesions, the variably sized spindle and epithelioid cells are entrapped in a dense, collagenous, and eosinophilic connective tissue. Cytologically, the cells of the Spitz nevus have prominent nuclei and ample wispy or foamy cytoplasm. The nucleus of the individual cell displays delicate chromatin, a fine nuclear margin, and a conspicuous, centrally placed, bluish nucleolus. In the cytoplasm, fine but haphazard melanin granules may be seen. More often than not, mitotic figures are noted and are occasionally abnormal; however, they are observed mainly in the superficial portion of the lesion. In this portion, the spindle and epithelioid cells are arranged in fascicles, the axes of which are perpendicular to the surface of the epidermis. As the cells extend into the reticular dermis, the fascicles diminish in size and break up to infiltrate as single cells in the deep reticular dermis. This phenomenon has been termed "maturation" and is not unique to Spitz nevus, but is also one of the features of benign acquired melanocytic nevi. Diminution in the size of the cells is concurrent with this phenomenon (Plate 33). Any deviation from these descriptions is regarded as atypical; however, extremely cautious interpretation of both architecture and cytology must be carried out before a label of benign or malignant is given to a doubtful lesion.

Pigmented Spindle Cell Nevus

The pigmented spindle cell nevus of Reed poses a greater difficulty in differentiation from cutanous malignant melanoma because this lesion is underrecognized and has many architectural features similar to those of primary cutaneous malignant melanoma.[56] Clinically, the pigmented spindle cell nevus appears as a pigmented dark brown or deep black papule over the lower extremities of females between the ages of 20 and 40 years[56]; however, skin colored or red, hemangioma-like lesions of this type have been observed. This tumor erupts suddenly and grows rapidly to stabilize at a diameter of 4–6 mm. Because of its unusual clinical appearance, pigmented spindle cell nevus is frequently excised to rule out cutaneous malignant melanoma.

Microscopically, the intraepidermal component of the pigmented spindle cell nevus is composed of multiple, sharply circumscribed nests of spindle-shaped nevus cells. The nests are arrayed along hyperplastic rete ridges and, in contrast to the haphazard disposition and variability of size and form of nests in malignant melanoma, tend to be rather regularly spaced and uniform in size. The cells possess open, ovoid nuclei with finely dispersed chromatin and small, dot-like, blue nucleoli. The cytoplasm is likewise ovoid and is vacuolated; it contains coarsely granular melanin. Lateral extension with loss of sharp demarcation, lentiginous melanocytic hyperplasia, and pagetoid spread are not characteristic, but may be seen, particularly in lesions arising in preteen years. If present, such features are not considered malignant if the cytologic characteristics of the cells are benign.

The papillary dermis is almost always involved. The cells in it are also nested, spindle-shaped and pigmented and exhibit the maturation effect described in the section dealing with the Spitz nevus. In some lesions, the dermal nevus cells form a large, expansile nodule that fills and thickens the papillary dermis. Such cases are mistakenly interpreted as malignant melanoma with a vertical growth phase. Mitoses are either few or numerous, but are invariably benign in character. The cytology of the cells comprising these nests is banal. A lymphocytic host response along with melanophages is uniformly observed. The papillary dermal collagen is increased and exhibits prominent vessels.

In short, the features that would differentiate the pigmented spindle cell nevus from a cutanous malignant melanoma include symmetry, the presence of the lymphoid infiltrates in a perivascular distribution rather than a band-like one, maturation of the dermal component, lack of fully evolved cytological atypia, a relatively uniform appearance of the spindle cells, and minimal mitotic activity.[56] Histological similarities between pigmented spindle cell nevus and melanoma are the lack of sharp lateral demarcation, the presence of lateral extension, lentiginous melanocytic hyperplasia, and pagetoid spread.[56] The pagetoid spread observed in pigmented spindle cell nevus is usually limited to the lower half of the epidermis, while this feature affects all levels of the epidermis in malignant melanoma.

CONCLUSION

By definite clinicopathological criteria, one is able to subdivide primary cutaneous malignant melanoma into four main subtypes:

1. superficial spreading melanoma,
2. lentigo maligna melanoma,
3. acral lentiginous melanoma,
4. nodular melanoma.

Among the various parameters included in the histopathologic reporting, tumor thickness is the single most important factor in predicting survival for patients with cutaneous malignant melanoma without regional lymph node involvement.

Several well-characterized variants of malignant melanoma are recognized. These do not quite fit into the four main subtypes of the more common melanomas and include the following:

1. desmoplastic and neurotropic melanoma,
2. amelanotic melanoma,
3. minimal deviation and borderline melanoma,
4. pedunculated melanoma,
5. balloon-cell melanoma,
6. regressed melanoma,
7. malignant blue nevus.

In recognizing malignant melanoma and its many variants, one must be aware of the benign simulants including the spindle and epithelioid cell nevus, or Spitz nevus, and the pigmented spindle cell nevus.

By emphasizing the fine distinctions among characteristics of these melanocytic neoplasms, we hope to reach a better understanding of pathogenesis, behavior, and therapy of melanoma.

REFERENCES

1. Mihm MC, and Googe PB. *Problematic Pigmented Lesions: A Case Method Approach*. Philadelphia: Lea and Febiger, 1990, 241–287.
2. Ackerman AB. Malignant melanoma: A unifying concept. *Hum Pathol* 11:591–595 1980.
3. Ackerman AB, and David KM. A unifying concept of malignant melanoma: Biologic aspects. *Hum Pathol* 17:438–440, 1986.
4. Clark WH. A classification of malignant melanoma in man correlated with histogenesis and biologic behavior. In: Montagna W. and Hu F (eds.) *Advances in Biology of the Skin, vol. 8, The Pigmentary System*. New York: Pergamon Press, 1967, 621–647.
5. Clark WH, From L, Bernardino EA, and Mihm MC. Histogenesis and biologic behavior of primary human malignant melanoma of the skin. *Cancer Res* 29:705–727, 1969.
6. Flotte TJ, and Mihm MC. Melanoma: The art versus the science of dermatopathology. *Hum Pathol* 17:441–442, 1986.
7. Clark WH, Elder DE, and Van Horn M. The biologic forms of malignant melanoma. *Hum Pathol* 17:443–450, 1986.
8. Clark WH, Elder DE, Guerry D, Epstein MN, Greene MH, and Van Horn M. A study of tumor progression: The precursor lesions of superficial spreading and nodular melanoma. *Hum Pathol* 15:1147–1165, 1984.
9. Price NM, Rywlin AM, and Ackerman AB. Histologic criteria for the diagnosis of superficial spreading malignant melanoma: Formulated on the basis of proven metastatic lesions. *Cancer* 38:2434–2441, 1976.
10. Clark WH, and Mihm MC. Lentigo maligna and lentigo maligna melanoma. *Am J Pathol* 55:39–53, 1969.
11. McGovern VJ, Mihm MC, Bailly C, Booth JC, Clark WH, Cochran AJ, Hardy EG, Hicks JD, Levene A, Lewis MG, Little JH, and Milton GW. The classification of malignant melanoma and its histologic reporting. *Cancer* 32:1446–1457, 1973.
12. Penneys NS. Microinvasive lentigo maligna melanoma. *J Am Acad Dermatol* 17:675–680, 1987.
13. Paladugu RR, Winberg CD, and Yonemoto RH. Acral lentiginous melanoma. A clinicopathologic study of 36 patients. *Cancer* 52:161–168, 1983.
14. Coleman WP, Loria PR, Reed RJ, and Krementz ET. Acral lentiginous melanoma. *Arch Dermatol* 116:773–776, 1980.
15. Balch CM, Murad TM, Soong SJ, Ingalls AL, Richards PC, and Maddox WA. Tumor thickness as a guide to surgical management of clinical stage I melanoma patients. *Cancer* 43:883–888, 1979.
16. Van der Esch EP, Cascinelli N, Preda F, Morabito A, and Bufalino R. Stage I melanoma of the skin: Evaluation of prognosis according to histologic characteristics. *Cancer* 48:1668–1673, 1981.
17. Breslow A. Thickness, cross-sectional areas and depth of invasion in the prognosis of cutaneous melanoma. *Ann Surg* 172:902–908, 1970.
18. Wanebo HJ, Woodruff J, and Fortner JG. Malignant melanoma of the extremities: A clinicopathologic study using levels of invasion (microstage). *Cancer* 35:666–676, 1975.
19. Eldh J, Boeryd B, and Peterson LE. Prognostic factors in cutaneous malignant melanoma in stage I: A clinical, morphological and multivariate analysis. *Scand J Plast Reconstr Surg Hand Surg* 12:243–255, 1978.
20. Drzewiecki KT, and Andersen PK. Survival with malignant melanoma: A regression analysis of prognostic factors. *Cancer* 49:2414–2419, 1982.
21. Day CL, Mihm MC, Lew RA, Kopf AW, Sober AJ, and Fitzpatrick TB. Cutaneous malignant melanoma: Prognostic guidelines for physicians and patients. *CA Cancer J Clin* 32:113–122, 1982.
22. Koh HK, Michalik E, Sober AJ, Lew RA, Day CL, Clark W, Mihm MC, Kopf AW, Blois MS, and Fitzpatrick TB. Lentigo maligna melanoma has no better prognosis than other types of melanoma. *J Clin Oncol* 2:994–1001, 1984.
23. Balch CM, Wilkerson JA, Murad TM, Soong SJ, Ingalls AL, and Maddox WA. The prognostic significance of ulceration of cutaneous melanoma. *Cancer* 45:3012–3017, 1980.
24. Schmoeckel C, and Braun-Falco O. Prognostic index in malignant melanoma. *Arch Dermatol* 114:871–873, 1978.
25. Huvos AG, Shah JP, and Miké V. Prognostic factors in cutaneous malignant melanoma. A comparative study of long term and short term survivors. *Hum Pathol* 5:347–357, 1974.
26. Day CL, Sober AJ, Lew RA, Mihm MC, Fitzpatrick TB, Kopf AW, Harris MN, Gumport SL, Raker JW, Malt RA, Golomb FM, Cosimi AB, Wood WC, Casson P, Lopransi S, Gorstein F, and Postel A. Malignant melanoma patients with positive nodes and relatively good prognosis: Microstaging retains prognostic significance in clinical stage I melanoma patients with metastases to regional nodes. *Cancer* 47:955–962, 1981.
27. Srivastava A, Laidler P, Hughes LE, Woodcock J, and Shedden EJ. Neovascularization in human cutaneous melanoma: A quantitative morphological and Doppler ultrasound study. *Eur J Cancer Clin Oncol* 22:1205–1209, 1986.
28. Srivastava A. Laidler P, Davies RP, Horgan K, and Hughes LE. The prognostic significance of tumor vascularity in intermediate-thickness (0.76–4.0 mm thick) skin melanoma: A quantitative histologic study. *Am J Pathol* 133:419–423, 1988.
29. Clark WH, Elder DE, Guerry D, Braitman LE, Trock BJ, Schultz D, Synnestvedt M, and Halpern AC. Model predicting survival in stage I melanoma based on tumor progression. *J Natl Cancer Inst* 81:1893–1904, 1989.
30. Conley J, Lattes R, and Orr W. Desmoplastic malignant melanoma (a rare variant of spindle cell melanoma). *Cancer* 28:914–936, 1971.
31. Reed RJ, and Leonard DD. Neurotropic melanoma: A variant of desmoplastic melanoma. *Am J Surg Pathol* 3:301–311, 1979.

32. Ackerman AB, and Godomski J. Neurotropic malignant melanoma and other neurotropic neoplasms in the skin. *Am J Dermatopathol* 6(Suppl.):63–80, 1984.
33. Kossard S, Doherty E, and Murray E. Neurotropic melanoma. A variant of desmoplastic melanoma. *Arch Dermatol* 123:907–912, 1987.
34. Kibbi AG, and Mihm MC. Malignant melanoma with desmoplasia and neurotropism. *J Dermatol Surg Oncol* 13:1204–1208, 1987.
35. Frolow GR, Shapiro L, and Brownstein MH. Desmoplastic malignant melanoma. *Arch Dermatol* 111:753-754, 1975.
36. Labrecque PG, Hu CH, and Winkelmann RK. On the nature of desmoplastic melanoma. *Cancer* 38:1205–1213, 1976.
37. Nakajima T, Watanabe S, Sato Y, Kameya T, Shimosato Y, and Ishihara K. Immunohistochemical demonstration of S100 protein in malignant melanoma and pigmented nevus, and its diagnostic application. *Cancer* 50:912–918, 1982.
38. Gibson LE, and Goellner JR. Amelanotic melanoma: Cases studied by Fontana stain, S-100 immunostain, and ultrastructural examination. *Mayo Clin Proc* 63:777–782, 1988.
39. Muhlbauer JE, Margolis RJ, Mihm MC, and Reed RJ. Minimal deviation melanoma: A histologic variant of cutaneous malignant melanoma in its vertical growth phase. *J Invest Dermatol* 80:63S–65S, 1983.
40. Phillips ME, Margolis RJ, Merot Y, Sober AJ, Reed RJ, Muhlbauer JE, and Mihm MC. The spectrum of minimal deviation melanoma: A clinicopathologic study of 21 cases. *Hum Pathol* 17:796–806, 1986.
41. Niven J, and Lubin J. Pedunculated malignant melanoma. *Arch Dermatol* 111:755–756, 1975.
42. Rosenberg L, Goldstein J, Ben-Yakar Y, and Mahler D. The pedunculated malignant melanoma: A misunderstood and neglected variant. *J Dermatol Surg Oncol* 7:123–126, 1981.
43. Schrader WA, and Helwig EB. Balloon cell nevi. *Cancer* 20:1502–1514, 1967.
44. Gardner WA, and Vazquez MD. Balloon cell melanoma. *Arch Pathol* 89:470–472, 1970.
45. Nathanson L. Spontaneous regression of malignant melanoma: A review of the literature on incidence, clinical features, and possible mechanisms. *Natl Cancer Inst Monogr* 44:67–76, 1976.
46. Pellegrini AE. Regressed primary malignant melanoma with regional metastases. *Arch Dermatol* 116:585–586, 1980.
47. Kelly JW, Sagebiel RW, and Blois MS. Regression in malignant melanoma. A histologic feature without independent prognostic significance. *Cancer* 56:2287–2291, 1985.
48. McGovern VJ, Shaw HM, and Milton GW. Prognosis in patients with thin malignant melanoma: Influence of regression. *Histopathology* 7:673–680, 1983.
49. Cooper PH, Wanebo HJ, and Hagar RW. Regression in thin malignant melanoma: Microscopic diagnosis and prognostic importance. *Arch Dermatol* 121:1127–1131, 1985.
50. Mishima Y. Cellular blue nevus. Melanogenic activity and malignant transformation. *Arch Dermatol* 101:104–110, 1970.
51. Rodriguez HA, and Ackerman LV. Cellular blue nevus: Clinicopathologic study of forty-five cases. *Cancer* 21:393–405, 1968.
52. Allen AC, and Spitz S. Malignant melanoma: A clinicopathological analysis of the criteria for diagnosis and prognosis. *Cancer* 6:1–45, 1953.
53. Goldenhersh MA, Savin RC, Barnhill RL, and Stenn KS. Malignant blue nevus. Case report and literature review. *J Am Acad Dermatol* 19:712–722, 1988.
54. Hernandez FJ. Malignant blue nevus: A light and electron microscopic study. *Arch Dermatol* 107:741–744, 1973.
55. Sagebiel RW, Chinn EK, and Egbert BM. Pigmented spindle cell nevus. Clinical and histologic review of 90 cases. *Am J Surg Pathol* 8:645–653, 1984.
56. Barnhill RL, and Mihm MC. Pigmented spindle cell naevus and its variants: Distinction from melanoma. *Br J Dermatol* 121:717–726, 1989.

Chapter 11

IMMUNOHISTOLOGY OF MELANOMA

Dirk J. Ruiter and Eva-Bettina Bröcker

INTRODUCTION

Monoclonal antibody technology has made possible the identification of many different antigens on tumors and on normal cells. Despite many efforts to detect tumor-specific antigens on human tumor cells, with the exception of a rare case, no such antigens have been described. Therefore, one should speak of "tumor-associated" instead of "tumor-specific" antigens. Tumor-associated antigens that play a role in the clinical management of patients are called tumor markers. They can be detected in cell preparations, tissue sections, and body fluids by immunocytology, immunohistology, and immunochemical assays, respectively. Although this chapter is mainly devoted to immunohistology of human melanocytic lesions, some aspects of immunocytology will also be discussed. Emphasis will be put on those markers shown to possess a value for the diagnosis and the assessment of prognosis in melanoma patients. Where appropriate the tumor biological or immunological background of melanoma-associated antigens is elucidated in order to put the clinical application in full perspective. Last, we will mention some future developments on the immunopathology of melanoma and precursor lesions.

MELANOMA-ASSOCIATED ANTIGENS

Melanoma-associated antigens can be classified according to their chemical nature, biological function, or (sub-)cellular distribution. Herlyn and Koprowski[1] have propagated a hybrid classification based on the chemical nature and the function of the antigens. They have distinguished gangliosides, oncofetal proteins, growth factor receptors, HLA antigens, pigmentation related antigens, extracellular matrix proteins, and other molecules.

For practical purposes and based on a large experience with the immunohistology of human melanocytic lesions, we have used a simplified classification.[2] This includes *differentiation antigens, progression antigens,* and *other antigens,* most of which are related to a known cellular function, but lack the distribution of the first two categories. A differentiation antigen should have a preference for all melanocytic lesions and not, or rarely, be detectable in other cell types or the corresponding tumors. The typical distribution of a melanocytic differentiation antigen is shown in Fig. 11-1A. Although all types of melanocytic lesions indicated show expression of

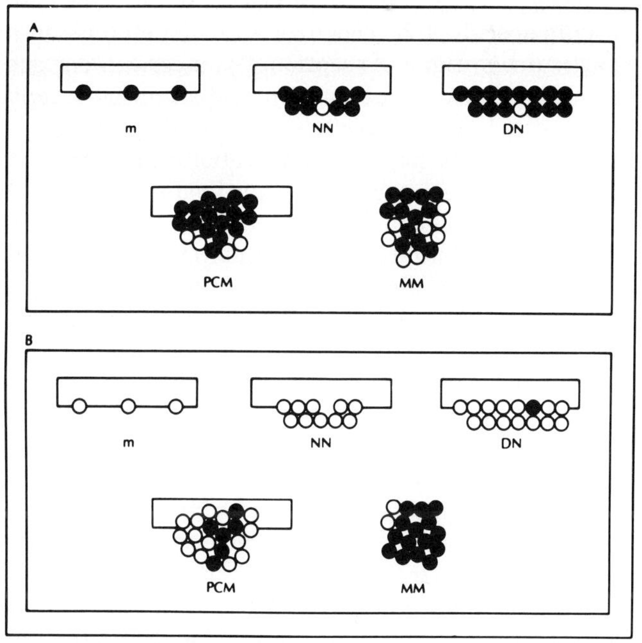

FIG. 11-1A. Distribution of a melanocytic differentiation antigen. B. Distribution of a melanocytic progression antigen. Closed circles represent positive cells. Boxes represent epidermis. m = melanocyte; NN = nevocellular nevus; DN = dysplastic nevus; PCM = primary cutaneous melanoma; MM = melanoma metastasis. (Reprinted with permission from the publisher from Current Opinion in Oncology. 1990; 2:377–387.)

the differentiation antigens, the expression in advanced primary melanoma and melanoma metastases may be only focally present or even lost, as a reflection of tumor heterogeneity induced by tumor progression. This phenomenon may hamper the efficacy of immunohistochemistry in the diagnostic procedure. A progression antigen should have a preference for a particular or only few stages of the process of neoplastic progression, for example for melanoma and not for nevocellular nevus. An example of the distribution of a progression antigen is given in Fig. 11-1B. The figure shows, in this case, that with increasing degree of malignancy the relative number of melanocytic cells expressing the antigen markedly increases.

DETECTION OF MELANOMA-ASSOCIATED ANTIGENS

For the detection of melanoma-associated antigens in cell preparations and tissue sections immunocytochemical and immunohistochemical procedures, respectively are used. In order to understand the possibilities and limitations of these procedures, a short discussion of the most important technical aspects is given, with emphasis on immunohistology.

The principle of immunohistology is the detection of antigens in tissue sections by antibodies, either monoclonal or polyclonal. Monoclonal antibodies are highly specific and recognize only one epitope on a particular antigen. Exceptionally, a certain epitope may be present on other, nonrelated antigens, and unexpected "cross"-reactions occur. Polyclonal antibodies mostly are raised in rabbits and are of a lower purity than monoclonal antibodies. Therefore, these antibodies should be extensively characterized by different immunological and immunochemical techniques, and they should be affinity purified.

To visualize the antigen-antibody reaction, the primary antibody (direct procedure) or a second or third antibody recognizing the former antibody (indirect procedure) are labeled with a fluorochrome, or an enzyme such as horse radish peroxidase, alkaline phosphatase, or glucose oxidase, or a complex containing enzyme-anti-enzyme or avidin-biotin. In order to enable optimal comparison of the staining signal with the morphological appearance, we do not use immunofluorescence in the study of melanocytic lesions. Instead, we employ a two- or three-step immunoperoxidase procedure with hematoxylin or nuclear green counterstaining. In order to avoid confusion of the melanin pigment with the brown staining product of the chromogen di-ethyl-amino-benzidine (D.A.B.), we use amino-ethylcarbazole (A.E.C.), which has a red color (Plates 34 and 35). Another possibility is to remove the melanin pigment with potassium permanganate and oxalic acid, which does not interfere with the immunoperoxidase staining, at least for the antigens tested. If double labeling is required, both A.E.C. and chloro-naphtol, which results in a blue color, are used.

Staining results are influenced by the sensitivity and the specificity of the procedure. Sensitivity can be defined as the minimal amount of antigen detectable. It is determined by the nature of the antigen, especially its stoichiometric properties, and is severely influenced by the fixation procedure. Unfortunately, most melanoma-associated antigens cannot be detected in routinely formaldehyde-fixed and paraplast-embedded tissue specimens, as this processing results in a reduced immunohistological reaction by cross-linking of antigenic determinants. On the other hand, some antigens even withstand the complete tissue processing. In some instances enzymatic pretreatment of sections with proteases, such as trypsin or pepsin, enables the immunohistological reaction in routinely fixed specimens. As most antigens, however, can be detected in acetone-fixed frozen sections, we advise sampling a representative paracentral slice from fresh and unfixed surgical specimens, quick-freezing and storing them at minus 80 grades Celsius or in liquid nitrogen. The working-up procedure for tissue preparation, which should not interfere with the conventional histopathological procedure, is illustrated in Fig. 11-2. It enables the optimal application of immunohistology

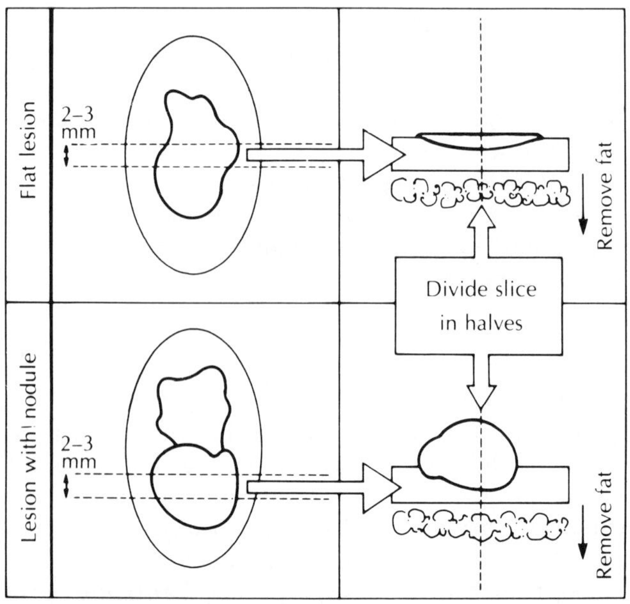

FIG. 11-2. Working up of a specimen with primary cutaneous melanoma lesions, either flat or nodular. Divide slice into halves, deep-freeze them immediately in OCT. compound, and store them at − 70°. (Reprinted with permission from the publisher from Curr Opin Oncol 2:377–387, 1990.)

whenever needed for diagnostic or prognostic purposes.[2]

Specificity of the immunohistological procedure can be defined as the degree of exclusivity for the antigen to which the antibody is directed. It is dependent on the purity of the antibody. As we have already discussed, monoclonal antibodies may give rise to unexpected reactions due to epitope sharing. Specificity in terms of a diagnostic test is also related to the nature of the antigen and its tissue distribution. To the best of our knowledge, none of the monoclonal antibodies described so far recognizing melanocytic differentiation antigens are absolutely specific for cells of the melanocytic lineage, and only few have a high degree of specificity (HMB-45 and NKI/beteb). The low specificity of most melanoma-associated antigens for the melanocytic lineage is caused by their chemical nature and function—for example gangliosides are expressed in all types of neuroectodermal cells, and growth factor receptors can be found in all sorts of tissues with regenerative capacity. Another explanation of the rather low degree of specificity of melanoma-associated antigens reported in recent studies, as compared to earlier ones, is the higher sensitivity of the immunohistological procedures more recently used.[3] Still another factor may be the higher level of awareness of possible unexpected reactions as a result of the experience in immunohistological studies gained during the last decade.

The interpretation of immunohistological slides requires knowledge of the technical procedures involved, the biology of the antigen to be detected, and the histopathology of the disease studied. We strongly recommend that, for diagnostic and prognostic purposes, the immunohistological findings are incorporated into one histopathological diagnosis, in which all the relevant clinical and pathological data has been integrated. As the antibodies used in histopathology are not specific for a certain cell type or tumor type, it has become practice to use a panel of different antibodies with a different reaction pattern. The application of such a panel will be elaborated in the section "Principles of Pathology Diagnosis."

Regarding the interpretation of the immunohistological staining signal, one has to pay attention to the distribution in various cells and tissues, to the staining intensity, and to the proportion of cells stained (of a given normal tissue or tumor). We score the staining intensity as +/− (weak), + (dull), + + (moderate), or + + + (marked). As the staining intensity may vary with the immunohistological procedure, it is mandatory to include a positive control. The proportion of tumor cells (or nevocellular nevus cells) is roughly estimated by two independent observers and expressed in one of the following categories: 0, 1–5 percent, 6–25 percent, 26–50 percent, 51–75 percent, 76–100 percent. Only cells with a staining intensity of + or more are scored. The categories correspond with the following terms: negative, sporadically positive, locally positive, occasionally positive, majority positive, large majority positive. In case of disagreement between the observers, consensus can be reached during revision of the slides. This approach has been reliable for us.

MELANOCYTIC DIFFERENTIATION ANTIGENS

Relevant properties of antibodies recognizing melanocytic differentiation antigens are summarized in Table 11-1. Only those antibodies that have been used for diagnostic purposes are included. Sensitivity is called "high" if 90 percent or more melanocytic lesions stained, "moderate" if between 50 and 90 percent, and low if less than 50 percent. Specificity is called "high" if only rarely other types of lesions stained, "moderate" if this is occasionally so, and "low" if it occurs frequently. The various antigens will be discussed separately in the following paragraphs.

S-100 Protein

S-100 protein is an acidic calcium-binding protein that was isolated from bovine brain extract. It was named S-100 protein because of its solubility in saturated ammonium sulfate solution at neutral pH. The protein is not only distributed abundantly in the nervous system of vertebrates, but also in several nonneural cells, such as melanocytes, Langerhans cells, chondrocytes, and myoepithelial cells. It is biochemically a mixture of three similar proteins, S-100a, S-100ab, and S-100b, that consist of alpha-alpha, alpha-beta, and beta-beta subunits, respectively.[4–6]

Rabbit polyclonal antibody against S-100 protein is commercially available through Dakopatts, Copenhagen, Denmark. This antibody has been used widely, and it is applicable on paraffin sections (Plate 34). Recently monoclonal antibodies against the alpha and beta subunits have been developed.[7] They are commercially available through Nihon Kontai Kenkyu Jo or JIMRO, Sakae-cho, Takasaki, Japan, and have been reported to be also applicable on paraffin sections.[7]

S-100 protein can be demonstrated in practically all types of melanocytic lesions, including amelanotic melanoma and its metastases.[4–6] The staining pattern is both intracytoplasmatic and intranuclear. Often, the majority of melanocytic cells stains, although a heterogeneous distribution may be seen. Based on its high sensitivity, the absence of S-100

TABLE 11-1
PROPERTIES OF ANTIBODIES RECOGNIZING MELANOCYTIC DIFFERENTIATION ANTIGENS

ANTIGEN	ANTIBODY	SENSITIVITY	SPECIFICITY	REMARKS
S-100 protein	Rabbit antiserum (Dakopatts)	High	Low	P + F
Neuron specific enolase	Rabbit antiserum (Dakopatts)	Low	Low	P + F
High molecular weight melanoma-associated antigen	225.28 S (Dr. S. Ferrone) or Mel.14 (Dr. S. Carrel)	High	Low	F
Gp 25-110	NKI/C3 (Sanbio)	Moderate	Moderate	P
Gp 100-7	HMB-45 (Enzo Labs)	High/moderate	High	P + F
Gp 100-7	NKI/beteb (Sanbio)	Moderate	High	F

Explanations of abbreviations:
F = applicable on frozen sections
P = applicable on paraffin sections

immunoreactivity in a poorly differentiated malignant tumor has been used as evidence against a diagnosis of melanoma. This high sensitivity is paired to a low specificity, as S-100 protein is detectable in a variety of other tumors, such as Schwannoma (often not detectable in malignant Schwannoma!), chondroma and chondrosarcoma, chordoma, benign and malignant myoepithelial tumors, and some carcinomas.

The distribution of the S-100 subunits in melanocytic lesions has not been studied widely. Recent observations of the S-100b subunit indicate a profile of a progression antigen and not that of a differentiation antigen.[7]

Neuron Specific Enolase (NSE)

Neuron specific enolase (NSE) is the most acidic isoenzyme of the glycolytic enzyme enolase. It is found in neurons, peripheral and central neuroendocrine cells, and tumors deriving from them.[8,9] It appears to be only occasionally detectable in melanocytic tumors, and it has a local staining pattern, which makes it unsuitable as a melanocytic differentiation marker.[8,9] Moreover, it can be detected in a variety of other tumors, resulting in a low specificity. Therefore, NSE is not being used as marker for the diagnosis of melanoma any more.

High Molecular Weight Melanoma-Associated Antigen (HMW-MAA)

The high molecular weight melanoma-associated antigen (HMW-MAA) is a chondroitin sulphate proteoglycan, consisting of two chains with a molecular weight of 420 and 250 kDa.[3,10–13] It is also known as melanoma proteoglycan. Functional studies suggest a role of the molecule in cell-substratum and cell-cell interactions. Many monoclonal antibodies against the HMW-MAA have been developed by several research groups.[3,10–13] Most of these are directed against distinct and spatially distant determinants. Our experience includes the monoclonal antibodies 225.28S, 763.74, and TP 41.2, produced by Dr. S. Ferrone (New York Medical College, Valhalla, NY, USA),[12] AMF-6 (later named NKI/M6), produced by Drs. J. de Vries and C. Figdor (The Netherlands Cancer Institute, Amsterdam, the Netherlands),[13] and Mel.14, produced by Dr. S. Carrel (Ludwig Institute, Epalinges, Switzerland).[11] For diagnostic purposes we have mostly used the antibodies 225.28S and Mel.14 because of their marked and consistent immunoreactivity.

The antigen can be detected reliably in frozen sections only. In normal human skin melanocytes are not stained, but cultured melanocytes do stain. However, basal keratinocytes, epithelial cells in the hair bulbs, smooth muscle cells in the arrector muscles and in the walls of blood vessels in frozen sections of normal skin also stain. In melanocytic lesions, the staining pattern is membranous and cytoplasmic. Often the staining is diffuse, although a heterogeneous pattern may be observed.

All types of melanocytic tumors stain, including a melanotic melanoma and metastases in a very high proportion of lesions tested. However, various types of tumors express HMW-MAA, including carcinomas and sarcomas, such as chondrosarcomas and leiomyosarcomas. Therefore, the antigen is of limited value as a melanocytic differentiation marker.

Glycoprotein 25-110 (NKI/C3 Antigen)

By developing monoclonal antibodies against melanoma one of the resulting hybridomas named NKI/C3 was found to react with melanocytic lesions in paraffin sections. Subsequent biochemical analysis revealed that it recognizes a glycoprotein with a heterogeneous distribution of gel filtration, ranging between 25 and 110 kDa.[14] It is conceivable that the glycoprotein exists in various degrees of glycosilation. The antibody is commercially available through Sanbio, Nistelrode, the Netherlands.

The antigen is detectable in the cytoplasm and by immunoelectron microscopy appears not to be associated with organelles such as melanosomes.[14] In paraffin sections of normal human skin it can be demonstrated in acinar cells of sweat glands and in mast cells; normal melanocytes are negative. Melanocytic tumor cells are markedly stained in a cytoplasmic pattern. Often a heterogeneous distribution is found, with preference for the junctional and subepidermal components in nevocellular nevus and primary melanoma.[15,16] Areas of necrosis markedly stain. The antibody should not be used in frozen sections, as herein a broad reactivity with nonmelanocytic cells is found. In comparison to S-100 protein and HMW-MAA, the proportion of melanocytic tumors stained is less,[17] especially regarding amelanotic melanoma. On the other hand, its specificity in paraffin sections is higher, although neuroendocrine tumors and occasional carcinomas and sarcomas have shown staining.[14,15]

HMB-45 Antigen

The HMB-45 antigen also was found by developing monoclonal antibodies against melanoma that were selected to be reactive on paraffin sections, most of which had been fixed in methanol-Carnoy's (Methacarn).[18] Sections obtained from buffered formaldehyde-fixed tissue also reacted. The nature of the antigen is not well known, although competition studies using the monoclonal antibody NKI/beteb suggest that a similar melanosomal antigen is recognized (see the next section). The antibody is commercially available through Enzo Labs, New York, NY 10013.

The antigen is detectable in junctional nevus cells but not in intradermal nevi, and in fetal and neonatal melanocytes but not in normal adult melanocytes.[18] The staining pattern is intracytoplasmic. Often a heterogeneous staining distribution is found. The degree of sensitivity was reported to be less than that of S-100 protein in one study[19] and higher in two others.[20,21] Based on an immunohistochemical study of a large panel of other malignant tumors, the specificity for melanoma has been claimed to be absolute.[18] Recently, however, reactivity with a few other cancer lesions has been found.[22] We still consider HMB-45 as highly valuable for the assessment of the diagnosis melanoma in case of a poorly differentiated malignant tumor, based on its high sensitivity and specificity.

Glycoprotein 100-107 (NKI/beteb Antigen)

Based on a similar approach, as used for NKI/C3, the monoclonal antibody NKI/beteb has been developed. The antigen recognized is a glycoprotein with a molecular weight of 100-107 kDa.[23] Immuno-electronmicroscopy has revealed that the antigen is situated within melanosomes. It can be detected in frozen sections of normal skin in melanocytes, and also in all types of melanocytic lesions tested.[23] Staining in paraffin sections is not consistent in our hands. The monoclonal antibody is commercially available through Sanbio, Nistelrode, the Netherlands.

Immunocompetition assays showed that KNI/beteb and HMB-45 recognize different epitopes of the same molecule.[23] The antigens have a similar tissue distribution in frozen sections. A distinct cytoplasmic staining pattern is seen (Plate 35). In our experience the degree of sensitivity is less than that of S-100 protein and the HMW-MAA, especially in case of amelanotic melanoma. Specificity is very high and comparable to that of HMB-45.

Other Antigens

Other antigens reported to have the profile of a melanocytic differentiation marker include the ganglioside GD3, and M-2-2-4 antigen, the melanosome-associated HMSA-1 and HMSA-2 antigens, the FKH-1 antigen, gp 57, the TA-99 antigen, the CF-21 antigen, the C-350 antigen, and the HMB-50 antigen.[1,2] These antigens are not discussed further, as they have been used only rarely for diagnostic purposes. The reasons for being used only rarely are a low sensitivity, a low specificity, or incomplete data on the tissue distribution.

USE OF ANTIBODIES RECOGNIZING MELANOCYTIC DIFFERENTIATION ANTIGENS IN IMMUNOHISTOLOGY AND IMMUNOCYTOLOGY

Principles of Pathology Diagnosis

The basis for pathology diagnosis remain conventional histology and cytology, which yield an unequivocal answer in the large majority of tumors, including those of the melanocytic lineage. Immunohistology and immunocytology are a very useful adjunct to the diagnostic repertoire of the pathologist in cases where the conventional examination gives no definite diagnosis. Antibodies recognizing melanocytic differentiation antigens can be used to identify poorly differentiated malignant lesions as being melanoma, and they also can be used to detect minimal amounts of melanoma cells in the vicinity of the primary tumor or at distant sites in case of a micrometastasis. Therefore, the clinical applications can be formulated as follows:

1. differential diagnosis of poorly differentiated malignant tumors,

2. microstaging of the primary tumor,
3. detection of micrometastases.

Based on the tissue distribution of melanocytic differentiation antigens, no contribution of immunohistology and immunocytology can be expected to discriminate between benign and malignant melanocytic lesions or to assess the prognosis in melanoma. For these purposes, antibodies recognizing melanoma-associated progression antigens may be useful. This is discussed in the section "Progression Associated Melanoma Antigens."

DIFFERENTIAL DIAGNOSIS OF POORLY DIFFERENTIATED MALIGNANT TUMORS

The differential diagnosis of such tumors include carcinoma, malignant lymphoma, sarcoma, and melanoma. In order to classify a tumor in one of these major diagnostic categories we use a panel of monoclonal antibodies recognizing various differentiation markers.[24] As the sensitivity and specificity of most of the antibodies used singly is not absolute, the combination of antibodies in such a panel yields a higher efficacy by accounting for the positive and negative staining results.[25] The composition of the panel used for the mentioned differential diagnosis is given in Table 11-2. In addition, the interpretation of the staining results is indicated in a global way. A tumor can be identified as an amelanotic melanoma with a high degree of certainty if it is positive for S-100, vimentin, and the gp 100–107, and negative for the other markers mentioned in Table 11-2. However, in some cases an aberrant expression of cytokeratins 8, 18, and 19 has been detected,[26,27] which complicates the interpretation of the immunohistological findings. This cytokeratin expression was confirmed by two-dimensional gel electrophoresis.[27] On the other hand, epithelial membrane antigen has not been found in melanoma lesions, although it can be expressed in the deeper portions of nevocellular nevi where spindle cells resembling perineural differentiation are present.[28] Another pitfall of immunohistology is the presence of tumor heterogeneity, with loss of the expression of differentiation markers in a part of the tumor or even in the whole tumor lesion.[29] Such cases are very difficult to classify with certainty. Extensive sampling of the tumor is important to be able to include the areas that yield diagnostic information. With these restrictions in mind the use of the panel mentioned in Table 11-2 can be recommended. It is not only applicable to cutaneous melanoma lesions, but also to those of the mucosae and uvea.

MICROSTAGING OF PRIMARY MELANOMA

The major parameter for the assessment of the microstage of primary melanoma lesions still is the Breslow thickness. For this purpose it is important to identify the lower border of the tumor. In some lesions, however, the lower border of the tumor is difficult to discern due to marked changes of inflammatory regression. Staining for S-100 in these lesions has been found helpful to visualize small groups

TABLE 11-2
PROPERTIES OF (MONOCLONAL) ANTIBODIES USED IN A PANEL FOR THE IMMUNOHISTOLOGICAL OR IMMUNOCYTOLOGICAL DIAGNOSIS OF POORLY MALIGNANT TUMORS

ANTIGEN	*ANITBODY*	*SOURCE*	*INTERPRETATION OF POSITIVE STAINING RESULT*
Cytokeratin[a]	PKE (P + F)	Eurodiagnostics	Carcinoma,
Cytokeratin 5 + 8	RCK 102 (F)	Eurodiagnostics	some sarcomas
Epithelial membrane antigen	Clone E29 (P + F)	Dakopatts	Carcinoma, some sarcomas and lymphomas
Vimentin[a]	PVI (P + F)	Eurodiagnostics	Sarcoma, lymphoma, melanoma, some carcinomas
Vimentin	RV202 (F)	Eurodiagnostics	
Leucocyte common antigen	clones 2B11 and PD 7/26 (P + F)	Dakopatts	Lymphoma
Desmin[a]	PDE (P + F)	Eurodiagnostics	Myosarcoma
Desmin	RD 301 (F)	Eurodiagnostics	
S-100 protein[a]	Anti S-100 A and B (P)	Dakopatts	Melanoma, various sarcomas, myoepithelial tumors, some carcinomas
Gp 100-107	HMB-45 (P + F)	Enzo Labs	Melanoma

Explanation of symbols:
[a] = polyclonal antibody
P = applicable on paraffin section
F = applicable on frozen section

of tumor cells surrounded by lymphocytes and macrophages.[16,17] Dendritic cells that also stain for S-100 can be discriminated from melanoma cells by their different morphology. In our experience, staining with NKI/C3 and NKI/beteb are less valuable for the visualization of the lower tumor border, as they preferentially stain the upper portions of the primary melanoma lesions.

DETECTION OF MICROMETASTASES

Cochran et al. have reported that the incidence of melanoma micrometastases in the regional lymph nodes of patients with clinical stage I melanoma is higher than has previously been appreciated.[30] For this purpose they used immunohistochemical staining for S-100 on more than 2200 lymph nodes derived from 100 patients, and found an incidence of 14 percent. Importantly, in none of the 14 patients metastases had been detected using conventional H&E staining. Furthermore, 6 of the 14 cases (41 percent) died of melanoma as compared to only 18 of the 86 (21 percent) without occult lymph node metastases.

In earlier studies using a similar approach, these authors have found[31] that in stage II melanoma patients microscopic foci of melanoma cells could be detected in 29 percent of ostensibly negative regional lymph nodes. These findings indicate that the detection of micrometastases by immunohistology: (a) is more sensitive than conventional histology and (b) is clinically relevant.

Immunocytological Applications

Using immunocytology on cell preparations of fine needle aspirates and effusions, it was found that a panel of monoclonal antibodies including anticytokeratin, antivimentin, NKI/C3, and NKI/beteb (Plate 35) is useful for a more accurate diagnosis of melanoma.[32] The authors showed a high sensitivity of the melanocytic differentiation antigens studied. However, as nonmelanoma cases were not included, no impression of the specificity of the marker pattern for the diagnosis of melanoma could be given. Using the monoclonal antibody HMB-45 and immunocytology other authors found a high specificity and sensitivity for melanoma.[33] Because in both series the majority of melanoma cases were at least in part melanotic, further studies containing mainly amelanotic melanoma cases should be undertaken in order to assess the efficacy of immunocytology in those cases that are difficult to diagnose.

PROGRESSION ASSOCIATED MELANOMA ANTIGENS

Establishment of primary melanoma from its precursor lesion and progression to a highly metastatic tumor was shown to be associated with stepwise expression of a variety of cell surface, cytoplasmic, or nuclear molecules.[1,34,35] Progression-associated melanoma antigens (PAMAs) either represent growth factor receptors, such as the receptor for nerve growth factor (NGF-receptor)[36,37] or epidermal growth factor (EGF-receptor),[38] or growth factor itself such as human angiogenic factor (HAF).[39] The transferrin receptor expressed on melanocytic tumors is an indicator of cytological dysplasia and, moreover, of malignant transformation.[40–42] Other PAMAs recently were shown to be adhesion molecules such as the glycoprotein A.1.43[34,35] which is identical with the integrin VLA-2,[43] and the 89 kDa glycoprotein P358,[35,44] which is identical whith the intercellular adhesion molecule-1 (ICAM-1).[45] Adhesion molecules may not only play a direct role in the process of metastasis[13,45] but also in the interaction with cell-mediated tumor cell lysis.[46] The function of the PAMA HLA-DR[34,35,47] on melanoma cells is not yet clear. The nuclear antigen Ki67[48] is expressed in cells having entered the cell cycle, and thus correlates with tumor growth. Some antigens associated with progression of melanoma that have been broadly tested in situ to prove their practical value for differential diagnosis between nevi and melanoma, and for prognostication of primary and metastatic melanoma are listed in Table 11-3. With the exception of HLA-DR and 25 F9 these PAMAs can be detected only in frozen sections.

DISTRIBUTION OF PAMAs IN MELANOCYTIC TUMORS

PAMAs in principle are defined by their absence or relatively low expression in benign melanocytic tumors and their presence or relatively high expression in malignant lesions. The frequency of PAMAs in melanocytic tumors of the skin is summarized in Table 11-4. The "sensitivity" and "specificity" of a single PAMA depends on the purpose it is used for. Only very few of the PAMAs listed in Tables 11-3 and 11-4 allow a clear-cut differential diagnosis between nevus and melanoma. For instance, only the *ABSENCE* of PAL-M1 speaks in favor of a benign lesion because it is broadly expressed in nearly 100 percent of malignant melanomas but also in 30 percent of dysplastic nevi (Table 11-4). Thus, its sensitivity is high but its specificity is low. Antigens that are very rare in nevi but only seldom expressed in early primary melanomas such as A.10.33[34] and Muc 18[35] have a high specificity, but their sensitivity is too low to regard them as useful markers for differential diagnosis. As shown later, the in situ determination of a panel of PAMAs rather than single markers of melanoma progression may be a useful approach to improve determination of dignity, and prognostication of melanocytic tumors.

TABLE 11-3
PROGRESSION-ASSOCIATED MELANOCYTIC ANTIGENS (PAMAs)

ANTIBODY	ANTIGEN	DIFFERENTIAL DIAGNOSIS	PROGNOSIS PRIMARY MELANOMA	PROGNOSIS METASTATIC MELANOMA
A-1-43	VLA-2	−	+ +	+
PAL-M1	Transferrin receptor	+ +	−	−
P358	ICAM-1	+	+	?
anti HLA-DR[o]	HLA-DR	+	+ +	+
anti HLA-A,B,C	HLA-A,B,C	−	?	+
Muc 18	113 kDa	(+)	?	?
A-10-33	?	(+)	+ +	−
20.4,200.3	NGF-Receptor	(+)	?	?
Q14[a]	130 kDa	+ +[a]	−	?
25F9[bo]	86 kDa	−	+	+

− = no value as a single marker
(+) = little value as a single marker
\+ = considerable value as a single marker
\+ + = high value as a single marker
[a] = only in lentiginous proliferations
[b] = on tumor infiltrating macrophages
[o] = applicable in formalin-fixed material
? = not known

A.1.43 (VLA-2)

By immunization with the highly malignant melanoma cell line A.375, a monoclonal antibody was generated by Brüggen and Sorg.[49] The antibody A.1.43 reacts with a glycoprotein of about 130 kDa which is constitutively expressed by keratinocytes of the basal cell layer and in Schwann cells.[50] Extensive *in situ* studies revealed that the antigen is progression-associated in melanocytic tumors.[34,35] The antigen is, however, not exclusively expressed in malignant melanoma but to a varying degree in melanocytic nevi (Table 11-4). It is associated with early metastatic spread when present in primary melanoma,[34] and with a poor prognosis when present in skin metastases.[51] As shown in Table 11-4, A.1.43 is more frequent in primary melanomas of stage II/III patients than in stage I patients.

Recently it was shown that the antibody A.1.43 reacts with the α-chain of the integrin VLA-2 which is a receptor for extracellular matrix proteins.[43] In nude mice, A.1.43 positive melanoma cell lines formed spontaneous metastases.[52] Thus, this well-characterized PAMA might be directly involved in the process of local invasiveness and metastatic spread of human melanoma.

PAL-M1 (Transferrin Receptor)

The antibody PAL-M1 was selected to discriminate between nevus and melanoma.[40] It is broadly expressed on the vast majority of primary and meta-

TABLE 11-4
FREQUENCY OF PAMAs IN CUTANEOUS MELANOCYTIC TUMORS POSITIVE/TESTED LESIONS[a] (PERCENTAGE)

PAMA	COMMON AQUIRED NEVI	HALO NEVI	DYSPLASTIC NEVI	CONGENITAL NEVI	SPINDLE CELL NEVI o	PRIMARY MELANOMA STAGE I	PRIMARY MELANOMA STAGE II/III
A.1.43	14/64(22)	0/22(0)	31/108(28)	16/44(36)	4/14(29)	101/318(32)	22/30(73)
PAL-M1	6/64(9)	0/24(0)	38/127(39)	9/44(20)	10/14(29)	119/126(94)	16/17(94)
P358	3/64(5)	2/22(9)	4/69 (6)	12/44(27)	3/10(30)	45/120(38)	10/11(90)
HLA-DR	1/64(2)	3/24(13)	11/137(8)	4/44(9)	2/14(14)	116/288(40)	23/29(79)
Muc 18	1/29(3)	0/22(0)	0/32 (0)	1/44(2)	3/11(27)	35/104(34)	9/10(90)
A.10.33	3/64(5)	0/24(0)	4/112(4)	0/44(0)	4/10(40)	35/235(15)	15/30(50)

[a]Data are derived from publications 34, 35, 40, 53, 56, 68, 81 and from unpublished cases of Spitz nevi and Reed's-tumors.

static melanoma[35,40] (Table 11-4), but occasionally also on nevus cells, in particular in dysplastic nevi,[35,40] where it was found correlated with the degree of dysplasia.[53]

Recently, PAL-M1 was shown to react with the transferrin receptor.[41] PAL-M1 is a good reagent to discriminate between benign and malignant lesions, because its absence indicates a benign tumor. The only exception is lentigo maligna where PAL-M1 also was absent in many lesions.[54]

P358 (ICAM-1)

In 1985, Holzmann et al. described a 89 kDa glycoprotein that discriminates between nevus and melanoma.[44] Later it was shown to be a PAMA that is induced in melanoma cells by IFN_{γ}.[35] Johnson et al. proved that the antigen recognized by the antibody P358 is identical with the intercellular adhesion molecule 1 (ICAM-1), which is the receptor for the lymphocyte function-associated molecule 1 (LFA-1).[45] In primary but not in metastatic melanoma, it is coexpressed with HLA-DR and is correlated with the degree of intratumoral T-cell infiltrates.[55] Interestingly, the antigen is quite frequent in congenital nevi with no evidence of its in situ-induction by T cell-derived lymphokines[56] (Table 11-4).

HLA-DR

The expression of MHC-class II molecules is induced by IFN_{γ} on a variety of cells including normal and malignant melanocytes.[57,58] While studies on isolated melanoma cells suggested that HLA-DR/DP/DQ antigens might be functionally active in the means of tumor defense mechanisms because of providing the structural condition for tumor cell-lymphocyte interactions,[59] immunohistological data more and more showed that class II MHC molecules, in particular HLA-DR antigens, are markers of melanoma progression and, independent from tumor thickness, are indicative of a poor prognosis in primary melanoma and in loco-regional melanoma metastases.[34,35,60,61] HLA-DR and -DQ antigen expression correlated with the amount of intratumoral T cells.[55,62] and with the presence of IFN_{γ} in primary melanomas.[55]

In metastases, HLA-DR antigens are found expressed without signs of in situ induction.[62] Systemic interferon treatment, however, in vivo increased the expression in soft tissue metastases.[63] In visceral metastases a loss of HLA-DR antigen expression together with a loss of HLA-A,B,C antigen expression was observed in situ.[34] The immunohistological determination of HLA-DR antigens in routinely fixed melanoma-specimen appears to be of great practical importance, since monoclonal antibodies are available that react with formaline resistant epitopes of the molecule[60,64,65] (Plate 36).

Muc 18

A monoclonal antibody against a surface molecule of 113 kDa has been described by Lehmann et al.[66] It is absent in melanocytic nevi and is expressed in increased frequency in melanomas in proportion to invasiveness and progression.[35] Recent studies revealed that the molecule belongs to the *Ig*-gene superfamily and shows homology to the N-CAM adhesion molecule.[67] The only cross-reaction of the antibody Muc 18 in frozen tissues are smooth muscles. The use of Muc 18 in a panel of antibodies against PAMAs may be of high practical importance for prognostication, although its sensitivity for differential diagnosis between nevus and primary melanoma as a single marker is low due to its rather rare expression in primary melanoma of the radial growth phase.[35]

A-10-33

The antibody A-10-33 was, like A-1-43, raised against the melanoma cell line A375.[49] The molecular nature of the antigen, which might be associated with the receptor for vitronectin (G.P. Tuszynski, unpublished) has yet to be finally analyzed. mAb A-10-33 strongly reacts with human blood vessel endothelium,[50] weakly with epidermis and epidermal appendages, and not with normal epidermal melanocytes. As shown in Table 11-4, it is found neither in congenital melanocytic nevi nor in most common acquired nevi, but it was found in Spitz nevi[68] and pigmented spindle cell tumors (Reed's) (unpublished). Its rare expression in primary melanoma was found associated with early metastatic spread,[34] and its more frequent expression in visceral melanoma metastases than in skin metastases[34] suggests that this antigen indicates highly aggressive melanoma cells. Like Muc 18, its sensitivity for differential diagnosis between nevus and melanoma is low because of its rare expression in stage I primary melanoma, although its determination is worthwhile in order to find potentially metastatic clones within a thin primary melanoma.

Q14 (130 kDa)

A transformation- and proliferation-associated glycoprotein of 130 kDa, which is expressed by a variety of human tumor cell lines has been described by Klein et al.[69] In situ we found it expressed homogeneously on melanoma, and heterogeneously on nevi (unpublished). Normal epidermal melanocytes were negative in all lesions tested. In contrast to benign lentiginous melanocytic proliferations, lentigo maligna proved to be Q14 positive.[54] Further immunohistological studies will show whether Q14 is a reagent to allow the determination of the dignity of lentiginous melanocytic proliferation in histologically difficult cases, such as acral and mucosal lentigines.

NGF-Receptor

Although the functional role of nerve growth factor (NGF) for growth and differentiation of melanocytes is yet unknown, expression of high affinity NGF-receptor (NGF-R) has been described on melanoma cells in vitro and in situ.[36,70] Normal epidermal melanocytes are NGF-R negative in situ, but can be positive in vitro, depending on culture conditions.[71] In situ we found NGF-R expressed mainly in malignant melanocytic proliferations, but no correlation to local invasiveness of primary melanoma was observed.[72] Interestingly, considerable NGF-R expression in nevi was restricted to potential melanoma precursor lesions, that is, dysplastic and congenital nevi.[72] It has yet to be determined whether NGF-R is a prognostic marker.

K-1-2

A melanocytic antigen, K-1-2, that decreases in the course of local and systemic melanoma progression[34,35] has been described by Suter et al.[73] It is expressed in nevi and early primary melanoma to about the same extent, thus the antibody K-1-2 is no reagent for discrimination between nevus and melanoma (Table 11-3). In metastatic melanoma, however, the presence of K-1-2 was found correlated with a more favorable prognosis.[51] The molecular nature of the antigen K-1-2 is not known. It is found, like NKI-beteb[23] and HMB 45,[18] in the cytoplasm of normal and malignant melanocytes, but the tissue distribution is different.

Other Antigens

A variety of other antigens that are positively or negatively correlated to melanoma progression have been described by various groups.[37,74–77] Most of them have been mainly studied in cultured cells. In situ, the proliferation-associated marker Ki67[48] has been studied in larger series of melanocytic tumors in order to find whether its immunohistological determination provides additional prognostic information.[42,78]

IMMUNOHISTOLOGY OF THE TUMOR INFILTRATES: PROGNOSTIC IMPLICATION

Local and systemic progression of melanoma is associated not only with changes in the antigen phenotype of tumor cells but also with changes in the composition and activation state of the inflammatory infiltrates.[55] A subset of tissue macrophages characterized by the expression of the 86 kDa protein 25 F9[79] has been found to be positively correlated with poor prognosis in primary and metastatic melanoma.[80] The antigen is detectable in routinely fixed paraffin-embedded material after a mild trypsinization of sections and incubation with the antibody overnight.[80]

PATTERN ANALYSES OF PAMAs FOR DIAGNOSTIC AND PROGNOSTIC PURPOSES

Due to tumor cell heterogeneity, which is not only a feature of malignant melanoma but also of benign nevi, the determination of a panel of PAMAs rather than the in situ determination of single markers provided information of dignity, risk of malignant transformation, and prognosis. Steijlen et al.[56] found single PAMAs more often expressed in congenital nevi than in common acquired nevi (Table 11-5). Five congenital nevi of the series developed a melanoma, and all of them coexpressed at least two out of six PAMAs studied. In halo nevi we occasionally found the IFN-induced PAMAs P358 and HLA-DR but no other PAMAs expressed. Coexpression of PAMAs was not observed in halo nevi.[81]

In stage I primary melanomas that metastasized within one year coexpression of at least four PAMAs were observed in the majority of cases (Table 11-6). Thus, the finding of more than one PAMA expressed in a melanocytic lesion indicates the risk of malignant transformation and metastatic potential. The prognosis of locoregional metastases was found cor-

TABLE 11-5
COEXPRESSION OF PAMAs IN MELANOCYTIC NEVI[56]

NUMBER OF PAMAs	COMMON ACQUIRED NEVI	CONGENITAL MELANOCYTIC NEVI
0–1	18/29 (97%)	35/44 (79%)
2–3	1[a]/29 (3%)	8[b]/44 (19%)
–6	0/29 (0%)	1[c]/44 (2%)

[a]Normal compound naevus of a melanoma patient
[b]Four of them with melanoma
[c]With melanoma

TABLE 11-6
EXPRESSION AND COEXPRESSION OF PAMAs IN PRIMARY MELANOMAS THAT METASTASIZED WITHIN ONE YEAR

PAMA	POSITIVE/TESTED	LESIONS (%)
A.1.43	13/16	(81)
PAL-M1	13/13	(100)
P358	13/15	(87)
HLA-DR	13/16	(81)
Muc18	11/14	(79)
A.10.33	11/16	(69)
NUMBER OF PAMAs		
0–1	0/12	(0)
2–3	1/12	(8)
4–6	11/12	(92)

related with the pattern of HLA-class I and class II antigen expression.[61] For better definition of a melanocytic lesion, a panel of several PAMAs rather than the determination of a single marker is required.

CONCLUSION

The immunohistological experience allow the following conclusions:

1. With the exception of lentigo maligna, the *lack* of PAL-M1 strongly suggests a benign tumor even if another PAMA is expressed.
2. The *presence* of PAL-M1 together with at least one other PAMA favors a malignant lesion.
3. The *lack* of the Q14 antigen in a lesion with lentiginous growth pattern strongly suggests a benign melanocytic proliferation.
4. A discrimination between Spitz/Reed nevi and primary melanoma with the help of immunohistology on frozen sections is not possible with the panel of PAMAs studied so far.
5. Coexpression of $\geq$ 2 PAMAs in congenital melanocytic nevi indicates risk of malignant transformation.
6. Coexpression of $\geq$ 4 PAMAs in primary melanoma indicates the risk of early metastases.

The immunohistological determination of the majority of PAMAs described here has been possible only in frozen sections. This reduces their practical application in routine histopathology. Further work should focus on the development of reagents against formaline-resistant epitopes on biologically interesting molecules. Another approach may be the development of probes in order to detect the responsible genes by in situ-hybridization.

REFERENCES

1. Herlyn M, and Koprowski H. Melanoma antigens. Immunological and biological characterization and clinical significance. *Annu Rev Immunol* 6:283–308, 1988.
2. Ruiter DJ. Pathology and case reports. *Curr Opin Oncol* 2:377–387, 1990.
3. Garin-Chesa P, Beresford R, Carrato-Mena A, Oettgen H, Old LJ, Melamed ML, and Rettig WJ. Cell surface markers of human melanoma. Immunohistochemical analysis of the gp 57, GD 3, and mel-CSPG antigenic systems. *Am J Pathol* 135:295–305, 1989.
4. Cochran AJ, Wen D-R, Herschman HR, and Gaynor RB. Detection of S-100 protein as an aid to the identification of melanocytic tumors. *Int J Cancer* 30:295–297, 1982.
5. Nakajima T, Watanabe S, Sato Y, Kameya T, Shimosato Y, and Ishihara K. Immunohistochemical demonstration of S-100 protein in malignant melanoma and pigmented nevus and its diagnostic application. *Cancer* 50:912–918, 1982.
6. Stefansson K, Wollmann R, and Jerkovic M. S-100 protein in soft-tissue tumors derived from Schwann cells and melanocytes. *Am J Pathol* 106:261–268, 1982.
7. Hyun Cho K, Hashimoto K, Taniguchi J, Pietruk T, Zarbo RJ, and An T. Immunohistochemical study of melanocytic nevus and malignant melanoma with monoclonal antibodies against S-100 subunits. *Cancer* 66:765–771, 1990.
8. Springall DR, Gu J, Cocchia D, Michetti F, Levene A, Levene MM, Marangos PJ, Bloom SR, and Polak JM. The value of S-100 immunostaining as a diagnostic tool in human malignant melanomas. *Virchows Arch A Pathol Anat Histopathol* 400:331–343, 1983.
9. Hachisuka H, Sakamoto F, Nomwra H, Mori O, and Sasai Y. Immunohistochemical study of S-100 protein and neuron specific enolase in melanocytes and the related tumors. *Acta Histochem* 89:215–223, 1986.
10. Bumol TF, and Reisfeld RA. Unique glycoprotein-proteoglycan complex defined by monoclonal antibody on human melanoma cells. *Proc Natl Acad Sci U S A* 79:1245–1249, 1982.
11. Carrel S, Accolla RS, Carmognola AL, and Mach J-P. Common human melanoma-associated antigen(s) detected by monoclonal antibodies. *Cancer Res* 40:2523–2525, 1980.
12. Giacomini P, Natali PG, and Ferrone S. Analysis of the interactions between human high-molecular weight melanoma-associated antigens and the monoclonal antibodies to three distinct antigenic determinants. *J Immunol* 135:696–702, 1985.
13. De Vries JE, Keizer GD, Te Velde AA, Voordouw A, Ruiter DJ, Rümke P, Spits H, and Figdor CG. Characterization of melanoma-associated surface antigens involved in the adhesion and motility of human melanoma cells. *Int J Cancer* 38:465–473, 1986.
14. Vennegoor C, Calafat J, Hageman Ph, Van Buitenen F, Janssen H, Kolk A, and Rümke Ph. Biochemical characterization and cellular localization of a formalin-resistant melanoma-associated antigen reacting with monoclonal antibody KNI/C3. *Int J Cancer* 35:287–295, 1985.
15. Van Duinen SG, Ruiter DJ, Hageman Ph, Vennegoor C, Dickersin GR, Scheffer E, and Rümke Ph. Immunohistochemical and histochemical tools in the diagnosis of amelanotic melanoma. *Cancer* 53:1566–1573, 1984.
16. MacKie RM, Campbell L, and Turbitt ML. The use of NKI/C3 monoclonal antibody in the assessment of benign and malignant melanocytic lesions. *J Clin Pathol* 37:367–372, 1984.
17. Hagen EC, Vennegoor C, Schlingemann RO, Van der Velde EA, and Ruiter DJ. Correlation of histopathological characteristic with staining patterns in human melanoma assessed by (monoclonal) antibodies reactive on paraffin sections. *Histopathology* 10:689–700, 1986.
18. Gown AM, Vogel AM, Hoak D, Gough F, and McNutt MA. Monoclonal antibodies specific for melanocytic tumors distinguish subpopulations of melanocytes. *Am J Pathol* 123:195–203, 1986.
19. Colombari R, Bonetti F, Zamboni G, Scarpa G, Marino F, Tomezzoli A, Capelli P, Menestrina F, Chilosi M, and Fiore-Donati L. Distribution of melanoma specific antibody (HMB-45) in benign and malignant melanocytic tumours. An immunohistochemical study on paraffin sections. *Virchows Arch A Pathol Anat Histopathol* 413:17–24, 1988.
20. Ordonez NG, Xiaolong J, and Hickey RC. Comparison of HMB-45 monoclonal antibody and S-100 protein in the immunohistochemical diagnosis of melanoma. *Am J Clin Pathol* 90:385–390, 1988.
21. Thomson W, and MacKie RM. Comparison of five antimelanoma antibodies for identification of melanocytic cells on tissue sections in routine dermatopathology. *J Am Acad Dermatol* 21:1280–1284, 1989.
22. Kornstein MJ, and Franco AP. Specificity of HMB-45. Letter to the editor. *Arch Pathol Lab Med* 114:450, 1990.
23. Vennegoor C, Hageman Ph, Van Nouhuys H, Ruiter DJ, Calafat J, Ringens PJ, and Rümke Ph. A monoclonal

antibody specific for cells of the melanocytic lineage. *Am J Pathol* 130:179–192, 1988.
24. Henzen-Logmans SC, Meyer CJLM, Ruiter DJ, Mullink H, Balm AJM, and Snow GB. *Cancer* 61:702–711, 1988.
25. Corwin DJ, and Gown AM. Review of selected lineage-directed antibodies useful in routinely processed tissues. *Arch Pathol Lab Med* 113:645–652, 1989.
26. Gatter KC, Ralfkiaer E, Skinner J, Brown D, Heryet A, Pulford KAF, Hou-Jensen K, and Mason DY. An immunocytochemical study of malignant melanoma and its differential diagnosis from other malignant tumours. *J Clin Pathol* 38:1353–1357, 1985.
27. Zarbo RJ, Gown AM, Nagle RB, Visscher DW, and Crissman JD. Anomalous cytokeratin expression in malignant melanoma: one- and two-dimensional Western blot analysis and immunohistochemical survey of 100 melanomas. *Mod Pathol* 3:494–501, 1990.
28. Cramer SF. Epithelial membrane antigen staining of melanocytic nevi. Correspondence. *Hum Pathol* 21:121–122, 1990.
29. Duray PH, Palazzo J, Gown AM, and Ohuchi N. Melanoma cell heterogeneity. A study of two monoclonal antibodies compared with S-100 protein in paraffin sections. *Cancer* 61:2460–2468, 1988.
30. Cochran AJ, Wen D-R, and Morton DL. Occult tumor cells in the lymph nodes of patients with pathological stage I malignant melanoma. An immunohistological study. *Am J Surg Pathol* 12:612–618, 1988.
31. Cochran AJ, Wen D-R, and Herschman HR. Occult melanoma in lymph nodes detected by antiserum to S-100 protein. *Int J Cancer* 34:159–163, 1984.
32. Angeli S, Koelma IA, Fleuren GJ, and Van Steenis GJ. Malignant melanoma in fine needle aspirates and effusions. An immunocytochemical study using monoclonal antibodies. *Acta Cytol* 32:707–712, 1988.
33. Walts AE, Said JW, and Shintaku IP. Cytodiagnosis of malignant melanoma. Immunoperoxidase staining with HMB-45 antibody as an aid to diagnosis. *Am J Clin Pathol* 90:77–80, 1988.
34. Bröcker EB, Suter L, Brüggen J, Ruiter DJ, Macher E, and Sorg C. Phenotypic dynamics of tumor progression in human malignant melanoma. *Int J Cancer* 36:29–35, 1985.
35. Holzmann B, Bröcker EB, Lehmann JM, Ruiter DJ, Sorg C, Riethmüller G, and Johnson JP. Tumor progression in human malignant melanoma: Five stages defined by their antigenic phenotypes. *Int J Cancer* 39:466–471, 1987.
36. Ross AH, Grob P, Bothwell M, Elder DE, Ernst CS, Marano N, Christ BFD, Slemp CC, Herlyn M, Atkinson B, and Koprowski H. Characterization of nerve growth factor receptor in neural crest tumors using monoclonal antibodies. *Proc Natl Acad Sci U S A* 81:6691–6695, 1984.
37. Herlyn M, Balaban G, Bennicelli J, Guerry D, Halaban R, Herlyn D, Elder DE, Maul GG, Steplewski Z, Nowell C, Clark WH, and Koprowski H. Primary melanoma cells of the vertical growth phase: Similarities to metastatic cells. *J Natl Cancer Inst* 74:283–289, 1985.
38. De Wit PEJ, Moretti S, Weterman MAJ, Defize BLHK, Van Muijen GNP, Gianotti B, and Ruiter DJ. Epidermal growth factor receptor is a progression marker in human melanocytic lesions. *Invest Dermatol* 99:168–173, 1992.
39. Frühbeis B, Zwadlo G, Bröcker EB, Schulze-Osthoff K, Hagemeier HH, Topoll H, and Sorg C. Immunolocalization of an angiogenic factor (HAF) in normal, inflammatory and tumor tissues. *Int J Cancer* 42:207–212, 1988.
40. Ruiter DJ, Dingjan GM, Steijlen PM, van Beveren-Hooyer M, de Graaff-Reitsma CB, Bergman W, van Muijen GNP, and Warnaar SO. Monoclonal antibodies selected to discriminate between malignant melanomas and nevocellular nevi. *J Invest Dermatol* 85:4–8, 1985.
41. Muijen GNP van, Ruiter DJ, Hoefakker S, and Johnson JP. Monoclonal antibody PAL-M1 recognizes the transferrin receptor and is a progression marker in melanocytic lesions. *J Invest Dermatol* 95:65–69, 1990.
42. Soyer HP, Smolle J, Smolle-Juettner FM, and Kerl H. Proliferation antigens in cutaneous melanocytic tumors—an immunohistochemical study comparing the transferrin receptor and the Ki67 antigen. *Dermatologica* 179:3–9, 1989.
43. Klein CE, Steinmayer TH, Kaufmann D, Weber L, and Bröcker EB. Identification of a melanoma progression antigen as integrin VLA-2. *J Invest Dermatol,* 96:281–284, 1991.
44. Holzmann B, Johnson JP, Kaudewitz P, and Riethmüller G. In situ analysis of antigens on malignant and benign cells of the melanocytic lineage: Differential expression of two surface molecules, gp75 and gp89. *J Exp Med* 161:366–377, 1985.
45. Johnson JP, Stade BG, Holzmann B, Schwäble W, and Riethmüller G. De novo expression of intercellular-adhesion molecule 1 in melanoma correlated with increased risk of metastasis. *Proc Natl Acad Sci U S A* 86:641–644, 1989.
46. Anichini A, Mortarini R, Berti E, and Parmiani G. Multiple VLA antigens on a subset of melanoma clones. *Hum Immunol* 28:119–122, 1990.
47. Bröcker EB, Suter L, and Sorg C. HLA-DR antigen expression in primary melanomas of the skin. *J Invest Dermatol* 82:244–247, 1984.
48. Gerdes J, Lemke H, Baisch H, Wacker HH, Schwab U, and Stein H. Cell cycle analysis of a cell proliferation-associated human nuclear antigen defined by the monoclonal antibody Ki-67. *J Immunol* 133:1710, 1984.
49. Brüggen J, and Sorg C. Detection of phenotypic differences on human malignant melanoma lines and their variant sublines with monoclonal antibodies. *Cancer Immunol Immunother* 15:200–205, 1983.
50. Suter L, Bröcker EB, Brüggen J, Ruiter DJ, and Sorg C. Heterogeneity of primary and metastatic human malignant melanoma as detected with monoclonal antibodies in cryostat sections of biopsies. *Cancer Immunol Immunother* 16:53–58. 1983.
51. Suter L, Bröcker EB, Ostmeier H, Schumann J, and Sorg C. Metastatic human melanoma. Phenotypic heterogeneity and antigen expression in relation to the clinical status. *J Cancer Res Clin Oncol* 115:459–464, 1989.
52. Muijen, v. GNP, Cornelissen LMHA, Jansen CFJ, Figdor CG, Johnson JP, Bröcker EB, and Ruiter DJ. Antigen expression of metastasizing and non-metastasizing human melanoma cells xenografted to nude mice. *Clin Exp Metastasis,* 9:259–272, 1991.
53. Hofmann-Wellenhof R, Hamm H, Kolde G, Ruiter DJ, Johnson JP, and Bröcker EB. Dysplastic nevi: Which are precursors of melanoma? (Abstr)*Arch Dermatol Res* 281:573, 1990.
54. Christian, E, Klein CE, Schwaaf A, Ruiter DJ, and Bröcker EB. Transformation-associated antigen in lentiginous melanocytic proliferations. (Abstr). *Arch Dermatol Res,* 283:51, 1991.
55. Bröcker EB, Zwadlo G, Holzmann B, Macher E, and Sorg C. The inflammatory infiltrates in huamn melanomas at different stages of tumor progression. *Int J Cancer* 41:562–567, 1988.
56. Steijlen PM, Hamm H, Erp v. PEJ, Johnson JP, Ruiter DJ, and Bröcker EB. Immunohistological evidence for the malignant potential of congenital melanocytic nevi. *J Invest Dermatol* 92:366–370, 1989.

57. Houghton AN, Thomson TM, Gross D, Oettgen HF, and Old LJ. Surface antigens of melanoma and melanocytes. Specificity of induction of Ia antigens by human interferon. *J Exp Med* 160:55–269, 1984.
58. Carrel S, Schmidt-Kessen A, and Giuffrè L. Recombinant interferon$_\gamma$ can induce the expression of HLA-DR and -DC or DR-negative melanoma cells and enhance the expression of HLA-ABC and tumor-associated antigens. *Eur J Immunol* 15:118–123, 1985.
59. Pollack MS, Chin-Louie J, and Moshief R. Functional characteristics and differential expression of class II DR, DS, and SB antigens on human melanoma cell lines. *Hum Immunol* 9:75–87, 1984.
60. Zaloudik J, Moore M, Ghosh AK, Mechl Z, and Rejthar A. DNA content and MHC class II antigen expression in malignant melanoma: Clinical course. *J Clin Pathol* 41:1078–1084, 1988.
61. Duinen SG van, Ruiter DJ, Bröcker EB, van der Velde EA, Sorg C, Welvaart K, and Ferrone S. Level of HLA antigens in locoregional metastases and clinical course of the disease in patients with melanoma. *Cancer Res* 48:1019–1025, 1988.
62. Vreeswijk H van, Ruiter DJ, Bröcker EB, Welvaart K, and Ferrone S. Differential expression of HLA-DR, DQ, and DP antigens in primary and metastatic melanoma. *J Invest Dermatol* 90:755–760, 1988.
63. Bröcker EB, Ruiter DJ, Stamm v. U, and Carrel S. Interferon α (IFNα) effects on melanoma cell phenotype *in vivo*. *J Invest Dermatol* 92:407, 1989.
64. Wilson BS, Herzig MA, and Lloyd RV. Immunoperoxidase staining for Ia-like antigens in paraffin-embedded tissues from human melanoma and lung carcinoma. *Am J Pathol* 115:102–108, 1983.
65. Sorg C, Bröcker EB, Zwadlo G, Redmann K, Feige U, Ax W, and Feller AC. A monoclonal antibody to a formaldehyde-resistant epitope on the nonpolymorphic constant part of the HLA-DR antigens. *Transplantation* 39:90–93, 1985.
66. Lehmann JM, Holzmann B, Breitbart EW, Schmiegelow P, Riethmüller G, and Johnson JP. Discrimination between benign and malignant cells of melanocytic lineage by two novel antigens, a glycoprotein with a molecular weight of 113,000 and a protein with a molecular weight of 70,000. *Cancer Res* 47:841–845, 1987.
67. Lehmann JM, Riethmüller G, and Johnson JP. MUC18, a marker of tumor progression in human melanoma, shows sequence similarity to the neural cell adhesion molecules of the immunoglobulin superfamily. *Proc Natl Acad Sci U S A* 86:9891–9895, 1989.
68. Hamm H, Happle R, and Bröcker EB. Multiple agminate spitz naevi: Review of the literature and report of a case with distinctive immunohistological features. *Br J Dermatol* 117:511–522, 1987.
69. Klein E, Ozer HL, Traganos F, Atzpodien J, Oettgen HF, and Old LJ. A transformation-associated 130- akD cell surface glycoprotein is growth controlled in normal human cells. *J Exp Med* 167:1684–1696, 1988.
70. Chesa PG, Rettig WJ, Thomson TM, Old LJ, and Melamed MR. Immuno-histochemical analysis of nerve growth factor receptor expression in normal and malignant human tissues. *J Histochem Cytochem* 29:577, 1981.
71. Peacocke M, Yaar M, Mansur CP, Chao MV, and Gilchrest BA. Induction of nerve growth factor receptors on cultured human melanocytes. *Proc Natl Acad Sci U S A* 85:5282–5286, 1988.
72. Bröcker EB, Magiera H, and Herlyn M. Nerve growth and nerve growth factor receptor expression in tumors of melanocytic origin. *J Invest Dermatol,* 96:662–665, 1991.
73. Suter L, Brüggen J, Bröcker EB, and Sorg C. A tumor-associated antigen expressed in melanoma cells with lower malignant potential. *Int J Cancer* 35:787–791, 1985.
74. Real FX, Houghton AN, Albino AP, Cordon-Cardo C, Melamed MR, Oettgen HF, and Old LJ. Surface antigens on melanomas and melanocytes defined by mouse monoclonal antibodies: Specificity analysis and comparison of antigen expression in cultured cell and tissues. *Cancer Res* 45:4401–4411, 1985.
75. Herlyn M, and Koprowski H. Melanoma antigens: Immunological and biological characterization and clinical significance. *Annu Rev Immunol* 6:283–308, 1988.
76. Elder DE, Rodeck U, Thurin J et al. Antigenic profile of tumor progression in human melanocytic nevi and melanomas. *Cancer Res* 49:5091–5096, 1989.
77. Houghton AN, Real FX, Davis LJ, Cordon-Cardo C, and Old LJ. Phenotypic heterogeneity of melanoma. Relation to the differentiation program of melanoma cells. *J Exp Med* 164:812–829, 1987.
78. Ostmeier H, and Suter L. The Ki-67 antigen in primary human melanomas—its relationship to mitotic rate and tumor thickness and its stability. *Arch Dermatol Res* 281:173–177, 1989.
79. Zwadlo G, Bröcker EB, Bassewitz v, DB, Feige U, and Sorg C. A monoclonal antibody to a differentiation antigen present on mature human macrophages and absent from monocytes. *J Immunol* 134:1487–1492, 1985.
80. Bröcker EB, Zwadlo G, Suter L, Brune M, and Sorg C. Infiltration of primary and metastatic melanomas with macrophages of the 25F9-positive phenotype. *Cancer Immunol Immunother* 25:81–86, 1987.
81. Van der Wiel-Miezenbeek JM, Steijlen PM. Bergmann W, Bröcker EB, Johnson J, and Ruiter DJ. Low frequency of melanoma-associated-progression-antigens in halo nevi. *J Invest Dermatol* 91:408, 1988.

Chapter 12

PATHOLOGICAL EVALUATION OF PRIMARY AND METASTATIC MELANOMA: IMPLICATIONS FOR STAGING, PROGNOSIS, AND TREATMENT

Alistair J. Cochran, Duan-Ren Wen, Zohreh Farzad, Ana-Maria A. Lana, Qing-Si Zeng, and Donald L. Morton

INTRODUCTION

Cutaneous malignant melanoma remains a comparatively infrequent form of malignancy, although there is evidence of a recent and continuing increase in its incidence.[1,2] There has been an associated increase in the number of deaths from melanoma, but the great majority (85–90 percent) of patients with cutaneous melanoma confined to the site of origin at the time of initial treatment are cured by wide excision of their primary tumor.[3] Management of patients with melanoma spread beyond the primary site remains less satisfactory. While some patients with melanoma metastatic to the regional lymph nodes are cured or achieve long term survival after therapeutic lymph node dissection, most eventually die of disseminated melanoma.[4–81] The situation is even worse when melanoma has spread to the viscera, a development which few, if any, patients survive and for which there is at present no effective therapy.[3]

To improve the clinical outcome for patients with metastatic melanoma, logical strategies are to diagnose the disease at as early a stage as possible, when the chance that metastatic spread has occurred is least, and to develop approaches for preventing or aborting the metastatic process. The natural history of melanoma may present special therapeutic opportunities. In contrast to some other forms of malignancy, for example breast cancer, the majority of melanoma patients (67 percent) who develop metastases, do so first in the regional lymph nodes,[9,10] and there is little evidence that clinically significant visceral spread is an inevitable or even frequent concomitant of nodal spread.

The management of patients with cutaneous melanoma overtly spread to the regional lymph nodes is well established. Few would argue against the view that the patient with melanoma that is clinically detectable in the regional nodes is most appropriately managed by "therapeutic" dissection of the group of nodes that contains metastatic melanoma.

In contrast there is a longstanding and unresolved debate over the most effective management of the patient whose lymph nodes are ostensibly negative on clinical assessment, but who has a primary melanoma, the characteristics of which, from previous experience, have been associated with the probability of concurrent or subsequent metastatic spread. Clinical assessment of the regional lymph nodes is a notoriously fallible method of identifying those individuals in whom early and limited spread of melanoma has occurred. In studies of lymph nodes removed from melanoma patients by elective lymph node dissection for "high risk" melanomas, up to 15 percent of patients were found, by microscopic examination of slides conventionally stained by hematoxylin and eosin, to have small deposits of metastatic melanoma in nodes that were evaluated as tumor-free on careful clinical assessment by experienced physicians.[11,12] Application of immunohistochemical techniques to nodes from the 85 percent of melanoma patients regarded as tumor-free on the basis of clinical evaluation and scrutiny of hematoxylin and eosin stained slides, identified small numbers of "occult" tumor cells in an additional 14 percent of patients.[12] Thus 29 percent of patients regarded as having melanoma confined to the primary site after standard clinical assessment, in fact, have metastases in the regional nodes, albeit that the extent of spread is extremely limited in some patients.

If lymph node dissection is effective in the management of melanoma spread to the regional nodes, it is likely to benefit individuals where the extent of tumor spread to the nodes is limited. At this stage the capacity of the surgeon to remove the metastatic tumor is maximal, and the likelihood that the tumor has spread to visceral metastatic sites, beyond the lymph nodes, is minimal. This simple fact has long been recognized, as has the need to develop techniques to identify those patients most likely to have subclinical spread of melanoma to the regional nodes. This need has led to major efforts to identify the characteristics of primary melanoma that are most often associated with the development of metastases. These efforts have achieved a degree of success in that the parameters that have been developed can identify *groups* of patients likely to develop metastases, but precision in assessment of prognosis on an *individual patient* basis remains less precise.

ASSESSMENT OF THE LIKELIHOOD OF METASTASES, BASED ON CHARACTERISTICS OF THE PRIMARY TUMOR

The main parameters that have been found useful are observations that index the size of the primary melanoma. Tumor size is a correlate of the time that the tumor has been present and of its capacity to grow progressively against the patient's tumor-inhibitory defenses. It is also likely that the longer a tumor is present the more probable it is that it will have developed the phenotypic characteristics necessary to allow the development of metastases (the metastatic phenotype).

This general association between the size of a primary melanoma and the likelihood of metastases has been known for many years. Tumor size was initially assessed by evaluating whether the tumor was superficial or deep,[13] or by examining the cross-sectional profile of the primary tumor (flat vs. convex vs. polypoid)[14] or evaluating whether the deepest invasive tumor cells lay above or below the sweat glands.[15]

The assessment was made more precise by Clark[16] who related the deepest invasive melanoma cells to standard anatomical landmarks of the skin: the dermo-epidermal junction, the papillary dermis, the interface between the papillary and the reticular dermis, the reticular dermis, and the subcutaneous fat (Fig. 12-1). This remains a practical approach because patients with tumors of more superficial Clark level (I–III) relatively seldom develop metastases compared to those with deeper level tumors (IV and V). The technique has biologic relevance, particularly in the separation of tumors above and below the dermo-epidermal junction or the papillary-reticular dermal interface. There are some practical lim-

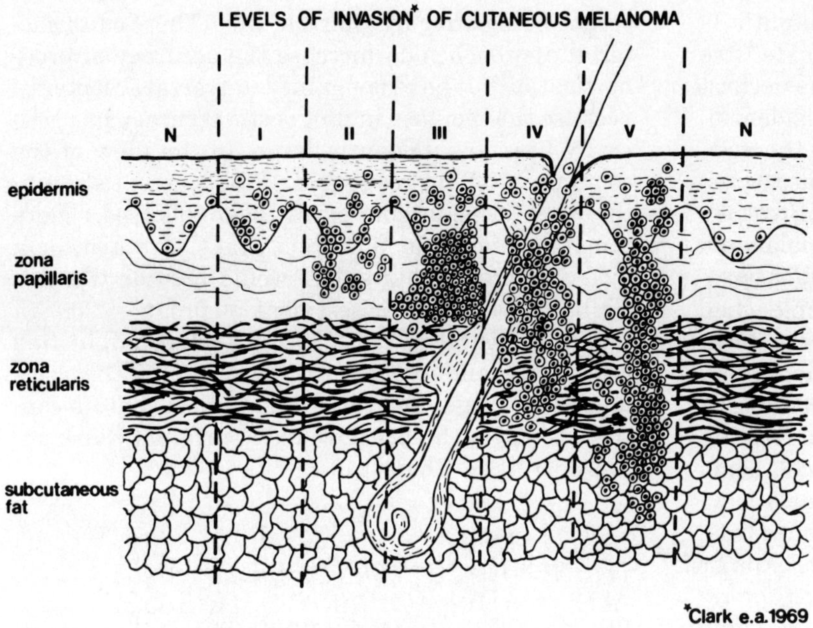

FIG. 12-1 Clark's technique for assessing the level of invasion of a primary malignant melanoma, relative to microanatomical levels of the skin.[16]

itations to its application.[17] The papillary dermis and the reticular dermis are difficult to separate in some body sites, such as the acral areas, because the papillary dermis is poorly developed. The reference landmarks may be obscured by the presence of a dense lymphoid infiltrate, by fibrosis, or by the cells of a preexisting nevus. In sites where there are abundant hair follicles, it may be difficult to separate direct invasion from extension down the stromal sheath of a hair follicle, and this may lead to overestimation of the depth of invasion.

Clark's approach has, to a degree, been replaced by the micrometer measured assessment of thickness described by Breslow,[18] which remains the most useful single microscopic feature that relates to prognosis. Tumor thickness is quantified to the nearest tenth of a millimeter with an ocular micrometer (Fig. 12-2), measuring from the top of the granular layer of the overlying epidermis or the base of a tumor ulcer, to the deepest contiguous invasive melanoma cell. There is an excellent direct correlation between tumor thickness and the probability of the development of metastases. Thickness measurements do not include subjacent satellites, foci of vascular invasion, or tumor sheathing epidermal appendages. The technique should not be uncritically applied, for example to tumors where the overlying epidermis is substantially thickened, as this will lead to an

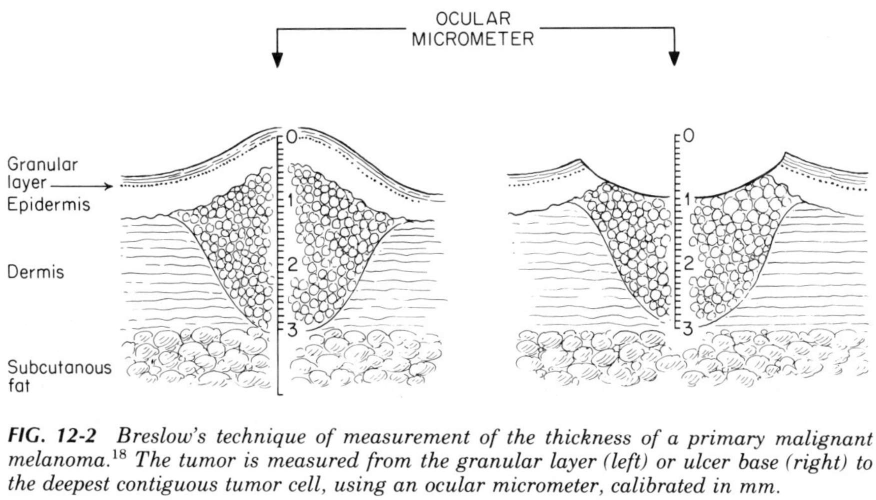

FIG. 12-2 Breslow's technique of measurement of the thickness of a primary malignant melanoma.[18] *The tumor is measured from the granular layer (left) or ulcer base (right) to the deepest contiguous tumor cell, using an ocular micrometer, calibrated in mm.*

overestimate of true tumor thickness and potentially to overtreatment. When there has been extensive regression, the measurement is made to the deepest tumor cell, being careful to avoid the misidentification of melanophages as tumor cells, and the measurement is qualified by the statement that regression is present. A major problem in applying Breslow's technique may be encountered when a melanoma coexists with, and blends with, cells showing nevocytic morphology. The problem is quite simple when a melanoma abuts a preexisting nevus, the measurement being made to the deepest melanoma cell. More difficult is the situation when melanoma cells blend with a population of nevocytoid cells. Here an attempt has to be made to separate a melanoma showing nevocytic differentiation from melanoma infiltrating a nevus. Assistance can be obtained from an examination of the nevocytic portion of the tumor under polarized light or in sections stained for reticulin, the reticulin framework generally being lighter around nevocytically differentiated melanoma cells than around true nevocytes. Another approach is to stain sections for the melanoma-associated epitope HMB45 (see the next section). This is present in most melanoma cells, including those that are nevocytically differentiated, and is absent from true intradermal nevocytes. If, after these approaches, doubt persists, the surgeon should be provided with a measurement that includes all the melanocyte-derived cells in the dermis, but should be advised of the nature of the dilemma.

Curiously, most errors in applying Breslow's technique come from simple mathematical mistakes in converting the micrometer measurement to mm or from attempting to use a microscope that has not been calibrated for use with the particular micrometer employed.

Other histologic characteristics of primary melanoma correlate with the likelihood of the development of metastases, but none have the power of the Breslow or Clark approaches. The most relevant of these observations include the micrometer-measured width of ulceration,[19] the frequency of mitotic figures.[14,20] the presence of tumor within blood or lymphatic vessels,[14,21] the presence of "microsatellites" and the presence and distribution of lymphohistiocytic infiltrates in the peritumoral area and within the area of the tumor.[15,22,23]

In addition to interest in single prognostic parameters, attempts have been made to increase the accuracy of prediction of clinical outcome by combining several clinical and pathological features into a prognostic score sheet or formula. We initiated this approach in 1968,[15] and its utility was confirmed by MacKie et al.[24] Since that time a number of other similar schemes have been presented,[25,26] the most recent being that by Clark et al.[22] These multifactorial approaches do increase the accuracy of prognostication but have not gained universal acceptance because the increase in prognostic accuracy has generally been insufficiently large, in the view of the community of surgeons and pathologists, to justify the often considerable extra labor involved. There remains a need for a system that, in return for a modest increment in effort, would provide the possibility of accurate assessment of prognosis *on an individual patient basis*. Such a system might find acceptance and practical application in the community at large. For the present, most centers continue to apply the Breslow and/or original Clark approaches. (See Chap. 14.)

EVALUATION OF THE SENTINEL LYMPH NODES: AN ALTERNATIVE TO PARAMETER-BASED PROGNOSIS IN DECIDING ON THE TREATMENT OF REGIONAL LYMPH NODES

We and others developed the capacity to identify small numbers of tumor cells in tissues, including lymph nodes.[27,28] We initially reported that S-100 protein was an operationally useful marker for benign and malignant cells of melanocytic lineage.[27,29] We then reported that in patients with melanoma spread to the regional lymph nodes, 40 percent of the nodes that lay close to overtly tumor-containing nodes and that were regarded as tumor-free on examination of sections stained with hematoxylin and eosin actually contain small numbers of tumor cells that are readily detectable in sections stained with antibodies to S-100 protein.[11] We next examined regional nodes excised electively from patients with high risk primary melanoma that was confined to the primary site on clinical examination and in whom standard histological evaluation of the lymph nodes had shown no tumor. Further sections from the nodes were stained, using antibodies to S-100 protein and the melanoma-associated epitopes, NKI/C3[20] and HMB45/50.[31] In 14 percent of these patients, evaluation of the sections stained immunohistochemically showed that one or more nodes contained tumor cells. It should be emphasized that this is in addition to the 15 percent of patients who, despite a negative clinical evaluation, were found to have tumor on conventional pathological assessment.[12] These studies were undertaken retrospectively and utilized formalin-fixed and paraffin-embedded material. To permit intraoperative evaluation of nodal tissues, we have developed a rapid immunohistochemical technique that, using standard frozen sections, allows an accurate assessment in 30 minutes of whether or not a node contains tumor.[32]

Techniques still needed to be developed to identify the regional nodes that were located nearest to primary melanoma on the relevant lymphatic pathway, the nodes that a priori are those most likely to contain metastatic tumor cells. We initially examined the lymphatic drainage of young cats, by injecting blue dye intradermally into the skin of the thighs and lower abdomen. The inguinal nodal area was surgically exposed, the passage of the dye along the lymphatics followed, and the nodes observed for the development of blue color. The routes and destinations of lymphatic drainage were remarkably constant and, when dye was injected into the same anatomic site, essentially identical from cat to cat.[33]

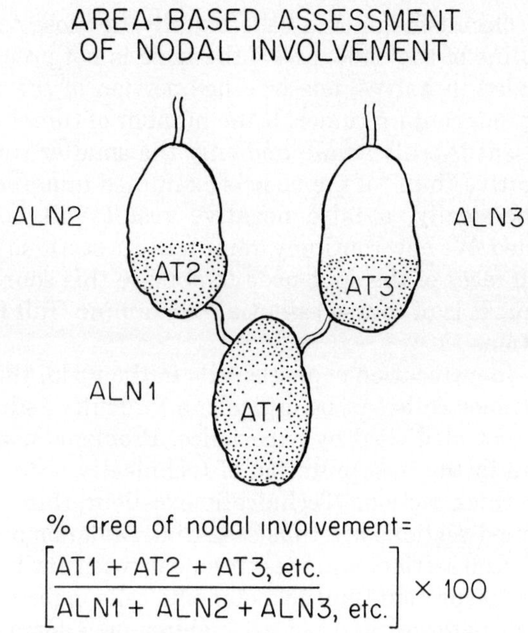

FIG. 12-3 Technique for assessing the proportional area of melanoma in a lymph node group. Tumor area and total area for each node are measured using planimetry or computer-assisted image analysis. The data from each node are summed, and aggregate tumor area is expressed as a percentage of aggregate tumor nodal area.

On the basis of these observations, the studies were extended to a series of melanoma patients. A marker dye was injected intradermally in the normal skin adjacent to primary melanoma, or the site of excision of biopsies of melanomas. The regional lymph nodes, confirmed as the site of lymphatic drainage by lymphoscintigraphy where appropriate, are surgically exposed and the afferent lymphatics examined for the passage of the marker dye. Lymph nodes that developed a blue coloration were excised with a 2 cm margin of surrounding tissue and sent immediately to pathology for frozen section examination and for rapid immunohistochemistry to identify any melanoma cells that were present. While pathological evaluation is in progress, the area of the primary tumor is widely excised. If the sentinel lymph nodes contain tumor a full lymphadenectomy is performed.

At least one dye-delineated sentinel node has been identified in 81 percent of the 243 patients managed in this manner. The success rate varied slightly with the site of the lymph nodes (groin, 89 percent, axilla, 78 percent), and as each surgeon gained experience with the technique (61–97 percent). Most patients had a single sentinel node, but 20 percent had two and 8 percent had three or more. A sentinel node was identified in 194 lymphadenectomy specimens and 40 (21 percent) contained metastatic melanoma. Tumor was identified in H & E stained sections in 23 instances (57 percent) and exclusively by immunohistochemistry in the remaining 17 (43 percent) (Figs. 12-3 and 12-4). Melanoma was identified in 62 of 3332 lymph nodes (2 percent). The metastases occurred exclusively in the sentinel lymph nodes in 47 patients (76 percent) but occurred in both the sentinel and nonsentinel nodes that lay within 2 cm of the sentinel node in 13 patients (21 percent). Metastases were found exclusively in nonsentinel nodes in only two patients (1 percent). These were among the earliest patients studied, before we appreciated how quickly dye passes from skin to sentinel nodes and then to nodes beyond. We have not encountered this problem in our most recent 200 patients and consider that these two patients are exceptional, reflecting our initial lack of knowledge of the kinetics of dye flow. We have not encountered any examples of skip metastases.

How accurately can we identify small numbers of melanoma cells intraoperatively? We compared our intraoperative evaluation of nodes, based on H & E frozen sections and rapid immunohistochemistry, with the evaluation of the nodes after formalin fixation, using H & E and immunostained sections. Exact concordance between the intraoperative evaluation and permanent preparations was achieved in 220 of 227 patients (97 percent). In 36 patients tumor cells were identified intraoperatively and confirmed in the permanent preparations (Fig. 12-3). Thus no false positive opinion was issued on the basis of frozen section interpretation. In 191 patients no tumor cells were identified intraoperatively, and the absence of tumor was confirmed in the final material in 184 (97 percent). In seven patients tumor was not identified intraoperatively, but was present in the final preparations, a false negative rate of 3 percent, a figure within the range of published false negatives for routine frozen sections (3–5 percent). Such errors usually arose from insufficient sampling of the regional nodal tissues when the frozen sections were prepared.

Occult melanoma cells usually lie close to the midline of the node, and if the node is not precisely divided in halves, one or other portion of the node may not contain tumor. If the number of tumor cells present is truly small, and only the smaller tumor-negative "half" of the node is examined immunohistochemically, a false negative result will be obtained. We now routinely immunostain sections from both faces of the split node to obviate this source of error. It is of course essential to examine "full face" sections.

Identification of single cells in the nodal tissues as tumor cells can be difficult; a difficulty reduced, but not abolished by experience. Problems usually arise in the interpretation of technically poor, usually thick sections. Technically excellent, thin, well-stained sections are thus essential. Melanoma cells in frozen sections stain less intensely with antibodies to S-100 protein than do melanoma cells in formalin-fixed material, and not all melanomas express the epitopes detected by the melanoma-directed monoclonal antibodies NKI/C3 and HMB45/50. Difficulties in intraoperative interpretation may thus be due to weak or absent staining of melanoma cells in frozen material.

Our current approach to the management of the patient with primary melanoma that is likely to metastasize is as follows: the draining node group is identified by scintigraphy and the sentinel lymph node, the node most likely to contain early metastases, is identified by its blue color after injection of dye into the skin around the primary tumor. The sentinel node and any immediately adjacent nodes are evaluated intraoperatively for the presence of tumor cells by standard H&E-stained frozen sections and rapid immunohistology. If the sentinel nodes contain tumor, a full lymphadenectomy is performed; if they are negative, no further nodes are removed. We consider that dye-directed biopsy of the sentinel lymph nodes is a simple and essentially non-morbid approach to identifying those patients most likely to benefit from lymph node dissection. We further believe that this approach is substantially more accurate than patient selection based on a consideration of prognosis-related characteristics of the primary tumor.

ASSESSMENT OF PROGNOSIS FOR THE PATIENT WITH MELANOMA SPREAD TO THE REGIONAL LYMPH NODES

The outlook for the patient with melanoma spread to the regional lymph nodes (stage II) stage IIb according to international staging has improved substantially in the recent past. Studies published in the 1950s and 1960s indicated that about 80 percent of such patients would die of further spread of their melanoma.[4,34] More recent reports have indicated that about 50 percent of patients with node-spread melanoma will be alive and tumor free on clinical examination 5 years after therapeutic lymph node dissection and that most patients who fall into this category will achieve long-term survival and die eventually of causes other than melanoma,[7,8] There is, therefore, a need for techniques that will accurately predict the likely outcome for the individual patient with stage II melanoma at the time of lymphadenectomy.

From studies of groups of patients with stage IIb melanoma, factors considered prognostically relevant have included disease free interval from primary excision to development of lymph node metastases,[35,36] thickness and width of ulceration of the primary tumor,[19] specific histologic subtypes of primary melanoma,[37] extent of spread of melanoma to the regional nodes (for example, clinically palpable node involvement versus histologically detectable node penetration), number of lymph nodes containing tumor,[7,38,39] and extension of the tumor through the lymph node capsule.[40,41]

In a study at UCLA of 150 patients with stage IIb melanoma, we found that the number of melanoma-containing lymph nodes correlated with outcome as follows: 47 percent of patients with 3 or fewer tumor-positive lymph nodes were 5-year survivors, whereas only 21 percent of those with tumor in 4 or more lymph nodes survived 5 years after lymphadenectomy.[7] Prospective application of this approach accurately predicted the likelihood of survival (85 percent correct), but substantially underestimated the chance of death from melanoma (40 percent correct). We consider that this unacceptably low accuracy indicates that the number of tumor-containing nodes is a very imprecise index of tumor burden. On this basis a patient who has three grossly enlarged, tumor-replaced nodes would be held to have the same prognosis as a patient who has three nodes containing microfoci of tumor in the subcapsular sinus.

We have extensively examined this practical dilemma,[42] and the following is a summary of our findings: Measurement of absolute tumor volume or tumor volume relative to the volume of the affected group of nodes would likely be the best indicator of risk of subsequent recurrence or death from melanoma, but measurements of this kind are not really practical for the working surgical pathologist. We then followed a line of reasoning similar to that which led Breslow to devise his highly successful micrometer-based thickness measurement as a means of predicting outcome for the patient with primary melanoma.[3] This encouraged us to investigate the measurement of aggregate lymph-nodal tumor *area* and aggregate nodal tumor *diameter* as correlates of tumor volume. Such approaches could be used instead of, or to supplement, the number of nodes containing tumor and other indicators of likely clinical outcome in stage IIb melanoma.

Using simple assessment of the number of nodes that contain tumor, 11 of 13 five-year survivors had tumor in 3 or fewer nodes and would have been predicted to survive—a predictive accuracy of 85 percent. Of the 15 patients who died of melanoma only 6 had tumor in 4 or more nodes and would have been predicted to die of melanoma—an accuracy of prediction of 40 percent (Table 12-1).

Using the same cohort of 28 patients, we examined the predictive accuracy of (1) assessing the area of lymph nodes occupied by tumor (Fig. 12-4) and (2) measuring the aggregate diameter of tumor in the lymph nodes (Plate 37). Patients in whom 15 percent or less of the total nodal area was occupied by tumor had a relatively favorable outcome. Those who had greater than 15 percent tumor replacement were more likely to die of melanoma. Using these parameters, 10 of the 13 patients who were tumor-free for more than 5 years were predicted as survivors—an accuracy of 77 percent; whereas 9 of the 15 who died of melanoma were regarded as having an unfavorable prognosis—an accuracy of 60 percent. Overall, assessment of tumor area correctly predicted outcome in 19 of the 28 patients—an accuracy of 68 percent.

Measurement of tumor area is time consuming and requires image analysis equipment. We

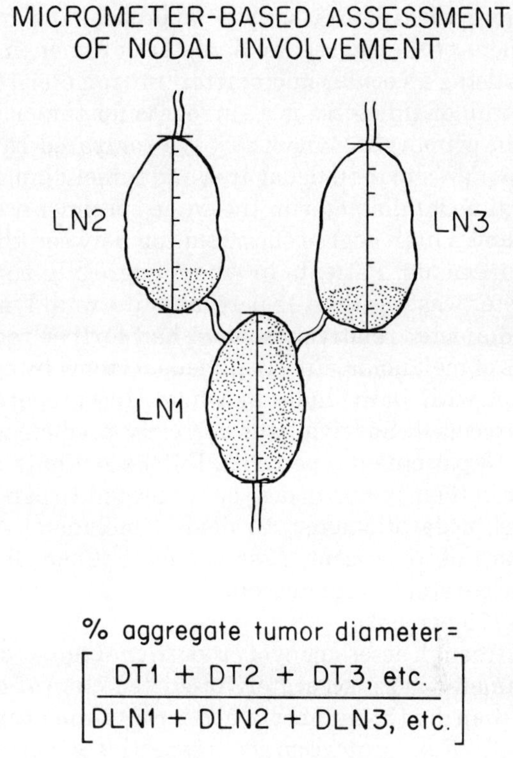

FIG. 12-4 Technique for assessing the proportional maximum diameter of melanoma in a lymph node group. Maximum tumor diameter and nodal diameter for each node are measured using a micrometer. The data from each node are summed, and aggregate tumor diameter is expressed as a percentage of aggregate nodal diameter.

TABLE 12-1
ACCURACY OF PREDICTION OF SURVIVAL OR DEATH IN STAGE II MELANOMA: A COMPARISON OF VARIOUS TECHNIQUES USED ALONE AND IN COMBINATION

		PREDICTION CORRECT[a]		
		SURVIVORS	MELANOMA DEATHS	BOTH
		NO. TOTAL (%)	NO. TOTAL (%)	NO. TOTAL (%)
A	Number of nodes with tumor	11/13 (85)	6/15 (40)	17/28 (61)
B	Area of tumor Tumor area node group	10/13 (77)	9/15 (60)	19/28 (68)
C	Maximum tumor diameter Maximum diameter node group	11/13 (85)	10/15 (67)	21/28 (75)
A + B		12/13 (92)	11/15 (73)	23/28 (82)
A + C		12/13 (92)	12/15 (80)	24/28 (86)[b]
B + C		10/13 (76)	11/15 (73)	21/28 (75)

[a]Prediction based on: A = favorable if number of nodes containing tumor ≤ 3; B = favorable if area of tumor in nodes < 15% of total nodal area; C = favorable if aggregate diameter of tumor in nodes < 15% aggregate nodal diameter; B + C = favorable if area of tumor and aggregate diameter of tumor < 15% nodal area and diameter; A + B = favorable if ≤ 3 lymph nodes positive for tumor and area of tumor < 15% of total nodal area; A + C = favorable if ≤ 3 lymph nodes positive and aggregate diameter of tumor < 15% of nodal diameter. (In all situations where these parameters are exceeded, prognosis is regarded as unfavorable.)
[b]Accuracy of prediction is significantly greater than that based on node number alone, $p < 0.05$.

therefore turned to a simpler approach, the measurement of the aggregate diameter of tumor in the nodes using an ocular micrometer (micrometer-measured tumor thickness is a surrogate for tumor volume in primary melanoma).[18] We compared ratios of tumor area to total nodal area and tumor diameter to total nodal diameter in the same specimens, and we found a high degree of correlation between these measurements. Patients in whom aggregate tumor diameter was less than 15 percent of the total lymph node diameter relatively seldom had further recurrences of melanoma after lymphadenectomy by comparison with individuals in whom this proportion was exceeded. Survival was correctly predicted for 11 of 13 patients (85 percent). Fifteen patients had tumor in their lymph nodes that exceeded 15 percent of total nodal diameter; 10 died of melanoma—an accuracy of 67 percent. Assessment of tumor diameter accurately predicted outcome in 21 of 28 patients (75 percent).

Although assessment of proportional tumor area or diameter more accurately predicted clinical outcome than did the number of nodes containing tumor (68 and 75 percent accuracy, respectively, relative to 61 percent), the increase in accuracy was not statistically significant and the level of accuracy fell short of ideal. We therefore examined the effectiveness of combining various techniques.

We examined combinations of the number of nodes containing tumor and aggregate tumor diameter. Prognosis was considered favorable with tumor in three or fewer nodes and aggregate tumor diameter less than 15 percent of total nodal diameter. By this combination, a favorable outcome was accurately predicted for 12 of 13 patients (92 percent accuracy) and fatal progression correctly forecasted for 12 of 15 individuals (80 percent accuracy)—an overall accuracy of 86 percent. This combination of techniques was a significantly better predictor of outcome than the number of tumor-containing lymph nodes alone or combinations of number of nodes and tumor area. The combination of number of nodes and tumor diameter more accurately predicted outcome for male and female patients and for patients who had removal of nodes from groin, axilla, and the cervical area.

Assessment of the number of lymph nodes that contain tumor, a widely used measure of prognosis, predicts the subsequent clinical course of patients with stage IIb melanoma with relative inaccuracy. This is especially true of attempts to predict an unfavorable outcome. We believe that this low accuracy is due to the inability of this approach to discriminate between nodes that are completely overrun by tumor and those that are only partly replaced. A similar prognosis would then be assigned to patients who had quite different volumes of tumor and hence numbers of tumor cells in the nodes.

The combination of number of tumor-containing nodes and tumor diameter provides enhanced accuracy of prognostication suggesting that tumor expansion within a lymph node and extension from node to node are different tumor attributes that are separately correlated with patient survival or death from melanoma.

The combined assessment of number of nodes containing tumor and the aggregate micrometer-measured diameter of tumor provide a very precise indication of subsequent tumor behavior. It is questionable whether a greater degree of precision could be obtained by using morphological features alone. Patients who die of their disease despite a relatively favorable lymph node profile may do so because of tumor characteristics that permit an unusually early, rapid, or extensive hematogenous dissemination. Such characteristics may not be detectable by examination of tumor cell morphology or pattern or extent of lymph node permeation.

At a practical level, when an attempt is being made to assess accurately prognosis for a patient with stage IIb melanoma, for example in stratification for clinical trials, we believe that assessment of the number of nodes containing tumor should be supplemented by data on the extent of nodal penetration, using micrometer-measured aggregate tumor diameter as a surrogate for tumor area and hence tumor volume. Combinations of immunohistologic approaches to detect occult tumor[11,12] with the standard morphologic parameters may yield additional accuracy; this possibility is currently under investigation.

NUCLEAR MEASUREMENTS OF METASTATIC MELANOMA CELLS AND PROGNOSIS

Recent reports of nuclear DNA ploidy analysis using flow and static DNA cytometry have defined inherent tumor nuclear aberrations, which provide additional prognostic information. For example, patients with stage I cutaneous melanoma that shows an aneuploid pattern have a lower survival than patients with diploid tumors.[43,44] Although flow cytometry has the advantages of high speed and accuracy, the requirement of at least 10,000 single cells may be difficult to meet when the study lesion is small. We believe that static DNA cytometry gives useful information and is particularly suitable for assessing morphometric and densitometric information in specific areas in tissue sections. Using static DNA cytometry therefore, a study was undertaken to characterize the nuclear DNA abnormalities in melanoma metastatic to lymph nodes and to evaluate the biologic significance of these findings.[44]

We studied 22 patients who had undergone lymph node dissection for clinically evident metastatic melanoma. In order to obtain a sufficient number of cells for DNA analysis, the three largest metastases were selected from each case. Paraffin blocks of these metastases and a section of normal skin as control were cut at 10 μm thickness, stained by the Feulgen method, and mounted with an immersion oil (refractive index, 1.494).

The nuclear DNA content (expressed in arbitrary units) and nuclear area were measured using a computerized digital imaging system.[46] The methods are described in detail in Zeng et al.[45]

In each case, the three metastatic lymph nodes were measured separately. All acceptable tumor cell nuclei were measured without selection, at least 100 nuclei when the metastasis was small, but usually 250 to 300 nuclei. At the completion of measurements, a DNA histogram of each metastasis was displayed and compared with that of 50 normal intermediate squamous cells of the skin serving as diploid (2N) controls. The mean, standard deviation (SD), and coefficient of variation (CV = 100 × SD/mean, expressed as a percentage) of control cells were computed for each specimen. The CV of control cells serves as an overall indicator of instrument sensitivity, operator consistency, and sample quality. Based on DNA histograms, we analyzed a variety of parameters, including: ploidy level (mean DNA/distal peak), ploidy patterns (diploid vs. polyploid, etc.), clonality and mean CV of DNA content of each metastasis.

Analysis of Ploidy

Of the cases tested 19 of the 22 were aneuploid (86 percent), including 16 with aneuploidy in all metastases, and 3 with aneuploidy in some and tetraploidy in other metastases. The remaining 3 cases (14 percent) had a tetraploid pattern in all metastases.

Number of Clones

There were 7 cases that had a single clone, and the remaining 15 cases had more than 1 clone. All 7 patients with a monoclonal tumor survived more than 14 months. Of the 15 patients with polyclonal tumors, 8 patients (53 percent) died within 14 months. This difference in survival rate is statistically significant ($P < .025$). Other investigators have published similar findings.

Mean Coefficient of Variation of DNA Content

All 7 patients whose mean CV of DNA content was less than 30 percent survived more than 14 months, whereas 8 of 15 patients (53 percent) with CV of DNA content greater than 30 percent died within 14 months ($P < .025$, Table 12-2). In patients whose

TABLE 12-2
MEAN COEFFICIENT OF VARIATION OF DNA CONTENT AND LENGTH OF SURVIVAL

CV OF DNA CONTENT (%)	SURVIVAL PERIOD <14 MO (%)	SURVIVAL PERIOD >14 MO (%)	TOTAL (%)
<30	0 (—)	7 (100)	7 (100)
>30	8 (53)	7 (47)	15 (100)

Fisher's test: $p < .025$

tumors showed a mean CV of DNA content that exceeded 30 percent, the tumors were more likely to be polyclonal.

Total Number of Metastases and Area of the Largest Metastasis

Multiple clones were found at a similar frequency in patients with fewer than and greater than 10 lymph node metastases. The area of the largest metastasis, which varied from 15 to 370 mm^2, correlated directly with the number of clones (Table 12-3). There was no correlation between survival rate and the total number of metastases or the area of the largest metastasis. It should, however, be noted that as all patients had more than three lymph nodes containing metastatic tumor they would, on this basis, fall into the unfavorable prognostic category described by (among others) Cohen et al.[39] and Callery et al.[7]

In our study, slightly over two-thirds of cases had more than one stem-cell line. This occurrence is associated with tumor volume rather than with the number of individual metastases. In renal cell carcinomas, polyclonality tends to occur in poorly differentiated tumors.[47]

Although the number of cases is small, eight of 15 patients with two or more clones of tumor cells in their metastases died within 14 months, whereas all seven patients with monoclonal metastases survived more than 14 months. Other investigators have noticed that patients with polyclonal tumors have a

TABLE 12-3
AREA OF LARGEST METASTASIS AND NUMBER OF CLONES

TUMOR SIZE (mm^2)	SINGLE CLONE (%)	POLYCLONAL (%)	TOTAL (%)
<41	4 (100)	0 (—)	4 (100)
>41	3 (17)	15 (83)	18 (100)

Fisher test: $p < .01$

worse prognosis compared with those with single clone tumors.[48,49] Sondergaard et al.[48] noticed an increase of mortality rate for melanoma patients with polyclonal tumors. The explanation for the rapid clinical course of some, but not all, patients with multiclonal metastases may relate to particular cytogenetic rearrangements, which influence metastatic potential and response to therapy. In a murine melanoma model, clones of cells with specific karyotypes are associated with widespread lung metastasis.[50,51]

In association with multiple clones and increasing aneuploidy, the DNA values tend to become widely scattered. Thus, it is not surprising that mean CV of DNA content also correlates with polyclonality and survival rate. Other parameters, such as 5N-ER, mean and CV of nuclear area, and total number of metastases, correlate to some extent with survival rate, but not at a formally significant level in this relatively small series of patients. In the case of number of nodes containing tumor, the patients in the series all had three or more lymph nodes that contained tumor and would be expected to have unfavorable evolution according to previous reports. The presence of multiple clones or a mean CV of DNA content greater than 30 percent is an indicator of a high chance of mortality during the first 14 months after lymph node dissection.

Although flow cytometry has the advantages of high speed and accuracy, the requirement of at least 10,000 single cells may be difficult to meet when the study lesion is small. As shown in this study, useful information can be obtained by a digital imaging system, which is particularly suitable for assessing morphometric and densitometric information in specific areas of interest in the tissue specimens.

EVALUATION OF LYMPH NODE DISSECTION SPECIMENS TO ASSESS COMPLETENESS OF LYMPH NODE DISSECTION

Recurrence of melanoma in the area of a lymph node dissection for melanoma overtly spread to the nodes is not infrequent and in most patients is a grave occurrence, rapidly followed by disseminated metastases and death. In many instances the regrowth occurs from tumor-containing nodes that were not removed at the initial lymphadenectomy. There is, therefore, a need for a method by which surgeons can assess the completeness of their node dissection. This requires meticulous examination of the dissection specimen to identify and count the number of lymph nodes present. From a study of 72 dissection specimens from melanoma patients,[52] we found the mean number of lymph nodes in the axilla to be 19 with a standard deviation of ± 7. For inguinal dissections the figures were 17 ± 5. We suggest that, when a full lymphadenectomy is intended, the specimen should contain a number of nodes close to the mean figures described above. This requires the operating surgeon to dissect all nodes in the area and the examining pathologist, appraised of the quality assurance significance of the number of nodes identified, to meticulously examine the specimen, if necessary, before and after formalin fixation of the tissues. We consider from clinical experience, operative observations, and pathology of individual patients referred to the John Wayne Clinic that recurrence in the site of a prior lymphadenectomy most often develops from nodes not excised during the initial operation. Studies are, however, required to determine the correct course of action when the number of nodes identified in the lymphadenectomy specimen is substantially below that expected. We need to determine the frequency with which local regrowth follows an observation of this kind to decide whether such patients require immediate reoperation to complete the lymphadenectomy, or local radiation therapy, or can reasonably be managed on a "wait and see" basis.

DIMINISHED NODAL IMMUNOCOMPETENCE AS A BASIS FOR THE DEVELOPMENT OF METASTASES

Since most nodes regional to melanoma do not contain tumor cells, we wondered whether the presence of occult tumor cells might indicate that affected nodes eradicate invading cells less effectively than normal nodes. We compared the reactivity of nodes near tumor with that of more remote nodes. In nodes draining melanoma, the main reaction is paracortical, with less activity in sinuses and relatively low B-follicular reactivity. Nodes nearest primary or nodal metastatic tumor show significantly less reaction than those further from tumor.[52] Stage-related variations in lymph node reactivity have also been observed by other workers[53–55] and have been correlated with clinical outcome.[69–71]

We sought an objective measure of paracortical activity. Interdigitating dendritic cells (IDC) of the paracortex are accessory antigen-presenting cells and increase in nodes reacting to T-dependent antigens, providing an accurately measurable index of paracortical activity. IDC express S-100 protein, HLA-DR, and the CD-1 marker.[56] Since S-100 protein is detectable in formalin-fixed, paraffin embedded material[57] and is a good marker for IDC,[58] we employed it in our studies. IDC can be separated from melanoma cells by cytology and differential staining with antimelanoma monoclonal antibodies. IDC were least frequent in the lymphoid portion of nodes partly replaced by melanoma (mean 38 ± 5, S.D., range

0–91), in tumor-free nodes close to tumor (32 ± 5, 0–99), and those further from tumor (30 ± 4, 0–52). They were most numerous in nodes in the middle of the nodal area (66 ± 9, 0–213). In nodes from outside the regional area IDC were infrequent (7 ± 2, 2–6). These data support the assessment of node reactions on H & E sections and confirm the reduced paracortical reactivity of nodes near tumor. That IDC are important in lung cancer is indicated by recent studies showing that the number of IDC in a lung cancer correlates with prognosis.[94–96]

To provide an indication of lymph node activity in vivo, single cell suspensions were prepared from recently excised nodes and assessed for their capacity spontaneously to incorporate thymidine[59] and generate migration-inhibiting lymphokines.[60] Both thymidine uptake and lymphokine generation were least in nodes nearest tumor. In the absence of exogenous stimulation the relative activity of these cell suspensions reflects the in vivo activity of the nodes from which they were prepared. To assess immunological activity in vitro, we cocultivated single cell suspensions from nodes with mitogens (PHA and CON A), alloantigens (one-way MLR) and interleukin-2.[59] We found significant variations in the strength of response of different individual nodes from a single node group to these stimuli. Individual nodes react as separate entities rather than as subunits of a uniformly reactive whole group (the node group). When we correlated reaction and nodal position, nodes closest to tumor were less reactive. The extent of reduction of response, correlated broadly with closeness of the node to tumor and amount of tumor present, being maximum in patients with stage II melanoma. These functional studies strongly support our histology and immunohistology-based concept that nodes located close to tumor are relatively immune-suppressed.

These studies indicate clearly that cellular immune responsiveness to a variety of stimuli is suppressed in nodes near tumor. If this immune suppression favors survival of tumor cells, it is likely that tumoristatic and tumoricidal activities of lymph node cells would also be affected. A recent paper by Mickel et al.[61] has shown NK cell suppression in nodes from patients with squamous carcinoma of the head and neck where the node contains a small focus of metastatic tumor. A spectrum of natural killer (NK) cell activity exists in the tumor draining nodes of patients with head and neck cancer, and the level of activity depends on degree and pattern of nodal tumor involvement. Our studies in progress are designed to assess variations in NK activity, lymphokine-activated killer (LAK) cell activity, and T cell mediated cytotoxicity in tumor-draining nodes.

Mechanism of Tumor-Proximate Nodal Immune Suppression

We have investigated changes in cellular composition of the immune-suppressed nodes and tumor-derived materials that modulate immunocyte function.

1. *Studies of the phenotypes of the cells comprising lymph node cell populations:* This approach has been used in breast cancer and other tumors.[62–64] Morton et al.[64] using two-color immunofluorescence flow cytometry with monoclonal antibodies, found that "changes in local-regional immunocompetent cell subsets may be related to metastasis of tumor to the regional nodes and progression of disease without being full reflected in the systemic circulation."

   We phenotyped lymphocytes from the nodes of melanoma patients, using two-color flow cytometry, seeking the markers CD2, CD3, CD4, CD8, CD19, CD45R, DR, CD11b, CD56, and CD25.[83] Data were analyzed according to stage of disease, presence or absence of tumor in the node and, in the case of tumor-free nodes, distance of the node from nearest tumor. Tumor involved nodes contained fewer $CD3^+$ total T cells and cells of the $CD4^+$ /$CD45R^+$ suppressor-inducer subset and increased Leu 19^+ NK cells. Comparison of tumor-free stage I and stage II nodes (Table 12-4) showed significantly increased $CD8^+$ cytotoxic/suppressor cells, ($p < 0.001$) and $CD56^+$ NK cells, ($p < 0.01$) in stage II nodes with a reduction in $CD4^+$ (helper/inducer) T cells ($P < 0.01$). The CD4/CD8 ratio in stage II (3.8 +/− 0.2) was less than half that of stage I nodes (8.5 +/− 0.5). When analyzed with respect to distance from nearest tumor, nodes closest to primary tumor contained fewer $CD19^+$ B cells in stage I disease. In stage II disease there was a progressive increase in $CD56^+$ NK cells in nodes closer to tumor and increases in $CD19^+$ B cells. Substantial changes in phenotypic profile occur in the lymphocytes of nodes regional to melanoma as the disease progresses from stage I to stage II and during the development of metastases. That changes occur in tumor-free nodes indicates that these changes precede the presence of tumor in the node and may even be essential to the metastatic process and disease progression.
2. *Suppressor cells in tumor-draining lymph nodes.* We examined suppressor T-lymphocyte activity using a Con A suppressor cell induction assay.[65–68] In all melanoma patients examined, the nodes nearest tumor contained most inducible suppressor cells. The response of indicator peripheral blood lymphocytes (PBL), admixed with

TABLE 12-4
DISTRIBUTION OF LYMPH NODE LYMPHOCYTE PHENOTYPES IN PATIENTS WITH STAGE I AND STAGE II MELANOMA

CELL MARKER	STAGE I (n = 21)	STAGE II (TUMOR FREE) (n = 19)	STAGE II (TUMOR POSITIVE) (n = 8)
CD2	77.0 ± 2.9[a]	68.6 ± 8.7	81.3[b]
CD3	74.5 ± 0.9	71.6 ± 3.9	47.6 ± 20
CD45R	65.9 ± 4.1	59.2 ± 9.1	45.4[b]
CD4	69.4 ± 1.3(a)	50.9 ± 2.1(a)	51.7 ± 7.9(a)
HLA DR	21.2 ± 2.2	22.0 ± 5.7	27.4 ± 8.5
CD19	10.6 ± 3.8	17.9 ± 2.1	17.6 ± 1.9
CD8	9.8 ± 0.2(b)	16.7 ± 0.7(b)	13.9 ± 5
CD11b	5.9 ± 0.1	10.3 ± 3.6	5.1[b]
CD56	1.9 ± 0.4(c)	7.1 ± 1.6(c)	6.5 ± 1.7
CD25	1.5 ± 0.4	0.8 ± 0.2	0.3[b]
CD4 CD45R	38.1 ± 2.7	34.7 ± 10.8	14.0[b]
CD4 DR	3.7 ± 0.2	2.3 ± 0.7	2.3 ± 1.1
CD4/CD8	8.5 ± 0.5	3.8 ± 0.2	5.2 ± 1.9

[a]Mean ± SE
[b]Single observation

The percentage of cells positive for each marker is shown. *n* = number of nodes examined. With the exception of the single observations, markers were assessed on all samples. Uninvolved stage II nodes had a lower percentage of $CD4^+$ cells ($P < 0.001$) (a) and a higher percentage of $CD8^+$ cells ($P < 0.001$) (b) and $CD56^+$ (Leu 19^+) NK cells ($P < 0.01$)(c) compared with stage I nodes. Tumor-involved stage II nodes were very similar to uninvolved stage II nodes, except that $CD3^+$ total T-cells were very variable in number.

induced suppressors, was reduced between 25 and 91 percent.[66] Similar studies show that breast cancer-draining nodes too contain suppressor cells, though at a generally higher level than in melanoma. Inducible suppressor activity was high in nodes at all levels of the axilla, suggesting that the suppressive influence of the cells of breast cancer is stronger than that of melanoma.[67]

Suppressor cells have previously been reported in human malignant disease[69–73] and in animal experimental tumors.[74,75] Cozzolino et al.[76] reported $T3^+$, $T8^+$, $OKMI^+$, Leu 7^+ cells, a phenotype associated with a subset of T-suppressor cells by Landay et al.[77] and Clement et al.[78] in lymph nodes containing metastatic human tumor. Removal of $T3^+$, $T8^+$, $OKMI^+$, Leu 7^+ cells from lymph node cell suspension allows the demonstration of a population of cells that undergoes blast transformation in the presence of IL-2 and autologous (but not allogenic) tumor cells.

3. *Tumor-derived materials that can immune-modulate lymph node cells.* The concurrence of immune suppression and increased numbers of inducible suppressor cells in nodes nearest tumor supports the likelihood that down-regulation of lymph node function is due to materials from tumor cells.

a. *Gangliosides.* We chose to study the immune-modulatory effects of gangliosides because tumor cells are rich in gangliosides, and in human and animal systems gangliosides modify lymphocyte function.[79] We examined gangliosides from human melanoma cells for their effect on the responses of lymphocytes to Interleukin-2 (IL-2). Ganglioside mixtures, representative of the ganglioside constitution of the melanoma cells, inhibited the response to IL-2 at high and moderate concentrations, but stimulated this response at low concentration. Purified GM2 or GD2 individually enhanced the response to IL-2, but GM3 or GD3 significantly inhibited it.[79] Gangliosides from melanoma cells thus affect lymphocyte functions fundamental to host-tumor interaction. There is excellent evidence from ganglioside extraction studies and thin layer chromatography of melanomas that the relative amounts of the different gangliosides vary from tumor to tumor.[80] Since different gangliosides individually increase or decrease lymphocyte activity, and the ganglioside composition of the cell membrane determines the mixture of gangliosides released into the tissue fluids, the net effect, up-regulation or down-regulation, of each different melanoma on adjacent lymphoid tissues is unique. The ganglioside content of melanoma, by up-regulating or down-regulating adjacent lymphoid tissues may determine whether or not node spread occurs and the timing of its occurrence.

b. *Prostaglandins* (PG). To assess the effects of PG, we utilized the fact that indomethacin inhibits the actions of PG including their capacity to suppress lymphocyte function. We exposed lymph node lymphocytes (LNL) from single lymph nodes to phytohemagglutinin (PHA) and compared lymphocyte proliferation in the presence and absence of indomethacin. In some experiments indomethacin had no effect on lymphocyte proliferation, but in others lymphocyte proliferation was significantly increased in the presence of indomethacin. In 45 percent of the node groups examined, reduced immune reactivity was associated with prostaglandin effects and was reversible by a prostaglandin inhibitor. In many patients the fact that immune suppression of the node nearest tumor is not released by indomethacin, in contrast to the response in nodes more remote from tumor, suggests that different mechanisms of suppression operate in different lymph nodes.[81]

c. *Melanoma-derived lipoprotein "antigens."* Melanoma-TAA is a 180–190 kDa melanoma-associated "antigen" secreted by the human melanoma cell line UCLA-SO-M14.[82] As a secreted tumor product, it could have reached the lymph nodes in vivo and we were interested in its effect on immunocyte functions. Melanoma-TAA suppresses human lymphocyte functions including the responses to PHA, anti-CD3, and tetanus toxoid (Stene M, in preparation). It has no effect on resting lymphocytes and a range of human tumor and nontumor tissue culture lines. Studies are in progress to identify the mechanism(s) involved in the interaction between melanoma-TAA and lymphocytes.

Since a variety of melanoma-cell products modulate immune function, some being up-regulatory and others down-regulatory, the regulatory influence exerted by each individual melanoma on adjacent lymphoid tissue reflects the uniquely proportioned mixture of active molecules released by it into the tissue fluids. The constitution of the cell membrane and the molecules that the tumor cell releases may change as the tumor evolves, and it is possible that the acquisition of an immune suppressive profile is an important component of the metastatic phenotype.

Tumor-product induced immune suppression provides two avenues of approach to therapy to prevent metastases. It may be possible to modify tumor cell characteristics to abort or diminish the suppressive effect. Alternatively, it may be practicable to protect or rescue susceptible lymphoid tissue from tumor product-induced suppression.

REFERENCES

1. Magnus K. Epidemiology of malignant melanoma of the skin. In: Veronesi U, Cascinelli N, Santinami M., (eds.), "*Cutaneous Melanoma: Status of Knowledge and Future Perspectives.*" Orlando, Fla.: Academic Press, 1987, 1–13.
2. Armstrong BK. Epidemiology of malignant melanoma: Intermittent or total accumulated exposure to the sun. *J Dermatol Surg Oncol* 14:835–847, 1988.
3. Balch CM, and Milton GW. Cutaneous melanoma. Philadelphia: J.B. Lippincott, 1985.
4. Cochran AJ. Malignant melanoma. A review of ten years experience in Glasgow, Scotland. *Cancer* 23:1190–1199, 1969.
5. Das Gupta TK. Results of treatment of 269 patients with primary cutaneous melanoma: A 5-year prospective study. *Ann Surg* 186:201–209, 1977.
6. Balch CM, Soong SJ, Murad T, et al. A multifactorial analysis of melanoma. III. Prognostic factors in melanoma patients with lymph node metastases (Stage II). *Ann Surg* 193:377–388, 1981.
7. Callery C, Cochran AJ, Roe DJ, Rees W, et al. Factors prognostic for survival in patients with malignant melanoma spread to the regional lymph nodes. *Ann Surg* 196:69–75, 1982.
8. Berdeaux DH, Meyskens F, Parks B, et al. Cutaneous malignant melanoma. II. The natural history and prognostic factors influencing the development of Stage II disease. *Cancer* 63:1430–1436, 1989.
9. Little JH, and Davis NC. Secondary malignant melanoma in lymph nodes: Incidence, time of recurrence, and mortality. *Aust N Z J Surg* 48:9–13, 1978.
10. O'Rourke MG, and Louis A. Metastasis in malignant melanoma. *Aus N Z J Surg* 52:154–158, 1982.
11. Cochran AJ, Wen D-R, and Herschman HR. Occult melanoma in lymph nodes detected by antiserum to S-100 protein. *Int J Cancer* 34:159–163, 1984.
12. Cochran AJ, Wen D-R, and Morton DL. Occult tumor cells in the lymph nodes of patients with pathological Stage I malignant melanoma. *Amer J Surg Pathol* 12:612–618, 1988.
13. Allen AC, and Spitz S. Malignant melanoma. A clinicopathological analysis of the criteria for diagnosis and prognosis. *Cancer* 6:1–45, 1953.
14. Little JH. Histology and prognosis in cutaneous malignant melanoma. In: Melanoma and Skin Cancer. Proceedings of the International Cancer Conference. Sydney, Australia: VCN Bligh, Government Printer, 1972, 107–120.
15. Cochran AJ. Histology and prognosis in malignant melanoma. *J Pathol* 97:459–468, 1969.
16. Clark WH, Jr. A classification of malignant melanoma in man correlated with histogenesis and biologic behavior. In: Montagna W, Hu F. (eds.). Advances in Biology of the Skin. The Pigmentary System, Vol. 8. London: Pergammon Press Ltd, 1967, 621–645.
17. Prade M, Sancho-Garnier H, Césarini J-P, and Cochran AJ. Difficulties encountered in the application of Clark classification and the Breslow thickness measurement in cutaneous malignant melanoma. *Int J Cancer* 26:159–163, 1980.
18. Breslow A. Thickness, cross-sectional areas and depth of invasion in the prognosis of cutaneous melanoma. *Ann Surg* 1902–1908, 1970.
19. Balch CM, Wilkerson JA, Murad TM, et al. The prognostic significance of ulceration of cutaneous melanoma. *Cancer* 45:3012–3017, 1980.
20. Schmoeckel C, Bockelbrink A, Bockelbrink H, et al. Low and high risk malignant melanoma. I. Evaluation of clinical and histological prognosticators in 585 cases. *Eur J Cancer* 19:227–235, 1983.
21. Larsen TE, and Grude TH. A retrospective histological study of 669 cases of primary cutaneous malignant melanoma in clinical stage I. The relation of cross-sectional profile, level of invasion, ulceration and vascular invasion to tumor type and prognosis. *Acta Path Microbiol Scand Sect A* 87:131–138, 1979.
22. Clark WH, Elder DE, Guerry D, Braitman LE, Trock BJ, Schulz D, Synnestvedt M, and Halpern AC. A model predicting survival in stage I melanoma based upon tumor progression. *J Natl Cancer Inst* 81:1893–1904, 1989.
23. Cochran AJ. Method of assessing prognosis in patients with malignant melanoma. *Lancet* 2:1062–1064, 1968.
24. MacKie RM, Carfrae DC, and Cochran AJ. Assessment of prognosis in patients with malignant melanoma. *Lancet* 2:455–456, 1972.
25. Vollmer RT. Malignant melanoma. A multivariate analysis of prognostic factors. *Pathol Annu* 24:383–407, 1989.
26. Soong S-J. A computerised mathematical model and scoring system for predicting outcome in melanoma patients. In: Balch CM, Milton GW (eds). *Cutaneous Melanoma.* Philadelphia: Lippincott, 1985, 353–367.
27. Gaynor R, Herschman HR, Irie RF, Jones PC, et al. S-100 protein: A marker for human malignant melanomas? *Lancet* 1:869–871, 1981.
28. Nakajima T, Watanabe S, Sato Y, Kameya T, and Shimosato Y. Immunohistochemical demonstration of S-100 protein in

human malignant melanoma and pigmented nevi. *Gann* 72:335–336, 1981.
29. Cochran AJ, and Wen D-R. S-100 protein as a marker for melanocytic and other tumors. *Pathology* 17:340–345, 1985.
30. Hagen EC, Vennegoor C, Schlingemann RO, Van der Velde ER, and Ruiter DJ. Correlation of histopathological characteristics with staining patterns in human malignant melanoma assessed by (monoclonal) antibodies reactive on paraffin sections. *Histopathology* 10:689–700, 1986.
31. Gown AM, Vogel AM, Heak D, Gough D, and McNutt MA. Monoclonal antibodies specific for melanocyte tumors distinguish subpopulations of melanocytes. *Amer J Path.* 123:195–203; 1986.
32. Morton DL, Wen D-R, Wong JH, Economou JS, Cagle LA, Storm FK, Foshag LJ, and Cochran AJ. Management of clinical stage I melanoma by selective lymphadenectomy: Technical aspects. *Arch Surg.* 127:392–399, 1992.
33. Cagle LA, Wong JH, and Cochran AJ. Dye-targeted lympadenectomy: A feline experimental model. In preparation.
34. Fortner JG, Woodruff J, Schottenfeld DM, and MacLean B. Biostatistical basis of elective node dissection for malignant melanoma. *Ann Surg* 186:101–103, 1977.
35. Karakousis CP, Seedig MK, and Moore R. Prognostic value of lymph node dissection in malignant melanoma. *Arch Surg* 115:719–22, 1980.
36. Dasmahapatra KS, and Karakousis CP. Therapeutic groin dissection in malignant melanoma. *Surg Gynecol Obstet* 156:21–4, 1983.
37. Day CL, and Lew RA. Malignant melanoma prognostic factors of: Elective lymph node dissection. *J Dermatol Surg Oncol* 11:233–9, 1985.
38. Nava M, Santinami M, Clemente C, et al. Prognosis of skin melanoma. *Eur J Surg Oncol* 9:366 (abstract), 1983.
39. Cohen MHL, Ketcham AS, Felix EL, et al. Prognostic factors in patients undergoing lymphadenectomy for malignant melanoma. *Ann Surg* 186:635–42, 1977.
40. Rayner CR. The results of node resection for clinically enlarged lymph nodes in malignant melanoma. *Br J Plast Surg* 34:152–6, 1981.
41. Singletary SE, Byers RM, Shallenberger R, et al. Prognostic factors in patients with regional cervical nodal metastases from cutaneous malignant melanoma. *Am J Surg* 152:371–5, 1986.
42. Cochran AJ, Lana AMA, and Wen D-R. Histomorphometry in the assessment of prognosis in Stage II malignant melanoma. *Amer J Surg Pathol* 13:600–604, 1989.
43. Kheir S, Bines SD, Vonroenn JH, et al. Prognostic significance of DNA aneuploidy in Stage I cutaneous melanoma. *Ann Surg* 207:455–461, 1988.
44. Buchner TH, Hiddeman W, Wormann B, et al. Differential pattern of DNA aneuploidy in human malignancies. *Pathol Res Pract* 179:310–317, 1985.
45. Zeng Q-S, Fu Y-S, and Cochran AJ. Nuclear DNA measurements of metastatic melanoma by a computerized digital imaging system. *Hum Pathol* 21:1112–1116, 1990.
46. Fu Y-S, Cheng L, Huang I, et al. DNA ploidy analysis of cervical condyloma and intraepithelial neoplasia obtained by punch biopsy. *Anal Quant Cytol Histol* 11:187–195, 1989.
47. Ljungberg B, Stenling R, and Roos G. DNA content in renal cell carcinoma with reference to tumor heterogeneity. *Cancer* 56:503–508, 1985.
48. Sondergaard K, Larsen KJ, Moller U, et al. DNA ploidy characteristics of human malignant melanoma analyzed by flow cytometry and compared with histology and clinical course. *Virchows Arch B Cell Pathol* 42:43–52, 1983.
49. Kallioniemi O, Blanco G, Alavaikko M, et al. Improving the prognostic value of DNA flow cytometry in breast cancer by combining DNA index and S phase fraction. *Cancer* 62:2183–2190, 1988.
50. Poste G, Doll J, Brown AE, et al. Comparison of the metastatic properties of B16 melanoma clones isolated from cultured cell lines, subcutaneous tumors, and individual lung metastases. *Cancer Res* 42:2770–2778, 1982.
51. Poste G, Tzeng J, Doll J, et al. Evolution of tumor cell heterogeneity during progressive growth of individual lung metastases. *Proc Natl Acad Sci USA* 79:6574–6578, 1982.
52. Cochran AJ, Pihl E, Wen D-R, Hoon DS, and Korn EL. Zoned immunosuppression of lymph nodes draining malignant melanoma. Histologic and Immunohistologic Studies. *J Natl Cancer Inst* 78:399–405, 1987.
53. Weidner F, Horstein OP, Hermanek P, and Wutz P. Early metastases in regional lymph nodes and prognosis of malignant melanoma. *Arch Dermatol Res* 256:167–177, 1976.
54. Weidner F. Comparative histological studies of regional lymph nodes of 201 melanoma patients. *Arch Dermatol Res* 266:161–175, 1979.
55. Pihl E, Jansson B, Schwartz MA, Malahy MA, Smith JL, Gutterman JV, and Hersh EM. Germinal center hyperplasia: An unfavorable immune response in recurrent malignant melanoma. *Pathology* 14:13–16, 1982.
56. Hoon DSB, Pihl E, Fairhurst MV, and Cochran AJ. Phenotype of paracortical dendritic cells in human lymph nodes. *Fed Proc* 1984 (abstract); 43:1435.
57. Gaynor R, Herschman HR, Irie RF, Jones PC, Morton DL, and Cochran AJ. S-100 protein: A marker for human malignant melanomas? *Lancet* 1:869–871, 1981.
58. Nakajima T, Watanabe S, Sato Y, Shimosata Y, Motoi M, and Lennert K. S-100 protein in Langerhans cells, interdigitating reticulum cells and histocytosis X cells. *Gann* 73:429–432, 1982.
59. Hoon DSB, Korn EL, and Cochran AJ. Variations in functional immunocompetence of individual tumor-draining lymph nodes in humans. *Cancer Res* 47:1740–1744, 1987.
60. Wen D-R, Hoon DSB, Chang C, and Cochran AJ. Variations in lymphokine generation by individual lymph nodes draining human malignant tumors. *Cancer Immunol Immunother* 30:277–282, 1989.
61. Mickel RA, Kessler DJ, Taylor JMG, and Lieshenstein A. Natural killer cell cytotoxicity in the peripheral blood, cervical lymph nodes and tumors of head and neck patients. *Cancer Res* 48:5017–5022, 1988.
62. Heindenreich W, Jagla K, Schussler J, Borner P, Dehnhard F, Kalden JR, Leibold W, Peter HH, and Deicher H. Immunological characterization of mononuclear cells in peripheral blood and regional lymph nodes of breast cancer patients. *Cancer* 43:1308–1313, 1979.
63. Eremin O, Roberts P, Plumb D, and Stephens JP. Human regional tumor lymph nodes. Alterations of microarchitecture and lymphocyte subpopulations. *Br J Cancer* 41:61–72, 1980.
64. Morton BA, Ramey WG, Paderon H, and Miler RE. Monoclonal antibody-defined phenotypes of regional lymph node and peripheral blood lymphocyte subpopulations in early breast cancer. *Cancer Res* 46:2121–2126, 1986.
65. Fineman MS, Mudawar FB, Geha RS. Characteristics and mechanisms of action of the concanavalin A-activated suppressor cells in man. *Cell Immunol* 45:120–132, 1979.
66. Hoon DSB, Bowker R, and Cochran AJ. Suppressor cell activity in human melanoma-draining lymph nodes. *Cancer Res* 47:1529–1533, 1987.
67. Hoon DSB, Bowker R, and Cochran AJ. Suppressor cell activity in human breast cancer-draining lymph nodes. *Surgical Res Comm* 9:167–176, 1990.
68. Catalona WJ, Ratliff TL, and McCool RE. Concanavalin A-

inducible suppressor cells in regional lymph nodes of cancer patients. *Cancer Res* 39:4372–4377, 1979.

69. Akiyami M, Bean MA, Sadamoto K, Takahashi Y, and Brankovan V. Suppression of the responsiveness of lymphocytes from cancer patients triggered by co-culture with autologous tumor-derived cells. *J Immunol* 131:3085, 1983.
70. Werkmeister J, McCarthy W, and Hersey P. Suppressor cell activity in melanoma patients. I. Relation to tumor growth and immunoglobulin levels in vivo. *Int J Cancer* 28:1–9, 1981.
71. Vose BM, Ferguson R, and Moore M. Mitogen responsiveness and inhibitory activity of mesenteric lymph node cells. Conditioned medium containing T cell growth factor reversed suppressor function. *Cancer Immunol Immunother* 13:105–111, 1982.
72. Mukherji B, Wilhelm SA, Guha A, Ergin MT. Regulation of cellular immune response against autologous human melanoma. I. Evidence for cell mediated suppression of in vitro cytotoxic immune response. *J Immunol* 136:1888–1892, 1986.
73. Mukhjerji B, Nashed AL, Guha A, and Ergin MT. Regulation of cellular immune response against autologous human melanoma. II. Mechanism of induction and specificity of suppression. *J Immunol.* 136:1893–1898, 1986.
74. Mills CD, and North RJ. Expression of passively transferred immunity against an established tumor depends on generation of cytolytic T cells in recipient. Inhibition by suppression T cells. *J Exp Med* 157:1448–1460, 1983.
75. North RJ, and Bursuker I. Generation and decay of the immune response to a progressive fibrosarcoma. I. Ly-1^+, 2^- suppressor T cells down regulate the generation of Ly-1^-, 2^+ effector T cells. *J Exp Med* 159:1295–1311, 1984.
76. Cozzolino F, Torcia M, Carossino AM, Giordani R, Selli C, Talini G, Reali E, Vovelli A, Postoia V, and Ferrarini M. Characterization of cells from invaded lymph nodes in patients with solid tumors. *J Exp Med* 166:303–318, 1987.
77. Landay A, Gartland GL, and Clement LT. Characterization of a phenotypically distinct subpopulation of Leu2^+ cells that suppress T cell proliferative responses. *J Immunol* 131:2757–2761, 1983.
78. Clement LT, Grossi CE, and Gartland GL. Morphologic and phenotypic features of the subpopulation of Leu-2^+ cells that suppress B cell differentiation. *J Immunol* 133:2461–2468, 1984.
79. Hoon DSB, Irie RF, and Cochran AJ. Gangliosides from human melanoma immunomodulate response of T cells to interleukin-2. *Cell Immunol* 111:410–419, 1988.
80. Tsuchida T, Morton DL, and Irie RF. Heterogeneity of gangliosides in human melanoma. *Proc Amer Assoc Cancer Res* 26:320 (abstract), 1985.
81. Cochran AJ, Hoon DSB, Korn EL, Ferraro A, and Stene M. Effect of indomethacin on the immunocompetence of human tumor-draining lymph nodes. *Fed Proc* 44:965 (abstract), 1985.
82. Gupta RK, and Morton DL. Studies of a melanoma tumor-associated antigen detected in the spent culture medium of a human melanoma cell line by allogeneic antibody. II. Immunobiologic characterization. *J Nat Cancer Inst* 72:75–82, 1984.
83. Farzad Z, Cochran AJ, McBride WH, Gray JD, Wong V, and Morton DL. Lymphocyte subset alterations in nodes regional to human melanoma. *Cancer Res* 50:3585–3588, 1990.
84. Bassett F, Soler P, Wyllie L, et al. Langerhans cells in a bronchioloalveolar tumor of lung. *Virchows Arch A Pathol Anat Histopathol* 362:315–320, 1974.
85. Watanabe S, Sato Y, Kodama T, et al. Immunohistochemical study with monoclonal antibodies on immune response in human lung cancer. *Cancer Res* 43:5883–5889, 1983.
86. Furukawa T, Watanabe S, Kodama T, et al. T-zone histiocytes in adenocarcinoma of the lung in relation to postoperative prognosis. *Cancer* 56:265–272, 1985.

Chapter 13

CLINICAL PRESENTATION OF PRIMARY CUTANEOUS MELANOMA

Natale Cascinelli and Stefano Zurrida

INTRODUCTION

Mass education campaigns and greater awareness on the part of general practitioners have resulted in increased and earlier diagnosis of cutaneous melanoma.[1] However, the number of cases that first come to the attention of the specialist in an advanced stage of development is still great. Early diagnosis and surgery is the only known way to cure the disease.[2,3,4] Thus, it is essential that cutaneous melanoma or other suspicious lesions be recognized early by primary physician and specialist alike. Otherwise, clinically unsuspected and unrecognized early melanoma will progress to a more unfavorable stage. Familiarity with the clinical appearance of suspicious lesions will also obviate unnecessary biopsy of low risk benign pigmented lesions. The aim of this chapter is to bring to the attention of the physician the clinical characteristics of the various types of melanoma to aid in early diagnosis. Possessing such skills is important to select patients judiciously for biopsy. Although instrumental aids such as dermatoscopy have recently been advocated, their use in clinical diagnosis is not yet widely practiced. The clinical appearance of a melanoma depends on its histogenesis and also on its stage of development. From a strictly clinical point of view it is possible to distinguish three variants of cutaneous melanoma; flat melanoma corresponding to histologic superficial spreading melanoma, nodular melanoma, and flat melanoma containing a nodular area.

FLAT MELANOMA

Flat melanoma is by far the commonest of the melanomas and may be found anywhere on the skin surface; it is more frequently localized on the trunk or the back in the male and on the lower limbs in the female. It is a pigmented lesion with greatest diameter nearly always exceeding 5 millimeters. Two phases of development may be discerned: a macular phase and a plaque phase.

Macular Phase (Non-Palpable Melanoma)

The macular phase corresponds to the so-called "thin melanoma," signifying a neoplasm in its initial proliferative phase with no clinical evidence of spontaneous regression. If localized on the trunk or limbs it is generally small (usually less than 6 mm), but may become much larger on the face, mucous membranes, palms, and plantar region of the foot. In this phase, the neoplasm is only modestly aggressive: appropriate surgical treatment results in cure in almost all cases. These completely asymptomatic lesions can only be recognized by a very careful examination of the skin.

There are several clinical characteristics alerting the physician to suspect flat cutaneous melanoma. Irregular outline or *asymmetry* is very common; *edges* are cleanly defined and irregularly indented with focal areas of outward proliferation giving the lesion an appearance resembling a map. The *color* varies from reddish-brown to black-brown with uneven distribution of pigment. The *diameter* of the lesion generally exceeds 5 to 6 millimeters[5] (Plates 38 and 39).

Plaque Melanoma (Palpable Melanoma)

Plaque melanoma, or palpable melanoma, is not necessarily a progression from the macular phase. The lesion appears slightly raised from the surface of the skin and varies from 5 millimeters to several centimeters in diameter (Plate 40). Morphologically it resembles the macular form although its characteristics are more accentuated. Lesions of this type have typically been present on the patient's skin for some time. As soon as they appear they increase rapidly in radial diameter and then stabilize and remain at that stage for a long period of time. Changes, if any, tend toward greater asymmetry rather than increased size. At this point, the history of change in nevi or evolution becomes an important consideration for biopsy. A lesion which the patient reports as having changed its appearance must always be regarded with suspicion. *Spontaneous Regression* is typical of this phase of melanoma. Within the pigmented area, usually hypopigmented, nearly normal, slightly atrophied areas of skin may appear, giving the lesion an annular or arcuate appearance (Plates 41 and 42). On occasion regression may be total leaving a hypopigmented area with the form of the original lesion.

Sites where flat melanoma has special characteristics are the face, the palmar and plantar regions, and under the nailbed.

FACE

Commonly found facial lesions are lentigo maligna or Hutchinson-Dubrehuil's lentigo. Most commonly afflicting old people, the lesion appears first as a macular phase melanoma which slowly spreads horizontally to reach a considerable size after several years (Plate 43). It usually has variegated color with conspicuous areas of regression and irregular, sometimes indistinct edges. The flat lesion may, after many years (10–20 years), develop circumscribed areas of vertical growth which present as one or more blue-black or achromic raised nodules, often with a raw, bleeding surface (Plate 44).

PALM, PLANTAR REGION, AND NAILBED

Melanoma is rare at these sites, comprising 3 to 15 percent of the extra-ocular melanomas[6] and constitutes, from a clinical and anatomopathological point of view, a distinct entity called *acral lentiginous melanoma* (ALM) (Plates 45 and 46). It affects the black skinned population more often than the white population and has a worse prognosis than melanomas at other sites because it may be more aggressive and generally is diagnosed late. The patient cannot explore these sites as easily as others and the thickness of the stratum corneum of the plantar region can hide the typical aspects of a melanotic lesion; these factors contribute to the late diagnosis. The lesion usually first appears as a flat phase melanoma which accentuates the adjacent cutaneous sulci and has irregular margins and pigmentation.

NODULAR MELANOMA

A nodular melanoma may appear on healthy skin on any part of the body, although it occurs most often on the covered skin of the trunk (Plate 47). Due to its rapid rate of vertical growth, a lesion will quickly take on first a papular then a nodular appearance, with a regular and smooth convex surface and a fleshy consistency. The border with healthy skin is always distinct. The lesion soon becomes eroded (ulceration), exuding serous and bloody fluids.

The pigmentation may be irregularly distributed or may be entirely lacking (amelanotic) in which case the neoplasm appears as a reddish firm nodule which is very difficult to diagnose because it can resemble other cutaneous neoformations such as pyogenic granuloma, angioma, vegetating squamous cell carcinoma, inflamed seborrhoeic keratosis, and so on. Close inspection, however, will frequently reveal a ring of pigment around its margin, in which case the term hypomelanotic melanoma would be more appropriate.

FLAT MELANOMA WITH NODULE

A nodular lesion will commonly appear within the confines of a flat melanoma in macular or plaque phase, although it usually does so years after the initial appearance of the primary flat lesion. Facial melanomas typically develop in this manner. This marks a new stage in the development of the neoplasm. The nodular component generally has a large base. Occasionally, the lesion may assume a polypoid appearance. Such lesions frequently become ulcerated and may bleed spontaneously or after very mild trauma (Plates 48 and 49). Nodules develop relatively late in the course of a superficial spreading melanoma, whereas in nodular melanoma the nodule is the first visible manifestation. It is thus important to recognize that a nodule within a flat pigmented area is not a nodular melanoma.

MELANOMA ASSOCIATED WITH A NEVUS

As well as developing on healthy skin, cutaneous melanoma may present on or near an established nevus (Plate 50). In persons with giant congenital melanotic nevi, the risk of developing cutaneous melanoma is thought to be approximately 6.3 percent,[8] although literature estimates vary from 2 to 31 percent. The risk of developing cutaneous melanoma seems directly related to the size of the congenital lesion. The melanoma appears as a raised area, usually the same color or darker than the nevus itself. The melanoma may grow quite rapidly and often becomes ulcerated. The appearance of a cutaneous melanoma associated with an acquired nevus is considered by some authors to be a chance occurrence[9] with only 5 percent of melanomas arising from such pre-existing lesions. However, other authors have demonstrated coexisting benign nevus cells within melanoma in a much higher percentage of cases (see Chapter 10). Occasionally, melanoma may develop in contiguity with acquired intradermal nevus (Plates 51 and 52), in which case the melanoma is seen to grow over the surface of the nevus. In the early stages, the clinical characteristic of the nevus remains evident and later the melanoma tends to completely obliterate the nevus which, however, remains palpable as a modest and irregular prominence.

DIFFERENTIAL DIAGNOSIS

The differential diagnosis of cutaneous melanoma is generally easy since the morphological characteristics of the neoplasm are distinct. The changes which become evident as the lesion develops are such as to accentuate these characteristics and render the diagnosis even easier.

In the initial stages, when the melanoma is not obvious and some of its clinical characteristics are not yet evident or are poorly developed, the diagnosis may be relatively difficult and the neoplasm may be mistakenly diagnosed as a benign melanocytic or other lesion. Accurate clinical diagnosis is vital in order to identify the skin neoplasms which must be removed and avoid unnecessary biopsy of large numbers of other pigmented benign lesions.

Cutaneous lesions which often resemble melanoma are as follows:

benign melanocytic lesions
pigmented basal cell carcinoma
seborrhoeic keratosis
thrombosed angioma
pyogenic granuloma
dermatofibroma

Acquired benign melanocytic lesions may simulate or precede melanoma. More than two-thirds of adult white-skinned people present at least one acquired nevus.[10] Absent at birth, acquired nevi increase in number until late middle age. They consist of nidi of histologically normal melanocytes which may be located in the dermal-epidermal transition zone (junctional or transition nevi), the dermis (dermal nevi), or both levels (compound nevi).

Junctional nevi appear as clearly circumscribed circular or oval small macular or slightly raised lesions of bronze or black color. They are randomly distributed over the surface of the body. *Dermal nevi* are more distinct than junctional nevi and often present as uniformly bronze color or brownish distinct dome-shaped papules. They are commonly present on the face and the neck. *Compound* nevi are slightly raised papular or nodular formations which may range from uniformly brown to uniformly black. They may present a smooth or verrucous surface and regular round or oval margins.

Dysplastic nevi are generally larger than ordinary acquired nevi; they are predominantly macular and often variegated in color. Typically, they have indistinct margins that merge imperceptibly with healthy skin. Some individuals may possess dozens of these lesions which at times appear so atypical as to be indistinguishable from melanomas. Dysplastic nevi have a malignant potential, particularly the familial type, where the risk of developing cutaneous melanoma is several hundred times greater than in the general population (see Chap. 9). *Blue nevus* presents as a uniformly blue- or blackish-colored smooth-surfaced nodule with regular margins and diameter rarely 1 centimeter. Size, contour, and color generally remain stable. Very rarely blue nevus may become malignant (see Chap. 9). While resembling a nodular melanoma there is almost never a history of rapid growth. *Sutton's nevus* (halo nevus) has a distinctive appearance. It is a brown or brownish raised lesion with a generally circular peripheral ring of depigmentation. This ring expands to as to bring about complete disappearance of the nevus. *Spitz's nevus or spindle cell and/or epithelioid nevus* presents as a nodular, small sized, regular lesion of black or brown coloration. It occurs typically in infants and children with no tendency to change in size. (See Chapter 9.)

A change in a nevus certainly requires further investigation. However, it is important to note that the normal life cycle of acquired nevi includes periods of development and regression, and these are not expressions of malignant transformation. Trauma, infection, and hormonal changes such as during puberty and pregnancy all tend to induce changes in the appearance of nevi. It is useful to bear in mind that acquired nevi only rarely develop into melanomas.

Pigmented basal cell carcinoma is generally a pearly or slightly translucent papule which may have superficial telangiectasia. The lesion typically develops on chronically sun-exposed body areas such as the trunk (in outdoor workers) and the face, growing relatively slowly. Sometimes a basal-cell carcinoma may be slightly pigmented and take on a bluish hue so as to induce the suspicion of a melanoma, especially when the lesion is ulcerated; in the majority of cases, however, the margin retains its characteristic pearly aspect.

Seborrhoeic keratoses vary in color and may be yellowish-brown, grey, or even black. They commonly occur in crops in middle aged or elderly people. The lesion is raised and the surface is cerebriform and has a waxy appearance.

Thrombosed angioma usually has a shiny smooth surface and is black or deep red in color with a surrounding area of inflammation in which dilated capillaries are frequently seen. They are tender on palpation.

Distinguishing *pyogenic granuloma* lesions from melanotic or hypomelanotic melanoma can be difficult by simple inspection; the patient's history here becomes very important (trauma to the site and very rapid growth). The commonest site is the digits.

Dermatofibroma is usually found on the extremities. The lesion is regular in shape and may be reddish-brown or dark. Its consistency is typically hard.

CONCLUSION AND FUTURE PERSPECTIVE

Although cutaneous melanoma is a relatively uncommon neoplasm, for several reasons it is increasingly attracting the attention of the physician and the public. Its incidence continues to increase and is thought to be doubling every 10 years.[11] In the United States, the rate of increase is about 10 percent annually with 27,300 new cases diagnosed in 1988.[12] This is a rate of increase second only to that of lung carcinoma in women and it is estimated that by the year 2000 one person per hundred will develop cutaneous melanoma. If the trend continues, melanoma will become one of the commonest neoplasms of light-skinned people and will affect men and women more or less equally at an average age that continues to decline.

The etiology of melanoma has not been completely elucidated. There is a diversity of hypotheses to explain the etiology of cutaneous melanoma, some of which, for example the solar radiation theory, have enormous social implications and have undoubtedly contributed to the interest of general public in this disease.

Educational campaigns have alerted people to the health issues; they become more aware of their physical state and increasingly recognize when something is not right; more often it is the patient who detects melanoma and brings it to the attention of the physician. Just as it is important to recognize early melanoma and other suspicious lesions to achieve a high-cure rate, it is also important to recognize benign lesions so as to minimize unnecessary biopsy and costs of diagnosis. Since the success of primary prevention is at present uncertain, the only way to reduce mortality from melanoma is to educate everyone, general practitioners, surgeons, and so on, in early diagnosis when the cure rate is almost 100 percent.

For these reasons we have been conducting a study involving the computer analysis of photographs of 300 pigmented skin lesions. The initial hypothesis was the supposition that the clinical diagnosis of melanoma is based almost exclusively on visual inspection by the clinician. The visual data are interpreted in the doctor's brain whose diagnostic ability depends very much on accumulated experience. We supposed that the visual system could equally well be a tele-camera and the interpretative organ a computer. The diagnostic data are transformed from clinical impressions informed by experience into logical formulae representing shape, margin surface, color, and so on, of the lesion. There appear to be two main possibilities for the future use of such a system: (1) to assist the inexperienced physician to diagnose melanoma by providing him or her with a tool for objectively and reliably measuring the characteristics of a lesion and estimating the risk of malignancy, and (2) to provide the expert clinician with additional diagnostic data, not perceived by the human eye, which will improve diagnostic accuracy.

REFERENCES

1. Doherty VR, and MacKie RM. Experience of a public education program on early detection of cutaneous malignant melanoma. *BMJ* 297:388–392, 1988.
2. Clark WH Jr, Elder DE, Guerry D IV, Epstein ME, Greene MH, and VanHorn M. A study of tumor progression: The precursor lesions of superficial spreading and nodular melanoma. *Hum Pathol* 17:1147–1165, 1984.
3. Maize JC, and Ackerman AB. *Pigmented Lesions of the Skin*. Lea & Febiger, Philadelphia: 1987, 75–77.
4. Veronesi U, Cascinelli N, and Santinami M. Prognostic factors in malignant melanoma. In: *Cutaneous Melanoma*. "Status of Knowledge and future perspective." London: Pergamon Press Ed, 1987, 99–110.
5. Friedman RJ, and Rigel DS. The clinical features of malignant melanoma. *Dermatol Clin* 3:271–283, 1985.
6. Magnus K. Prognosis in malignant melanoma of the skin. Significance of stage of disease, anatomical site, sex, age and period of diagnosis. *Cancer* 40:389–397, 1977.
7. Mackie RM. Which moles matter? The association between

melanocytic nevi and malignant melanoma. *Br J Dermatol* 105:607–609, 1981.

8. Rhodes AR, Wood WC, Sober AJ, and Mihm MC. Non-epidermal origin of malignant melanoma associated with gigantic congenital nevocellular nevus. *Plast Reconstr Surg* 67:782–790, 1981.
9. Maize JC, and Ackerman AB. Histologic simulators of malignant melanoma. In: *Pigmented Lesions of the Skin.* Philadelphia: Lea & Febiger, 1987, 225–269.
10. Kraemer KH, Greene M, Tarone R, Elder DE, Clark WH Jr, and Guerry D IV. Dysplastic nevi and cutaneous melanoma risk. *Lancet* 2:1076–1077, 1983.
11. Elwood JM, and Lee JAH. Recent data on the epidemiology of melanoma. *Semin Oncol* 2:149–154, 1975.
12. Handley WS. The pathology of melanotic growths in relation to their operative treatment. *Lancet* 1:996–1003, 1970.
13. Cristofolini M, Zumiani G, Boi S, and Piscioli F. Community detection of early melanoma. *Lancet* 1:18, 1986.

Chapter 14

THE INFLUENCE OF PROGNOSTIC FACTORS ON MELANOMA MANAGEMENT

W. H. McCarthy and H. M. Shaw

INTRODUCTION

A large number of prognostic factors for melanoma have been proposed. For the practicing oncologist, the task is to identify those factors useful in optimizing the management of patients presenting with specific patterns of primary or recurrent melanoma. Management includes choice of appropriate therapy, accurate counseling of the patient and relatives, expert surgery when surgery is the treatment of choice, and intervention at the earliest possible time for metastatic melanoma. A much smaller list of prognostic factors influence these management tasks directly. Prognostic factors can thus be classified as: (a) immediately useful, (b) indirectly useful, or (c) currently of interest but not influencing management at the present time.

IMMEDIATELY USEFUL PROGNOSTIC FACTORS

Stage of Disease at First Presentation

Clinical staging of melanoma has a clear influence on management. Until recently, melanoma patients were classified into three stages according to the extent of disease at first presentation.

Stage I	Melanoma localized to primary lesion site
Stage II	Metastases in regional lymph nodes
Stage III	Distant melanoma metastases

This staging system for melanoma has now been superseded by agreement between the Union Internationale Contre le Cancer (UICC) and the American Joint Committee on Cancer (AJCC). The new classification provides the best differentiation of patients into stages that are evenly distributed and significant for prognosis.[1,2] The main difference between the old and new system lies in the classification of patients with lymph node metastases. In the previous system, stage II indicated the patient had involved lymph nodes. In the UICC/AJCC staging system, lymph node involvement is now stage III. The UICC/AJCC staging system is shown in Table 14.1.

For stage III disease, prognosis has been shown to be related to the degree and number of lymph nodes involved.[3–5] In patients undergoing elective lymph node dissection, the survival for those patients with microscopic involvement of only part of a single lymph node is only slightly lower than for patients with primary lesions of similar thickness and no lymph node involvement. However, once involvement of more that one node occurs, the prognosis deteriorates markedly. Analysis of a large number of studies relating prognosis to the degree

TABLE 14-1
UICC/AJCC STAGING SYSTEM

PRIMARY TUMOR (pT)	
pTX	Primary tumor cannot be assessed.
pTO	No evidence of primary tumor.
pTis	Melanoma in situ (atypical melanotic hyperplasia, severe melanotic dysplasia), not an invasive lesion (Clark's level I).
pT1	Tumor 0.75 mm or less in thickness and invades the papillary dermis (Clark's level II).
pT2	Tumor more than 0.75 mm but not more than 1.5 mm in thickness and/or invades to papillary-reticular interface (Clark's level III).
pT3	Tumor more than 1.5 mm but not more than 4 mm in thickness and/or invades the reticular dermis (Clark's level IV).
pT3a	Tumor more than 1.5 mm but not more than 3 mm in thickness.
pT3b	Tumor more than 3 mm but not more than 4 mm in thickness.
pT4	Tumor more than 4 mm in thickness and/or invades the subcutaneous tissue (Clark's level V) and/or satellite(s) within 2 cm of the primary tumor.
pT4a	Tumor more than 4 mm in thickness and/or invades the subcutaneous tissue.
pT4b	Satellite(s) within 2 cm of primary tumor.
LYMPH NODE (N)	
NX	Regional lymph nodes cannot be assessed.
NO	No regional lymph node metastasis.
N1	Metastasis 3 cm or less in greatest dimension in any regional lymph node(s).
N2	Metastasis more than 3 cm in greatest dimension in any regional lymph node(s) and/or in-transit metastasis.
N2a	Metastasis more than 3 cm in greatest dimension in any regional lymph node(s).
N2b	In-transit metastasis.
N2c	Both (N2a and N2b).
DISTANT METASTASIS (M)	
MX	Presence of distant metastasis cannot be assessed.
MO	No distant metastasis.
M1	Distant metastasis.
M1a	Metastasis in skin or subcutaneous tissue or lymph node(s) beyond the regional lymph nodes.
M1b	Visceral metastasis.

STAGE GROUPING			
Stage I	pT1	NO	MO
	pT2	NO	MO
Stage II	pT3	NO	MO
	pT4	NO	MO
Stage III	Any pT	N1,N2	MO
Stage IV	Any pT	Any N	M1

of nodal involvement by metastatic melanoma indicates the presence of a single lymph node is associated with around 50 percent survival at 5 years and 35 percent survival at 10 years. For patients with two or three nodes involved, the prognosis falls to 40 percent at 5 years and 20 percent at 10 years. For patients with more than three lymph nodes, the survival is less than 30 percent at 5 years and no more than 10 percent at 10 years. It is interesting to note, that even with four or more nodes involved, a small number of patients survive longer than 10 years.[6–8]

For the surgical oncologist, these figures determine the surgical approach to the patient with melanoma. The question of elective lymph node dissection is extensively canvassed in the surgical literature. Most surgeons agree that a subset of patients exists in whom elective lymph node dissection will clearly improve survival, that is, those patients with minimal tumor involvement of a single node detected histologically but not palpable clinically, have a good prognosis even if the primary tumor is between 1.5 and 4.00 mm thick. Their survival will be similar to patients with tumors of this thickness and uninvolved lymph nodes, that is, around 75 percent at 5 years. Once a single node is fully involved, the prognosis will fall to 50 percent. Thus, the aim for the future is to identify those patients with tumors in this intermediate range who already have minimal lymph node involvement and to undertake elective lymph node dissection in this subset only. At the present time it is not possible to identify this subset, so elective node dissection is practiced by a large number of melanoma centers. Various studies indicate occult nodal metastases will be found in approximately 20 percent of patients with intermediate thickness melanoma. However, the incidence of clinically occult nodal metastases in patients with lesions > 1.5 mm thick undergoing elective lymph node dissection is 36 percent when more intense scrutiny of the nodes and the use of S100 to identify small clumps of tumor cells was undertaken.[6,7] Many studies have indicated that a policy of elective lymph node dissection in the group of patients with intermediate thickness lesions (1.5 mm to 4 mm) will provide a significant therapeutic advantage with survival rates improved by at least 25 percent.[9,10] The major objections to this policy of elective lymph node dissection has been summarized recently by Cady.[11]

Two large studies, one from the Mayo Clinic and the other from the WHO Melanoma Group, reported no benefit from elective lymph node dissection for stage I patients with melanoma of the extremities. However, both these studies have been severely criticized by proponents of elective lymph node dissection.[10] At present, two large prospective evaluations of elective lymph node dissection patients with tumors of intermediate thickness are in the process of accrual in the United States and Europe.

Extranodal extension of tumor in resected lymph

node specimens is of bad prognostic significance.[12] This finding may influence the surgical oncologist to suggest radiotherapy to the dissected field for these patients. As yet there are no studies to confirm the value of this approach, but some evidence is available by extrapolation. Overgaard et al.[13] have indicated that radiation will give the same outcome for head and neck tumors as elective lymph node dissection, suggesting that radiation can control tumor in lymph nodes without the need for surgical resection. Also, tumor cell spillage, which is likely in patients with extranodal spread may be rendered innocuous by the addition of radiation in the postoperative period.

Breslow Thickness/Clark's Levels

Breslow thickness is now the most important histological prognostic factor in the choice of therapy for primary melanoma. Tumor thickness is related to the risk of local recurrence, to the risk of lymphatic involvement, and to the risk of hematogenous dissemination. In most centers, therapeutic approaches to patients with melanoma are based primarily on the tumor thickness measurement.

The observations of Alexander Breslow[14,15] have largely superseded Clark's level of invasion. Breslow thickness is defined as the maximum vertical dimension of the tumor in millimeters measured with an ocular micrometer from the top of the granular cell layer of the epidermis to the deepest invasive tumor cell excluding periappendigeal and perifollicular regions. In ulcerated tumors, the measurement is taken from the ulcer base. The greater accuracy and comparability of the Breslow thickness make this measurement more accurate than level of invasion. Clark levels have been shown to vary by as much as 30 percent, that is, the concordance between groups of pathologists examining the same tumor is only approximately 70 percent. The concordance for Breslow thickness is very high, usually exceeding 90 percent.[16] Clark's levels do not provide useful prognostic information for polypoidal lesions, which seldom penetrate beyond level 3 no matter how thick they are. There is, however, a close correlation between tumor thickness and survival for these types of lesions.[17]

There may be some residual prognostic significance available through the Clark levels, which is independent of the Breslow thickness measurement. Sober et al. suggested for some subsets of melanomas, levels are the best predictors of deaths within 24 months.[18] In this series, lesions between 0.76 mm and 1.69 mm in thickness had a far higher than expected mortality if the lesions were also noted to reach level 4 in the dermis. The same conclusions were confirmed by other authors.[19]

If tumors are placed into five main Breslow groups, that is, < 0.76 mm, 0.76 mm to 1.50 mm, 1.51 mm to 2.50 mm, 2.51 mm to 4.00 mm, and > 4.00 mm, there is a close correlation of thickness with survival[20] (Fig. 14-1). However, the relationship between thickness and prognosis is not exactly linear in that there is a small subset of thin melanomas that are at high risk of metastasis. Similarly, there is a group of patients with thick melanomas that does not have the expected survival outcome. Slingluff et al. reported a series of 681 patients with primary tumors < 0.75 mm thick with a 4.8 percent risk of recurrence.[21] The patients at greatest risk were men with axial lesions, and tumors with severe regression, or invading to Clark level 4 or greater. In the Sydney Melanoma Unit series, 7.3 percent of patients with lesions < 0.75 mm thick developed recurrences. The recurrent tumors were those that were ulcerated, reached Clark level 3 or 4, or showed increased mitotic activity.[22] Since most of these recurrences developed either around the primary lesion site or at regional lymph nodes, a wider local excision and careful monitoring of the lymph nodes, perhaps with ultrasound[23] as well as clinical appraisal is appropriate for thin lesions with these histopathological criteria. Elder et al. have proposed that those melanomas capable of metastasis may be recognizable by a small vertical growth phase even though they are thin by Breslow measurements.[24]

In the subset of thick tumors (> 6 mm) that do not metastasize with 10 years, it has been difficult to determine any prognostic variable that is helpful in isolating this group of patients.[25] None of the standard histological prognostic criteria nor the use of immunological markers or DNA ploidy studies

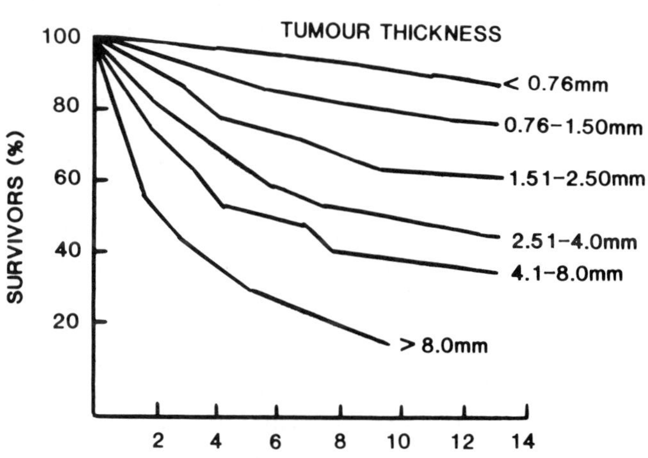

FIG. 14-1 Survival according to tumor thickness in 2627 patients with melanoma localized to the primary lesion site.

revealed any way of predicting those patients with thick tumors who would survive beyond 10 years.

The surgical oncologist should expect the pathologist to provide both Breslow thickness and level of invasion in the histopathological report. The surgeon may then choose to treat rather more aggressively and follow up rather more carefully those lesions, which though relatively superficial on Breslow thickness, reach Clark level 4 or 5 in the dermis.

A common pattern of surgical practice for stage I melanoma, which is the pattern used by the Sydney Melanoma Unit, is as follows:

1. < 0.76 mm: Local excision with a margin of 0.50 to 1.0 cm (1.0 cm preferred if achievable without skin grafting or local flaps).
2. 0.76 mm to 1.50 mm: Wide excision with margins increasing from 1 cm to 3 cm as the tumor thickness increases.
3. 1.51 mm to 4.00 mm: Wide excision with elective lymph node dissection except for melanomas occurring on the legs of women In women, elective lymph node dissection is not undertaken until the tumors are > 2 mm in thickness.
4. > 4.00 mm: Wide excision and elective lymph node dissection. It is appreciated that the undertaking of lymph node dissection in this group may offer only marginal advantage to the patient in terms of survival. However, the majority of these patients will present with lymph node involvement if wide excision only is undertaken.[26] The policy of elective dissection at the time of the primary removal aims to obviate a second expensive and time-consuming admission to hospital at a later date for removal of involved lymph nodes. In this group, the lymph node recurrence rate for nondissected patients exceeds 60 percent.[26] The long term survival in these patients is relatively poor (10 to 15 percent) even after therapeutic lymph node dissection, since hematogenous spread usually supervenes quite rapidly.

Tumor Volume

In developing his theory about the significance of tumor thickness, Breslow maintained that thickness was, in fact, a crude estimate of tumor volume.[14] Recently, it has been demonstrated that tumor volume may be related to prognosis.[27] Lesions with a reconstructed volume of > 200 mm^3 or more had a significantly worse 5 year survival rate (11 percent) than those with a tumor volume < 200 mm^3 (90 percent). Thus, tumor volume appeared to be a more powerful predictor of outcome than thickness.

Further attempts have been made to design computer-based systems for developing physical three-dimensional morphology of the primary melanoma. When vertical growth of a superficial melanoma commences, the underside surface area of the tumor becomes elongated from the region of vertical growth. A method of computing the underside surface area to tumor volume ratio as a measure of the irregularity of the tumor surface has recently been developed.[28] Tumors with a higher ratio of area to surface appear to have a poor prognosis. This factor may be important in the future as the most accurate histological prognostic variable.

Histogenetic Type

The histogenetic classification of the tumor no longer has a large influence on the management of melanoma. Since the pioneering work of Wallace Clark in 1969 revealing the high degree of correlation between level of penetration of the tumor with survival and surgical outcome, the purely histogenetic classification of superficial spreading, nodular, and acral lentiginous melanoma has become far less important. Nonetheless, some useful prognostic information is retained in differentiating among lentigo maligna and desmoplastic neurotrophic melanoma and the other three classifications. Some reports continue to indicate that acral lentiginous melanoma also has a worse prognosis than superficial spreading and nodular melanoma. The Sydney Melanoma Unit regards lentigo maligna melanoma as a more benign disease than the other melanoma classifications.[29] Accordingly, local surgery of the primary lesion is less radical than for the other melanomas, and elective lymph node dissection is seldom undertaken for thicker lentigo maligna melanoma. Desmoplastic neurotrophic melanoma has a higher risk of local recurrence than tumors of comparable Breslow thickness.[30] For the surgical oncologist, a diagnosis of acral lentiginous or desmoplastic neurotrophic melanoma should suggest the need for wider margins of resection. A margin of 5 cm, where possible, is used at the Sydney Melanoma Unit.

Microscopic Satellitosis

Microscopic satellitosis is defined as the presence of malignant melanocytes within 0.5 cm of the primary lesion separated from the main body of tumor by normal reticular dermal collagen or subcutaneous fat. There is no doubt this is a bad prognostic sign, Day et al. reporting a 46 percent decrease in 5 year survival patterns with microscopic satellitosis.[31] Harrist et al. found 53 percent of patients with microscopic satellitosis had occult nodal metastases, while only 12 percent of patients without microscopic satellitosis had occult nodal metastases.[32] Kelly et al. documented the increased frequency of local recurrence when microscopic satellites are detected.[33] From this it is obvious the presence of microscopic satellitosis justifies more radical local excision of the primary tumor and elective node dissection regardless of the thickness of the primary tumor.

Ulceration

Ulceration of the primary lesion is an important adverse prognostic factor for consideration by the surgical oncologist and thus indicates a more aggressive approach to both the primary tumor and the lymph nodes. Studies on the effect of ulceration on survival from melanoma suggest ulceration should be regarded as additive to the decisions based on tumor thickness alone, for example, a tumor measuring 1.3 mm in thickness should be placed in the next prognostic group in determining therapeutic approach.[34,35]

Mitotic Rate

Mitotic rate, the number of mitoses per square millimeter, is an important histological prognostic factor, which must be considered by the surgical oncologist. Ten year survival rates in patients with one or less mitoses per high-power field was 87 percent compared to 64 percent for lesions with two or more mitoses per high-power field.[28] Schmoeckel and Braun-Falco have developed a mitotic index by multiplying the lesion thickness by the number of mitoses.[36] Patients having a mitotic index of 0 to 10 have a 5 year disease-free survival of 64 percent compared with 21 percent for patients with lesions with a mitotic index > 10. Kopf et al. noted that an even greater differentiation can be achieved when 18 is used as the discriminator in the mitotic index.[37] They found that 5 year survival rates for patients with a mitotic index over 18 was 23 percent, while it was 85 percent for those with an index of < 18. Shaw et al. found that a high-mitotic rate was predictive of a poor prognosis in patients with thin lesions.[22] Thus, mitotic rate will be utilized by the surgical oncologist in counseling the patient about the likely outcome of therapy for his melanoma. However, as yet it is not clear how this feature should influence the decision on width of excision or the need for prophylactic elective lymph node dissection. It appears likely that mitotic rate is more closely related to hematogenous dissemination than to local recurrence or lymph node involvement.

Anatomical Site

The BANS area is the region on the upper back, the posterior arms, the posterior and lateral parts of the neck, and the posterior part of the scalp. Originally, tumors on the BANS area of the body were considered to be associated with a worse prognosis[38] but subsequent studies have not confirmed this finding.[39–42] Recently, Weinstock et al. using meta-analysis of six other BANS studies, concluded that these anatomical sub-sites do have a poorer prognosis but large numbers of cases are needed to demonstrate this disadvantage.[43] The studies of the Sydney Melanoma Unit involving more than 4000 cases did not reveal BANS location as a prognostic variable (Shaw et al., unpublished). Although surgical oncologists may ignore the BANS location of the tumor in choosing optimal therapy, consideration should be given to the fact that axial sites in general have a poorer prognosis than extremity sites, independent of tumor thickness.[20]

Some cutaneous and all mucosal sites have a particularly poor prognosis. The cutaneous sites are the sole, the palms, the scalp, the ears, and under the nail beds.[44–46] Studies relating to the palms, scalp, and ears are based on too few cases to determine the extent of prognostic disadvantage of these sites. However, subungual melanoma has been shown to have a worse prognosis than other melanomas of the limbs and trunk with a higher incidence of lymph node involvement at the time of primary presentation.[46] This increase in lymph node involvement is not entirely dependent on the primary tumor thickness. Even if the nodes appear clinically negative, in our opinion, subungual melanoma should in almost all instances warrant elective lymph node dissection as well as appropriate local amputation of the affected digit.

The commonest mucosal sites for melanoma are the anus, the vulval region, and the mouth. Almost all melanomas in these areas are detected late in their progression and overall survival is 10 to 35 percent.[47–49] Studies comparing node dissection with local removal only of the lesion reveal no difference in survival.[50,51] Abdominoperineal resection for anal melanoma does not improve survival over local resection only.[49,53] The surgical oncologist may thus be content with wide local resection of these lesions and a watchful policy on the draining lymph nodes.

Age of Patient

The age of the patient is not an independent prognostic determinant. It has been clearly shown that older patients, in general, do as well as younger patients with comparable tumor thickness. Older patients tend to present later in the course of the disease and therefore have thicker, more ulcerated tumors.[54,55] Acral lentiginous melanoma is more common in older patients and in these patients, after correction for thickness, there is still a subset in which the diagnosis of an acral lentiginous melanoma does worsen the prognosis.[56]

The extremes of age may, of course, influence the choice of surgery for specific patients. It is certainly unnecessary to undertake radical surgery for patients whose life expectancy is measured in months or a few years. However, experience at the Sydney

Melanoma Unit has indicated that those patients who are fit enough to undergo standard treatment for melanoma based on the tumor thickness measurement should indeed have that therapy. In many instances where lymph node dissection is appropriate and treatment of the primary lesion only is undertaken, the patient will return within 3 years with involved lymph nodes necessitating therapeutic lymph node dissection when the patient is older. In general, it is advised that whenever possible the appropriate treatment should be applied independent of the patient's age.

The same observations can be made in relation to children. Unpublished studies at the Sydney Melanoma Unit have indicated the outcome of treatment of melanoma in children under 12 years is better if standard treatment is applied, that is, those patients whose tumors warrant lymph node dissection should have that lymph node dissection. Prognosis in children who have been adequately treated is similar to that in adults with lesions of comparable thickness. In contrast, early reports in the literature on childhood melanoma indicated a poor prognosis. This was probably a reflection of the fact that it was previously believed that melanoma did not occur in childhood, so these patients almost invariably presented for treatment at an advanced stage of the disease.[57,58]

Gender of Patient

Virtually all studies indicate women patients do better than men. However, not all studies indicate that gender is an independent prognostic variable. In general, women first present for treatment with tumors less thick and less ulcerated than the tumors in men.[59] Also, lesions in women tend to be located on prognostically favorable sites, such as the upper and lower limbs, while male lesions are concentrated more on axial sites.[60] In summary, all these factors bestow a more favorable prognosis for women.[61] However, the female superiority in survival cannot be fully explained by these differences at first presentation. Women still retain some prognostic advantage in multivariate studies.[20,62] However, gender does not greatly influence the management of melanoma. At the Sydney Melanoma Unit, the better prognosis for women with melanomas on the extremities influences the decision for elective node dissection. Node dissection is not undertaken until the tumor thickness is > 2.00 mm. Hormonal influences are often queried by female patients. Menopause, oral contraceptives, and pregnancy have all been considered as deleterious prognostic factors. However, a wide range of studies have concluded that hormonal influences have little or no influence on outcome from melanoma. Certainly they do not influence the choice of management policy.

Biopsy Techniques

PRIMARY LESION

Much debate has centered on the effect of initial biopsy on subsequent tumor behavior. Rampen, in a series of 84 patients, showed a 16 percent worsening of 5-year survival in patients who initially had an incisional biopsy versus an excisional biopsy.[63] He suggested that this difference may be due to malignant cells being spread during biopsy procedure. However, his series was not stratified by tumor thickness. Subsequent studies[64] have revealed no difference in prognosis when related to type of initial biopsy. Examination of 5000 melanomas in New South Wales by McCarthy et al. indicated that initial biopsy was only significantly correlated with subsequent recurrence when the tumor was thicker than 3 mm.[65]

Nevertheless, on general grounds it would seem desirable for the surgical oncologist to perform an excisional biopsy wherever possible. Not only is the theoretical risk of dissemination of tumor cells by the incisional biopsy obviated, but the task of the pathologist to report other prognostic variables is made considerably easier when he or she is provided with the entire tumor. Prior excisional biopsy followed by delayed wider excision has been shown to be a safe procedure.[66]

LYMPH NODE

There is as yet little evidence to indicate any deleterious effects of needle versus excisional biopsy of involved lymph nodes. However, at the Sydney Melanoma Unit, a substantial number of patients who have had previous excisional node biopsy for diagnosis of metastatic melanoma, have subsequently recurred in the scar of the node biopsy or in the node resected area after definitive resection. This has not occurred where needle biopsy was undertaken nor if node dissection was undertaken without preliminary biopsy of any type. It would, therefore, seem prudent at the present time for the surgical oncologist to use needle biopsy wherever possible, pending more detailed study of this prognostic factor.

Width of Primary Lesion Excision and Closure Policy

Many attempts have been made to determine the most appropriate width of excision for primary melanomas. Narrow margins (1 cm) seem perfectly safe for thinner lesions < 1.0 mm.[67,68] However, the most recent WHO study[69] has suggested that significant differences in local recurrence and survival rates do occur for tumors > 1.5 mm in thickness if narrow excision is undertaken as the definitive treatment. It is, therefore, prudent for surgical oncologists to adequately clear all diagnosed invasive melanomas with a minimum margin of 1 cm. For thick tumors, the risk of local recurrence is considerably higher. In Zeitels' study,[68] there was a significant difference in local recurrence rates for lesions > 1 mm thick when margins were < 2 cm (11.5 percent) than when margins were > 2 cm (2.1 percent). At the Sydney Melanoma Unit, lesions < 1 mm in thickness are excised with a 1 cm margin. For lesions between 1.00 and 2.00 mm thick, a minimum margin of 3 cm is used. For very thick tumors, (> 2 mm), a 5 cm margin is utilized where possible.[67] The type of closure following the wide excision is unimportant in terms of local recurrence or survival. Where possible, primary closure or local flaps may be preferred to extensive skin grafting for cosmetic reasons. However, either approach will give satisfactory results in terms of prevention of local recurrence.

Adequacy of Lymph Node Dissection Technique

The competence of the surgeon will determine to a large extent the outcome of surgery for all forms of cancer. This is particularly relevant in considering the treatment of melanoma and specifically in the treatment of metastatic melanoma in the lymph nodes. Melanoma cells have a particular ability to regrow in scars, to grow well in fat, and to seed into the surrounding lymph channels and veins if tumor spillage occurs during surgery. For many surgeons, policies on melanoma management are developed from their experience with breast cancer patients, and thus, inadequate and inappropriate dissections are sometimes performed, particularly in the axilla, but also in the groin. In some parts of the world, surgeons have not been taught the principles of adequate cancer surgery, that is,

1. removal of all malignant tissue with the maximum possible surrounding cuff of normal tissue,
2. meticulous avoidance of lymphatic leak,
3. adequate hemostasis,
4. control of the proximal and distal lymphatics early in the surgical procedure,
5. sharp dissection where ever possible,
6. adequate exposure of the dissection field at all times during the operative procedure,
7. cytotoxic washout of residual cavities,
8. en bloc resection of all lymph nodes in the affected field,
9. incontinuity resection of biopsy scars,
10. distal to proximal dissection,
11. suction drainage of cavities,
12. incontinuity resection of the primary lesion site and the nodes where possible.

Many of the descriptions of axillary, inguinal, and neck node dissections in published literature clearly breach one or more of these important techniques.

Extensive experience of one of the authors (McCarthy) on operating on patients with recurrence reveals the main inadequacies in axillary dissection are related to incomplete exposure of the whole axilla by not dividing the pectoralis major, failure to remove the pectoralis minor leaving behind pectoral and subpectoral lymph nodes, failure to resect the lymph node situated laterally in the angle between the subscapular vessels and the axillary vein, and breaching of lymphatic channels during the surgery, allowing tumor cells to spill into the wound.

Clearly, it is incumbent on the surgeon who undertakes dissection for clinically obvious melanoma in lymph nodes to be appropriately trained in radical dissection of the whole lymph node field. "Node picking" operations are totally inappropriate for patients with melanoma in the lymph nodes.

Follow-up Pattern

A regular pattern of follow-up is an important part of melanoma management. Follow-up is designed to detect early recurrences, either by the patient or the doctor and to maintain the patient's positive outlook. The pattern of follow-up of the Sydney Melanoma Unit is based on the presumption that local, in transit, and nodal recurrences can be more effectively managed if detected at the earliest manifestation. Using a mathematical model, McCarthy et al. have determined this system of follow-up, which may detect these recurrences.[70]

1. Thin melanomas < 1 mm: six monthly for 2 years then yearly for 5 years.
2. Intermediate thickness melanomas 1 to 3 mm: four monthly for 2 years, six monthly for 3 years, and yearly for 10 years.
3. Thick melanomas > 3 mm: four monthly for 3 years, six monthly for 3 years, and yearly for 10 years.

Although nearly all (95 percent) recurrent melanoma occurs within 8 years of definitive therapy,[70] recurrences after 10 years develop in 0.98 percent to 6.7 percent of patients.[71–74] However, one series[75] recorded 25 percent of patients developing late recurrences. This emphasizes the importance of the continual annual follow-up beyond 10 years, if completely accurate records are to be maintained and these recurrences detected.

Local Recurrence

Local recurrence after removal of a primary melanoma or after removal of lymph nodes is of serious prognostic significance. Urist et al. reported 5-year disease-free survival of only 34 percent in those patients with local recurrence.[76] Reintgen et al. noted recurrent disease in 35.9 percent of 4185 with clinical stage I melanomas.[77] In this study, 10-year survival rates for those who did not have a local recurrence was 88 percent compared to 42 percent for those who had local relapse. Certainly, the likelihood of ultimate cure decreases if melanoma is not completely excised at initial definitive therapy. This factor is essentially the determinant of the current practice of width of excisions related to tumor thickness.

INDIRECTLY USEFUL PROGNOSTIC FACTORS

Clinical Appearance of Tumor

With the exception of clinically visible satellite lesions, the appearance of the melanoma has become largely irrelevant. The blue color once thought to be of prognostic significance is now known to be due to the depth of the melanocytes in the dermis. Amelanotic melanoma is often regarded as more dangerous but the poorer prognosis of the amelanotic melanoma is simply due to the inability of the clinician to diagnose this tumor until it is well advanced. When Breslow tumor thickness is taken into account, the presence or absence of pigment does not influence the management of the melanoma patient.[78]

Clinically visible satellitosis is a very important prognostic sign and does influence management. Visible satellitosis is associated with a high risk of recurrence unless very wide excision is undertaken. In many centers visible satellitosis is an indication for postoperative radiotherapy to the primary site.

The presence of an inflammatory halo has no predictive value for the surgical oncologist.

Regression

Regression is defined as areas of degeneration with inflammatory infiltrate and fibrosis beneath the primary tumor accompanied by vascular proliferation and ectasia. A wide variety of views have been expressed on the importance of regression of the primary tumor.[79,80] However, in the most recent large reviews of prognostic factors in patients with thin lesions, regression does not emerge as an independent variable.[22,81–83] P. Hersey (unpublished observations) has provided an elegant rationale for the differing reports of the value of regression in preventing tumor growth. He postulates that regression may be stimulated by either free antigen from the primary melanoma or tumor cells themselves in the lymph nodes. If the regression phenomenon is stimulated by antigen alone, then prognosis will be better. If regression is stimulated by the presence of tumor cells in the lymph nodes, then the outcome will be worse. Overall, the two factors will balance making it difficult to determine in any individual patient whether regression is a prognostic determinant. At the present time, regression of the primary lesion plays little part in the decision-making of the surgical oncologist.

Lymphocytic Response to Tumor

The intensity of the postinflammatory response is judged by the presence of accumulations of lymphocytes surrounding the base and periphery of the tumor. The intensity of the response is inversely correlated with tumor thickness.[37,84] However, after controlling for tumor thickness, intensity of the response does not correlate with survival. Recently, Elder and Clark noted that plasma cells are more likely to be found in the infiltrate of thicker tumors and have postulated that these cells may be producing antibodies that block the antigenic sites on the melanoma cells leading to local immunological tolerance.[85] However, such postulates, while providing a lucid explanation of the phenomenon, do not influence the surgical oncologist in the choice of therapy.

Cellular Subtype in the Vertical Growth Phase

While the most important parameter to prognosis relates to the vertical growth of the melanoma, some recent studies have suggested the melanocytes of the radial growth phase are different from those in the vertical component. Day et al. have indicated that patients with a vertical nodular growth phase comprised of well-differentiated spindle cells had a 100 percent survival rate over a period of 8 years.[86] When epithelioid or small cells with granular cytoplasm arranged in prominent nests were present, the 100-month survival was 49 percent. This implies that the epithelioid cell subtype in the vertical growth phase conveys a poor prognosis. However, this study did not take into account the close correlation between cell type and tumor thickness. McGovern et al. and Ronan et al. did not find that cell type was an independent prognostic factor.[78,35] At present, these findings need further evaluation and do not influence management.

Association with a Nevus

Friedman et al. have reported that melanomas associated with acquired melanocytic nevi have a better prognosis than those which appear to arise de novo (95 percent 5-year survival with nevus and 85 percent survival without nevus). In the New York University series, this finding was confirmed with a 10-year survival rate of 89 percent for lesions associated with a histologically determined nevus against 77 percent for those without a nevus. They postulated that the difference may be due to a greater proportion of nodular melanomas arising de novo than superficial spreading melanomas and that the thicker melanomas may obliterate a previously existing nevus.[87] Nonetheless, the association of melanoma with a nevus does not influence the surgical oncologist in management decisions.

Racial Origin of Patient

Although the melanomas of the Negroid and Oriental races have a significantly worse prognosis than those of Caucasians, this is essentially because the tumors are diagnosed at a more advanced stage and most of the tumors are on the sole and of the acral lentiginous variety.[88] It is likely that the worse prognosis of these tumors is related to greater thickness at the time of diagnosis and not to racial origin. Racial origin per se does not influence the management of melanoma.

Skin Type of Patient

Suggestions have been made that those melanoma patients who are unable to produce a tan and burn easily, that is, skin type 1, have a poor prognosis. There are no specific studies confirming these observations. A similar comment can be made about the role of sunlight as a factor potentiating the development of metastases after adequate treatment of the primary. There are now many observations indicating ultraviolet damage to the skin adversely influences both skin immunity and systemic immunity.[89–91] However, it has as yet to be determined if excessive exposure to sunlight following removal of a primary melanoma adversely influences the recurrence rate. As a matter of prudence, therefore, the practicing surgical oncologist must heed these laboratory findings and suggest to the patient that it is a sensible precaution to limit sunlight exposure after surgery for melanoma.

Immunological Status of Patient

A four times higher than normal incidence of melanoma in immune-suppressed patients, particularly those who have had organ transplantation, has been observed.[92] This excess is much lower than the incidence of squamous and basal cell carcinomas in these patients. Furthermore, immuno-compromised patients may be expected to have tumors that will behave more aggressively because of their depleted immune status. These factors will influence the management by indicating a need for more frequent follow-up of these patients.

The advent of AIDS in the community can provide a dilemma for the surgical oncologist managing the patient with melanoma. Melanoma patients who are seropositive for the Human Immune Deficiency Virus (HIV) may have palpable lymph nodes due to the virus. As yet, there is insufficient experience of melanoma in AIDS patients to determine an optimal management policy.[93] At the Sydney Melanoma Unit, Melanoma Unit, lymph nodes are not electively dissected in seropositive patients or those with frank AIDS unless the patient has palpable nodes that are proven by needle biopsy or frozen section to contain melanoma. In this situation, a routine node dissection (with appropriate infection control procedures) is undertaken. To date, healing has been normal in the seropositive patients. It is too early to determine if the long-term outcome for these patients is comparable to seronegative patients.

Psychosocial Factors

Psychosocial factors do not in general influence the management of melanoma. However, delay in seeking attention for cutaneous melanoma is correlated positively with tumor thickness. Lack of knowledge about melanoma and low socio-economic status are associated with thicker tumors.[94] The physician with an understanding of the psychological responses to melanoma patients can play an important part in public, individual, and family education programs and thus can influence the mortality of melanoma in the community by encouraging preventative behavior and early presentation for diagnosis.

Some preliminary evidence suggests that "stoicism" and feelings of hopelessness/helplessness are negatively correlated with survival.[95] It thus behoves the oncologist providing optimal care for his or her patients to present positive attitudes and to involve the patient in all phases of the decision process relating to the proposed management program.

Prognostic Models

Various authors have attempted to develop prognostic models for patients with melanoma. After the initial attempt by Mackie et al. in 1972 to produce a prognostic model using 11 prognostic factors,[96] more advanced multivariate analysis routines have been developed. Despite the multiplicity of prognostic factors, the one variable that appears consistently in all prognostic models is tumor thickness. In one model, Rigel et al. divided the 5-year survival period into an early interval (1 to 24 months after presentation) and a later interval (25 to 60 months). Factors that appear to dominate prognosis were derived for both the early and later time intervals. By determining which of the prognostic variables were present and adding the points associated with those factors, a predicted probability of survival was computed for the 1- to 24- and 25- to 60-month intervals.[97] Soong has developed a similar and perhaps easier prognostic model using 11 clinical and pathological parameters.[98] The predictive model was derived from a well-known formulation of the proportional hazard model proposed by Cox. The validity of the model was tested not only on the data from which it was developed but also on the large Sydney Melanoma Unit series. A stepwise procedure was used to select a subset of factors that best predicted survival rates. The dominant factors selected included: tumor thickness ($p < 0.00001$), ulceration ($p = 0.00001$), anatomical site ($p = 0.00001$), surgical treatment ($p < 0.0001$), level of invasion ($p = 0.0001$), and pathological stage ($p < 0.0001$). The mathematical model (expressed in terms of the estimated survival function) obtained through this procedure was:

$$\hat{S}(t) = [\hat{S}_0(t)]^{exp(x\hat{\beta})}$$

where

$$\begin{aligned} X\hat{\beta} = {} & 0.3216 \times (\text{Tumor Thickness} - 2.6164) \\ & + 0.9013 \times (\text{Ulceration} - 0.2561) \\ & - 0.9408 \times (\text{Surgical Treatment} - 0.3826) \\ & + 0.6455 \times (\text{Lesion Location} - 0.5210) \\ & + 1.1370 \times (\text{Pathologic Stage} - 1.0346) \\ & + 0.4399 \times (\text{Level of Invasion} - 3.3592) \end{aligned}$$

and $\hat{S}_0(t) =$ the estimated baseline survival function.

The following numerical values were assigned to: (a) ulceration (0 = present; 1 = absent), (b) surgical treatment (0 = wide local excision and regional lymph node dissection, (c) lesion location (0 = axial; a = extremity).

The computer program for this mathematical model can generate a prognostic summary analysis for an individual patient based on the patient's presenting characteristics. To illustrate this application, one can consider the case of a clinical stage I male patient with an extremity, nonulcerated melanoma of thickness 1.2 mm invading to Clark level III. The estimated risk for isolated metastatic melanoma in regional nodes in this patient is 21 percent and metastatic melanoma at distant sites is 11 percent. Ten-year survival rates with and without elective lymph node dissection are 89 percent and 68 percent respectively.

Clark et al. have recently developed a model testing 23 attributes[99] and incorporating the steps of tumor progression as well as multiple tumor attributes. Both backward and forward stepwise model building was used to arrive at the final six independent prognostic variables:

1. mitotic rate,
2. tumor-infiltrating lymphocytes,
3. tumor thickness,
4. anatomical site of primary melanoma,
5. gender of patient,
6. histologic regression.

Table 14-2 shows survival probabilities 8 years after definitive therapy for all combinations of attributes generated by this model.

TABLE 14-2
PROBABILITIES OF 8-YEAR SURVIVAL

			WOMEN				MEN			
			EXTREMITY		AXIAL		EXTREMITY		AXIAL	
MITOTIC RATE (mm²)	TIL[a]	REGRESSION	TT1	TT2	TT1	TT2	TT1	TT2	TT1	TT2
0	Brisk	Absent	1.0	.99	1.0	.98	1.0	.98	.99	.95
		Present	1.0	.99	.99	.95	.99	.96	.96	.86
	Nonbrisk	Absent	1.0	.98	.98	.94	.99	.95	.96	.84
		Present	.99	.95	.96	.85	.97	.88	.89	.66
	Absent	Absent	.99	.94	.95	.82	.96	.85	.86	.60
		Present	.96	.86	.87	.61	.89	.67	.69	.35
0.1–6.0	Brisk	Absent	1.0	.98	.98	.94	.99	.95	.95	.84
		Present	.99	.95	.96	.84	.97	.87	.88	.65
	Nonbrisk	Absent	.99	.95	.95	.82	.96	.86	.87	.61
		Present	.96	.86	.87	.62	.90	.68	.70	.36
	Absent	Absent	.95	.83	.84	.57	.87	.63	.65	.31
		Present	.88	.64	.66	.32	.71	.38	.40	.14
> 6.0	Brisk	Absent	.99	.94	.95	.81	.96	.85	.86	.60
		Present	.96	.85	.86	.61	.89	.67	.68	.35
	Nonbrisk	Absent	.95	.84	.84	.57	.88	.63	.65	.31
		Present	.88	.64	.66	.32	.72	.38	.40	.14
	Absent	Absent	.85	.59	.61	.28	.67	.33	.34	.12
		Present	.68	.34	.35	.12	.42	.15	.16	.04

[a]Tumor infiltrating lymphocytes
TT1 = < 1.70 mm
TT2 = ⩾ 1.70 mm

Because of all of these models' high degrees of predictability, they have already been successfully applied in a clinical setting for patient evaluation and treatment management. The surgical oncologist may find prognostic models of use in planning follow-up patterns.

PROGNOSTIC FACTORS NOT YET USEFUL IN MANAGEMENT

DNA Ploidy

DNA ploidy is yet to be established as an independent predictor of survival. Kheir el al. found that aneuploidy is an independent predictor for survival for tumors < 1.5 mm and for tumors > 3 mm thick.[100] However, Zalovdik et al. failed to find an association between ploidy and prognosis in patients with nodular melanoma.[101] Similarly, Zardawi et al. were unable to show clearly that flow cytometry had sufficient predictive value in distinguishing thin melanomas that metastasized from those that did not, due to the great variability between samples.[102] Gattuso et al. also found that ploidy was not significant when stratified for tumor thickness.[103] Further studies in this area are needed to resolve this problem. At present, the surgical oncologist cannot use this variable in decision-making relating to the patient with melanoma.

HLA-DR Expression

Considerable interest has been evident recently in HLA-DR antigens in melanoma. Intensity of expression of these antigens is correlated positively with thickness and depth of invasion. Several studies have suggested that an increased expression of HLA-DR and decreased expression of HLA A,B, and C indicate a significant adverse effect on survival outcomes. This factor remains true after controlling for thickness.[104-107] However, these factors do not help in making decisions about patient management at present.

Surface Gangliosides

A high level of expression of GD2 on a primary melanoma may indicate a more biologically aggressive tumor with a poor prognosis, but the role of any of the prominent glycolipids on the surface of melanoma cells has yet to be fully developed.[108] For the present, these immunological parameters are not helpful in determining the management of the patient with melanoma.

Growth Factor Receptors

Many growth factor receptors are present on melanocytes, and they are expressed in various densities at various stages of tumor progression. EGF and NGF receptors increase with tumor progression. The significance of this is not known at present. These markers may soon be potentially useful as prognostic indicators, with high levels of these factors indicating an aggressive tumor, which may need to be treated more aggressively. Some growth factors may be useful in identifying those thin tumors with few mitoses that metastasize.[109] These theoretical concepts do not as yet influence the approach of the surgical oncologist.

Antibody Responses

Recent studies have suggested elevated levels of circulating antigen complexes may be directly related to a poorer prognosis. Rossen et al. and Gupta and Morton have reported the presence of tumor-associated antigens or immune complexes correlating well with the higher recurrence rate.[110,111] Jones et al. reported that elevated levels of IGM against melanoma oncofetal antigen is associated with an increased disease-free interval.[112] Werkmeister et al. noted that patients whose melanoma cells were reactive with a melanoma-associated antiserum had a longer disease-free period.[113] Further studies will be necessary to elaborate these complex reactions between the host and tumor. At the present time, antibody responses are not useful in determining an approach to the clinical management of the patient with melanoma.

Nuclear Volume

Recent developments within the field of stereology allow unbiased, objective, and reproducible estimation of the three-dimensional, shape independent nuclear volume from histological sections. Sorenson concludes that stereologic estimation of tumor volume may be a powerful prognostic predictor in the near future.[114] At present this factor has not been used in management decisions.

PROGNOSTIC FACTORS FOR DISSEMINATED DISEASE

There are few favorable prognostic factors for stage IV disease. The site of hematogenous dissemination is important in the therapeutic decision-making, but in general stage IV patients have a very limited survival. The best the surgical oncologist can hope to achieve in this situation is prolongation of life rather than long-term survival. Balch et al. and Khadra et al. have shown the longest survival intervals in patients with disseminated disease are achieved in those patients in whom isolated or small numbers of metastases can be resected.[20,115] This applies to subcutaneous, pulmonary, small bowel, retroperitoneal, and cerebral metastases. In each of these situations where complete resection is possible, long-term survival can occur, and prolongation of life exceeds that provided by chemotherapy or other therapeutic modalities.

CONCLUSION

For the practicing oncologist, only a limited number of prognostic variables are currently useful in deciding how to manage the patient with any stage of melanoma progression. For stage I melanoma, the major prognostic variable is clearly tumor thickness. After determining the tumor thickness, small additional input to the therapeutic decision is made by the mitotic index, the presence of ulceration, and the defining of microscopic satellites. Patients with subungual melanoma, acral lentiginous melanoma on the sole, desmoplastic neurotrophic melanoma, clinically visible satellites, or local recurrence will require more radical surgery for the primary tumor and in most cases elective lymph node dissection. The principles of good cancer surgery must be borne in mind when treating patients with suspected or pathologically proven lymph node metastases. The lymph nodes must be extirpated neatly, cleanly, and completely, leaving a tumor-free sterile field. The presence of in transit metastases after excision of primary melanoma will indicate the need for radical excision of the metastases and an elective lymph node dissection, if this has not already been performed. In these patients, consideration should be given to isolation perfusion therapy. For visceral metastases, the anatomical site and resectability of the metastases will determine the approach of the surgical oncologist. (Table 14-3)

TABLE 14-3
SUMMARY OF ESTABLISHED FAVORABLE AND UNFAVORABLE PROGNOSTIC FACTORS

FAVORABLE
Independent factors
Disease confined to primary lesion site
Tumor thickness < 0.75 mm or volume < 200 mm^3 not exhibiting a vertical growth phase
No tumor ulceration
No invasion of tumor past papillary dermis
Low tumor mitotic rate
No clinical or microscopic satellites around tumor
Lentigo maligna melanoma histogenetic type
Extremity location of primary tumor
Adequate elective lymph node dissection in selected subgroups of patients
Dependent factors
Female gender
Young age
UNFAVORABLE
Independent factors
Disease not confined to primary lesion site and occurring in multiple unresectable sites
Tumor thickness > 2.00 mm or volume > 200 mm^3 exhibiting a vertical growth phase
High tumor mitotic rate
Presence of either clinical or microscopic satellites around tumor
Desmoplastic neurotrophic or acral lentiginous histogenetic types
Axial, mucosal, or ocular location of primary tumor
Dependent
Male gender
Old age

REFERENCES

1. Ketcham AS and Balch CM. Classification and staging systems. In: Balch CM, Milton GW, Shaw HM, and Soong SJ (eds). *Cutaneous Melanoma. Clinical Management and Treatment Results Worldwide.* Philadelphia: Lippincott, 1985, 55–62.
2. Ghussen F, Kruger I, and Groth W. The value of current staging systems for melanoma of the extremities. *Cancer* 66:396–401, 1990.
3. Day CL, Sober AJ, Kopf AW, Lew RA, Mihm MC, Hennessey P, Golomb FM, Harris MN, Gumport SL, Raker JW, Malt RA, Cosimi AB, Wood WC, Roses DF, Gorstein F, Postel A, Grier WRN, Mintzis MN, and Fitzpatrick TB. A prognostic model for clinical stage I melanoma of the upper extremity. *Ann Surg* 193:436–440, 1981.
4. Cascinelli N, Vaglini M, Nava M, Santinami M, Marolda R, and Rovini D. Prognosis of skin melanoma with regional node metastases (stage II). *J Surg Oncol* 25:240–247, 1984.
5. Roses DF, Provet JA, Harris MN, Gumport SL, and Dubin N. Prognosis of patients with pathologic stage II cutaneous malignant melanoma. *Ann Surg* 210:103–107, 1985.
6. Cochran AJ, Lana AMA, and Wen DR. Histomorphometry in the assessment of prognosis in stage II malignant melanoma. *Am J Surg Pathol* 13:600–604, 1989.
7. Morton D. Current management of malignant melanoma. *Ann Surg* 212:123–124, 1990.
8. Cochran AJ, Wen DR, and Morton DC. Occult melanoma in the lymph nodes of patients with pathological stage I malignant melanoma. *Am J Surg Pathol* 12:612–618, 1988.
9. McCarthy WH, Shaw HM, and Milton GW. Efficacy of elective lymph node dissection in 2347 clinical stage I malignant melanoma patients. *Surg Gynecol Obstet* 161:575–580, 1985.
10. Balch CM, Cascinelli N, Milton GM, and Sim FH. Elective lymph node dissection: Pros and cons. In: Balch CM, Milton GW, Shaw HM, and Soong SJ (eds.), *Cutaneous Melanoma. Clinical Management and Treatment Results Worldwide* Philadelphia: Lippincott, 1985, 131–157.
11. Cady B. "Prophylactic" lymph node dissection in melanoma: Does it help? *J Clin Oncol* 6:2–4, 1988.
12. Bevilacqua RG, Coit DG, Rogatko A, Younes RN, and Brennan MF. Axillary dissection in melanoma. *Ann Surg* 212:125–131, 1990.
13. Overgaard J, Zucali R, Bentzen SM, and Kenda R. The role of radiotherapy in the treatment of melanoma. In: Cascinelli N, Santinami M, and Veronesi U (eds.). *Cutaneous Melanoma. Biology and Management.* Milano: Masson, 1990, 257–272.
14. Breslow A. Thickness, cross-sectional areas and depth of invasion in the prognosis of cutaneous melanoma. *Ann Surg* 172:902–908, 1970.
15. Breslow A. Tumor thickness, level of invasion, and node dissection in stage I cutaneous melanoma. *Ann Surg* 182:572–575, 1975.
16. Heenan PJ, Matz LR, Blackwell JB, Kelsall GRH, Singh A, Ten Saldam REJ, and Holman CDJ. Inter-observer variation between pathologists in the classification of cuta-

neous malignant melanoma in Western Australia. *Histopathology* 8:717–729, 1984.
17. McGovern VJ, Shaw HM, and Milton GW. Prognostic significance of a polypoid configuration in malignant melanoma. *Histopathology* 7:663-672, 1983.
18. Sober AJ, Day CL, Fitzpatrick TB, Lew RA, Kopf AW, and Mihm MC. Early death from clinical stage I melanoma. *J Invest Dermatol* 80:50s–52s, 1983.
19. Kelly JW, Sagebiel RW, Clyman S, and Blois MS. Thin level IV melanoma. A subset in which level is the major prognostic indicator. *Ann Surg* 202:98–103, 1985.
20. Balch CM, Soong SJ, Shaw HM, and Milton GW. An analysis of prognostic factors in 4000 patients with cutaneous melanoma. In: Balch CM, Milton GW, Shaw HM, and Soong SJ (eds.). *Cutaneous Melanoma. Clinical Management and Treatment Results Worldwide.* Philadelphia: Lippincott, 1985, 321–352.
21. Slingluff CL, Vollmer RT, Reintgen DS, and Seigler HF. Lethal "thin" malignant melanoma: Identifying patients at risk. *Ann Surg* 208:150–161, 1988.
22. Shaw HM, McCarthy WH, McCarthy SW, and Milton GW. Thin malignant melanoma and recurrence potential. *Arch Surg* 122:1147–1150, 1987.
23. Prayer L, Winkelbauer H, Gritzmann N, Winkelbauer F, Helmer M, and Pehamberger H. Sonography versus palpation in the detection of regional lymph-node metastases in patients with malignant melanoma. *Eur J Cancer* 26:827–830, 1990.
24. Elder DE, Guerry D, Epstein MN, Zehngebot L, Lusk E, Van Horn M, and Clark WH. Invasive malignant melanoma lacking competence for metastasis. *Am J Dermatopathol* 6(Suppl 1):55–61, 1984.
25. Rivers JKR, McCarthy SW, Shaw HM, Jones AS, Glasziou P, Doran TJ, and McCarthy WH. Patients with thick melanomas surviving at least ten years: Histological, cytometric, and HLA analyses. *Histopathology* 18:339–346, 1991.
26. Balch CM. The role of elective lymph node dissection in melanoma: Rationale, results, and controversies. *J Clin Oncol* 6:163–172, 1988.
27. Friedman RJ, Rigel DS, and Kopf AW. Tumor volume as a prognostic factor in patients with melanoma. *J Am Acad Dermatol* (in press).
28. Rigel DS, Sober AJ, and Friedman RJ. Prognostic factors influencing survival in persons with malignant melanoma. In: Friedman RJ, Rigel DS, Kopf AW, Harris MH, and Baker D (eds.), *Cancer of the Skin*. Philadelphia: WB Saunders, 1991, 198–206.
29. McGovern VJ, Shaw HM, Milton GW, and Farago GA. Is malignant melanoma arising in a Hutchinson's melanotic freckle a separate disease entity? *Histopathology* 4:235–242, 1980.
30. Smithers BM, McLeod GR, and Little JH. Desmoplastic, neural transforming and neurotropic melanoma: A review of 45 cases. *Aust N Z J Surg* 60:967–972, 1990.
31. Day CL, Harrist TJ, Gorstein F, Sober AJ, Lew RA, Friedman RJ, Pasternack BS, Kopf AW, Fitzpatrick TB, and Mihm MC. Malignant melanoma. Prognostic significance of "microscopic satellites" in the reticular dermis and subcutaneous fat. *Ann Surg* 194:108–221, 1981.
32. Harrist TJ, Rigel DS, Day CL, Sober AJ, Lew RA, Rhodes AR, Harris MN, Kopf AW, Friedman RJ, Golomb FM, Cosimi AB, Gorstein F, Malt RA, Wood WC, Postel A, Hennessey P, Gumport SL, Roses DF, Mintzis MM, Raker JW, Fitzpatrick TB, and Mihm MC. Microscopic satellites are more highly associated with regional lymph node metastasis than is primary melanoma thickness. *Cancer* 53:2183–2187, 1984.
33. Kelly JW, Sagebiel RW, Calderon W, Murillo L, Dubin RL, and Blois MS. The frequency of local recurrence and microsatellites as a guide to re-excision margins for cutaneous malignant melanoma. *Ann Surg* 200:759–763, 1984.
34. McGovern VJ, Shaw HM, Milton GW, and McCarthy WH. Ulceration and prognosis in cutaneous melanoma. *Histopathology* 6:399–407, 1982.
35. Ronan SG, Han MC, and Das Gupta TK. Histologic prognostic indicators in cutaneous malignant melanoma. *Semin Oncol* 15:558–565, 1988.
36. Schmoeckel C and Braun-Falco O. Prognostic index in malignant melanoma. *Arch Dermatol* 114:871–873, 1978.
37. Kopf AW, Gross DF, Rogers GS, Rigel DS, Hellman LF, Levenstein M, Wolkvitch B, Friedman RJ, Roses DF, Bart RS, and Gumport SL. Prognosis index for malignant melanoma. *Cancer* 59:1236–1241, 1987.
38. Day CL, Mihm MC, Sober AJ, Harris MN, Kopf AW, Fitzpatrick TB, Lew RA, Harrist TJ, Golomb FM, Postel A, Hennessey P, Gumport SL, Raker JW, Malt RA, Cosimi AB, Wood WC, Roses DF, Gorstein R, Rigel D, Friedman RL, and Mintzis MM. Prognostic factors for melanoma patients with lesions 0.76–1.69 mm in thickness. *Ann Surg* 195:30–34, 1982.
39. Woods JE, Taylor WF, Pritchard DJ, Sim FH, Ivins JC, and Bergstralh EJ. Is the BANS concept for melanoma valid? *Am J Surg* 150:452–455, 1985.
40. Cascinelli N, Voglin M, Bufalino R, and Morabito A. BANS-A cutaneous region with no prognostic significance. *Cancer* 57:441–444, 1986.
41. Rogers GS, Kopf AW, Rigel DS, Levenstein ML, Friedman RJ, Harris MN, Golomb FM, Hennessey P, Gumport SL, Roses DF, and Mintzis MM. Influence of anatomic location in prognosis of malignant melanoma: Attempt to verify the BANS model. *J Am Acad Dermatol* 15:231–237, 1986.
42. Meyskens FL, Berdeaux DH, Parks B, Tong T, Loescher L, and Moon TE. Cutaneous malignant melanoma, natural history and prognostic factors, influencing survival in patients with stage I disease. *Cancer* 62:1207–1214, 1988.
43. Weinstock MA, Morris BT, Lederman JS, Bleicher P, Fitzpatrick TB, and Sober AJ. Effects of BANS location on the prognosis of clinical stage I melanoma: New data and meta-analysis *Br J Dermatol* 119:559–565, 1988.
44. Sober AJ, Day CL, Fitzpatrick TB, Lew RA, Kopf AW, and Mihm MC. Factors associated with death from melanoma from 2 to 5 years following diagnosis in clinical stage I patients. *J Invest Dermatol* 80:53s–55s, 1983.
45. Wanebo HJ, Cooper PH, Young DV, Harpole DH, and Kaiser DL. Prognostic factors in head and neck melanoma. Effects of lesion location. *Cancer* 62:831–837, 1988.
46. Milton GW, Shaw HM, and McCarthy WH. Subungual melanoma: A disease entity separate from other forms of cutaneous melanoma. *Australas J Dermatol* 26:61–64, 1985.
47. Hoyt DJ, Jordan T, and Fisher SR. Mucosal melanoma of the head and neck. *Arch Otolaryngol Head Neck Surg* 115:1096–1099, 1989.
48. Bradgate MG, Rollason TP, McConkey CC, and Powell J. Malignant melanoma of the vulva: A clinicopathological study of 50 women. *Br J Obstet Gynaecol* 97:124–133, 1990.
49. Slingluff CL, Vollmer RT, and Seigler HF. Anorectal melanoma: Clinical characteristics and results of surgical management in twenty-four patients. *Surgery* 107:1–9, 1990.
50. Davidson T, Kissin M, and Westbury G. Vulvo-vaginal melanoma—should radical surgery be abandoned? *Br J Obstet Gynaecol* 94:473–476, 1987.
51. Rose PG, Piver MS, Tsukada Y, and Lau T. Conservative therapy for melanoma of the vulva. *Am J Obstet Gynecol* 159:52–55, 1988.

52. Reid GC, Schmidt RW, Roberts JA, Hopkins MP, Barrett RJ, and Morley GW. Primary melanoma of the vagina: A clinicopathologic analysis. *Obstet Gynecol* 74:190–199, 1989.
53. Ross M, Pezzi C, Pezzi T, Meurer D, Hickey R, and Balch C. Pattern of failure in anorectal melanoma. *Arch Surg* 125:313–316, 1990.
54. Shaw HM, McCarthy WH, and Milton GW. Melanoma: differing clinical patterns in older men and women. *Geriatric Medicine Today* 4:31–43, 1985.
55. Karjalainen S and Hakulinen T. Survival and prognostic factors in patients with skin melanomas. A regression model analysis based upon nationwide cancer registry data. *Cancer* 62:2274–2280, 1988.
56. Ho VC and Sober AJ. Prognostic factors for cutaneous melanoma. In: Ferrone S (ed.). *Human Melanoma.* Berlin: Springer-Verlag, 1990, 308–322.
57. Reintgen DS, Vollmer R, and Seigler HF. Juvenile malignant melanoma. *Surg Gynecol Obstet* 168:249–253, 1989.
58. Roth ME, Grant-Kels JM, Kuhn MK, Greenberg RD, and Hurwitz S. Melanoma in children. *J Am Acad Dermatol* 22:265–274, 1990.
59. Shaw HM, McGovern VJ, Milton GW, Farago GA, and McCarthy WH. Histological features of tumors and the female superiority in survival. *Cancer* 45:1604–1608, 1980a.
60. Shaw HM, McGovern VJ, Milton GW, Farago GA, and McCarthy WH. Malignant melanoma: Influence of site of lesion and age of patient in the female superiority in survival. *Cancer* 46:2731–2735, 1980b.
61. O'Doherty CJ, Prescott RJ, White H, McIntyre M, and Hunter JA. Sex differences in presentation of cutaneous malignant melanoma and in survival from stage I disease. *Cancer* 58:788–792, 1986.
62. Reintgen DS, Seigler HF, and McCarty KS. Sex related survival differences in instances of melanoma. *Surg Gynecol Obstet* 159:367–372, 1984.
63. Rampen FH, Van Horten WA, and Jop WC. Incisional procedures and prognosis in malignant melanoma. *Clin Exp Dermatol* 5:313–320, 1980.
64. Chanda JJ and Callen JJ. Adverse effect of melanoma incision. *J Am Acad Dermatol* 13:519–522, 1985.
65. Roberts G, Martyn AL, Dobson AJ, and McCarthy WH. Tumour thickness and histological type in malignant melanoma in New South Wales. *Pathology* 13:763–770, 1981.
66. Landthaler M, Braun-Falco O, Leitl A, Konz B, and Holzel D. Excisional biopsy as the first therapeutic procedure versus primary wide excision of malignant melanoma. *Cancer* 64:1612–1616, 1989.
67. Milton GW, Shaw HM, and McCarthy WH. Resection margins for melanoma. *Aust N Z J Surg* 55:225–226, 1985.
68. Zeitels J, La Rossa D, Hamilton R, Synnestvedt M, and Schultz D. A comparison of local recurrence and resection margins for stage I primary cutaneous melanoma. *Plast Reconstr Surg* 81:688–693, 1988.
69. Veronesi U, Cascinelli N, Adamus J, Balch C, Bandiera D, Barchuk A, Bufalino R, Craig P, De Marsillac J, Durand JC, Van Geel AN, Holstrom H, Hunter JA, Jorgensen OG, Kiss B, Kroon B, Lacour J, Lejeune F, Mackie R, Mechl Z, Mitrov G, Morabito A, Nosek H, Panizzon R, Prade M, Santi P, Van Slooten E, Tomin R, Trapeznikov N, Tsanov T, Urist M, and Wozniak KD. Thin stage I primary cutaneous malignant melanoma. Comparison of excision with margins of 1 or 3 cm. *N Engl J Med* 318:1159–1162, 1988.
70. McCarthy WH, Shaw HM, Thompson JF, and Milton GW. Time and frequency of recurrence of cutaneous stage I malignant melanoma: Guidelines for follow-up. *Surg Gynecol Obstet* 166:497–502, 1988.
71. Briele HA, Beattie CW, Ronan SG, Chaudhuri PK, and Das Gupta TK. Late recurrence of cutaneous melanoma. *Arch Surg* 118:800–803, 1983.
72. Shaw HM, Beattie CW, McCarthy WH, and Milton GW. Late relapse from cutaneous stage I malignant melanoma. *Arch Surg* 120:1155–1159, 1985.
73. Callaway MP and Briggs JC. The incidence of late recurrence (greater than 10 years): An analysis of 536 consecutive cases of cutaneous melanoma. *Br J Plast Surg* 42:46–49, 1989.
74. McEwan L, Smith JG, and Matthews JP. Late recurrence of localized cutaneous melanoma: Influence on follow-up policy. *Plast Reconstr Surg* 86:527-534, 1990.
75. Crowley NJ and Seigler HF. Late recurrence of malignant melanoma. *Ann Surg* 212:173–177, 1990.
76. Urist MM, Balch CM, Soong SJ, Shaw HM, Milton GW, and Maddox WA. The influence of surgical margins and prognostic factors predicting the risk of local recurrence in 3445 patients with primary cutaneous melanoma. *Cancer* 55:1398–1402, 1985.
77. Reintgen DS, Vollmer R, Tso CY, and Seigler HF. Prognosis for recurrent stage I malignant melanoma. *Arch Surg* 122:1338–1342, 1987.
78. McGovern VJ, Shaw HM, Milton GW, and Farago GA. Cell type and pigment content as prognostic indicators in cutaneous malignant melanoma. In: Ackerman AB (ed.). *Pathology of Malignant Melanoma.* New York: Masson, 1981, 327–332
79. McGovern VJ, Shaw HM, and Milton GW. Prognosis in patients with thin malignant melanoma: Influence of regression. *Histopathology* 7:673–680. 1983.
80. Ronan SG, Eng AM, Briele HA, Shioura NN, and Das Gupta TK. Thin malignant melanomas with regression and metastases. *Arch Dermatol* 123:1326–1330, 1987.
81. Kuehnl-Petzoldt C, and Fischer S. Tumor thickness is not a prognostic factor in thin melanoma. *Arch Dermatol Res* 279:487–488, 1987.
82. Shaw HM, McCarthy SW, McCarthy WH, Thompson JF, and Milton GW. Thin regressing malignant melanoma: Significance of concurrent regional lymph node metastases. *Histopathology* 15:257–265, 1989.
83. Jones SK, Pocock PV, and Briggs JC. Tumor thickness is not a prognostic factor in thin melanoma. *Arch Dermatol Res* 281:81–82, 1989.
84. McGovern VJ, Shaw HM, Milton GW, and Farago GA. Lymphocytic infiltration and survival from malignant melanoma. In: Ackerman AB (ed.). *Pathology of Malignant Melanoma.* New York: Masson, 1981, 341–344.
85. Elder DE and Clark WH. Malignant melanoma. In: Thiers BH and Dobson RL (eds.). *Pathogenesis of Skin Disease.* New York: Churchill Livingstone, 1986, 446–447.
86. Day CL, Harrist TJ, Lew RA, and Mihm MC. Classification of malignant melanoma according to histologic morphology of melanoma nodules. *J Dermatol Surg Oncol* 8:874–878, 1982.
87. Friedman RJ, Rigel DS, Kopf AW, Lieblich L, Lew R, Harris MN, Roses DF, Gumport SL, Ragaz A, Waldo E, Levine J, Levenstein M, Koenig R, Bart RS, and Trau H. Favorable prognosis for malignant melanomas associated with acquired melanocytic nevi. *Arch Dermatol* 119:455–462, 1983.
88. Reintgen DS, McCarty KM, Cox E, and Seigler HF. Malignant melanoma in black American and white American populations. A comparative review. *JAMA* 248:1856–1859, 1982.
89. De Fabo EC, and Noonan FP. Mechanism of immune suppression by ultraviolet irradiation in vivo. *J Exp Med* 157:84–98, 1983.

90. Kripke ML. Immunology and photocarcinogenesis. *J Am Acad Dermatol* 14:149–155, 1986.
91. Rivers JK, Norris PG, Murphy GM, Chu AC, Midgley G, Morris J, Morris RW, Young AR, and Hawk JLM. UVA sunbeds: Tanning, photoprotection, acute adverse effects and immunological changes. *Br J Dermatol* 120:767–777, 1989.
92. Sheil AGR, Flavel S, Disney APS, and Mathew TH. Cancer in dialysis and transplant patients. *Transplant Proc* 17:195–198, 1985.
93. Tindall B, Finlayson R, Mutimer K, Billson FA, Munro VF, and Cooper DA. Malignant melanoma associated with human immunodeficiency virus infection in three homosexual men. *J Am Acad Dermatol* 20:588–591, 1989.
94. Shaw HM, McGovern VJ, Milton GW, and Farago GA. Cutaneous malignant melanoma: Occupation and prognosis. *Med J Aust* 1:37–38, 1981.
95. DiClemente RJ, and Temoshok L. Psychosocial factors associated with prognostic indicators, progression, psychophysiology, and tumor-host response in cutaneous malignant melanoma. In: Nathanson L (ed.) *Basic and Clinical Aspects of Malignant Melanoma*. Boston: Martinus Nijhoff, 1987, 141–154.
96. Mackie RM, Carfrae DC, and Cochran AJ. Assessment of prognosis in patients with malignant melanoma. *Lancet* 2:455–456, 1972.
97. Rigel DS, Rogers GS, and Friedman RJ. Prognosis of malignant melanoma. *Dermatol Clin* 3:309–314, 1985.
98. Soong SJ. A computerized mathematical model and scoring system for predicting outcome in melanoma patients. In: Balch CM, Milton GW, Shaw HM, and Soong SJ (eds.). *Cutaneous Melanoma: Clinical Management and Treatment Results Worldwide*. Philadelphia: Lippincott, 1985, 353–367.
99. Clark WH, Elder DE, Guerry D, Braitman LE, Trock BJ, Schultz D, Synnestvedt M, and Halpern AC. Model predicting survival in stage I melanoma based on tumor progression. *J Natl Cancer Inst* 81:1893–1904, 1989.
100. Kheir SM, Bines SD, Vonroenn JH, Soong SJ, Urist MM, and Coon JS. Prognostic significance of DNA aneuploidy in stage I cutaneous melanoma. *Ann Surg* 207:455-461, 1988.
101. Zalovdik J, Moore M, Ghosh AK, Mechl Z, and Rejthan A. DNA content and MHC class II antigen expression in malignant melanoma: Clinical course. *J Clin Pathol* 41:1078–1084, 1988.
102. Zardawi IM, Jarvis L, Hersey P, Francis L, Shaw H, and Grace J. DNA ploidy in thin melanoma. *Pathology* 20:243–246, 1988.
103. Gattuso P, Reddy V, Solans E, Kathuria S, Aranha GV, Jacobs HK, and Walloch J. Is DNA ploidy of prognostic significance in stage I cutaneous melanoma? *Surgery* 108:702–709, 1990.
104. Ruiter DJ, Bhan AK, Harrist TJ, Sober AJ, and Mihm MC. Major histocompatibility antigens and mononuclear inflammatory infiltrate in benign nevomelanocytic proliferations and malignant melanoma. *J Immunol* 129:2808–2815, 1982.
105. Natali PG, Cavaliere R, Bigotti A, Nicotra MR, Russo C, Ng AK, Giacomini P, and Ferrone S. Antigenic heterogeneity of surgically removed primary and autologous metastatic human melanoma lesions. *J Immunol* 130:1462–1466, 1983.
106. Broker EB, Suter L, Bruggen J, Ruiter DJ, Macher E, and Sorg C. Phenotypic dynamics of tumor progression in human malignant melanoma. *Int J Cancer* 35:29–35, 1985.
107. Van Duinen SG, Ruiter DJ, Brocker EB, Van der Velde EA, Sorg C, Welvaart K, and Ferrone S. Level of HLA antigens in locoregional metastases and clinical course of the disease in patients with melanoma. *Cancer Res* 48:1019–1025, 1988.
108. Herlyn M, Clark WH, Rodeck U, Mancianti L, Jambrosic J, and Koprowski H. Biology of disease: Biology of tumor progression in human melanocytes. *Lab Invest* 56:461–474, 1987.
109. Kaudewitz P, Braun-Falco O, Ernst M, Landthaler M, Stolz W, and Gerdes J. Tumor cell growth fractions in human malignant melanomas and the correlation and histopathologic tumor grading. *Am J Pathol* 134:1063–1068, 1989.
110. Rossen RD, Crane MM, Morgan AC, Giannini EH, Giovanella BC, Stehlin JS, Twomey JJ, and Hersh EM. Circulating immune complexes and tumor cell cytotoxins as prognostic indicators in malignant melanoma: A prospective study of 53 patients. *Cancer Res* 43:422–429, 1983.
111. Gupta RK and Morton DL. Clinical significance and nature of circulating immune complexes in melanoma patients. *Contemp Top Immunobiol* 15:1–53, 1985.
112. Jones PC, Sze LL, Liu PY, Morton DL, and Irie PF. Prolonged survival for melanoma patients with elevated IgM antibody to oncofetal antigen. *J Natl Cancer Inst* 66:249–254, 1981.
113. Werkmeister JA, Edwards A, McCarthy WH, and Hersey P. Prognostic significance of expression of antigens on melanoma cells. *Cancer Immunol Immunother* 9:233–240, 1980.
114. Sorenson FB. Objective histopathologic grading of cutaneous malignant melanomas by stereologic estimation of nuclear volume. *Cancer* 63:1784–1798, 1989.
115. Khadra M, Thompson JF, Milton GW, and McCarthy WH. The justification for surgical treatment of metastatic melanoma of the gastrointestinal tract. *Surg Gynecol Obstet* 171:413–415, 1990.

Chapter 15

PREVENTION AND EARLY DIAGNOSIS OF PRIMARY SKIN MELANOMA

G. Roderick McLeod

INTRODUCTION

Malignant melanoma is a tumor with rapidly increasing incidence, and there is no evidence that the rate of increase is slowing. The incidence varies widely in geographical areas according to latitude, and the cutaneous disease is largely confined to white-skinned communities (see Chap. 1 Epidemiology of Melanoma).

Studies conducted by the Queensland Melanoma Project, established by Dr. Neville Davis in 1963, showed an annual incidence of melanoma in tropical and subtropical Queensland[1] eight times higher than that recorded in Great Britain.[2] A retrospective analysis of 498 cases treated in Queensland teaching hospitals between 1951 and 1963 revealed a 5-year survival rate of about 50 percent and a 10-year survival rate of nearly 40 percent,[3] denying the widely held view that malignant melanoma was almost invariably a fatal disease. A prospective study showed that survival rates were increased when the primary lesions were diagnosed and treated at an early level of invasion.[4,5] A genetic relationship in the heritability of liability to develop melanoma was demonstrated.[6,7] The relationship of sunlight exposure to the occurrence of melanoma was explored and direct and indirect effects were postulated.[8] An educational pamphlet was prepared to increase medical student and doctor awareness of melanoma and the need for early diagnosis. First published in Australia, this was subsequently reprinted and distributed in New Zealand, Great Britain, the USSR and in a modified form in the United States.

Malignant melanoma, if nonmelanoma skin cancers are excluded, is the fourth most common cancer in Australia and the third most common in the tropical and subtropical state of Queensland, where the annual incidence has risen steadily from 16.5 per 100,000 in 1966 to 45 per 100,000 in 1988, and is still increasing.[9] The incidence of melanoma in Europe is lower at about 8 per 100,000 annually, but rising. In some states of the United States where sunlight hours and outdoor activity are high, the incidence lies between the European and Australian rates.

Early Diagnosis

With the increasing incidence of melanoma worldwide and identification of factors which indicate a better prognosis has increased, measures to decrease the morbidity and mortality of melanoma are being undertaken. At first, action was mainly aimed at increasing awareness of both physicians and patients with the aim of achieving earlier diagnosis and treatment, but now preventive measures to reduce the incidence of melanoma are also being promoted.

METHODS USED TO IMPROVE EARLY DIAGNOSIS

The only evidence to date of improved 10-year survival rates for malignant melanoma has been the result of treatment of the lesions at an earlier stage in their development. Patients with thin melanomas as measured by the Breslow method[10] have a higher survival rate than do those with thicker lesions.[11] Efforts to improve survival rates are best concentrated on diagnosing and treating the primary lesions when thin. Improving the proportion of thin lesions diagnosed requires a variety of measures which are mainly concerned with education.[12,13]

EDUCATION FOR HEALTH PROFESSIONALS

The extent to which educational activities are pursued will depend on the potential significance of the morbidity and mortality from melanoma in a given country or region. Intensive activity is easily justified in areas with a population susceptible to melanoma and a high incidence of the disease such as Australia, New Zealand, Israel, and parts of the United States. Where the incidence is rising to significant levels as in Europe and some of the more northern states of the United States, professional and public education are necessary. In countries where cutaneous melanoma is rare, other health priorities will supervene and continuing melanoma education will be considered less necessary. The discussion which follows covers measures that may be utilized according to need.

As the need for programs to inform people of the symptoms and signs of early melanoma and the need to obtain medical advice about suspicious lesions became known, educational methods have been developed for the purpose. Initially, color brochures on the differential diagnosis of pigmented skin tumors were produced and distributed to practicing physicians, health workers, and medical students. These were readily accepted and the interest shown caused improved and expanded versions to be produced. Funding and distribution of these brochures came from pharmaceutical companies and the popular medical press. Additional help also came from the regional Cancer Society and the state run health education unit. The high-quality productions provided by the American Cancer Society and the Skin Cancer Foundation in the United States, and others including one from Germany, are good examples of a useful educational medium.

Cinema films on the differential diagnosis of pigmented skin tumors were very useful in the early part of the program used by the Queensland Melanoma Project but these are now largely replaced by videotape productions.

Dedicated television channels, either satellite or cable, used for educational purposes, are available in many countries for postgraduate and undergraduate education usage. These can be used for refresher and update programs on early diagnosis and treatment of melanomas, and for panel discussions which can include audience participation by telephone. These have proven very useful in the large area of Australia which is sparsely populated with many small towns and physicians working in isolation from colleagues.

A pigmented lesion or melanoma clinic at major centers provides a focus for inquiry from interested physicians and health workers, and in answering questions the opportunity for providing advice and encouragement for early diagnosis and prompt appropriate treatment is valuable.

EDUCATION OF THE PUBLIC ABOUT MELANOMA

Dermatologists as well as surgical oncologists will have to play an important role in increasing public awareness about melanoma. This is important to establish an early diagnosis program. Following are some of the methods for public education which may be utilized effectively.

The first aim in public education about pigmented skin tumors is to encourage seeking advice and treatment early. The message should be that early treatment of suspicious lesions allows a better prospect of cure. To this should be added the advice that early lesions require less radical treatment measures. Family physicians and health professionals must maintain their own awareness and be prepared to act when the indications are present.

The choice of educational medium will depend on availability and cost, as most programs are controlled by limitations of funds. In areas where the risk is high all measures should be used to reach the various age groups, but some media have more impact than do others. The wide variety of media used for melanoma programs in Australia will give ideas for planning of educational efforts elsewhere, though cultural differences between countries may alter the importance of any specific medium.

Access to newspapers and popular magazines is often the most easily obtained publicity, and is best used at the start of the season when holidays and outdoor activities are most popular. Other print media can include posters placed in medical waiting rooms, in public buildings, railway stations, and public transport vehicles. The warning signs of new or changing moles need to be emphasized.

Television has proven to be the most effective way of reaching the public and increasing the number of persons seeking early advice. This was clearly demonstrated when the Sydney Melanoma Unit presented, on a high rating national current affairs program, the story of a young man who was dying with metastatic melanoma.[13] A subsequent presentation after the death of the patient repeated and expanded the story and had considerable emotional impact. A noticeable increase in new patient numbers was evident after the first program with a further increase after the sequel (Figs. 15-1 to 15-4). The number of new primary melanomas removed in the state of Queensland in the 3 months after the program was twice the number removed in the corresponding 3 months of the previous year. When the programs were repeated 2 years later, a similar increase in new case presentations occured. This means that a large proportion of the increased number of new cases must have presented earlier than they otherwise would have, with consequent improvement in prognosis. Patient comment about this publicity, and about another program from the Queensland Melanoma Project with a similar emotional impact, shows the immediate and continuing effect of this educational medium.

Broadcast radio programs are another good method of increasing public awareness, and the popularity of talk-back programs allows audience questions and participation which helps to reinforce the message.

Educating the children about the dangers of excess sun exposure which may cause both nonmelanoma skin cancer or melanoma in later life is important. Visits by Cancer Foundation educators have proven successful, in conjunction with a national multimedia campaign which tells them to "slip on a shirt, slop on some sunscreen, and slap on a hat."

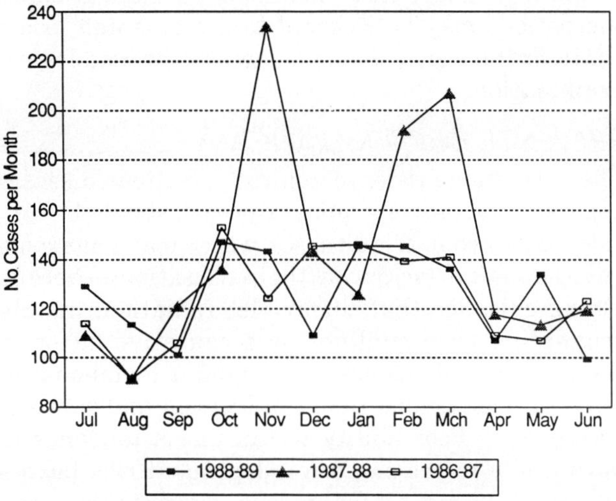

FIG. 15-1. *Increase in total number of melanomas excised after TV programmes on melanoma—October 1987 and February 1988 (Queensland).*

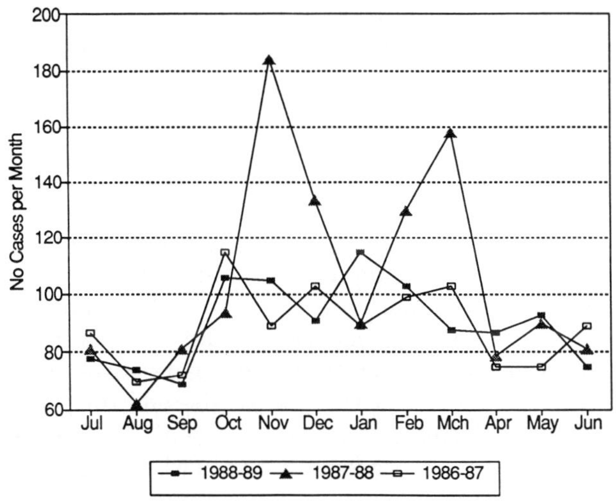

FIG. 15-2. *Increase in invasive melanomas up to 1 mm (Breslow)—October 1987 and February 1988 (Queensland).*

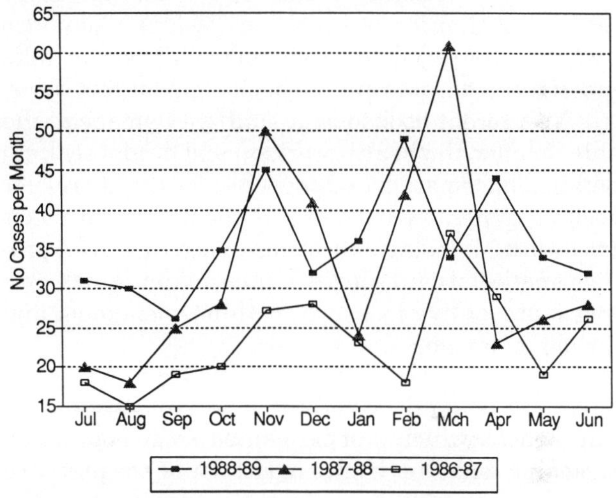

FIG. 15-3. *Increase in invasive melanomas greater than 1 mm (Breslow)—October 1987 and February 1988 (Queensland).*

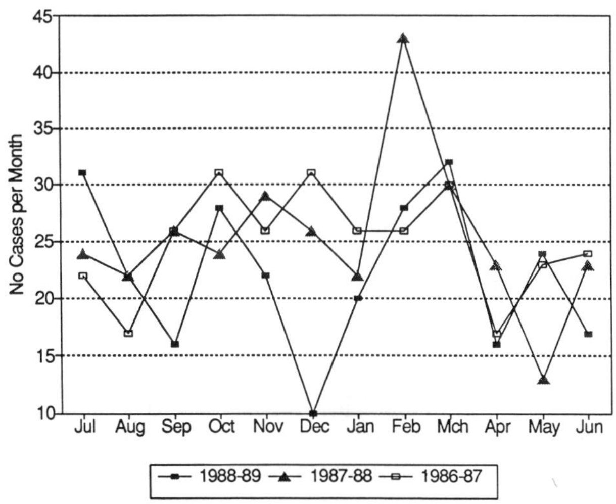

FIG. 15-4. *Increase in situ melanomas—October 1987 and February 1988 (Queensland).*

The Slip Slop Slap campaign with a theme song has been most effective. Efforts have also been made to encourage the provision of covered space in school grounds and planting of shade trees for protection of children during lunch breaks, rather than have them out in the strong midday sun. Sport should be delayed until the less sunny part of the day, and sport clothing should provide protection. Topical sunscreens should be provided for use before outdoor activities. These are all measures for high sunshine areas where the precautions are necessary.

Patients who have been successfully treated for melanoma can become a source of information for their relatives and friends. They are aware of the changes they saw in their own lesions and should be taught the warning signs. They will often take the role of lay adviser to others and encourage early medical evaluation of suspicious lesions. They also can be encouraged to teach their children to take protective measures and to check them for risk signs.

Two recent books about sunlight damage to the skin, one for the health workers and others seeking detailed information and the other for the lay reader seeking general advice are available.[14,15] In countries with high skin cancer incidence these can provide another useful source of information which promotes preventive measures both for melanoma and for nonmelanoma skin cancers.

POPULATION SCREENING

The benefit which can be gained from population screening for the evidence of risk for or the presence of melanoma will depend on the incidence of the disease in the community and the number of cases which will be identified early, or prevented, by participation in a screening program. Countries where there is a high incidence of melanoma may be able to justify population screening to detect high-risk individuals and early melanoma,[13] but the cost of a screening program may not be justified where melanoma is of low or moderate incidence.

Selective screening of people who have fair skin which burns easily, have high-mole counts, or who have a family or personal history of melanoma is valuable. These people are at increased risk of dysplastic nevus syndrome and melanoma, and the act of screening itself will work as an educational tool.

Short-term low-budget screening exercises are useful advertising tools, and focus community thoughts on sunlight protection and checking for suspicious lesions. These sessions are held in Queensland as part of Skin Cancer Awareness week, and at sea-side resorts in holiday periods. The number of probable melanomas identified in this way has been low, but solar keratoses and nonmelanoma skin cancers are seen more frequently.

Several technological methods have been developed as potential aids to diagnosis of pigmented skin lesions. They may become useful as aids to screening as well as in the diagnosis of difficult lesions. Photographic and video imaging, sometimes with computer analysis of the images, are being studied in several centers. Thermography and infrared reflectance, doppler and ultrasound, and cutaneous microscopy are also of interest. Wolff[16] presented a study of epiluminescence microscopy and demonstrated a marked improvement in the diagnostic accuracy using this technique. The hand dermatoscope which has become available in the last 2 years is a simple office tool which may help the specialist, rather than the family doctor, achieve better diagnostic accuracy.[17] For the family doctor who is trying to diagnose early melanoma, if there is doubt, the patient may be referred to a pigmented lesion clinic, or the lesion should be excised for histological examination.

PREVENTION OF MELANOMA

The first line of defense against infectious diseases is prevention, and a similar approach should be considered for neoplastic diseases, which may have some environmental factors in their causation. There is strong evidence that ultraviolet radiation, mainly originating from sunlight, is a causative factor in the increased incidence of malignant melanoma in fair-skinned persons living in tropical and subtropical areas.[18] Poor ability to tan and a tendency to burn easily in the sun are independent risk factors for melanoma.[19,20] Other evidence suggests that even limited sunburn in early childhood or youth may initiate the process for melanoma in later years.[18] If we can protect the children from excess ultraviolet radiation until adult life, it should be possible to reduce the risk of their developing malignant melanoma (see Chaps. 1 and 8).

Identification of high-risk individuals allows the provision of education and surveillance for these people. They should be taught to cover themselves with clothing and a hat and to use a topical sunscreen on all exposed skin. Clothing should be of material which gives the best protection from ultraviolet radiation. Colored rather than white cloth is better and thick weaves with little or no synthetics are best. Wet material allows more ultraviolet rays through, so a waterproof topical sunscreen should be used under shirts when swimming. We recommend screens which filter both UVA and UVB, with the addition of an infrared reflector of titanium pigment. With these screens filtration is adequate to allow up to 90 minutes in the tropical or subtropical sun in any 24-hour period, but advice is given to reduce this period where possible. In the Queensland climate, the use of topical sunscreens with a sun protection factor of less than 15+ is not advised. Fortunately, many of the patients identified as having high risk are already aware that they cannot tolerate sun exposure and accept the recommended protection. Compliance is less readily obtained in adolescents where peer pressure promotes the acquisition of a sun tan.

Patients at high risk of developing malignant melanoma include members of families with a history of melanoma, patients who have had a previous melanoma, persons with an increased number of nevi, and persons with dysplastic nevus syndrome.[21] Careful history taking will usually reveal any family or personal history of melanoma. Examination of the patient will produce evidence of the clinical entity of dysplastic nevus syndrome or of a high-mole count. Persons who have positive findings should be advised of the risks and counseled about preventive measures to be taken. They should also be advised to inform their close relatives of the possiblity of increased risk of developing melanoma, and to check their children. Meeting with the family physician concerning identification of high-risk individuals and continuation of surveillance will maintain patient awareness and encourage adherence to the need for sunlight protection and review of new or changing lesions.

The genetic mechanisms which predispose to dysplastic nevi and malignant melanoma have not yet been clearly identified. When they are known, genetic manipulation techniques may be developed to reduce the incidence of melanoma in high-risk individuals.[22] Meanwhile, the proposals of Fitzpatrick et al.[21] for an international cooperative effort to combat the increase in melanoma incidence give a guide to the available ways to take action.

CONCLUSIONS

The only way of improving prognosis available at present is to diagnose and treat the primary lesions when they are early and thin. There is belief that the incidence of melanoma could be reduced by measures aimed at identifying persons at high risk, teaching how to reduce melanoma promoting factors, and arranging regular surveillance of their lesions. Preventive measures should reduce the number of melanomas occurring in high-incidence countries, and early diagnosis will reduce the death rate. This can and must be done.

REFERENCES

1. Davis NC, Herron JJ, and McLeod GR. Malignant melanoma in Queensland. Analysis of 400 skin lesions. *Lancet* II:407–410, 1966.
2. Bodenham DC, and Lloyd OC. The diagnosis and treatment of malignant melanoma of the skin. Postgrad. *Med J* 39:278, 1963.
3. McLeod R, Davis NC, Herron JJ, Caldwell R, Little JH, and Quin RL. A retrospective survey of 498 patients with malignant melanoma. *Surg Gynecol Obstet* 126:99–108, 1968.
4. McLeod GR, Beardmore GL, Little JH, Quinn RL, and Davis NC. Results of treatment of 361 patients with malignant melanoma in Queensland. *Med J Aust* 1:1211–1216, 1971.
5. McLeod GR. Malignant melanoma in Queensland. Five year results for 361 patients. Proceedings of the Fifth World Congress of Plastic and Reconstructive Surgery. Melbourne: Butterworth 1971, 20–26.
6. Wallace DC, Exton LA, and McLeod GR. Genetic factor in malignant melanoma. *Cancer* 27:1262–1266, 1971.
7. Wallace DC, Beardmore GL, and Exton LA. Familial malignant melanoma. *Ann Surg* 177:15–20, 1973.
8. Davis NC. Sunlight and melanomas. *Lancet* 1:803, 1971.
9. MacLennan R, Green AC, McLeod GRC, and Martin NG. Increasing incidence of cutaneous melanoma in Queensland. *JNC*1 84:1427–1432, 1992.
10. Breslow A. Thickness, cross-sectional areas and depth of invasion in the prognosis of cutaneous melanoma. *Ann Surg* 172:902, 1970.
11. McLeod GR. Melanoma in Queensland Australia: Experience of the Queensland Melanoma Project. In Balch CM, and Milton GW (eds.) *Cutaneous Melanoma. Clinical Management and Treatment Results Worldwide.* Philadelphia: Lippincott, 1985, 379–387.
12. MacKie RM, and Doherty VR. Educational activities aimed at earlier detection and treatment of malignant melanoma in a moderate risk area. In: Elwood JM (ed.) *Pigment Cell* Vol 9 Basel: Karger 1988, 140–152.
13. McCarthy WH, and Rivers JK. Can early melanoma be diagnosed? In: Cascinelli N, Santinami M, and Veronesi U (eds.) *Cutaneous Melanoma Biology and Management.* Milan: Masson, 1990, 113–123.
14. Emmett A. *The Bare Facts. The Effect of Sun on Skin.* Sydney: Williams and Wilkins, 1988.
15. Emmett A. *Your Skin and the Sun.* Sydney: Simon and Schuster, 1990.
16. Wolff K. Can clinical diagnosis be improved (abstract). Scientific session. Second international conference on melanoma. Venice, 1988, 49.
17. Braun-Falco O, Stolz W, Bilek P, Merkle T, and Landthaler M. The dermatoscope. A simplification of epiluminescence microscopy of pigmented skin changes. *Hautarzt* 41:131–136, 1990.
18. Lancaster HO. Some geographical aspects of the mortality from melanoma in Europeans. *Med J Aust* 1:1082, 1956.
19. Holman CD, and Armstrong BK. Pigmentary traits, ethnic origin, benign nevi and familial history as risk factors for cutaneous malignant melanoma. *J Natl Cancer Inst* 72:257–266, 1984.
20. Green A, Siskind V, Bain C, and Alexander J. Sunburn and malignant melanoma. *Br J Cancer* 51:393–397, 1985.
21. Fitzpatrick TB, Rhodes AR, Sober AJ, and Mihm MC. Primary malignant melanoma of the skin: The call for action to identify persons at risk: To discover precursor lesions: To detect early melanomas. In: Elwood JM (ed.), *Pigment Cell* Vol 9 Basel: Karger, 1988 110–117.
22. Traupe H, and Macher E. Classical and molecular genetics of malignant melanoma and dysplastic naevi. In: Elwood JM, (ed.), *Pigment Cell* Vol 9 Basel: Karger, 1988 77–94.

Chapter 16

TREATMENT OF PRIMARY MELANOMA

F. Kristian Storm, David M. Mahvi

Diseases desperate grown
By desperate applicance are reliev'd,
Or not at all.

William Shakespeare (1564–1616)
Hamlet, IV, iii, 9

HISTORIC PERSPECTIVE

Other than whether or not to perform a prophylactic lymphadenectomy for high risk lesions, perhaps no topic in the treatment of melanoma has engendered more controversy and heated debate than the distance of radial reexcision (wide excision) necessary to prevent locally recurrent disease. The standard "5-centimenter rule" is attributed to the Hunterian lecture of 1907 given by Dr. Sampson Handley as reported in *Lancet*[1] and has been promulgated since that time. But, in fact, Handley recommended a skin margin of only "1 inch" (2.5 cm) and that the subcutaneous tissue margin be extended to "2 inches" (5 cm) in order to adequately remove the subdermal lymphatics potentially involved in centrifugal tumor permeation. While often quoted incorrectly in major texts as the first histopathologic investigation supporting a 5 cm margin of grossly normal tissue around a primary melanoma, Handley's recommendations, while not only arbitrary, were in reality based on an autopsy study of a single patient with recurrent melanoma that probably originated from a metastatic focus within an inguinal lymph node. These facts notwithstanding, conscientious surgeons in good faith adopted the 5 cm rule and, for inexplicable reasons, also included a 5 cm margin of overlaying normal skin. In support of this theoretical margin, entrenched for decades in the surgical literature, however, a disturbing potential field effect up to 4 to 5 cm surrounding primary tumors was demonstrated in the early 1970s by Wong[2] who found evidence of melanocytic activation and by Cochran[3] who recorded abnormal distributions of melanocytes, both occurring within this distance of grossly normal skin.

While it was Neville Davis, coordinator of the Queensland Melanoma Project, who in 1976 first proposed that the size of the resection margin should be determined by factors known to influence prognosis,[4] the first to scientifically question the 5 cm rule was the late Alexander Breslow in 1977.[5] Breslow, along with Steven Macht, was apparently disturbed by such *excessively radical treatment* for thin melanoma, particularly in view of his earlier observations suggesting that neither metastases nor local recurrences developed in patients in whom tumors were less than 0.76 mm thick and that for thicker lesions the rate of metastases was directly proportional to the measured depth of invasion.[6,7] This notion was substantiated by similar findings reported by Hansen and McCarten,[8] Wanebo and colleagues,[9] and by Breslow's personal communication with Wallace Clark at that time. Credit must be given to Breslow, a surgical pathologist, for stimulating scientific studies that have subsequently produced sufficient data for reasonable recommendations to be made concerning the preferred treatment of primary melanoma.

While the extent of surgery advised in the literature has ranged from 2 cm[10] up to 15 cm[11], until the results of ongoing prospective randomized trials are known, most experts have adopted a philosophy of "reasonableness" based on retrospective knowledge. It seems clear that limited excision for high-risk lesions carries an unacceptably high incidence of local recurrence, that local recurrence portends a grave prognosis, and that wide reexcision of the biopsy site may prevent this life-threatening complication.

RATIONALE FOR REEXCISION

Results of Simple Excision

The incidence of local recurrence in patients with invasive melanoma treated with observation after biopsy, electrodesiccation, or minimal or limited excision are shown in Table 16-1. Wilson[12] found 57 percent local recurrence after biopsy alone ($n = 49$) compared to 3 percent treated by wide reexcision ($n = 73$). McNeer and Cantin[13] found 58 percent local recurrence after electrodesiccation ($n = 69$). After limited surgery, various authors[13–15] found local recurrences of 27 to 37 percent ($n = 517$). Thus, simple excision alone is contraindicated as definitive therapy for invasive primary melanoma, as it results in an unacceptably high incidence of local recurrence.

Prognosis After Local Recurrence

Locally recurrent melanoma is defined as "wound recurrence," "satellitosis"—within 5 cm of the primary, and "intransit metastases"—extending beyond 5 cm from the primary, which may be intradermal or subcutaneous, or any combination of these features. Patients exhibiting locally recurrent disease carry a grave prognosis, with 55 to 86 percent dead within 5 years.[13,14,16–20] Urist et al.[36] reported that local recurrence in 95 patients treated with local wide reexcision resulted in half the patients being dead within 3 years. Storm and Morton[21] found that, even with effective subsequent local therapy (limb perfusion) and complete local control of more extensive recurrent disease, 60 percent of patients were dead within 2 years ($n = 16$). These studies indicated a high likelihood of subsequent systemic disease in patients with locally recurrent melanoma, the implication being that such local recurrences metastasize to distant sites more frequently than primary melanomas and subsequently kill the patient.

TABLE 16-1
RESULTS OF SIMPLE EXCISION

AUTHOR (REF)	TREATMENT TYPE	NO. PTS.	LOCAL RECURRENCE (%)
Wilson[12]	Biopsy only	49	28 (57%)
McNeer and Cantin[13]	Electrodesiccation	69	40 (58%)
Jones et al.[14]	Simple excision	49	19 (37%)
Cochran[15]	Simple excision	92	23 (27%)
McNeer and Cantin[13]	Simple excision	376	103 (27%)
Totals		635	213 (34%)

LOCAL RECURRENCE AFTER REEXCISION

Incidence

The overall incidence of locally recurrent melanoma after reexcision of the biopsy site is shown in Table 16-2, and approaches 3 percent (range 0–6 percent) from combined series ($n = 7736$). Urist et al.[36] analyzed the 3445 cases amassed from the University of Alabama and the Sydney Melanoma Unit (New South Wales) and found that increasing tumor thickness was the most significant predictor of local recurrence (Table 16-3). The deeper the lesion the more locally aggressive was its nature. Kelly et al.[41] found that the presence of microsatellites (discrete tumor nests separate from the main body of the tumor) correlated with local recurrence, which was dependent on tumor thickness. There were no microsatel-

TABLE 16-2
OVERALL INCIDENCE OF LOCAL RECURRENCE AFTER REEXCISION

AUTHOR (REF)	DATE	NO. PTS.	LOCAL RECURRENCE (%)
Breslow and Macht[4]	1977	62	0 (0%)
Das Gupta[22]	1977	269	8 (3%)
Milton[23]	1977	224	4 (2%)
Pitt[24]	1977	509	31 (6%)
Veronesi et al.[25]	1977	395	8 (2%)
Balch et al.[26]	1979	287	9 (3%)
Cascinelli et al.[27]	1980	593	24 (4%)
Goldman[28]	1980	160	0 (0%)
Bagley et al.[29]	1981	103	6 (6%)
Kenady et al.[30]	1982	202	8 (4%)
Elder et al.[31]	1983	109	0 (0%)
Golomb[32]	1983	223	5 (2%)
Roses et al.[33]	1983	658	7 (1%)
Schmoeckel et al.[34]	1983	105	3 (3%)
Cosimi et al.[35]	1984	49	0 (0%)
Kelly et al.[41]	1984	343	3 (1%)
Urist et al.[36]	1985	3445	95 (3%)
Totals		7736	211 (2.7%)

TABLE 16-3
LOCAL RECURRENCE BY PRIMARY TUMOR THICKNESS[36]

TUMOR THICKNESS (mm)	NO. PTS.	INCIDENCE LOCAL RECURRENCE, %[a]
< 0.76	707	0.2% ± 0.2%
0.76–1.5	721	2.1% ± 0.7%
1.5–3.99	907	6.4% ± 1.1%
⩾ 4.0	291	13.2% ± 3.2%

[a]Five-year minimum follow-up; eight-year median follow-up; mean ± standard deviation

lites seen in association with tumors < 1.0 mm thickness, 2/91 (2 percent) with tumors 1.0 to 1.9 mm, 4/34 (12 percent) with 2.0 to 2.9 mm, and 22/60 (37 percent) with ≥ 3.0 mm primary lesions. The presence of tumor ulceration, advanced age, and certain anatomic sites (foot 11.6 percent, hand 11.1 percent, lower extremity 4.7 percent, head and neck 4.4 percent, upper extremity 1.6 percent, trunk 1.2 percent) have also correlated with likelihood of local recurrence.[36]

Time to Recurrence

In 95 patients with local recurrence,[36] the median time to recurrence for lesions 0.76 to 1.49 mm thickness was 2.3 years; for 1.5 to 3.9 mm, 1.5 years; and for ≥ 4.0 mm, 0.7 years.

PREVENTION OF LOCALLY RECURRENT DISEASE

Various reviews have evaluated the role of the two major variables—tumor thickness and surgical margin—on local disease control. While not randomized and retrospective in nature, a rather clear picture emerges from these studies, which depict reasonable margins of reexcision that will achieve local disease control in the majority of patients. It is emphasized, however, that currently available data do not predict the *minimum safe margin* for any particular patient.

In Situ Melanoma

In situ melanoma, also termed Clark's level I melanoma, is best classified as Atypical Melanocytic Hyperplasia (AMH) since it is a noninvasive lesion that is not known to recur locally or distantly after adequate reexcision. As shown in Table 16-4, no recurrences have been observed after limited excision of these intraepithelial melanocytic growths (n = 220), while biopsy alone resulted in 3/3 recurrences that were invasive melanoma.

TABLE 16-4
LOCAL RECURRENCE OF IN-SITU MELANOMA (AMH) BY MARGIN OF EXCISION

AUTHOR (REF)	DATE	TUMOR DESCRIPTION	RESECTION MARGIN (cm)	NO. PTS.	LOCAL RECURRENCE (%)
Kelly[41]	1984	in situ	≤ 1/2	3	3 (100%)
McLeod[37]	1985	in situ	1/2–1	105	0 (0%)
Roses[33]	1983	in situ, < 0.5 mm	≥ 1	115	0 (0%)
Totals				223	3 (1%)

Thin Melanoma (< 1.0 mm)

The incidence of local recurrence of thin melanomas by margin of excision is shown in Table 16-5. In primary tumors with less than 1.0 mm depth of invasion, the overall local recurrence rate appears exceedingly low, 6/1663 (0.3 percent) from combined series. The few recurrences that have been observed generally occurred in patients with the wider excision margins suggesting that these were biologically more aggressive tumors or were, more likely, incorrectly microstaged.

Thick Melanoma (≥ 1.0 mm)

The incidence of local recurrence of thick melanomas by margin of excision is shown in Table 16-6. With primary tumors ≥ 1.0 mm depth of invasion, the overall incidence of local recurrence after wide excision was 62/1724 (3.5 percent) from combined series.

Of the 825 patients treated with "more than 3 cm" margins there were 24 (2.9 percent) local recurrences; of 374 treated with "5 cm" margins there were 14 (3.7 percent) recurrences; and of 525 treated with margins "between 3 cm and 5 cm" there were 24 (4.5 percent) local recurrences.

TABLE 16-5
LOCAL RECURRENCE OF THIN MELANOMA (< 1.0 mm) BY MARGIN OF EXCISION

AUTHOR (REF)	DATE	TUMOR THICKNESS (mm)	INCIDENCE LOCAL RECURRENCE BY RESECTION MARGIN (cm) <1/2	1/2–1	1–2	2–3	>3
Breslow and Macht[4]	1977	< 0.76	0/14	0/6	0/15	0/15	0/15
Balch et al.[26]	1979	< 0.76		0/3	0/5	0/3	0/25
Elder et al.[31]	1983	< 0.76			0/16	0/10	0/17
Golomb[32]	1983	< 0.85		0/11	0/64	0/68	0/59
Cascinelli et al.[27]	1980	< 1.0		0/6	0/12	0/31	1/38
Kelly et al.[41]	1984	< 1.0		1/48	1/130	1/84	0/81
Urist et al.[36]	1985	< 1.0			0/580	1/115	
Roses et al.[33]	1983	0.51–1.0					1/192
Totals			0/14	1/74	1/822	2/326	2/427

TABLE 16-6
LOCAL RECURRENCE OF THICK MELANOMA (≥ 1.0 mm) BY MARGIN OF EXCISION

AUTHOR (REF)	DATE	RESECTION MARGIN (cm)	NO. PTS.	LOCAL RECURRENCE (%)
Cascinelli et al.[27]	1980	> 3	497	16 (3.2%)
Golomb[32]	1983	> 3	223	5 (2.2%)
Schmoeckel et al.[34]	1983	> 3	105	3 (2.9%)
Goldman[28]	1980	3–5	160	0 (0%)
Roses et al.[33]	1983	3–5	365	24 (6.5%)
Das Gupta[22]	1977	5	150	10 (7.0%)
Milton[23]	1977	5	224	4 (2.0%)
Totals			1724	62 (3.5%)

TABLE 16-7
RECOMMENDED EXCISION MARGINS

TUMOR DEPTH (mm)	MINIMUM NORMAL TISSUE MARGIN (cm)	PREFERRED NORMAL TISSUE MARGIN (cm)[a]
in situ	1/2–1 cm	≥ 1 cm
< 1.0 mm	> 1 cm	≥ 2 cm
≥ 1.0 mm	3 cm	> 3, up to 5 cm

[a]If anatomically feasible

RECOMMENDATIONS FOR EXTENT OF EXCISION MARGINS

Tables 16-4, 16-5, and 16-6 show the incidence of local recurrence by extent of excision for in situ (level I melanoma, AMH), thin (< 1.0 mm) and thick (≥ 1.0 mm) primary melanomas, respectively. Since these tables only summarize different retrospective noncontrolled studies, statistical analyses or comparisons of these data cannot apply. All suffer from the potential of selection bias; were worse appearing lesions treated more aggressively? Moreover, different investigators use a different criterion (often not stated) for their "measurement of excision margin," as examples: that stated by the surgeon in the operative note; the fresh specimen measured by the pathologist; the fixed specimen measured by the pathologist; or some measurement stated on the pathology report. A recent study by Morton and Storm (unpublished) indicates that a freshly excised skin specimen shrinks in size up to 1 cm from that measured on the patient and up to 2 cm if the patient's skin is *prestretched* prior to measurement, with another centimeter shrinkage after 24 hours in formalin. Most studies are also unclear as to whether the margin of normal tissue taken during biopsy was incorporated in the overall measurement, or whether the wide excision measurement was made from the biopsy scar as is common practice. Thus, some studies may have underestimated the margin of normal tissue actually excised. These problems notwithstanding, recommendations can be made in an attempt to prevent local recurrence while preserving as much normal tissue as is reasonably safe (Table 16-7).

In situ melanoma is virtually curable with simple reexcision and a narrow margin of normal tissue (Table 16-4). Limited reexcision is warranted for thin melanomas, < 1.0 mm (Table 16-5), and a wide reexcision is mandated for thicker lesions, ≥ 1.0 mm (Table 16-6). The preferred recommendations (Table 16-7) should be used where anatomically feasible, and in patients with deeper lesions, advanced age, or primary tumors displaying ulceration or microsatellites. Because of confounding factors that may have underestimated the actual margins excised in the studies to date, the preferred recommendations incorporate margins consistent with reasonable tissue preservation and local disease control in the majority of patients.

RECOMMENDATIONS ON FASCIAL EXCISION

Handley's[1] original diagram depicting the technique of wide excision incorporated 2-inch (5 cm) margins of underlaying fascia in order to remove potentially contaminated subdermal lymphatics. Surgeons have embraced this philosophy (along with the "5 cm rule" for skin) for more than three quarters of this century.

Olsen[38] retrospectively compared groups of 31 versus 36 patients who had fascia excised or left intact and found no statistical difference in the incidence of local recurrence, but subsequent development of regional metastases in 45 percent and 14 percent, respectively. She postulated that the fascia posed a lymphatic barrier and found that intradermal or subcutaneous injections of a vital dye were never observed within subfascial lymphatics but subfascial dye injection did result in surface tissue staining, implying some type of one-way valve mechanism toward the surface. She believed that fascia removal could potentially contaminate subfascial lymphatics and result in regional nodal metastases. However, Neville Davis, reviewing the Queensland experience in this regard, could not confirm Olsen's clinical impression of increased nodal metastases after fascial excision.[4]

Kenady et al.[30] retrospectively reviewed sites of first recurrence in sequential groups of patients where the fascia was either excised ($n = 107$) or left intact ($n = 95$). There were 3 (3 percent) local and 21 (20 percent) regional node recurrences in the excision group, and 5 (5 percent) local and 24 (25 percent) regional recurrences in the nonexcision group, a trend favoring fascia excision. Unfortunately, no hard data exist to indicate the need for fascial excision; however, conversely, no data exist concerning the safety of nonremoval. In the studies addressing local control (Tables 16-5 and 16-6), the extent of fascial excision is most frequently not stated but has been presumed to be the same as the skin and subcutaneous tissue margin (or slightly greater). Pragmatically speaking, advancement flaps and partial-thickness skin engraftment are facilitated by excision of the underlaying deep fascia, and fascia removal generally assures complete removal of the potentially contaminated deep biopsy margin. Therefore, in the absence of compelling safety data to the contrary, fascia removal during wide excision is preferred.

TREATMENT OF MULTIPLE PRIMARY MELANOMA

Beardmore and Davis[39] reporting on the Queensland experience found 57/1444 (3.9 percent) patients who developed more than one primary melanoma. Second tumors usually developed within 5 years, usually occurred in a different area, and were usually less invasive than the first tumor. Moseley et al.[40] reviewed 712 consecutive patients with the diagnosis of melanoma and found 38 (5.3 percent) with more than one primary (range 2–8); 32 percent had synchronous primaries; and 45 percent had second primaries diagnosed within the first year. Microstaging indicated that 83 percent had a subsequent melanoma equally or less invasive than the original. Survival analysis of patients with multiple primary tumors projected 100 percent alive at 5 years and 75 percent alive at 10 years. While such patients had to have survived their first tumor to remain at risk for a subsequent melanoma, the presence of a second tumor did not necessarily appear to adversely affect overall prognosis. It is, therefore, recommended that each such tumor be treated independently according to its individual degree of invasion (Table 16-7).

TECHNICAL NOTES

Operative Management of Biopsy Site

Patients are frequently referred for definitive therapy with a freshly closed biopsy incision. The biopsy site should be left undisturbed and sutures—if present—allowed to remain in place during wide excision. The very small risk of infection is accepted in lieu of possible tumor cell contamination via weeping suture tracts. At times it may be desirable to additionally suture a sterile gauze barrier over the biopsy site if anticipated tissue manipulation could result in dehiscence of the biopsy incision.

Method of Wide Excision

Wide excision removes a 360 degree portion of normal skin, subcutaneous tissue, and underlying fascia surrounding the melanoma site as depicted in Fig. 16-1. The margin should be measured radially at multiple points from the epicenter of the biopsy site (or edge of any remaining tumor) and recorded on the pathology submission form and operative report. It is most efficacious to *prestretch the skin* and perform measurement for margins while the skin is under tension. This simple maneuver will frequently gain 1 to 2 cm on the overall wound and will frequently allow primary closure of otherwise larger defects. The specimen should be removed en bloc and oriented for the pathologist with a silk suture (e.g., "stitch at 12 o'clock, superior"). During subfascial resection directly beneath the biopsy site, extreme care should be given to assess fascial integrity. If there is evidence of suture material, scar, or inflammation suggesting prior violation of the fascia, this dissection plane should be carefully closed, the field reprepped and draped, and using new gloves and instruments a deeper dissection plane should be utilized incorporating a portion of uninvolved underlaying normal muscle margin.

Advancement Flap Closure of Wide Excision Site

Wide excision sites invariably on the trunk and occasionally on the extremity can be closed primarily by utilizing advancement skin flaps. Two methods giving excellent cosmetic results are shown in Fig. 16-2. In Fig. 16-2A, the circular wide excision site is incorporated within an extended angled-ellipse; adjacent skin and subcutaneous tissue are then un-

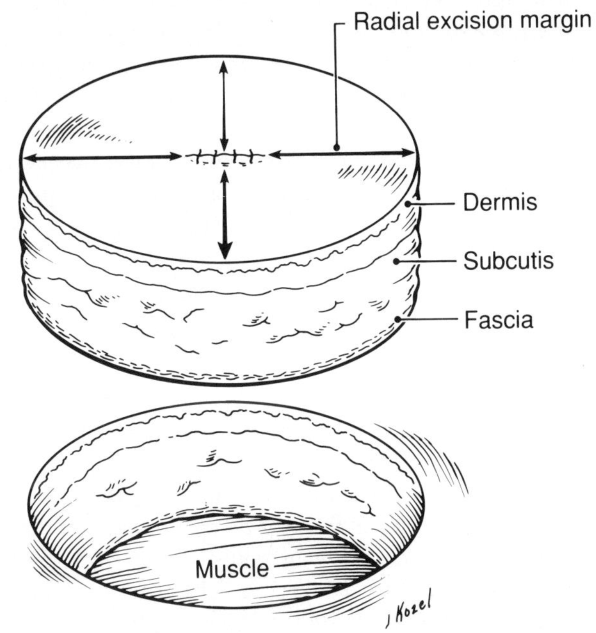

FIG. 16-1. *Method of wide excision: A 360-degree margin of normal skin, subcutaneous tissue, and underlaying fascia are resected en bloc.*

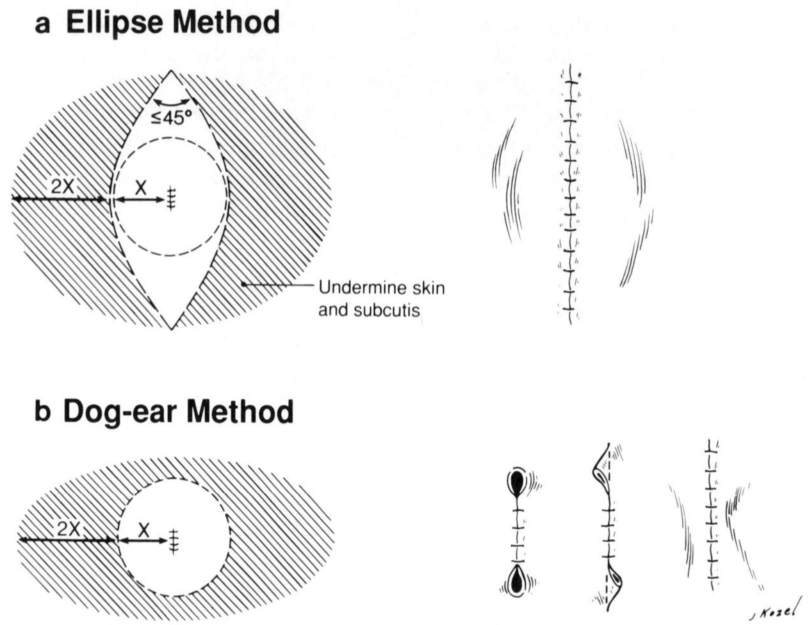

FIG. 16-2. Advancement flap closure of wide excision site. A, Ellipse method: Wide excision is formed into an angled ellipse with angles ≤ 45 degrees, undermined, and closed in layers. B, Dog-ear method: The circular wide excision site is closed after undermining and mobilizing adjacent tissue. The redundant skin at the ends of the wound are tailored, excised, and closed. In each case, closed-suction drains should always be used.

dermined for a distance of approximately twice the radical excision margin, and the wound closed in layers under minimal tension. As long as the angles at the ends of the ellipse are ≤ 45 degrees, a "dog-ear" will not occur.

Alternately, in cases where one does not have the luxury of additional tissue to form an angled-ellipse, one may close the circular wide excision site after undermining the surrounding tissue (Fig. 16-2B). The "dog-ears" that are created are tailored, excised, and closed in line with the remainder of the wound.

Major wound closures employing advancement flaps should utilize meticulous hemostasis, should always employ a closed drainage system, and should have sutures left in place for 14 to 21 days.

Skin Graft Closure of Wide Excision Site

Skin grafts are usually necessary for wide excision sites on the extremities and often for face and scalp locations. As shown in Fig. 16-3, once the specimen is removed, the skin is sewn to the edge of the underlaying fascia with absorbable sutures (Fig. 16-3A). The removal of an additional portion of subcutaneous tissue at this margin or the formation of an inward beveled edge of resection facilitates a smoother defect (Fig. 16-3B). A split-thickness skin graft of 12/1000 to 18/1000th inch is placed in the defect, tailored, and sutured to the skin with 3–0 long-silk sutures (Fig. 16-3C). The skin graft is covered first with a single layer of vaseline or xeroform impregnated fine-mesh gauze and then by a bolster of cotton saturated with sterile saline and mineral oil. The cotton is compressed and manipulated to conform to the defect, and the long silk sutures tied tightly over the bolster (Fig. 16-3D). In general, no fenestrations are made in the graft. Some surgeons prefer to staple the graft to the wound edges; some prefer dental "cigarette" bolsters affixed to the wound edges and treat the graft open. Only minimal extremity mobilization is allowed. The bolster is removed in 5 to 7 days.

Truncal Melanoma

Wide excisions on the trunk can be invariably closed with some form of advancement or rotation flap. In general, incisions on the upper torso should be oriented diagonally and those on the low back or pubis oriented horizontally to best facilitate adjacent skin mobilization and closure (Fig. 16-4). Undermining beyond the skin attachments at the spinal raphe is frequently necessary to achieve adequate tissue mobilization for excisions near the midline. When performing wide excisions of the back, it is important to place the patient prone on the operating table with arms down at their sides to allow skin closure without tension. Sutures in back skin should remain for 3 to 4 weeks. Skin grafts should be avoided in trunkal excisions where the likelihood of engraftment and cosmetic results are poor.

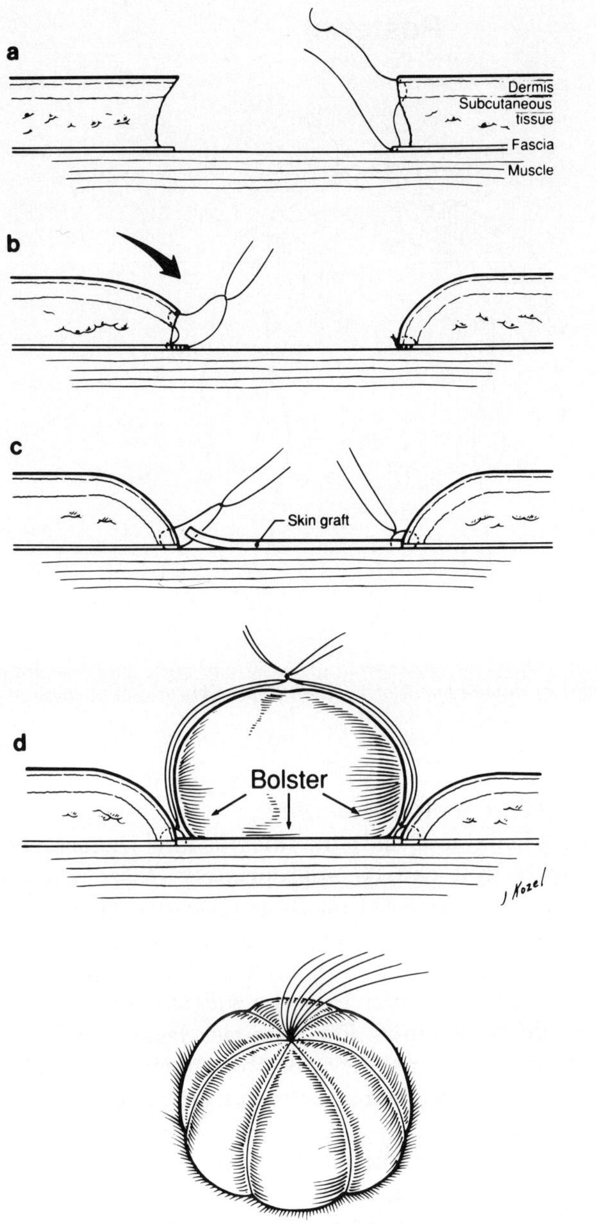

FIG. 16-3. Skin graft closure of wide excision site. A, Skin edge is approximated to fascia edge; B, tailoring the subcutaneous tissue facilitates smooth contour; C, skin graft placed in defect and sutured to skin edge with long silk; and D, cotton bolster placed and sutures tied over bolster for 5 to 7 days.

Female Breast Melanoma

Wide excision of lesions on the female breast is best accomplished by radially oriented angled-elliptical incisions, which do not displace the nipple on closure (Fig. 16-5A). The superficial mammary fascia should be removed as the deep margin of resection, with or without a wedge of subadjacent breast tissue to facilitate a cosmetic closure (Fig. 16-5B). Since subdermal breast skin lymphatics do not traverse mammary tissue, mastectomy is never warranted in the treatment of primary melanoma arising on breast skin.

Subungual Melanoma of the Thumb or Finger

Subungual melanoma is a virulent neoplasm warranting amputation of all or part of the affected digit (Fig. 16-6). Subungual lesions should always be biopsied and the diagnosis of melanoma confirmed prior to any form of amputative surgery.

Lesions of the thumb can often be treated with transection proximal to the IP joint which preserves a prehensile stump. In advanced thumb lesions, amputation at the M-P joint is required, with plastic surgical reconstruction by policization (transfer) of the index finger in selected patients.

Subungual melanomas of the fingers should be treated with either resection proximal to the DIP joint or ray-amputation. In such lesions, the vocation and cosmetic outcome are factors that influence the extent of amputation. In vocations where hand strength (grip, twist) is necessary, the width of the hand should be preserved by leaving all metacarpals intact, even if a gap or finger stump remains. In vocations where digital touch is important (e.g., typing) a finger stump often impedes dexterity warranting ray-amputation. If cosmesis is an important criterion, ray-amputation of fingers 2, 3, 4, or 5 is usually best.

In cases where a portion of the digit is to be preserved, the bone should be cut back several millimeters from the skin incision, and a volar pad created for coverage and to provide sensation (Fig. 16-6B).

Subungual Melanoma of the Toes

In the treatment of these virulent tumors functional outcome precedes cosmetic concerns (Fig. 16-7). Tumors of the nailbed of the great toe should be managed by amputation at the M-P joint with preservation of the metatarsal head. Subungual melanoma of the small toe should be treated with amputation of the digit and the head of the metatarsal bone. Tumors of the remaining toes are best managed with digit amputation with preservation of the metatarsal head to preserve width of the bearing surface of the foot.

Web-space Melanoma of the Hand or Foot

Treatment of web-space melanomas should be guided by the depth of invasion of the lesion and the presence or absence of tumor ulceration. On both the hand (Fig. 16-8A) and foot (Fig. 16-8B) high-risk lesions are best treated with ray-amputation of adjacent digits. For thin lesions without ulceration, appropriate limited reexcision and skin grafting should be considered as performed on similar lesions at other sites.

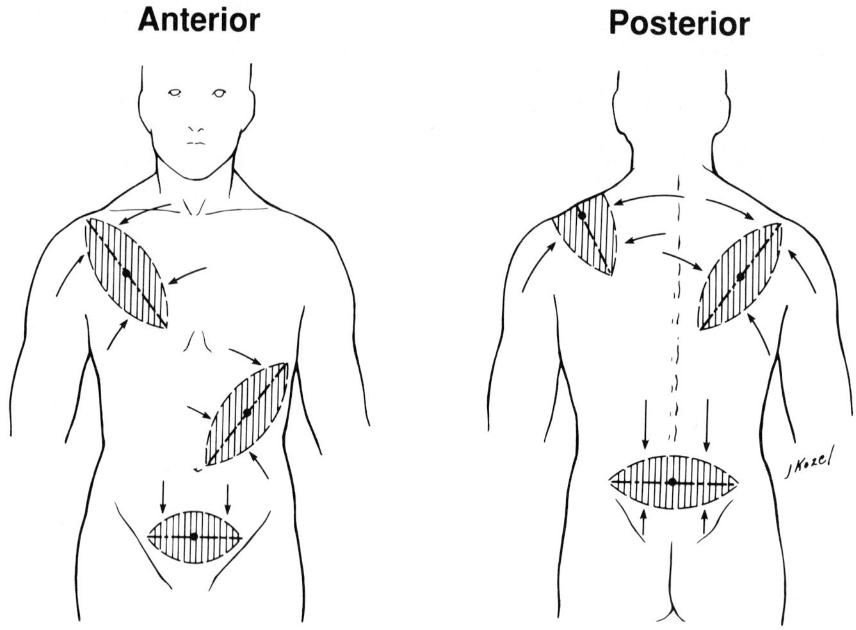

FIG. 16-4. Wide excision of truncal melanoma. Diagonal orientations are utilized for upper torso incisions and horizontal orientations for pubic or low back incisions. Truncal excisions can invariably be closed by advancement or rotation flaps. Skin grafts in these areas should be avoided.

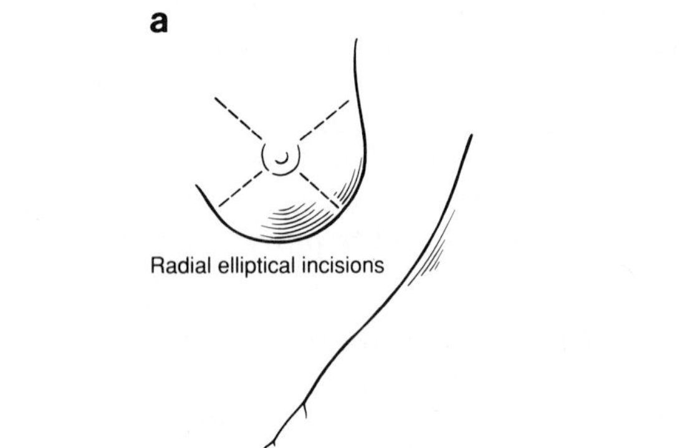

FIG. 16-5. Wide excision of female breast melanoma. A, Radially oriented elliptical incisions are utilized that do not displace the nipple on closure; and B, the deep margin of excision should include the superficial mammary fascia, with or without a wedge of breast tissue as best facilitates cosmetic closure. Mastectomy is never warranted.

Face and Scalp Melanoma

Most facial and scalp melanomas lend themselves to defects that can be appropriately closed with advancement or rotation flaps. Because of anatomic restrictions, it is often impossible to achieve preferred margins of excision based upon tumor microstaging, in which case the widest margin feasible should be attained. For high-risk lesions, a 2 to 2.5 cm margin is usually possible, particularly if the skin is prestretched and the margin measured under tension.

Lesions are frequently encountered on the malar eminence and preauricular cheek skin. In such cases, a shield-shaped wide excision is performed with the defect closed by skin from the pre- and postauricular areas employing a "cloverleaf" advancement flap (Fig. 16-9).

Skin grafts also provide an excellent means of coverage and a satisfactory cosmetic result on facial wounds, and they may be considered the first choice on scalp defects where the graft is affixed to the galea.

Ear Melanoma

Many historical texts advocated auriculectomy as treatment for melanoma of the ear, which is currently thought to be excessive and unwarranted ablative surgery in the majority of cases. Fortunately, most lesions of the ear occur on the helix or posterior skin and can be successfully managed with some form of wide excison and reconstruction (Fig. 16-10). The tragus and particularly the ear proper

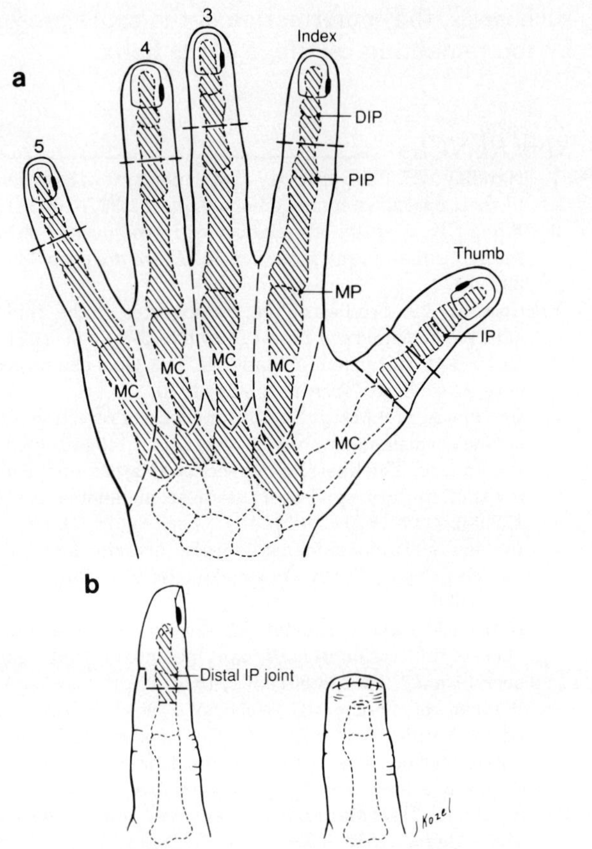

FIG. 16-6. *Subungual melanoma of the thumb or finger. Amputation is required for adequate therapy of these virulent lesions, a, The thumb may be amputated proximal to the IP joint, or at the M-P joint with reconstruction by transfer of the index finger in selected patients. Lesions of the fingers may be treated by amputation proximal to the DIP joint, or by ray-amputation, depending on vocational requirements and cosmetic considerations. In cases where a portion of the digit is preserved, a volar flap will provide coverage and sensation, b.*

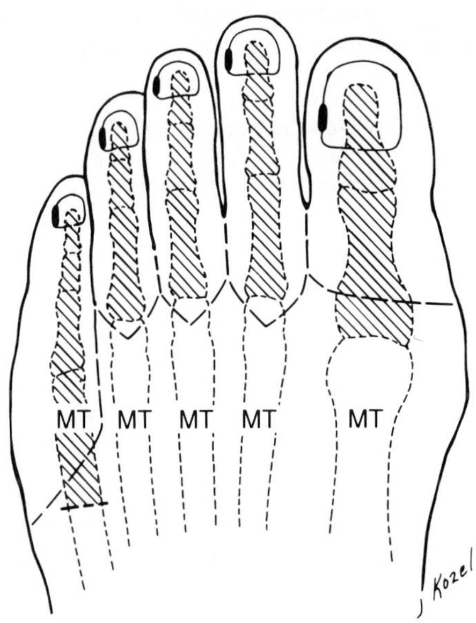

FIG. 16-7. *Subungual melanoma of the toes. Subungual melanoma of the toes should be treated with amputative surgery. The metatarsal head should be preserved on the great toe and for digits 2, 3, and 4 to preserve width of the bearing surface.*

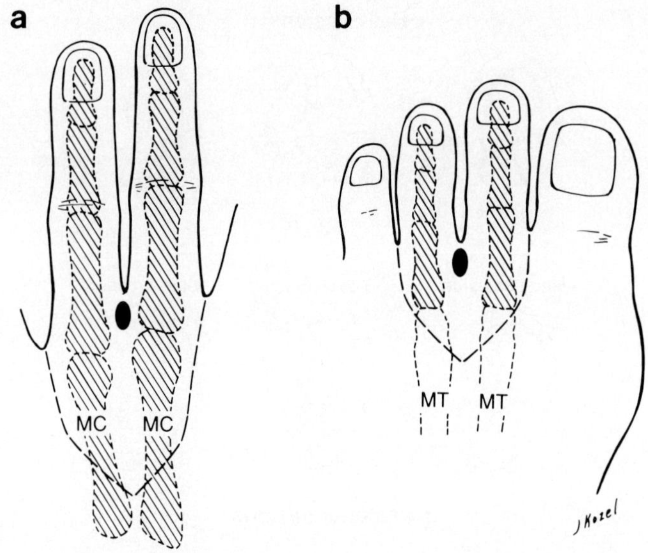

FIG. 16-8. *Web-space melanoma of the hand or foot. Treatment should be guided by tumor microstaging. High-risk lesions of the hand (a) or foot (b) should be treated with ray-amputation of adjacent digits. Low-risk lesions may be treated with appropriate limited reexcision and skin grafting.*

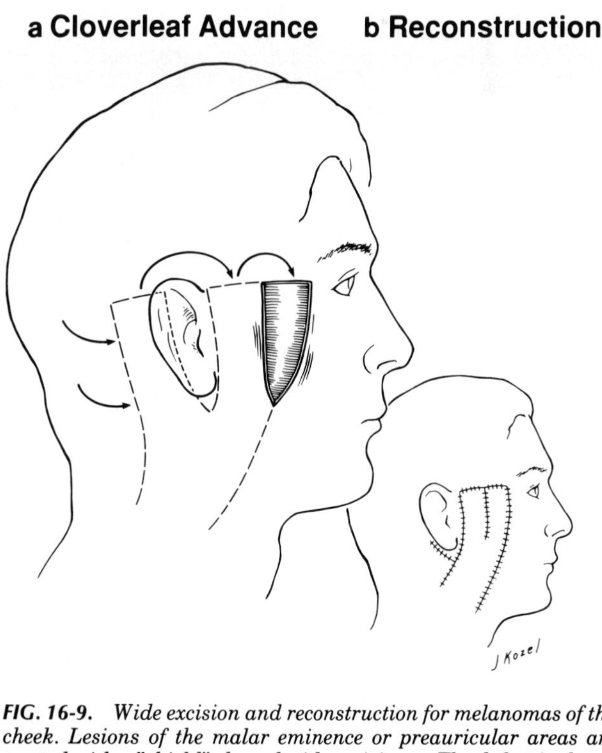

FIG. 16-9. *Wide excision and reconstruction for melanomas of the cheek. Lesions of the malar eminence or preauricular areas are treated with a "shield" shaped wide excision, a.* The defect is closed by a "cloverleaf" advancement flap utilizing pre- and postauricular skin, *b.* A small skin graft may be required in the resulting scalp defect.

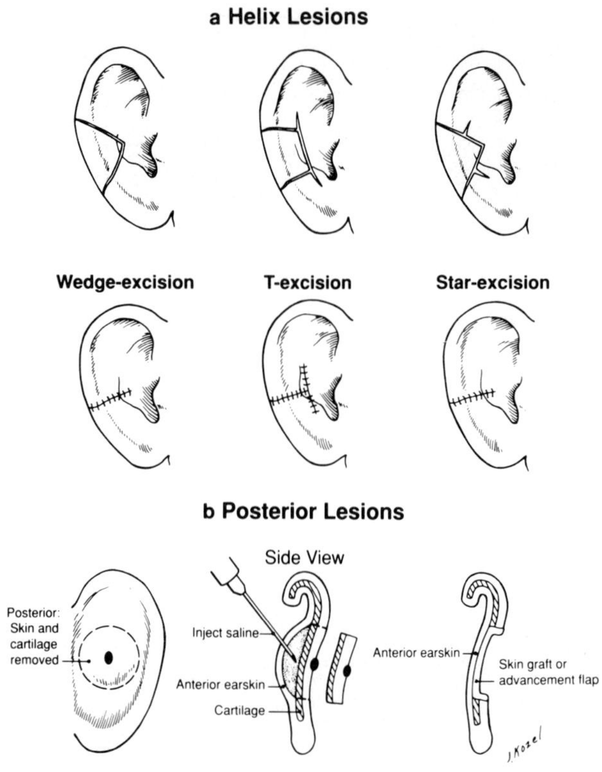

FIG. 16-10. *Ear melanoma. Most melanomas of the ear occur on the helix or posterior skin and can be managed by wide excision rather than auriculectomy. Helix lesions (A) are treated by either wedge, T- or star-excisions, though the latter two methods have improved cosmetic results. Lesions of the posterior ear (B) are treated with wide excision of the skin and underlaying cartilage, with the plane between the anterior skin and cartilage facilitated by the injection of saline to create a potential space. The defect can be closed with either a skin graft or advancement of local scalp.*

perform important functions in hearing and prevention of external otitis, as well as providing an important appendage for optical aids. Ear prostheses are uniformly unsatisfactory. For these reasons it is desirable to leave a portion of ear, if at all possible, to do so safely.

For lesions of the helix (Fig. 16-10a) either wedge-excision, T-excision, or star-excision is usually feasible. One of the latter two excision methods is often preferred to avoid "cupping" of the ear on closure of the defect, which often occurs after extensive wedge-shaped excisions.

Lesions of the posterior ear skin can often be managed by wide excision of posterior skin and cartilage, and skin grafting (Fig. 16-10b). The cartilage acts as an impenetrable deep barrier to tumor extension. The anterior ear skin is preserved and is separated from the cartilage by injecting saline to create a potential space. The wide excision is performed with the cartilage resected as the deep margin; the defect is either skin-grafted or closed with a local advancement flap of postauricular scalp. In such cases, the conformation of the ear is preserved by the remaining cartilage of the helix.

REFERENCES

1. Handley WS. The pathology of melanotic growths in relation to their operative management. *Lancet* 1:927–1003, 1907.
2. Wong CK. A study of melanocytes in the normal skin surrounding malignant melanomata. *Dermatologica* 141:215–225, 1970.
3. Cochran AJ. Studies of the melanocytes of the epidermis adjacent to tumors. *J Invest Dermatol* 57:38–43, 1971.
4. Davis NC. Cutaneous melanoma: The Queensland experience. *Curr Probl Surg* 13:28–31, 1976.
5. Breslow A, and Macht SD. Optimal size of resection for thin cutaneous melanoma. *Surg Gynecol Obstet* 145:691–692, 1977.
6. Breslow A. Thickness, cross-sectional areas and depth of invasion in the prognosis of cutaneous melanoma. *Ann Surg* 172:902–908, 1970.
7. Breslow A. Tumor thickness, level of invasion and node dissection in Stage I cutaneous melanoma. *Ann Surg* 182:572–575, 1975.
8. Hansen MG and McCarten AB. Tumor thickness and lymphocyte infiltration in malignant melanoma of the head and neck. *Am J Surg* 128:557–561, 1974.
9. Wanebo HJ, Fortner JG, Woodruff J, et al. Selection of optimum surgical treatment of stage I melanoma by depth of microinvasion: Use of the combined microstage technique (Clark-Breslow). *Ann Surg* 182:302–315, 1975.
10. Southwick HW. Malignant melanoma—how much surgery? *Minn Med* 47:1333, 1964.
11. Hines RW, Bodenham DC, Lloyd OC, et al. Malignant melanoma of the skin, In: S. Taylor (ed.), *Recent Advances in Surgery,* 7th ed. London: Churchill, 1969, 145.
12. Wilson R. Malignant melanoma—A follow-up study. *Surg Obstet Gynecol* 66:29–31, 1958.
13. McNeer G, and Cantin J. Local failure in the treatment of melanoma. *Am J Roentgen Rad Ther Nucl Med* 99:790–808, 1967.
14. Jones WM, Williams WJ, Robert MM, et al. Malignant melanoma of the skin: Prognostic value of clinical features and the role of treatment in 111 cases. *Br J Cancer* 22:437–451, 1968.
15. Cochran AJ. Malignant melanoma: A review of 10 years experience in Glasow, Scotland. *Cancer* 23:1190–1199, 1969.
16. Shingleton WW, Siegler HF, Stocks LH, et al. Management of recurrent melanoma of the extremity. *Cancer* 35:574–579, 1975.
17. Elias EG, Didolkar MS, Goel IP, et al. A clinicopathologic study of prognostic factors in cutaneous malignant melanoma. *Surg Gynecol Obstet* 149:17–21, 1979.
18. Storm FK, Sparks FC, and Mortion DL. Treatment of melanoma of the lower extremity with intralesional BCG and hyperthermic perfusion. *Surg Gynecol Obstet* 149:17–21, 1979.
19. Karakousis CP, and Holyoke ED. Biologic behavior and treatment of intransit metastases of melanoma. *Surg Gynecol Obstet* 150:29–32, 1980.
20. Milton GW, Shaw HN, Farago GA, et al. Tumor thickness and the site and time of first recurrence in cutaneous malignant melanoma (Stage I). *Br J Surg* 67:543–546, 1980.
21. Storm FK, and Morton DL. Value of therapeutic hyperthermic limb perfusion in advanced recurrent melanoma of the lower extremity. *Amer J Surg* 150:32–35, 1985.
22. Das Gupta TK. Results of treatment of 269 patients with primary cutaneous melanoma. A five-year prospective study. *Ann Surg* 186:201–209, 1977.

23. Milton GW. Malignant melanoma of the skin and mucous membranes. Edinburgh: Churchill-Livingston, 1977.
24. Pitt TTE. Aspects of surgical treatment for malignant melanoma. The place of biopsy and wide excision. *Aust N Z J Surg* 47:757–766, 1977.
25. Veronesi U, Adamus J, Bandiera DC, et al. Inefficacy of immediate node dissection in stage I melanoma of the limbs. *N Engl J Med* 297:627–630, 1977.
26. Balch CM, Murad TM, Soong S-j, et al. Tumor thickness as a guide to surgical management of clinical stage I melanoma patients. *Cancer* 43:883–888, 1979.
27. Cascinelli N, van der Esch EP, Breslow A, et al. Stage I melanoma of the skin. The problems of resection margins. *Eur J Cancer* 16:1079–1085, 1980.
28. Goldman LI. Decisions in the management of cutaneous malignant melanoma. *Semin Oncol* 7:370–375, 1980.
29. Bagley FH, Cady B, Lee A, et al. Changes in clinical preservation and management of malignant melanoma. *Cancer* 47:2126–2134, 1981.
30. Kenady DE, Brown BW, and McBride CM. Excision of underlying fascia with a primary malignant melanoma. Effect on recurrence and survival rates. *Surgery* 92:615–618, 1982.
31. Elder DE, Guerry D, Heiberger RM, et al. Optimal resection margin for cutaneous malignant melanoma. *Plast Reconstr Surg* 71:66–72, 1983.
32. Golomb FM. Editorial discussion for "Optimal resection margin for cutaneous melanoma." *Plast Reconstr Surg* 71:76–78, 1983.
33. Roses DF, Harris MN, Rigel D, et al. Local and intransit metastases following definitive excision for primary cutaneous malignant melanoma. *Ann Surg* 198:65–69, 1983.
34. Schmoeckel C, Bockelbrink A, Bockelbrink H, et al. Low- and high-risk malignant melanoma. III. Prognostic significance of the resection margin. *Eur J Cancer Clin Oncol* 19:245–249, 1983.
35. Cosimi AB, Sober AJ, Mihn MC, et al. Conservative surgical management of superficially invasive cutaneous melanoma. *Cancer* 53:1256–1259, 1984.
36. Urist MM, Balch CM, Soong S-j, et al. The influence of surgical margins and prognostic factors predicting the risk of local recurrence in 3445 patients with primary cutaneous melanoma. *Cancer* 55:1398–1402, 1985.
37. McLeod GR. Management of melanoma in situ. In: Charles M. Balch (ed.), *Surgical Approaches to Cutaneous Melanoma, Pigment Cell,* Vol 7. Basel: Karger, 1985, 1–7.
38. Olsen G. The malignant melanoma of the skin. New theories based on a study of 500 cases. *Acta Chir Scand* (Suppl) 365:128–136, 1966.
39. Beardmore GL, and Davis NC. Multiple primary cutaneous melanomas. *Arch Dermatol* 111:603–609, 1975.
40. Moseley HS, Giuliano AE, Storm FK, et al. Multiple primary melanoma. *Cancer* 43:939–944, 1979.
41. Kelly JW, Sagebiel RW, Calderon W, et al. The frequency of local recurrence and microsatellites as a guide to reexcision margins for cutaneous malignant melanoma. *Ann Surg* 200:759–863, 1984.

Chapter 17

ELECTIVE LYMPH NODE DISSECTION

Richard Essner and Donald L. Morton

Wide excision (WE) is the generally accepted treatment for primary cutaneous melanoma. Over 90 percent of patients will survive at least 5 years after surgical removal of melanomas confined to the primary site.[1–3] Deaths from melanoma are primarily due to visceral metastases. The most common route for metastatic spread is through the lymphatics to the regional lymph nodes.[4,5] Thus, removing nodal metastases may prevent the spread of tumor to distant sites.

Lymphadenectomy (LND) is currently the only effective treatment for melanoma metastatic to regional lymph nodes. *Therapeutic* LND (TLND) is generally recommended for local control of disease in patients with clinically suspicious nodes or pathologically proven metastases to regional lymph nodes (American Joint Committee on Cancer [AJCC] Stage III). However, by the time regional lymph nodes are palpable, 70 to 85 percent of the patients will have distant micrometastases, which eventually lead to death.[4,6–8] Even though the 10-year survival rate following TLND is only 15 to 30 percent,[3,9–11] the alternative of *elective* LND (ELND), that is, prophylactic removal of nodes having no clinical evidence of disease but a high risk of microscopic metastases, remains a source of heated controversy.

HISTORICAL PERSPECTIVE

The concept of ELND in conjunction with melanoma surgery was first proposed in 1892. In his lecture "Melanotic Cancerous Disease," Herbert L. Snow advocated wide excision and routine ELND as the most effective means to avoid lymphatic spread.[12]

> The danger lies in the diffusion of malignant cell particles from this primary focus; these always implicate the nearest lymph glands, which intercept them for a time. Eventually they pass beyond such "traps" into the blood current; then death with multiple visceral metastases ensues. Palpable enlargement of these glands is unfortunately but a late symptom of deposit therein; by the time it occurs there is almost always implication of deeper organs or tissues. We thus see the utter futility of operative measures which are addressed to the primary lesion only, as also the harm of irritating any growing wart by such pernicious procedures as the application of the ligature or of silver nitrate. We further see the paramount importance of securing, whenever possible, the perfect eradication of those lymph glands which will necessarily be first infected; before enlargement takes place radical removal of such organs in the axilla, groin, surface regions of the neck, etc., before they have undergone appreciable increase in bulk, is a safe and easy measure, which, under the conditions indicated, should never be neglected.

At the turn of the century, Frederic Eve reviewed the London Hospital's experience with 45 cases of cutaneous melanoma.[13] He echoed Snow's views in an emphatic endorsement of ELND for cutaneous melanoma: "The treatment of melanoma of the skin can be given in few words, that is, free excision or amputation, in accordance with the position and extent of the disease. The removal of the nearest chain of lymphatic glands, whether palpably enlarged or not, should never be omitted; for it may be taken as a matter of certainty that in the great majority of cases they are infected." Eve's colleague, William Sampson Handley, at the London Hospital in 1907 delivered two Hunterian Lectures in which he described the centrifugal permeation of melanoma from the primary lesion through the regional lymphatics and blood vessels.[14] Although his observations were based on a single cadaver, he advocated regional ELND and WE of the primary to control proliferation of disease. Importantly, Handley recognized the possibility of multiple drainage patterns for certain primary melanomas, concluding that "it is imperative to remove, along with the primary growth, the *two* sets of glands corresponding to the two lymphatic areas involved."

One year after Handley's Hunterian Lectures

were published, J. Hogarth Pringle emphasized the importance of regional lymph glands in the dissemination of melanoma[15]: "melanotic tumours have a remarkable tendency to develop secondary nodules here and there along the course of the lymph vessels themselves, which lead from the primary tumour to the nearest lymph glands." To deal with these nodes, Pringle proposed in continuity or en bloc dissection: "A radical extirpation of the disease will be most certainly ensured by excision of the tumour, with a good zone of healthy skin around it and a somewhat larger zone of the underlying subcutaneous tissue and of the deep fascia, with a broad strip of subcutaneous fascia up to and including the nearest anatomical group of glands at least; and all that is removed should be in one continuous strip as far as is possible."

Pringle's technique was rediscovered in 1945 by George T. Pack, who with his co-workers recommended in continuity dissection of the primary tumor, regional lymph nodes, and intervening lymphatic plexus.[16] Pack reported a 42 percent incidence of occult metastases in regional lymph nodes, commenting:

> The same surgeon who will invariably perform a radical mastectomy or an abdominoperineal rectal resection for cancers in these locations apparently is content to perform the most limited type of excision for malignant melanoma of the skin. This tumor tends to recur locally with such a high frequency and to metastasize to regional nodes with such a high incidence that it is imperative for every surgeon . . . to realize the extreme importance of applying radical surgical principles.

In a subsequent report in 1952, Pack's group linked ELND to improved survival, citing a 27 percent improvement in the 5-year cure rate when regional nodes were routinely removed.[17] However, the vast experience in the surgical management of melanoma during ensuing years has led to two distinct and conflicting evaluations of the efficacy of ELND.[1,4,5,11,18–25] Underlying this conflict is the problem of determining which patients might benefit from ELND. In 1965, Menhert and Heard were the first to present data justifying the value of LND for deeper lesions.[26] However, Breslow subsequently reported that tumor thickness rather than depth of invasion should be used as the criterion for ELND.[27,28]

CONTROVERSY ABOUT ROUTINE ELND

Support for ELND comes primarily from retrospective or nonrandomized studies reporting that the long-term survival of ELND patients is approximately 25 percent higher than that of patients undergoing TLND[6,7,10,29–33] (Table 17-1). Advocates of ELND believe that although not all patients will benefit from the procedure, those with limited tumor burden in the regional lymph nodes can be protected from the untimely progression of disease. The incidence of unsuspected micrometastases in the regional lymph nodes ranges from 15 to 50 percent.[4,5]

TABLE 17-1
FIVE-YEAR SURVIVAL OF MELANOMA PATIENTS WITH SUBCLINICAL REGIONAL NODE METASTASES (CLINICAL STAGE I) VERSUS CLINICALLY PALPABLE REGIONAL METASTASES (CLINICAL STAGE II)

INVESTIGATORS	CLINICAL STAGE I (%)	CLINICAL STAGE II (%)	DIFFERENCE
McNeer and Das Gupta, 1964	52	19	33
Cohen et al., 1977[a]	55	38	17
Das Gupta, 1977	69	20	49
Balch et al., 1981	48	24	24
Callery et al., 1982	48	36	12
Roses et al., 1985	44	20	24
Morton et al., 1991[a]	59	43	16
Average	54	28	26

[a]Data beyond 5 years.

Opponents of ELND advocate a "wait and see" policy, arguing that only 20 percent of patients with AJCC Stages I and II disease have occult metastases, and thus, 80 percent would be subjected to unnecessary surgery. They also argue that immediate LND may trap metastases that are "in transit" between the primary tumor and the regional lymph nodes, thereby increasing the rate of locoregional failure. Some authors state that removal of the regional lymph basins may favor hematogenous spread of any residual tumor cells. Others believe that the presence of regional lymph node metastases is a marker for systemic disease; delaying LND would therefore not adversely affect outcome.

The debate surrounding ELND is focused in the following issues: (1) Does removal of micrometastases from regional lymph nodes have a significant impact on the course of the disease? (2) Can we accurately identify those patients who are at high risk for nodal metastases but are unlikely to have systemic disease? (3) Finally, does removal of regional lymph nodes at the same time as the primary tumor improve the staging of those patients at risk for metastatic disease?

THEORETICAL BENEFITS OF ELND

Support for ELND is based on the theory that melanoma metastasizes in a predictable and sequential fashion from the primary site, through the lymphatics, to the regional lymph nodes, from which it travels to distant sites. The goal of removing the regional lymph nodes at the same time as the primary tumor is to eliminate a potential source of metastasis early in the natural history of the disease when the tumor to host relationship favors the host. Some investigators believe that even those patients without documented regional node involvement may benefit from ELND. They argue that the absence of micrometastases in the biopsied nodes may be partially explained by sampling error or insensitivity of routine H and E staining. Cochran and colleagues recently reported an additional 14 percent incidence of micrometastases in regional lymph nodes examined by immunohistological techniques, as compared to routine staining methods.[34,35] Heller and associates detected a 22 percent increase in regional micrometastases by cell culturing methods.[36]

Overall, 50 percent of patients who undergo regional LND for micrometastases will survive 5 years, compared to only 15 to 30 percent of patients with palpable disease.[3,9–11] Investigators from the Sydney Melanoma Unit and the University of Alabama found that patients with subclinical disease fared better following LND than those with clinical evidence of disease, even when matched by the number of nodes involved.[5] The opponents of ELND agree that the outcome of patients undergoing LND for microscopic nodal disease is better than that of patients presenting with multiple bulky regional nodes. Their main concern is that patients without nodal involvement may be subjected to unnecessary surgical morbidity and/or expense. Still, the survival advantage of patients treated by ELND has been demonstrated in a number of studies.[2,23,31,37–39]

SELECTION ON THE BASIS OF PROGNOSTIC INDICATORS

Patients most likely to benefit from ELND are those with subclinical lymph node metastases; patients whose disease is confined to the primary site will gain little from this procedure, since WE is sufficient for a high rate of cure.

A number of prognostic factors can be used to distinguish which clinically negative patients are at risk for harboring occult nodal disease or distant metastases.[6,27,40–45] Tumor thickness, Clark level of invasion, site of the primary, presence of ulceration or regression pattern of growth, and gender can serve as relative markers for the aggressive nature of the primary.

Tumor thickness can be used as a quantitative method for determining the risk of regional and distant metastases, as suggested by Balch[5] (Table 17-2 and Fig. 17-1). Thin (< 0.76 mm) melanomas are usually associated with localized disease, for which ELND would probably not be helpful.[2,3,5] By contrast, up to 60 percent of patients with intermediate-thickness (0.76–4 mm) melanomas have occult regional metastases. These patients also have a relatively low (< 20%) risk of developing distant metastases and, therefore, would theoretically benefit from ELND. Thick (> 4 mm) melanomas are associated not only with a high risk of regional metastases but also with 70 percent likelihood of distant disease. In this case, treatment of the regional nodes can only be palliative; survival is determined by control of distant disease.

The anatomical site of the primary is also an important factor for determining the risk of regional disease and the potential benefit of ELND. Patients with melanoma arising on the extremities generally have a more favorable prognosis than those with primaries arising on the trunk or head and neck.[5,39,46–49] Melanomas arising on the heels and palms (acral lentiginous melanoma) are more aggressive than those originating on other extremity sites, and these patients may benefit from ELND.

Primary melanomas of the head and neck are

TABLE 17-2
RELATIONSHIP BETWEEN MICROSTAGE OF PRIMARY MELANOMA, INCIDENCE OF REGIONAL LYMPH NODE METASTASES AND LONG-TERM SURVIVAL IN 5196 PATIENTS

TUMOR MICROSTAGE	NUMBER OF PATIENTS	LYMPH NODE METASTASES (%)	5-YEAR SURVIVAL (%)	10-YEAR SURVIVAL (%)
Breslow Thickness				
<0.76 mm	1061	8	98	97
0.76–1.5 mm	1167	20	91	85
1.51–3.99 mm	1166	36	71	64
≥4.0 mm	324	57	46	41
Clark Level				
I/II	1084	9	98	97
III	1600	24	87	82
IV	1403	37	72	64
V	198	53	53	44

1992 data from the melanoma database of the John Wayne Cancer Institute, Santa Monica, CA.

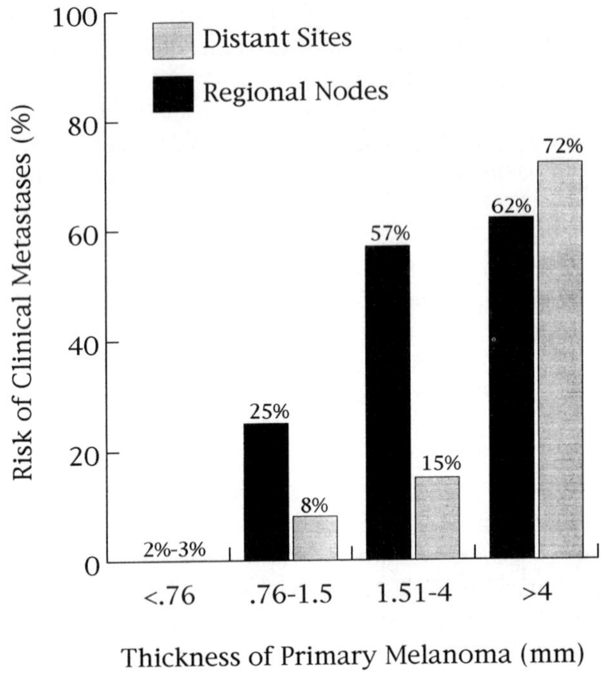

FIG. 17-1 Estimated biologic risk that melanoma micrometastases will become clinically evident in regional nodes (within 3 years) and at distant sites (within 5 years). (Adapted from Balch et al.[5])

considered more aggressive than melanomas of the extremities.[39] Most surgeons recommend TLND for patients with head or neck primaries that are accompanied by clinically suspicious nodes or biopsy-proven nodal disease. Some recommend ELND for all clinical Stage I patients having primary lesions of intermediate thickness or Clark level of invasion. However, 65 to 90 percent of these patients will not have histopathologic evidence of nodal disease; they will therefore, have risked the potential complications of radical neck surgery (including functional deficits and/or disfigurement) without experiencing any benefit from this procedure. On the other hand, the aggressive nature of head and neck primaries is a strong argument for an aggressive surgical approach. Although there are as yet no relevant prospective studies, in 1984 Urist and colleagues[39] reviewed survival data for 534 head and neck melanoma patients from the University of Alabama and the Sydney Melanoma Unit. After 5 years of follow-up, 72 percent of patients who underwent WE plus ELND for intermediate-thickness (1.5–3.99 mm) primaries were still alive, compared to only 45 percent of those who were initially treated by WE alone. Similarly, Hansen and McCarten found that ELND provided a survival benefit for patients with head and neck primaries thicker than 1.5 mm.[50]

The growth pattern of the primary lesion is an indicator of tumor aggressiveness. Ulceration and the presence of tumor regression both indicate more aggressive primary lesions and may be used as factors indicating ELND. Lentigo maligna melanoma (LMM) is generally regarded as having a low potential for metastasis, while nodular melanoma (NM) spreads at a much faster rate. Urist and colleagues found that 81 of the 534 patients with melanoma arising on the head and neck had histologic growth patterns of LMM.[39] These patients had significantly higher 5-year survival rates than patients with superficial spreading melanoma (SSM) or NM; however, survival data were not corrected for depth of the primary. Still, these data suggest that ELND is more likely to be beneficial in patients with SSM or NM rather than LMM.

Women may have a survival advantage and reduced risk of metastases. As shown in Table 17-3, the biologic potential for metastasis is low for women with extremity primaries.[5] The patient's age, general health, and other medical problems should also be used in deciding for or against ELND.[45,51]

IMPORTANCE OF ACCURATE STAGING

ELND affords the surgeon the best means of accurately staging melanoma and thereby identifying those patients who could benefit from adjuvant therapies.[2] Most clinical trials of adjuvant therapy will

TABLE 17-3
ESTIMATED RISK OF REGIONAL AND DISTANT MICROMETASTASES ACCORDING TO THE PATIENT'S SEX AND THE PRIMARY MELANOMA'S LOCATION AND THICKNESS

LOCATION	RISK OF REGIONAL MICROMETASTASES (%)	RISK OF DISTANT MICROMETASTASES (%)
Female Extremity		
<0.76 mm	2	1
0.76–1.49 mm	5–7	7–10
1.5–3.99 mm	7–19	10–24
≥4 mm	0	48
Male Extremity		
<0.76 mm	2	2
0.76–1.49 mm	22–24	22–24
1.5–3.99 mm	24–29	24–34
≥4 mm	0	70
Female Axilla		
<0.76	8	10
0.76–1.49 mm	14–17	21–29
1.5–3.99 mm	17–21	29–41
≥4 mm	0	60
Male Axilla		
<0.76 mm	9	14
0.76–1.49 mm	27–28	29–32
1.5–3.99 mm	28–30	32–45
≥4 mm	0	79

Adapted from Balch et al.[5]

only admit patients with proven regional or distant metastases. ELND can be used to identify patients with subclinical metastatic disease, who are eligible for these trials and most likely to benefit.

RESULTS OF NONRANDOMIZED AND RETROSPECTIVE STUDIES OF ELND

Many large, long-term, retrospective studies from single or multiple institutions have demonstrated a small but significant survival advantage in patients undergoing WE plus ELND for clinical Stage I melanomas of intermediate Clark level or Breslow thickness.[2,23,31,37,38] A large, nonrandomized, prospective study by the Sydney Melanoma Unit demonstrated improved survival following ELND in patients with intermediate lesions (0.76–4.0 mm) arising on the extremities, trunk, or head and neck.[38] ELND had a particularly high potential benefit in men with extremity primaries and in patients with axial primaries.

A similar but retrospective study from the University of Alabama also demonstrated a survival advantage in those patients with axial and extremity primaries who were treated by WE plus ELND versus WE alone.[2] In 1983 Reintgen and colleagues reported the Duke University series of 613 patients treated with WE or WE plus ELND.[23] Patients in the ELND group fared significantly better than those treated by WE alone. Although tumor thickness, presence of ulceration, and primary site (trunk versus extremity) were significant, only ELND was an independent indicator of improved prognosis. A mathematical model derived from their data was used to predict a survival advantage of up to 40 percent over 5 years in those patients with deep, ulcerated primaries who underwent ELND.

In 1991, Morton and associates at the John Wayne Cancer Institute reviewed their experience with 1134 melanoma patients whose disease had spread to regional lymph nodes.[31] Univariate analysis indicated that the number of involved nodes, gender, site of the primary (extremity versus trunk), and depth could be used to determine a patient's prognosis (Table 17-4). ELND was performed in those patients with primaries thicker than 0.65 mm. Survival rates of 5 and 10 years were significantly better for those patients who underwent LND for occult metastases than for those undergoing LND for clinically evident disease.

TABLE 17-4
UNIVARIATE AND MULTIVARIATE ANALYSIS OF PROGNOSTIC FACTORS USED TO PREDICT SURVIVAL OF MELANOMA PATIENTS WITH LYMPH NODE METASTASES (AJCC STAGE III)

	P-VALUE	
FACTOR	UNIVARIATE	MULTIVARIATE
Number of positive nodes	.0001	.0001
Breslow thickness	.0487	.0334
0.76–4 mm	.0016	.0942
≥4 mm	.2960	*
Sex	.0103	.0627
Age	.0670	*
Location of primary		
Extremity	.0104	.0059
Head and neck	.1845	*
Trunk	.1168	*
Unknown	.0876	*
Synchronous versus metasynchronous	.0170	*
Clark level	.3685	*
Adjuvant immunotherapy	.4118	*

*$P \geq 0.1$
Adapted from Morton et al.[31]

RESULTS OF COMPLETED RANDOMIZED TRIALS

Two important prospective randomized trials, one by Veronesi and WHO colleagues[11,25,53,54] and the other by the Mayo Clinic,[24] have helped clarify the benefits of ELND, but many questions still remain. Veronesi's group studied 553 clinical Stage I patients with melanoma confined to the distal two-thirds of the extremity.[25] Following WE of the primary lesion, 267 (48%) underwent immediate dissection of the nodes; the other 286 (52%) underwent LND only when clinically positive nodes were discovered. The two groups were matched according to major prognostic factors.

The WHO group observed no statistically significant survival benefit for patients who had undergone ELND versus TLND. The only patients to experience a benefit from ELND were those with Clark level IV lesions of intermediate depth (specifically 1.0–1.9 mm and 3–3.9 mm). These patients had a 10 percent better 5-year survival rate (20% at 10 years) than did similar patients treated by TLND. Because of the small number of patients in this subset of the trial, however, this survival advantage did not achieve statistical significance. The WHO study was also limited by the predominance (85%) of women in the trial. We now know that women with extremity lesions represent a highly favorable subset of patients and that the benefits of ELND will probably not be evident in these patients. In addition, the WHO trial was initiated prior to our understanding that tumor thickness, Clark level, and ulceration are important prognostic indicators. Therefore, patients were not stratified according to these variables, and the potential advantages of ELND may have been lost.

An important finding of the WHO study is that while only 14 percent of patients with primaries from 2 to 3.9 mm had regional lymph node metastases at the time of ELND, 40 percent of patients with equivalent-thickness lesions eventually required delayed LND for development of clinical node disease. This discrepancy confirms that the true incidence of regional lymph node involvement is underestimated, and offers strong support for the theory that some patients with subclinical disease may not be identified by routine pathologic exam.

Results of the WHO study were analyzed to determine the significance of the various prognostic indicators. By multivariate analysis, increasing tumor thickness and ulceration were found to have a negative influence on survival. Tumor thickness was fairly well distributed among patients in both groups. However, there was a maldistribution of patients with ulcerated primaries (52% versus 19%) treated with ELND. This discrepancy in patient groups likely had a negative impact on the survival of the ELND group.

The data were re-evaluated to determine low, intermediate, and high risk for recurrence. The intermediate group consisted of 60 patients treated by WE alone or WE plus ELND. At 10 years of follow-up, those patients who had undergone ELND had a 22 percent improvement in survival.[5] This difference was nearly significant. The potential benefit of ELND may have been obscured by the small size of this subgroup of patients. A larger randomized study should be undertaken to address this question.

The WHO investigators found a 10-year survival rate of 15 to 20 percent in those patients treated by TLND.[11] This means that up to 80 percent of these patients had distant microscopic disease by the time they developed clinical regional disease. These results demonstrate a significant decrease in survival compared to those patients treated by ELND.

In a Mayo Clinic study, 171 patients with AJCC Stages I and II melanoma were prospectively randomized into three groups: immediate excision of the regional lymph nodes (54 patients), delayed lymphadenectomy (55 patients), and no lymphadenectomy (62 patients).[24] Patients with primaries arising on the head and neck or axial trunk were excluded. The results showed no significant difference in total survival or metastasis-free survival among the three treatment groups. The 10-year survival rates were 85 percent when the nodes were left intact, 87 percent when the nodes were immediately removed, and 91 percent if a delayed LND was performed. The only factors significantly related to survival were tumor thickness and growth pattern. These results must, however, be considered cautiously since the majority of the primary lesions in this study were low-risk thin lesions with little likelihood of recurrence.

The limitations of both the WHO and Mayo studies may have obscured the benefit of immediate LND. Evaluation of prognostic variables such as microstaging, anatomic site, ulceration, and sex can identify patients at substantial risk for harboring microscopic metastatic disease.

Two new randomized trials are currently being conducted to determine the efficacy of ELND. The Intergroup Melanoma Protocol includes those patients with melanomas of intermediate thickness (1–4 mm) arising on both the trunk and extremity sites. Four treatment arms have been designed. Wide excision, comparing 2-cm to 4-cm margins, is performed alone or in combination with ELND in those patients with clinically negative regional basins. All patients with trunk melanomas have preoperative lymphoscintigraphy and all nodal basins are resected. Those patients with more than two drainage basins or bilateral cervical lymph node basins are ineligible for this study.

A second trial is being conducted by the WHO to determine the role of ELND in those patients with melanoma of the trunk. Patients with lesions arising within 2 cm of the midline are excluded. Patients are randomized to WE (3-cm margins) alone or in conjunction with ELND.

IDENTIFICATION OF THE LYMPH BASIN DRAINING THE PRIMARY MELANOMA

One of the concerns regarding the management of the regional lymph nodes in those patients considered for ELND is determining the pathway of drainage from ambiguous sites. Melanomas arising on the extremities have fairly predictable lymphatic drainage to the axillary or inguinal lymph basins.[55] Primaries arising on the trunk and on the head and neck are generally less predictable, making it difficult to determine which lymph node basin is at risk. Historically, ELND was avoided in patients with truncal melanoma because of the high risk of complications involved in performing multiple cervical, axillary, or inguinal lymphadenectomies in one patient.

MELANOMAS OF THE TRUNK

Drainage is often ambiguous when melanoma arises on the axial skin of the trunk, particularly near the midline or belt line. Because melanomas in these locations may drain to one or more lymphatic areas, it is important to define precisely the drainage pattern before undertaking LND. Sappey, drawing a line 2-cm wide around the trunk just above and below the umbilicus, determined that lesions arising above this line generally drain to the axillary nodes, while those below drain to the inguinal nodes. Recent work at the University of South Florida demonstrates that the drainage pattern from truncal primaries is more ambiguous than originally expected from the studies by Sappey, and up to 59 percent of the lymph node dissections may be misdirected if based on classical anatomical descriptions.[56] However, some midline lesions, especially those of the umbilical area or midline of the back, may drain to both axillary and inguinal basins.[55,57] The importance of lymphoscintigraphy in these sites cannot be overemphasized.

MELANOMA OF THE HEAD AND NECK

Lesions on the anterior scalp or face typically drain to the parotid lymph nodes and then to the ipsilateral cervical chain.[46] Those primaries on the posterior scalp drain to the occipital, postauricular, or posterior cervical lymph basins.

LYMPHOSCINTIGRAPHY

Cutaneous lymphoscintigraphy was initially introduced as a method to identify lymphatic drainage patterns from ambiguous sites such as the head and neck or trunk. In 1953, Sherman and Ter-Pogossian used interstitial injection of radioactive colloid gold (198 Au) in a gelatin solution to document the lymphatic flow from cutaneous sites.[58] In 1977, Robinson and associates used 198 Au to demonstrate the variability in lymphatic drainage pathways from the trunk or proximal portion of an extremity.[57,59] However, because of the high local exposure of radiation from 198 Au, technetium (99Tc) labeled dextran and human serum albumin have become the preferred agents for lymphoscintigraphy.[60] A number of studies have demonstrated the drainage pathways from primary lesions on the trunk. In all, approximately 50 percent of primaries will drain to multiple lymphatic basins or have pathways that are not predictable by standard anatomical description.[55,56] Although lymphoscintigraphy indicates which regional lymph basins drain cutaneous melanomas, it does not indicate whether or not the patient has nodal metastases.

INTRAOPERATIVE LYMPHATIC MAPPING AND SELECTIVE LYMPHADENECTOMY

Morton and associates have developed a minimally invasive intraoperative method to identify clinical Stage I melanoma patients with nodal micrometastases, who are most likely to benefit from immediate LND.[32] Hypothesizing that a primary melanoma drains initially to a single lymph node, the "sentinel node," from which it spreads, they developed the technique of intraoperative lymphatic mapping. Using this mapping technique with selective LND (SLND), surgeons can select those patients who are clinically Stage I but pathologically Stage III for immediate LND (in this case, TLND).

The technique of mapping with SLND begins with the identification of the regional lymph node basin into which the primary lesion drains. Ambiguous drainage is determined preoperatively by lymphoscintigraphy. Once the lymph basin is identified and general or local anesthesia has been administered, 0.5 to 1 ml of a vital dye, such as patent blue-V or isosulfan blue, is injected intradermally with a 25-gauge needle at the site of the primary melanoma. Injections are repeated every 20 minutes during the procedure. If the primary lesion has already been removed, the injection is made on either side of the incision scar. Gentle massaging of the injection sites moves the dye through the lymphatics. A small incision is made over the lymph basin into which the lesion is expected to drain, as determined by technetium lymphoscintigraphy, and the skin flap closest to the primary melanoma is dissected free of underlying tissue. The lymphatic channel, stained by the dye, can thus be visually identified, and by careful dissection it can be followed to the blue-stained sentinel node. The node is marked with a suture, excised, and sent for immediate frozen-section examination. After changing gloves and instruments, the surgeon excises the primary melanoma with radial margins of 2 to 3 cm. If metastasis is found in the frozen section, regional LND is carried out in standard fashion. Examination by immunohistochemical staining is preferred because it detects lymph node metastases at a higher frequency than does examination of conventional material.[34,35] However, if the sentinel node does not contain micrometastases, the procedure is halted and the patient is spared the costs and potential morbidity associated with regional LND.

Morton and colleagues recently reported their 4-year experience with intraoperative lymphatic mapping and SLND.[32] They were able to identify the sentinel node in 194 (82%) of 237 regional LND specimens. Of these specimens, 40 (21%) had metastases in at least one node. As expected, the overall incidence of metastases was significantly lower in patients with lesions thinner than 1.50 mm (9.8% versus 36.9% for lesions $\geq$ 1.5 mm). The incidence of metastases was one of 2.73 procedures when the lesions were thicker than 1.5 mm, but only one of every 10.2 procedures when the lesions were thinner than 1.5 mm. In the initial portion of the study, all patients underwent regional LND following identification of the sentinel node. Only 2 (0.06%) of 3079 nonsentinel nodes from 194 lymph basins were the exclusive site of metastases, a false-negative rate of 1 percent. At the time the study was reported, none of the patients with tumor-negative sentinel nodes had developed regional recurrence.

A number of technical aspects are important to the success of this procedure. Patent blue dye must be injected intradermally in order to avoid passage of dye through the deeper lymphatic channels along the veins. Extreme caution should be used when elevating the skin flaps, to prevent transection of lymphatic channels. The dye must be injected only in small volumes, and dye injection should be repeated every 20 minutes to prevent color loss from the sentinel node as dye progresses from this node to second-echelon nodes.

The highest success rate in identifying the drainage basins has been from primary lesions on the trunk or leg that drained to inguinal nodes. The sentinel node was located in 89 percent of groin dissections, 81 percent of cervical dissections, and 78 percent of axillary dissections. A sentinel lymph node was least often identified for primary lesions of the upper extremity, either on the arm draining to the axilla (68%) or on the shoulder draining to the neck (67%).

Complications associated with the use of dye for intraoperative mapping were infrequent and of little significance. All patients reported the presence of dye in their urine during the first 24 hours following the procedure. Only two patients had staining of the skin from residual dye. Overall, the rate of wound infection, seroma, and wound necrosis was less than 5 percent.

COMPLICATIONS OF LND

Most complications associated with LND are related to the wound itself, including infection, flap necrosis, seroma, and temporary nerve dysunction.[8,20,47,61–64] Although the complications are usually short term, they may prolong hospitalization. The severity and type of complication is related to the site of the node dissection. Generally, for example, there is minimal morbidity associated with axillary and neck dissections and rarely functional deficits. Axillary node dissection produces significant arm edema in approximately 1 percent of patients and wound seroma and infection relatively infrequently. Radical inguinal node dissection may, however, produce significant edema. This is particularly true when the iliac and obturator nodes are removed with the inguinal nodes and those of the femoral triangle. It is a debilitating complication for approximately 2 to 10 percent of patients. Urist and associates reported that 26 percent of patients experienced leg edema for 6 months or longer following dissection of inguinal nodes, but that only 8 percent suffered significant functional deficit.[8] Karakousis and colleagues reported no long-term edema in patients following axillary dissection.[63]

CONCLUSION

Support for ELND is based on the theory that melanoma metastasizes in a predictable and sequential fashion from the primary site through the lymphatics to the regional lymph nodes and then to distant sites. Rarely does metastatic disease bypass the regional lymph basins. For the past two decades there has been active debate in the literature regarding the efficacy of ELND. Support for the procedure is based on numerous retrospective and nonrandomized trials. The data do suggest that patients with intermediate-depth primary lesions may have an improved survival following the procedure. Up to 10 to 15 percent of patients may benefit from ELND. The results of the two randomized, prospective trials demonstrate a small survival advantage in those patients who underwent ELND. However, these trials were flawed by a sample size that may have been inadequate to prove statistical significance. Recently, Morton and associates reviewed their long-term follow-up of over 5000 patients treated at the John Wayne Cancer Institute.[65] Only 2.5 percent of patients had late (> 10 years) recurrences. Significantly, half of these relapses occurred in nodal basins not managed with ELND. The long-term follow-up of other groups may support the notion that ELND is necessary to prevent these late recurrences.

Morton and colleagues have introduced intraoperative lymphatic mapping and SLND as a minimally invasive technique to identify subclinical lymph node metastases in clinical Stage I melanoma patients and thereby limit regional LND to those patients for whom it is most appropriate.

Until the results of the newest randomized trials are completed and the technique of lymphatic mapping is standardized, we advocate ELND for clinical Stage I melanoma patients with intermediate-depth primary melanomas and those that are ulcerated or regressed. ELND provides a small but significant survival advantage in select patients but more importantly defines those patients who may be candidates for adjuvant therapies. Lymphoscintigraphy is used preoperatively for lesions arising on the axial trunk or head and neck. If no more than two lymph basins are identified, then ELND is performed.

Surgery is the mainstay of therapy for malignant melanoma. Numerous reports advocate the use of ELND. Newer methods of treatment including chemo- and immunotherapy are promising, but until an effective systemic therapy has been identified the regional lymph nodes should be managed by ELND.

REFERENCES

1. Balch CM, Murad TM, Soong SJ, Ingalls AL, Richards PC, and Maddox WA. Tumor thickness as a guide to surgical management of clinical stage I melanoma patients. *Cancer* 43:883–888, 1979.
2. Balch CM, Soong SJ, Milton GW, Shaw HM, McGovern VJ, Murad TM, McCarthy WH, and Maddox WA. A comparison of prognostic factors and surgical results in 1,786 patients with localized (stage I) melanoma treated in Alabama, USA, and New South Wales, Australia. *Ann Surg* 196:677–684, 1982.
3. Balch CM, Soong SJ, Murad TM, Ingalls AL, and Maddox WA. A multifactorial analysis of melanoma. II. Prognostic factors in patients with stage I (localized) melanoma. *Surgery* 86:343–351, 1979.
4. Balch CM. The role of elective lymph node dissection in melanoma: Rationale, results and controversies. *J Clin Oncol* 6:163–172, 1988.
5. Balch CM, Milton GW, Cascinelli N, and Sim FH. Elective lymph node dissection: Pros and Cons. In Balch CM, Houghton AN, Milton GW, et al (eds.), *Cutaneous Melanoma,* 2d ed. Philadelphia: JB Lippincott, 1992, 345–366.
6. Balch CM, Soong SJ, Murad TM, Ingalls AL, and Maddox WA. A multifactorial analysis of melanoma. III. Prognostic factors in melanoma patients with lymph node metastases (stage II). *Ann Surg* 193:377–388, 1981.
7. Roses DF, Provet JA, Harris MN, Gumport SL, and Dubin N. Prognosis of patients with pathologic stage II cutaneous melanoma. *Ann Surg* 201:103–107, 1985.
8. Urist MM, Maddox WA, Kennedy JE, and Balch CM. Patient risk factors and surgical morbidity after regional lymphadenectomy in 204 melanoma patients. *Cancer* 51:2152–2156, 1983.
9. Calabro A, Singletary SE, and Balch CM. Patterns of relapse in 1001 consecutive patients with melanoma nodal metastases. *Arch Surg* 124:1051–1055, 1989.
10. Cohen MH, Ketcham AS, Felix EL, Li SH, Tomaszewski MM, Costa J, Rabson AS, Simon RM, and Rosenberg SA. Prognostic factors in patients undergoing lymphadenectomy for malignant melanoma. *Ann Surg* 186:635–642, 1977.
11. Veronesi U, Adamus J, Bandiera DC, Brennhovd IO, Caceres E, Casinelli N, Claudio F, Ikonopisov RL, Javorski VV, Kirov S, Kulakowski A, Lacour J, Lejeune F, Mechl Z, Morabito A, Rodé I, Sergeev S, Slooten E v, Szczygiel K, Trapeznikov NN, and Wagner RI. Stage I melanoma of the limbs. Immediate versus delayed node dissection. *Tumori* 66:373–396, 1980.
12. Snow HL. Melanotic cancerous disease. *Lancet* 2:872–874, 1892.
13. Eve F. A lecture on melanoma. *The Practitioner* 70:165–174, 1903.
14. Handley WS. The pathology of melanotic growths in relation to their operative treatment: Lecture I & II. *Lancet* 1:927–935, 996–1003, 1907.
15. Pringle JH. A method of operation in cases of melanotic tumours of the skin. *Edinburgh Med J* 23:496–499, 1908.
16. Pack GT, Scharnagel I, and Morfit M. The principle of excision and dissection in continuity for primary and metastatic melanoma of the skin. *Surgery* 17:849–866, 1945.
17. Pack GT, Gerber DM, and Scharnagel IM. End results in the treatment of malignant melanoma. A report of 1190 cases. *Ann Surg* 136:905–911, 1952.
18. Cochran AJ, Wen DR, and Morton DL. Management of the regional lymph nodes in patients with cutaneous malignant melanoma. *World J Surg* 16:214–221, 1992.
19. Crowley NJ, and Seigler HF. The role of elective lymph node dissection in the management of patients with thick cutaneous melanoma. *Cancer* 66:2522–2527, 1990.
20. Gumport SL, and Harris MN. Results of regional lymph node dissection for melanoma. *Ann Surg* 179:105–108, 1974.
21. Holmes EC, Moseley HS, Morton DL, Clark W, Robinson D, and Urist MM. A rational approach to the surgical management of melanoma. *Ann Surg* 186:481–490, 1977.
22. Milton GW, Shaw HM, Cascinelli N, Santinami M, and Belli F. Elective lymph node dissection for melanoma: Two perspectives. *World J Surg* 16:203–213, 1992.
23. Reintgen DS, Cox EB, McCarty KS Jr, Vollmer RT, and Seigler HF. Efficacy of elective lymph node dissection in patients with intermediate thickness primary melanoma. *Ann Surg* 198:379–385, 1983.
24. Sim FH, Taylor WF, Pritchard DJ, and Soule EH. Lymphadenectomy in the management of stage I malignant melanoma: A prospective randomized study. *Mayo Clin Proc* 61:697–705, 1986.
25. Veronesi U, Adamus J, Bandiera DC, Brennhovd IO, Caceres E, Casinelli N, Claudio F, Ikonopisov RL, Javorski VV, Kirov S, Kulakowski A, Lacour J, Lejeune F, Mechl Z, Morabito A, Rodé I, Sergeev S, Slooten E v, Szczygiel K, Trapeznikov NN, and Wagner RI. Inefficacy of immediate node dissection in stage I melanoma of the limbs. *N Engl J Med* 297:627–630, 1977.
26. Menhert JH, and Heard JL. Staging of malignant melanomas by depth of invasion: A proposed index to prognosis. *Am J Surg* 110:168–176, 1965.
27. Breslow A. Tumor thickness, level of invasion and node dissection in stage I cutaneous melanoma. *Ann Surg* 182:572–575, 1975.
28. Breslow A. Thickness, cross-sectional areas and depth of invasion in the prognosis of cutaneous melanoma. *Ann Surg* 172:902–908, 1970.
29. Callery C, Cochran AJ, Roe DJ, Rees W, Nathanson SD, Benedetti JK, Elashoff RM, and Morton DL. Factors prognostic in patients with malignant melanoma spread to the regional lymph nodes. *Ann Surg* 196:69–75, 1982.
30. Das Gupta TK. Results of treatment of 265 patients with primary cutaneous melanoma: A five-year prospective study. *Ann Surg* 186:201–209, 1977.
31. Morton DL, Wanek L, Nizze JA, Elashoff RM, and Wong JH. Improved long-term survival after lymphadenectomy of melanoma metastatic to regional nodes: Analysis of prognostic factors in 1134 patients from the John Wayne Cancer Clinic. *Ann Surg* 214:491–499, 1991.
32. Morton DL, Wen DR, Wong JH, Economou JS, Cagle LA, Storm FK, Foshag LJ, and Cochran AJ. Technical details of intraoperative lymphatic mapping for early stage melanoma. *Arch Surg* 127:392–399, 1992.
33. McNeer G, and Das Gupta TK. Prognosis in malignant melanoma. *Surgery* 56:512–518, 1964.
34. Cochran AJ, Wen DR, and Morton DL. Occult tumor cells in the lymph nodes of patients with pathological stage I malignant melanoma: An immunohistological study. *Am J Surg Pathol* 12:612–618, 1988.
35. Cochran AJ, Wen DR, and Herschman HR. Occult melanoma in lymph nodes detected by antiserum to S-100 protein. *Int J Cancer* 34:159–163, 1984.
36. Heller R, Becker J, and Wasselle J. Detection of submicroscopic lymph node metastases in patients with melanoma. *Arch Surg* 126:1455–1460, 1991.
37. McCarthy WH, Shaw HM, and Milton GW. Efficacy of elective lymph node dissection in 2,347 patients with clinical stage I malignant melanoma. *Surg Gyn Obstet* 161:575–580, 1985.

38. Milton GW, Shaw HM, McCarthy WH, Pearson L, Balch CM, and Soong SJ. Prophylactic lymph node dissection in clinical stage I cutaneous malignant melanoma: Results of surgical treatment in 1319 patients. *Br J Surg* 69:108–111, 1982.
39. Urist MM, Balch CM, Soong SJ, Milton GW, Shaw HM, McGovern VJ, Murad TM, McCarthy WH, and Maddox WA. Head and neck melanoma in 534 clinical stage I patients. A prognostic factors analysis and results of surgical treatment. *Ann Surg* 200:769–775, 1984.
40. Soong SJ, Shaw HM, Balch CM, McCarthy WH, Urist MM, and Lee JY. Predicting survival and recurrence in localized melanoma: A multivariate approach. *World J Surg* 16:191–195, 1992.
41. Balch CM, Murad TM, Soong SJ, Ingalls AL, Halpern NB, and Maddox WA. A multifactorial analysis of melanoma: Prognostic histopathological features comparing Clark's and Breslow's staging methods. *Ann Surg* 188:732–742, 1978.
42. Day CL Jr, Mihm MC Jr, Lew RA, Harris MN, Kopf AW, Fitzpatrick TB, Harrist TJ, Golomb FM, Postel A, Hennessey MD, Gumport SL, Raker JW, Malt RA, Cosimi AB, Wood WC, Roses DF, Gorstein F, Rigel D, Friedman RJ, Mintzis MM, and Sober AJ. Prognostic factors for patients with clinical stage I melanoma of intermediate thickness (1.51–3.99 mm). A conceptual model for tumor growth and metastasis. *Ann Surg* 195:35–43, 1982.
43. Day CL Jr, Mihm MC Jr, Sober AJ, Harris MN, Kopf AW, Fitzpatrick TB, Lew RA, Harrist TJ, Golomb FM, Postel A, Hennessey P, Gumport SL, Raker JW, Malt RA, Cosimi AB, Wood WC, Roses DF, Gorstein F, Rigel D, Friedman RJ, and Mintzis MM. Prognostic factors for melanoma patients with lesions 0.76–1.69 mm in thickness. An appraisal of "thin" level IV lesions. *Ann Surg* 195:30–34, 1982.
44. Esch EP vd, Cascinelli N, Preda F, Morabito A, and Bufalino R. Stage I melanoma of the skin: Evaluation of prognosis according to histologic characteristics. *Cancer* 48:1668–1673, 1981.
45. Soong SJ. A computerized mathematical model and scoring system for predicting outcome in patients with localized melanoma. In Balch CM, Houghton AN, Milton GW, et al (eds.), *Cutaneous Melanoma,* 2d ed. Philadelphia: JB Lippincott, 1992, 200–212.
46. Byers RM. Cervical and parotid node dissections. In Balch CM, Houghton AN, Milton GW, et al (eds.), *Cutaneous Melanoma,* 2d ed. Philadelphia: JB Lippincott, 1992, 376–383.
47. Coit DG, and Brennan MF. Extent of lymph node dissection in melanoma of the trunk or lower extremity. *Arch Surg* 124:162–166, 1989.
48. Essner R, Wong JH, Economou JS, and Morton DL. Prognostic significance of melanoma arising in the scalp. *Am J Surg* 156:314–317, 1988.
49. Karakousis CP, Emrich LJ, Driscoll DL, and Rao U. Survival after groin dissection for malignant melanoma. *Surgery* 109:119–126, 1991.
50. Hansen MG, and McCarten AB. Tumor thickness and lymphocyte infiltration in malignant melanoma of the head and neck. *Am J Surg* 128:557–569, 1974.
51. Block GE, and Hartwell SW. Malignant melanoma: A study of 217 cases. Part I: Epidemiology. *Ann Surg* 154:74–87, 1961.
52. Morton DL, Foshag LJ, Hoon DSB, Nizze JA, Famatiga E, Wanek LA, Chang C, Davtyan DG, Gupta RK, Elashoff R, and Irie RF. Prolongation of survival in metastatic melanoma after active specific immunotherapy with a new polyvalent melanoma vaccine. *Ann Surg* 216:463–482, 1992.
53. Veronesi U, Adamus J, Bandiera DC, Brennhovd IO, Caceres E, Casinelli N, Claudio F, Ikonopisov RL, Javorski VV, Kirov S, Kulakowski A, Lacour J, Lejeune F, Mechl Z, Morabito A, Rodé I, Sergeev S, Slooten E v, Szczygiel K, Trapeznikov NN, and Wagner RI. Delayed regional lymph node dissection is stage I melanoma of the skin of the lower extremities. *Cancer* 49:2420–2430, 1982.
54. W.H.O. Collaborating Centres for Evaluation of Methods of Diagnosis and Treatment of Melanoma (Chairman U. Veronesi): Metastatic spread of stage I melanoma of the skin. *Tumori* 69:449–454, 1983.
55. Lamki LM, and Logic JR. Defining lymphatic drainage patterns with cutaneous lymphoscintigraphy. In Balch CM, Houghton AN, Milton GW, et al (eds.), *Cutaneous Melanoma,* 2d ed. Philadelphia: JB Lippincott, 1992, 367–375.
56. Norman J, Cruse CW, Espinosa C, Cox C, Berman C, Clark R, Saba H, Wells K, and Reintgen D. Redefinition of cutaneous lymphatic drainage with the use of lymphoscintigraphy for malignant melanoma. *Am J Surg* 162:432–437, 1991.
57. Robinson DS, Sample WF, Fee HJ, Holmes EC, and Morton DL. Regional lymphatic drainage in primary malignant melanoma of the trunk determined by colloidal gold scanning. *Surg Forum* 28:147–148, 1977.
58. Sherman A, and Ter-Pogossian M. Lymph node concentration of radioactive colloid gold following interstitial injection. *Cancer* 6:1238–1240, 1953.
59. Fee HJ, Robinson DS, Sample WF, Graham LS, Holmes EC, and Morton DL. The determination of lymph shed by colloidal gold scanning in patients with malignant melanoma: A preliminary study. *Surgery* 84:626–632, 1978.
60. Wanebo HJ, Harpole D, and Teates CD. Radionuclide lymphoscintigraphy with technetium 99m antimony sulfide colloid to identify lymphatic drainage of cutaneous melanoma at ambiguous sites in the head and neck and trunk. *Cancer* 55:1403–1413, 1985.
61. Baas PC, Koops HS, Hoekstra HJ, Bruggen JJ v, Weele LT, and Oldhoff J. Groin dissection in the treatment of lower-extremity melanoma, short-term and long-term morbidity. *Arch Surg* 127:281–286, 1992.
62. Finck SJ, Giuliano AE, Mann BD, and Morton DL. Results of ilioinguinal dissection for stage II melanoma. *Ann Surg* 196:180–186, 1982.
63. Karakousis CP, Heiser MA, and Moore RH. Lymphedema after groin dissection. *Am J Surg* 145:205–208, 1983.
64. Shaw JHF, and Rumball EM. Complications and local recurrence following lymphadenectomy. *Br J Surg* 77:760–764, 1990.
65. Guenther JM, Wanek L, and Morton DL. Low incidence of melanoma recurrences after ten years. Presented at the March 1993 Annual Meeting of the Society of Surgical Oncology, Los Angeles, Calif.

Chapter 18

MANAGEMENT OF REGIONAL LYMPH NODE METASTASES*

Michael A. Warso and Tapas K. Das Gupta

MANAGEMENT OF REGIONAL LYMPH NODE METASTASES

The propensity for melanoma to metastasize to the lymph nodes is well-known. Numerous studies[1–4] have detailed the increasing incidence of lymph node metastases associated with increasing stage and thickness of the primary tumor.[1] The incidence ranges from up to 10 percent in tumors less than 0.75 mm to about 67 percent in tumors greater than 4.00 mm in thickness. Balch in 1980 reported that, for thin melanomas (less than 1.50 mm), the incidence of lymph node metastases is under 10 percent.[4] This was further broken down by Holmes et al.,[1] who reported an incidence of lymph node metastases of 15 percent in lesions 0.77 to 1.50 mm thick. Incidence of metastases increases progressively, both by Clark's level and Breslow thickness. The percentage of patients with pathologically positive nodes by the time their melanoma reaches Clark's level V is 58 to 90 percent.[1–3] Similarly, the percentage of metastases in patients with melanomas greater than 4.00 mm in thickness and positive regional nodes is 67 percent.[5] Overall, in several studies, the incidence of patients with clinical Stage I melanoma who develop regional nodal metastases ranges from 15 to 32 percent.[5–8]

There are several other factors which have been shown to be predictive of the development of lymph node metastases. In general, these parallel the factors which are known to be of prognostic value in terms of overall survival (see Chap. 14, The Influence of Prognosis Factors on Melanoma Management). Sex, either by itself or in combination with age, was a factor in the studies done by Berdeaux et al.[5] and Eastwood and Baker.[7] Other indices which have been shown to be of variable importance include the presence of ulceration, the histologic type, and pathologic features.

Once lymph node metastases are apparent, other factors can be used to determine the relative risk of recurrence (see Chapter 14). These include the amount of disease in the regional nodes, that is, whether it is microscopic or macroscopic and the number of positive nodes, and the presence of extranodal disease. Overall survival in the presence of lymph node metastases largely depends on the clinical stage of the patient and whether the nodal dissection was performed electively or therapeutically. Fortner et al.[8] in 1977 reported a 10-year survival of 42 percent in patients with positive nodes discovered at the time of elective node dissection, compared to only 6 percent in those patients who required a therapeutic dissection for clinically positive disease. Das Gupta[2] in the same year reported that 35 of 51 patients (69 percent) who had negative nodes clinically, but were pathologically positive, survived 5 years. This is con-

*From *Malignant Melanoma: The Approach of the Surgical Oncologist*

trasted with only a 13 percent survival if the nodes were clinically positive. In general, other published studies report similar figures. In 1977, however, the NCI reported a 50 percent incidence of 10-year survival in the presence of clinically positive lymph nodes[3] (Table 18-1).

Several controversies surround the procedure of lymph node dissection in melanoma. Those aspects which are of specific concern to the Surgical Oncologist include the timing of regional lymphadenectomy, the extent of dissection, and the management of regional nodes in cases where the primary tumor is in an area of ambiguous drainage. Elective lymph node dissection and dissection for cutaneous melanoma arising in areas of ambiguous lymphatic drainage are covered in other chapters (see Chap. 17, Elective Lymph Node Dissection). In general, we continue to recommend prophylactic lymph node dissection for intermediate thickness melanoma (1.00 to 4.00 mm) when the probability for microscopic metastasis is the highest in the nodes without high chance of systemic spread and will perform simultaneous dissections of two nodal groups in cases of ambiguous drainage. In all cases where lymph node dissections are performed for melanoma, there should be a total removal of the lymphatic tissue, because the operation is being performed for therapeutic reasons. Especially in the presence of a palpable lymph node, the majority of patients will have multiple involved lymph nodes.[13,14]

TABLE 18-1
SURVIVAL AFTER THERAPEUTIC LYMPH NODE DISSECTION

5-YEAR SURVIVAL		*10-YEAR SURVIVAL*	
REFERENCE	%	*REFERENCE*	%
5	44	8	6
2	13	3	50
9	20	9	12
10	19		
11	13		
12	23		

COMPLICATIONS

As in most series reported for other conditions, the incidence of complications secondary to lymph node dissections depends on the site and extent of dissection. Overall, the most common complication is the presence of a postoperative lymphatic collection, or "seroma." For all sites, the second most common complication was reported to be nerve dysfunction by Urist et al.[15] in 1983. The report by Bland et al.[16] reaffirms the fact that a significant number of patients suffer local complications. Their rates, by site, are 37 percent for the neck, 50 percent for the axilla, and 59 percent for superficial groin dissection. The factors which contributed to a higher incidence of complications were age greater than 50 and obesity, especially in the group undergoing a cervical node dissection. Most series report a mortality rate of or close to zero percent. The rate of complications unrelated to the local operation has been reported to be 6.4 percent and includes other infections, myocardial infarctions, and pulmonary embolism.[15]

The data must be examined in a site-specific manner to fully understand the problem of complications. Although cervical node dissections do not usually result in postoperative edema, there is another series of problems unique to the site. As the type of operation performed changes from a classical radical neck dissection to a modified operation with preservation of the spinal accessory nerve, the incidence of morbidity from resection of vital structures decreases, especially the problems related to nerve dysfunction. Urist et al.[15] reported an incidence of nerve dysfunction of 19 percent, compared to a 21 percent incidence of transient nerve dysfunction reported by Vaglini et al.[17] when a superficial parotidectomy was added to the procedure. The other common complications range from 0 to 4 percent for infection, 0 to 10 percent for skin slough, and 3.4 to 17 percent for fluid collections. Long-term complications occur in a minority of the patients.[15,16,18]

Seromas are by far the most common complication after axillary dissection for melanoma, occurring in about 26 to 30 percent of the patients.[16,19] Other common complications are distinctly less prevalent. Necrosis of the edges of the skin flaps almost never occurs, and wound infection appears to be a problem in fewer than 10 percent in most reports,[1,15,19] although Bland et al. report flap necrosis and wound infection in 18 of 87 patients.[16] The incidence of postoperative pain varies significantly between different reports.[15,19] Edema of the arm is relatively uncommon, ranging from 1 to 12 percent, and is not disabling in any patients in these studies.

The most striking fact about the complications following groin dissection is the higher incidence of postoperative edema. The incidence of edema appears to be the same whether an inguinal or ilioinguinal nodal dissection has been performed, ranging from 22 to 41 percent. McCarthy et al. report a six times higher incidence in patients undergoing an ilioinguinal dissection compared to a superficial groin dissection.[20] However, most cases of edema appear to be mild to moderate, with only 10 percent experiencing any alteration in lifestyle due to the operation. Only two series reported any incidence of severe edema, and in both instances it was only 2 percent.[15,23] Those complications which are common

TABLE 18-2
COMPLICATIONS IN GROIN DISSECTION

REFERENCE	INFECTION (%)	SEROMA (%)	FLAP NECROSIS (%)	EDEMA (SEVERE) (%)
SUPERFICIAL				
15	5	23	2	26 (2)
21	18	24	12	29 (0)
22	5	12	7	23 (0)
ILIOINGUINAL				
21	18	18	14	41 (0)
22	16	8	7	25 (0)
23	10	28	19	22 (2)

to node dissections at other sites occur with similar frequencies, and, except for Holmes et al.,[1] who report that the majority of their major complications occurred in patients undergoing an ilioinguinal node dissection, most series show no differences related to the extent of the dissection. Wound infections occur in 5 to 18 percent, fluid collections in 8 to 28 percent, and flap necrosis in 2 to 19 percent of the patients.[1,15,21–23] This amounts to some form of wound-related complication in up to 47 percent of the patients.[16] The incidence of wound complications is related partially to technique and, thus, can be reduced with attention to detail and experience, as can be seen by comparing two series done at different times in the same institution[21,22] (Table 18-2).

In general, while there are complications associated with complete node dissection, these are manageable and rarely result in functional impairment.

SPECIAL CONSIDERATIONS

Head and Neck

Although there is a great deal of controversy surrounding the efficacy of elective lymph node dissection for cutaneous melanoma of the head and neck, there is agreement that, in the presence of clinically involved nodes, a dissection should be performed. It is important in these cases to pay special attention to the technique, as up to 13 percent of patients may have recurrence within the operative field.[24] We have identified those areas that should be of specific concern as those near the base of the skull and the infraparotid area.[25]

The completeness of the lymph node dissection is important due to the possibility of so-called "skip" metastases. Although Roses et al.[26] reported involvement in the draining nodes closest to the primary in all patients, we have failed to verify these findings and have several patients with skip metastases.[25]

It is known that the lymphatic drainage of certain cutaneous areas of the face and scalp includes the nodes within the parotid gland. These areas include the eyelid, posterior cheek, anterior ear, and frontal and temporal scalp. Vaglini et al.[17] have specifically looked at the advisability of removing the intraparotid nodes when a melanoma arises in any of these sites. Their review showed that, of 16 patients who had cutaneous primaries in the areas mentioned and palpable nodes, 31 percent had involvement of the intraparotid nodal group. Conversely, 27 percent of the patients who had clinical evidence of disease in the intraparotid lymph nodes had metastases elsewhere in the neck. These results make a strong case for adding a superficial parotidectomy to the neck dissection in those cases where the primary site is one of those at risk. (see Fig. 18-1.)

Groin

Most commonly, patients with groin node metastases will present with palpable nodes along the femoral vessels, which would be removed by a superficial groin dissection. The therapeutic benefit of adding an iliac and obturator dissection has been questioned. In patients with pathologically negative superficial groin nodes, the possibility of pelvic nodal disease is still present. Das Gupta[2] reported that, in the presence of negative femoral nodes, 7 of 74 patients still had positive iliac nodes, and Coit and Brennan[27] report a similar situation in only 3 percent of their patients. In general, however, those factors which are predictive of metastases to the

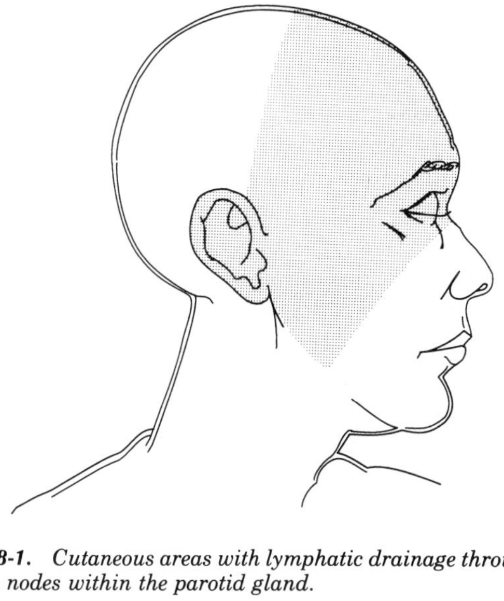

FIG. 18-1. *Cutaneous areas with lymphatic drainage through the lymph nodes within the parotid gland.*

pelvic nodes are the clinical stage of the patient, the pathologic status of Cloquet's node, and the number of positive superficial nodes.[27] The percentage of patients with positive iliac nodes increases from between 12 and 15 percent with one node positive to about 50 percent when more than three nodes are positive below the inguinal ligament.[27,28]

Although the prognosis of patients with positive pelvic nodes is poor, the presence of metastases in the iliac nodes is by no means fatal. Only McCarthy et al.[20] report no survivors among their patients with positive pelvic nodes. The highest survival rate reported is 30 percent at 5 years,[22] although most investigators reported survival in the range of 3 to 9 percent.[27–29]

We believe that all patients undergoing a lymph node dissection for palpable disease on the groin should have a complete ilioinguinal dissection. This dissection must entail removal of the obturator as well as the iliac nodes: these can be positive in up to 23 percent of patients with positive pelvic nodes and may be the only site of disease in some.[30]

Axilla

The technique of axillary node dissection is a common knowledge, but there are still points that should be made in reference to nodal dissection for melanoma. It is important to perform a complete axillary dissection, extending from the latissimus dorsi muscle all the way to the chest wall and encompassing all three levels as well as the supra-axillary fat pad, for total nodal clearance.[31]

Removal of the pectoralis minor muscle is required only when necessary for exposure and ease of dissection. The need to excise portions of the muscles, the long thoracic nerve, or the thoracodorsal nerve should be limited to rare instances where it is required for total removal of the tumor.

CONCLUSIONS

Palpable nodal metastases from a cutaneous melanoma should be treated with a complete dissection of the nodal group involved. Morbidity can be kept to a minimum with proper attention to technique and postoperative care. In the presence of the disease in the femoral nodes, a radical groin dissection should be performed. Neck dissection for melanoma arising in the appropriate areas of the scalp and face should take into consideration the removal of intraparotid lymph nodes.

REFERENCES

1. Holmes EC, Moseley HS, Morton DL, Clark, W, Robinson D, and Urist, MM. A rational approach to the surgical management of melanoma. *Ann Surg* 481–490, 1977.
2. Das Gupta TK. Results of treatment of 269 patients with primary cutaneous melanoma: A five-year prospective study. *Ann Surg* 186:201–209, 1977.
3. Cohen MH, Ketcham AS, Felix EL, Li S, Tomaszewski M, Costa J, Rabson AS, Simon RM, and Rosenberg SA. Prognostic factors in patients undergoing lymphadenectomy for malignant melanoma. *Ann Surg* 186:635–642, 1977.
4. Balch CM. Surgical management of regional lymph nodes in cutaneous melanoma. *J Am Acad Dermatol* 3:511–524, 1980.
5. Berdeaux, DH, Meyskens FL Jr, Parks B, Tong T, Loescher L, and Moon TE. Cutaneous malignant melanoma. *Cancer* 63:1430–1436, 1989.
6. Balch CM, Murad TM, Soong S, Ingalls AL, Richards PC, and Maddox WA. Tumor thickness as a guide to surgical management of clinical stage I melanoma patients. *Cancer* 43:883–888, 1979.
7. Eastwood J, and Baker TG. Cutaneous malignant melanoma in West Yorkshire: A prospective study of recurrence and prediction of lymph node metastases. *Br J Cancer* 50:35–43, 1984.
8. Fortner JG, Woodruff J, Schottenfeld D, and MacLean B. Biostatistical basis of elective node dissection for malignant melanoma. *Ann Surg* 186:101–103, 1977.
9. Roses DF, Provet JA, Harris MN, Gumport SL, and Dubin N. Prognosis of patients with pathologic stage II cutaneous malignant melanoma. *Ann Surg* 201:103–107, 1985.
10. McNeer G, and Das Gupta T. Prognosis in malignant melanoma. *Surgery* 56:512–518, 1964.
11. Gumport SL, and Meyer HW. Treatment of 126 cases of malignant melanoma: Long term results. *Ann Surg* 150:989–992, 1959.
12. Southwick HW, Slaughter DP, Hinkamp JF, and Johnson FE. The role of regional node dissection in the treatment of malignant melanoma. *Ann Surg* 85:79–85, 1962.
13. Balch CM, Soong S, Murad TM, Ingalls AL, and Maddox WA. A multifactorial analysis of melanoma: III. Prognostic factors in melanoma patients with lymph node metastases (stage II). *Ann Surg* 193:377–387, 1981.
14. Kane M, McClay E, and Bellet RE. Frequency of occult residual melanoma after excision of a clinically positive regional lymph node. *Ann Surg* 205:88–89, 1987.
15. Urist MM, Maddox WA, Kennedy JE, and Balch CM. Patient risk factors and surgical morbidity after regional lymphadenectomy in 204 melanoma patients. *Cancer* 51:2152–2156, 1983.
16. Bland KI, Klamer TW, Polk HC Jr, and Knutson CO. Isolated regional lymph node dissection: Morbidity, mortality and economic considerations. *Ann Surg* 193:372–376, 1981.
17. Vaglini M, Belli F, Santinami M, and Cascinelli N. The role of parotidectomy in the treatment of nodal metastases from cutaneous melanoma of the head and neck. *Eur J Surg Onc* 16:28–32, 1990.
18. Turkula LD, and Woods JE. Limited or selective nodal dissection for malignant melanoma of the head and neck. *Am J Surg* 148:446–448, 1984.
19. Harris MN, Gumport SL, and Maiwandi H. Axillary lymph node dissection for melanoma. *Surg Gynecol Obstet* 135:936–940, 1972.
20. McCarthy JG, Haagensen CD, and Herter FP. The role of groin dissection in the management of melanoma of the lower extremity. *Ann Surg* 179:156–159, 1974.
21. Dasmahapatra KS, and Karakousis CP. Therapeutic groin dissection in malignant melanoma. *Surg Gynecol Obstet* 156:21–24, 1983.
22. Karakousis CP, Emrich LJ, Rao U. Groin dissection in malignant melanoma. *Am J Surg* 152:491–495, 1986.

23. Harris MN, Gumport SL, Berman IR, and Bernard RW. Ilioinguinal lymph node dissection for melanoma. *Surg Gynecol Obstet* 136:33–39, 1973.
24. Byers RM. The role of modified neck dissection in the treatment of cutaneous melanoma of the head and neck. *Arch Surg* 121:1338–1341, 1986.
25. Briele HA, Walker MJ, and Das Gupta TK. Melanoma of the head and neck. *Clin Plast Surg* 12:495–504, 1985.
26. Roses DF, Harris MN, Grunberger I, and Gumport SL. Selective surgical management of cutaneous melanoma of the head and neck. *Ann Surg* 192:629–632, 1980.
27. Coit DG, and Brennan MF. Extent of lymph node dissection in melanoma of the trunk or lower extremity. *Arch Surg* 124:162–166, 1989.
28. Finck SJ, Giuliano AE, Mann BD, and Morton DL. Results of ilioinguinal dissection for stage II melanoma. *Ann Surg* 196:180–186, 1982.
29. Fortner JG, Booher RJ, and Pack GT. Results of groin dissection for malignant melanoma in 220 patients. *Surgery* 55:485–494, 1964.
30. Karakousis CP. Ilioinguinal lymph node dissection. *Am J Surg* 141:299–303, 1981.
31. Karakousis CP, and Rao U. Axillary node dissection in malignant melanoma. *Surg Gynecol Obstet* 152:507–509, 1981.

Chapter 19

MANAGEMENT OF LOCAL RECURRENCE, SATELLITES, AND IN TRANSIT METASTASES OF THE LIMBS WITH ISOLATION PERFUSION

H. Schraffordt Koops, B.B.R. Kroon, and F.J. Lejeune

INTRODUCTION

The principle of regional perfusion using cytostatic drugs resulted from a study by Klopp et al. in 1950,[1] who found that pain was alleviated and tumor size reduced when small doses of nitrogen mustard (chlormethine) were injected into the regional arterial blood flow. The best results were obtained when venous return from the area involved was blocked. In 1959, Creech et al.[2] combined this procedure with extracorporeal circulation, using a pump oxygenator.

In 1960, Stehlin et al.[3] reported 116 regional perfusions performed at the MD Anderson Hospital in Houston. The majority of patients had tumors of the extremities; the remainder had tumors of the pelvic region and the head and neck area. Luck[4] discovered that melphalan (L-phenylalanine mustard) was the most active agent to inhibit the growth of malignant melanoma in mice; this has since been the agent of choice for perfusions. In 1967, Cavaliere et al.[5] laid the foundation for perfusions under hyperthermia when they described the selective susceptibility of cancer cells to high temperatures.

Favorable results with regional limb perfusion have been reported by numerous investigators.[6–28] Perfusion of melanomas located in other parts of the body is not possible because leakage to the systemic circulation could become excessive and the advantage of regional perfusion—high local dosage of the cytostatic agents without systemic toxic reactions—is lost.

INDICATIONS FOR PERFUSION

The first indication for perfusion has historically been the in-transit metastases not amenable to surgery. The response rate is such that it has already been recognized for 30 years as a limb salvage procedure. Since good results were obtained in stage II, IIIA, and IIIAB of malignant melanoma, attempts have been made to use isolation perfusion to reduce the rate of recurrence and to improve survival in high-risk primary cases.

Indications for perfusion in clinical stage I patients are determined by microstaging (level and thickness). Perfusion may be indicated for patients with high-risk tumors such as melanomas with a Clark level IV or V invasion and a Breslow thickness of > 1.5 mm. Retrospective studies in these groups of patients however, gave conflicting results.[7,8,19] The value of adjuvant perfusion in stage I patients is now being tested in a prospective phase III randomized clinical trial (under auspices of the EORTC and WHO). In our opinion, the prognosis for the patients with a tumor thickness of < 1.5 mm is so good and the risk of local recurrence so small that excision without perfusion should suffice.

PERFUSION TECHNIQUE

General endotracheal anesthesia is used. Lower limb perfusions are performed via the external iliac artery and vein; the vessels are approached through the retroperitoneal space (Fig. 19-1). A lymph node dissection is first performed. The value of this procedure is that it removes the iliac and obturator lymph nodes and permits full exposure of the vessels to be cannulated. For iliac perfusion, the inferior epigastric, deep circumflex iliac vessels, and obturator vein are ligated or clipped, and the internal iliac artery is temporarily occluded. These vessel occlusions are a prerequisite for obtaining optimal isolation of the lower limb.

The patient is heparinized (3.3 mg/kg body weight), and after 2 minutes the vessels are occluded.

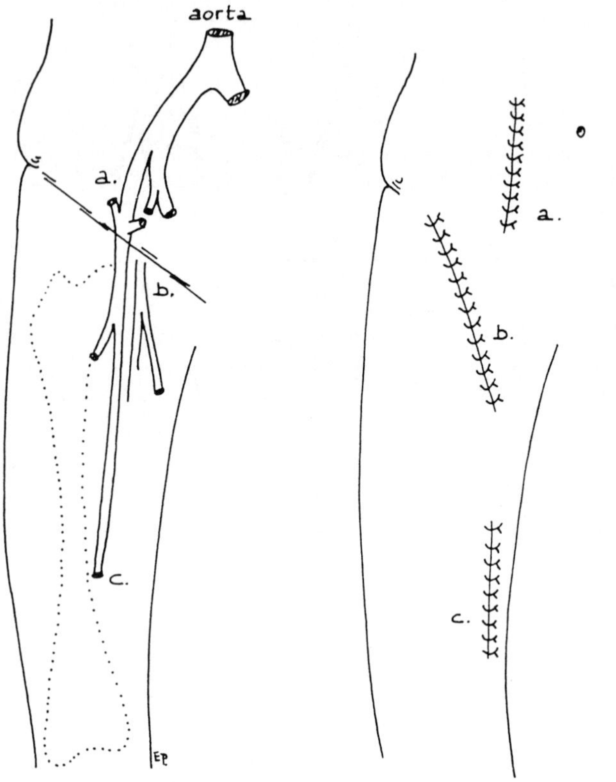

FIG. 19-1. *Technique of lower extremity perfusion. a = iliac perfusion via the external iliac artery and vein, b = lymph node dissection and femoral perfusion, c = popliteal perfusion.*

Flexible vinyl catheters are introduced into the external iliac artery and vein (Fig. 19-2).

Collateral vessels of the skin, especially those situated posteriorly, are occluded with the aid of a bandage. A pin is inserted into the iliac crest and a rubber bandage is twisted around this pin and the upper thigh. The tips of the catheters should be located just caudal to this bandage. The isolated limb is given an artificial circulation by means of an extracorporeal circuit containing a pump oxygenator and a heat exchanger (Fig. 19-3). The required flow rates for perfusion have to depend on limb volume, vessel size, and the calibre of the catheters. In the past few years, it was learned from experiments on the dogs that tissue perfusion during extracorporeal circulation differs from that in the nonperfused limb.[29] Adequate tissue oxygenation could be maintained only when the perfusion pressure was not lower than 15 mm Hg below systemic mean arterial pressure. During the past years, high flow rates (up to about 1200 ml/min) have been tested in the Groningen hospital with less toxicity and better tissue perfusion. Consequently, the dosage of cytostatic drugs could be increased. An additional advantage of high flows is that high tissue temperatures are attained more

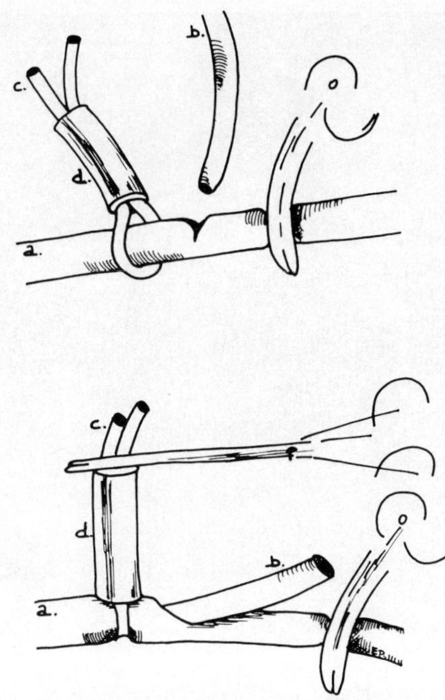

FIG. 19-2. *Technique of catheter cannulation into the vessel. a = vessel, b = catheter, c = rubber tape, d = rubber tubings.*

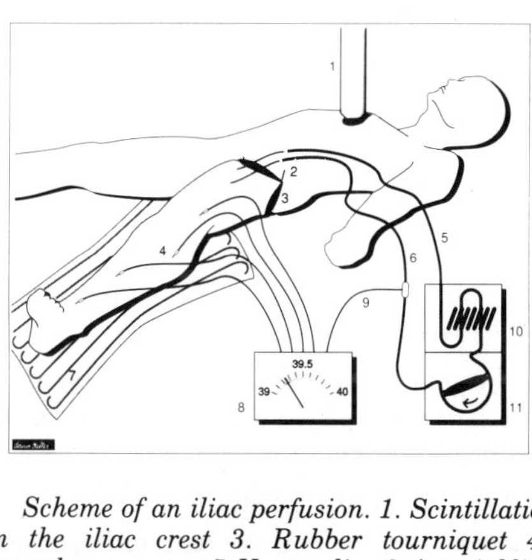

FIG. 19-3. *Scheme of an iliac perfusion. 1. Scintillation detector 2. Pin in the iliac crest 3. Rubber tourniquet 4. Muscle/subcutaneous thermometers 5. Venous line 6. Arterial line 7. Warm water blanket 8. Temperature measurement 9. Temperature arterial blood 10. Bubble oxygenator and heat-exchanger 11. Single roller pump.*

quickly. Inadequate low flow rates are usually the result of improper placement of the catheters or malpositioning of the tourniquet and can be corrected by proper adjustment.

Limb temperatures are monitored by four thermistor probes inserted through the skin into the subcutaneous tissue and the muscles of the upper and lower half of the leg. The administration of the drug is started when the subcutaneous tissue temperature of the lower part of the leg reaches 38°C. External heat loss is prevented by wrapping the limb in a sterile water circulation blanket adjusted to the required temperature. In cytostatic perfusion we prefer not to exceed tissue temperatures of 40°C.

Any leakage to the systemic circulation must be monitored carefully, due to the extremely high-drug concentration in the isolated region (for Melphalan for instance up to 20-fold the maximum tolerated concentration systematically can be attained locally). For this purpose a small calibration dose of ^{131}I-albumin is injected into the systemic circulation, while a larger dose is injected into the perfusate (10 times the calibration dose). Leakage from the perfusion region to the remainder of the body is indicated by the increase of radioactivity in the systemic circulation, measured by means of a scintillation detector placed over the heart. Unexpected excessive leakage can be detected quantitatively, and immediate corrective measures can be taken.

The cytostatic is injected either into the oxygenator or gradually into the arterial line (for example during one circulation time of the circuit) so that mixing can occur quickly. At completion of the perfusion, a wash-out is performed to remove drug and toxic end products from the isolated area. The tourniquet is released, the catheters are withdrawn, and the vessels repaired. The heparinization is reversed with protamine sulfate. At completion of the operation, a prophylactic fasciotomy of the lateral compartment of the lower leg is performed in some institutes to prevent compression of nerves as a result of muscle edema.[30]

For femoral perfusions, the catheters are introduced immediately below Poupart's ligament; this technique is used only after an inguinal lymph node dissection. For popliteal perfusion, the catheters are introduced at the level of the adductor canal. The technique for femoral and popliteal perfusion is the same as that for an iliac perfusion.

For upper limb perfusion the proximal portion of the axillary artery and vein is exposed (Fig. 19-4). An axillary lymph node dissection is performed because follow-up examination of the axilla has been difficult and unreliable due to the presence of scar tissue caused by the perfusion operation. With the aim of occluding collateral vessels of the skin, a pin is inserted into the head of the humerus, and a rubber bandage is twisted around this pin and the upper arm. Introduction of the catheters into the brachial vessels may be considered when a second perfusion becomes necessary.

It is our practice to perfuse arm and leg locations for 60 minutes after the cytostatic drug has been injected.

Anticoagulation is begun the day after perfusion and continued until the patient can walk normally. Antibiotics are not routinely given.

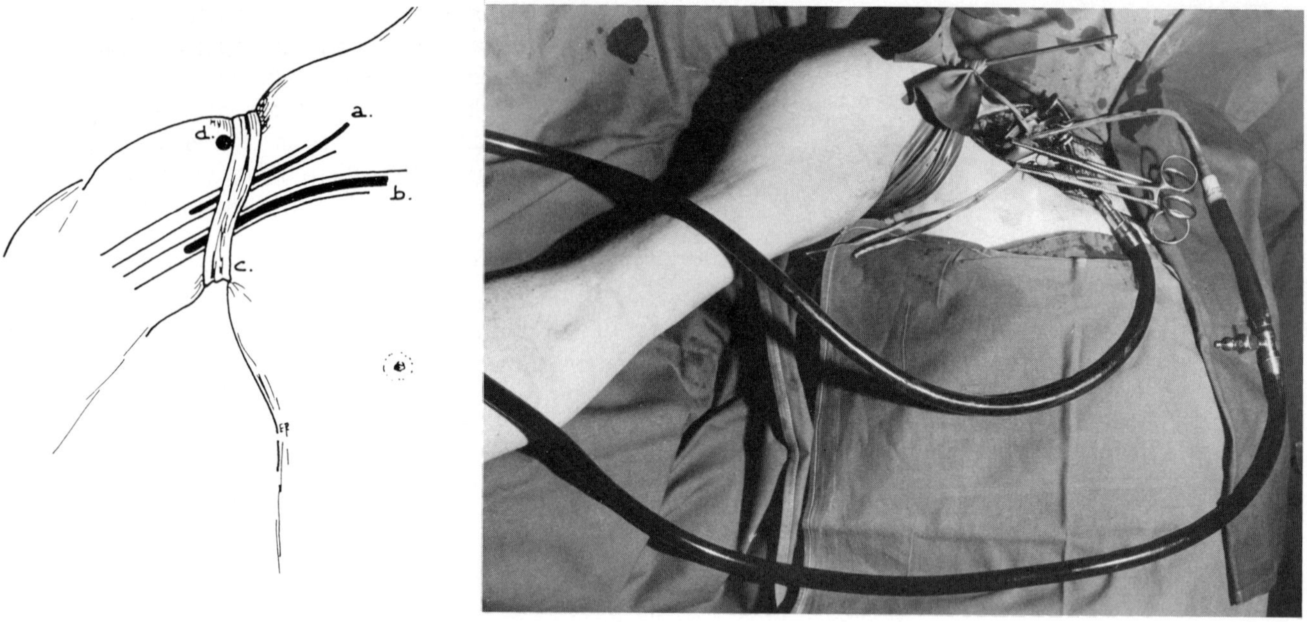

FIG. 19-4. *Technique of upper extremity perfusion. a = arterial catheter, b = venous catheter, c = Esmarch bandage, d = Steinmann pin in the head of the humerus.*

CHEMOTHERAPEUTIC AGENTS

Melphalan (L-phenylalanine mustard) is the drug most widely used for regional perfusion for melanoma, either alone or in combination with other drugs. Melphalan was originally selected for perfusion therapy since phenylalanine, a metabolite of melanin, is thought to deliver the attached cytotoxic alkylating radicals into the melanin-producing neoplastic cell.[4]

In our institutes and for current international protocols, the melphalan dosage is calculated on the basis of the limb volume, which is determined by immersion of the limb in water. Using this method, the toxic reactions of the skin appear to be remarkably less variable than what was formally experienced when the dose was calculated on the basis of total body weight. The latter method, namely, does not take into account the wide variation of limb volumes that can be found for the same body weight.[31] On the basis of a grading system for toxic reactions of the normal tissues, a melphalan dose of 10 mg/l perfused tissue has proved to be the maximum dose that is well tolerable. It is advised to perfuse regions smaller than 3.5 litres (mostly arms in which toxicity was indeed experienced to be less) with a larger dose of melphalan: 13 mg/l perfused tissue. This dose has been shown to give the same drug toxicity into small tissue volumes as the 10 mg/l dose in larger volumes.[32] An alternative and more precise way for cytostatic dosimetry is based on the calculation of the perfusate volume—that is, volume of the limb vascular bed + extracorporeal volume—according to the hematocrit method.[33] With this it was shown that for lower limb perfusions the dose of 10 mg/l will provide a mean melphalan concentration of 40 μg/ml of perfusate and that for upper limb perfusions using a melphalan dose of 13 mg/l, this concentration is 20 μg/ml. Details of this alternative dosimetric method are described in Chap. 21.

COMPLICATIONS

A tissue reaction of the extremity is seen about 2 days after perfusion. In most cases, the perfused extremity is red, warm, and slightly edematous. The red discoloration fades to brown which gradually, over about 3 months, turns to light brown. After about 6 months, there is no visible evidence of the changes due to perfusion. In a few cases, other local manifestations are seen (e.g., temporary loss of nails, drying or blistering of skin of palms or soles, and inhibition of hair growth on the extremity). These reactions and other local manifestations must all be taken as normal to be expected side effects of the cytostatic treatment. With increased experience and improvement of isolation techniques, the true complication of severe bone marrow depression (i.e., leucopenia and thrombocytopenia) no longer occurs in our patients.

The most common vascular complications described in the literature are thrombophlebitis, venous thrombosis, and pulmonary emoblism. It seems plausible that large heparin doses used during our perfusions and postoperative anticoagulant medication limit these complications, because they are very uncommon in our patients.

During the period 1965 to 1985, 295 stage I patients were treated in Groningen with 347 perfusions. Three patients died; two had diffuse intravascular coagulation of unknown origin a few hours after perfusion; another died of cerebral hemorrhage some days after perfusion. Two patients developed pulmonary embolism long after operation (7 and 8 months, respectively), and one of these was fatal. In two patients, amputation of the lower extremity was necessary because of serious burns following hyperthermic perfusion. These complications were seen only in the initial few years of perfusion experience.

THERAPEUTIC PERFUSION IN STAGE II, IIIA, AND IIIAB PATIENTS

To assess the value of a chemotherapeutic treatment modality, the method should first be tried in situations where measurable disease can be used to supply objective response evaluation. However, because most surgeons have excised all tumors present in the limb at the time of perfusion, thereby concentrating their attention on the end-point of survival, these data are rather scarce. In the literature on perfusion with melphalan in melanoma, an average remission rate—complete plus partial—of approximately 80 percent is described. Perfusions performed at the beginning of the perfusion era show lower remission rates. This may be attributed not only to the fact that most of these perfusions were probably performed under hypothermia, a condition which probably interferes with the effectiveness of chemotherapy, but also because the perfusion technique (e.g., flow rates, dosimetry, isolation) lacked its present sophistication. It is interesting to note that the response rate of normothermic perfusions (tissue temperatures between 37 and 38°C) (Plate 39) seems to be similar to that of perfusions performed under mildly hyperthermic conditions (tissue temperatures between 39 and 40°C).[34]

Survival rates after perfusion for patients with local recurrences, satellites, or in-transit metastases range from 29 to 80 percent, at 5 years and from 23 to 63 percent at 10 years, with a tendency to better survival in stage II patients and a worse survival in stage IIIAB patients (Table 19-1).[12,28,35–39]

For patients treated with surgery alone, 5-year survival rates vary from 9 to 50 percent, with one author reporting a better survival rate for patients with stage II disease.[40–43] During the period 1966 to 1986 in Groningen, 110 patients with local recurrence, satellites, or in-transit metastases (14 local recurrences, 22 satellites, 47 in-transit metastases, 27 recurrences with lymph node metastases) were treated exclusively by a combination of regional perfusion and wide excision. The total group included 89 females and 21 males. In 93 patients the tumor was localized in the leg, while 17 had a tumor of the arm. Melphalan was used as cytostatic and, since 1974, actinomycin-D as well as melphalan have been

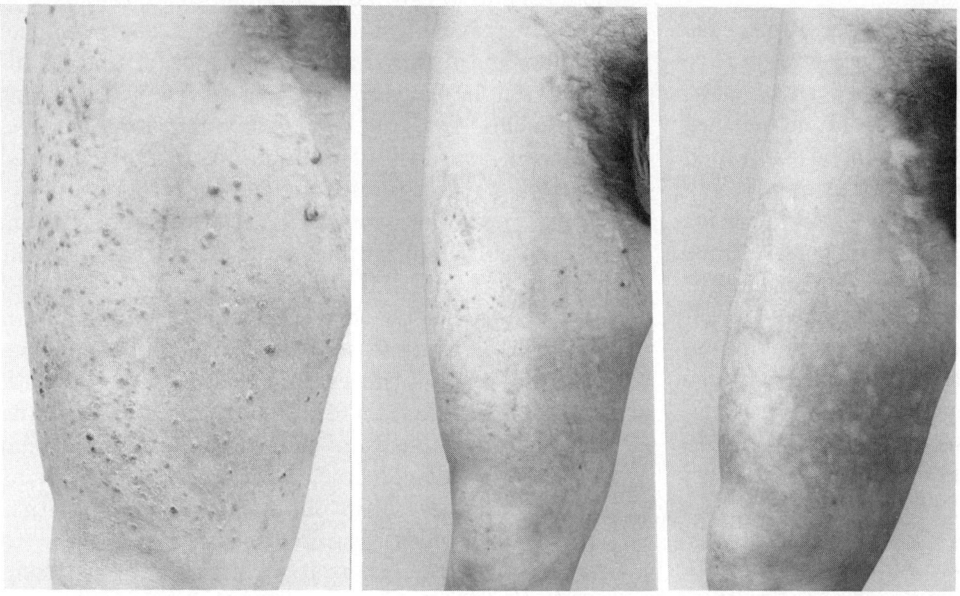

FIG. 19-5. In 1973 a 34-year-old man with intransit metastases of a malignant melanoma of the right upper leg with inguinal lymph node metastases was treated with an iliac perfusion. Six weeks later he had a groin dissection and femoral perfusion. After the perfusions all intransit metastases diminished. Left photograph 1 month after perfusion and groin dissection; middle photograph 13 months after perfusion, right photograph 29 months after perfusion. Patient is alive without recurrence in 1990.

TABLE 19-1

RESULTS OF REGIONAL PERFUSION IN PATIENTS WITH LOCAL RECURRENCE (II), IN-TRANSIT METASTASES (IIIA), AND LOCAL RECURRENCE AND/OR IN-TRANSIT METASTASES + POSITIVE LYMPH NODES (IIIAB)

AUTHOR	YEAR	CYTOSTATICS	NUMBER OF PATIENTS	LOCAL RECURRENCE RATE PERCENTAGE IN THE PERFUSED LIMB	5-YEAR SURVIVAL RATE (%)			10-YEAR SURVIVAL RATE (%)		
					II	IIIA	IIIAB	II	IIIA	IIIAB
Krementz et al.[12]	1985	Melphalan	182	—	64	35	31	58	28	28
Shiu et al.[35]	1986	Nitrogen mustard	18	—	—	50	38	—	—	—
Hartley and Fletcher[37]	1987	Melphalan	39	—		58[a]	29		44[a]	29
Stehlin et al.[38]	1988	Melphalan	117	—	75	70	36	—	50	23
Baas and Schraffordt Koops[28]	1988	Melphalan ± actinomycin-D	110	38	74	67	40	63	45	34
Di Filippo et al.[36]	1989	Melphalan	116	—	80	55	35	—	—	—
Santinami et al.[39]	1989	Melphalan (dacarbazin, cisplatin)	106	—	—	51	35	—	—	—

[a]Hartley and Fletcher did not discriminate between stage II and IIIA.

added to the perfusion fluid. Of the 110 patients, 42 (38 percent) developed a recurrence in the perfused extremity. The interval between perfusion and recurrence in the perfused extremity ranged from 1 to 96 months (mean 25 months). The 5-year disease-free and actuarial survival for these 110 patients is 35 and 61 percent, respectively. The 5-year disease-free survival for stage II is 58 percent, for stage IIA 27 percent, and for stage IIIAB 21 percent. The 5-year actuarial survival for stage II is 74 percent, for stage IIIA 67 percent, and for stage IIIAB 40 percent.[28]

No firm conclusions can be drawn from these results since recurrence rates after surgery alone are not available, and the seemingly improved survival after perfusion may be purely a result of patient selection. This patient selection may be explained by the fact that patients receiving perfusion possibly form a selected group, where the biological behavior of the tumor is characterized by a low potential for distant metastases (as only patients without distant metastases at the time of limb recurrence are selected for perfusion). The majority of melanoma experts, however, hold the view that, because of perfusion, uncontrollable locoregional disease necessitating amputation, sometimes encountered in the past, is seldom seen anymore.

REPEAT PERFUSIONS

The drawback of the perfusion method is the fact that fractionation and protraction of the treatment, well known in systemic chemotherapy, by which the difference of tolerance between normal and malignant cells increases, is difficult to realize.

Both the duration of drug circulation (at most a few hours) and the number of repeat perfusions (at most three) have their limits due to technical reasons. In order to explore the value of primary multiple perfusions, one of us (Kroon) recently reported on about four patients with locally inoperable melanoma confined to the lower leg, who were treated with three perfusions, each lasting 1 hour.[44] The melphalan dosage used was three times 7.5 mg/l on each occasion. On the basis of tumor biology, an interval of 3 weeks was chosen. Although this treatment schedule resulted in three complete remissions, it did not prove feasible in terms of patient tolerance. A double perfusion schedule is therefore being investigated in patients with measurable recurrent disease. For the first perfusion in this schedule a relatively low dose of melphalan, 6 mg/l perfused tissue, is given to reduce toxicity and thereby allowing an interval of 3 weeks. At the second perfusion, the dose of melphalan is 9 mg/l. Tumor tissue is left in situ, with the intention of removing it 6 to 12 weeks after the second perfusion in order to obtain histological response confirmation. Preliminary results indicate that this regimen is tolerated well with acceptable toxicity. So far, 22 patients are evaluable for response and in 14 of them a complete remission was achieved (64 percent), in three the remission was partial, whereas in five patients a no-change situation was observed[44] (Fig. 19-5).

Recently, one of us (Schraffordt Kroops) compared two groups of patients with local recurrence, satellitosis, and/or in-transit metastasis of the leg. One group of 37 patients had one and the other group of 56 patients had two perfusions. The interval between two perfusions in this schedule was 6 weeks and the cytostatic drugs used were melphalan (1.0–1.5 mg/kg body weight) and actinomycin-D (0.014 mg/kg body weight). After a 5-year follow-up there was no statistically significant difference in recurrence in the perfused extremity and survival between the patients treated with one and those given two perfusions.[18] Objective response data of these patients cannot be given, as the recurrent disease was excised at the moment of perfusion.

In Brussels, 24 patients were perfused twice because of recurrence after first perfusion for stage IIIA or IIIAB melanoma. Although disease-free survival was poor (4 percent at 4 years), the crude survival of these patients was unexpectively high (67 percent at 5 years). These findings favor the hypothesis that remaining melanoma cells after perfusion may undergo differentiation process with diminished biological aggressivity.[16]

Options to improve results for the future could be a combination of perfusion with repeat infusion treatments, or tourniquet infusions.[45] Although initial reports concerning this last method were hopeful, no new clinical data have appeared in recent years.

TISSUE TEMPERATURE

Since it is known that the specific cell killing effect of heat is obtained only at temperatures above 41.5°C, the benefit of the widely used so-called mild hyperthermia (tissue temperatures between 39 and 40°C) must still be queried.[13] True hyperthermia, that is, tissue temperatures above 41.5°C, is not often applied in cytostatic perfusion treatment because although encouraging antitumor effects were achieved, an unacceptably high toxicity was encountered. However, it should not be forgotten that the tissue temperatures in these perfusions were very high (up to 43.5°C), that the periods during which the hyperthermia was given were long (up to 4 hours), and that the physiological conditions in the perfused limb were, in many cases, probably not optimal.[5,27] It is interesting that in recent studies similarly encouraging response data were reported from cytostatic perfusions performed at tissue temperatures between 40.5 and 42°C ("borderline" hyperthermia).[25,36]

In Amsterdam, therefore, it was decided to explore the benefit of cytostatic perfusion at tissue temperatures between 41 and 42°C. This hyperthermia was applied during the whole hour of cytostatic perfusion. The drug melphalan was chosen in a dose of 10 mg/l perfused tissue, and the drug was only introduced into the perfusate at the moment that all tissues had reached a temperature of 41°C. Only patients with advanced disease were entered into this treatment schedule. During perfusion, care was taken for optimal physiological conditions, monitored by frequent blood gas analysis. Although the addition of this "borderline" true hyperthermia pointed at improved efficacy (Plate 40), the toxicity encountered was so severe that the experiment had to be stopped. It was concluded that adding "borderline" true hyperthermia to cytostatic perfusion enhances the efficacy; however, the simultaneous combination of these two treatment modalities gives an unacceptable toxicity. To diminish this toxicity, dose reduction of either one or both treatment modalities do not seem to be a good option, because by so doing the optimum therapeutic ratios would no longer be maintained. Therefore, at this moment we are studying the effect of administrating both treatment modalities in an additional way, separating heat and melphalan by means of a repeat perfusion.[46–48] The rationale of this schedule is that the first perfusion, a true hyperthermic one (for 2 hours tissue temperatures between 42 and 43°C) without cytostatics, will reduce the anoxic center of the tumor, whereas the second, a normothermic one, lasting 1 hour and with the optimum dose of 10 mg melphalan/liter perfused tissue, performed 1 week later, will attack the residual well-circulated periphery. The first results indicate that this combined schedule is feasible. When carefully performed, the toxicity of the first hyperthermic perfusion is negligible. The toxicity of the normothermic one appears to be similar to that of a melphalan perfusion alone. So far, all patients treated have shown tumor regression.

PERFUSION WITH DRUGS OTHER THAN MELPHALAN

In some studies, objective responses to perfusion with drugs other than melphalan are described.[13] It appears that none of the cytostatics tried (DTIC,[8,26,49] cisplatin,[6] nitrogen mustard[35]), however, are as effective as melphalan, either as a single agent or in combination. The combination of melphalan with other drugs such as thiotepa,[12,50] actinomycin-D,[18] and nitrogen mustard,[12] likewise, does not increase the number of remissions. Some publications indicate that cisplatin should not be used with tissue temperatures over 40°C, because otherwise severe nerve damage may occur.[6] Perfusions with the mouse monoclonal antibody R24 were described by Coit et al.[51] Twelve patients with unresectable in-transit metastases underwent 13 perfusions. One patient demonstrated a major clinical response at 10 weeks after perfusion, lasting for 5 months.

Recently, one of us (Lejeune) found very impressive responses of in-transit metastases during a combination of high dose recombinant tumor necrosis factor alpha (rTNFα) with interferon-gamma (IFN-gamma) and melphalan.[52] (See Chap. 20.)

TABLE 19-2
QUALITY CONTROL OF THE PERFUSION TRIAL EORTC 18832/WHO 15

INSTITUTION:
DATE OF VISIT:
NUMBER OF PATIENTS INTRODUCED IN THIS TRIAL:
1984: 1985: 1986: 1987: 1988: 1989: 1990: 1991:

CODES USED: 1 = correct: data correct
2 = deviation: data incorrect but without influence on the trial outcome
3 = incorrect: data incorrect, with possible influence on the trial outcome

CODE		ILIAC PERFUSION
_____		randomization
_____		previous treatment within 6 weeks
_____		volume measurement of leg
_____		tumor location at or distal of middle of the thigh
_____		heating blanket water supply
_____		para-iliac lymph node dissection
_____		inguinal lymph node dissection
_____		inguinal + para-iliac + obturator lymph node dissection
_____		ligation epigastric and circumflex vessels
_____		ligation obturator vein
_____		temporary closure of internal iliac artery
_____		heparinization (3.3 mg or 200 μ per kg body weight)
_____		introduction canulae through the external iliac vessels
_____		tip of the canulae reaching the common femoral artery
_____	Ch	canulae diameter
_____		rubber tourniquet
_____	min	first anoxic period < 5 min, 5–10 min, 10–20 min, > 20 min
_____		dosage melphalan, prepared just before use, injected as bolus into the oxygenator
_____	°C	temperature blood at introduction cytostatic drug
_____	°C	temperature of blood 0–10 min
_____	°C	temperature of blood 10–60 min
_____		4 needle thermistor probes in right position
_____	°C	temperature subcutaneous tissue below knee at time 0
_____	°C	temperature subcutaneous tissue (below knee) 0–10 min
_____	°C	temperature subcutaneous tissue (below knee) 10–60 min
_____		blood gas monitor in order to check pO_2, pCO_2, PH
_____	min	second anoxic period < 15 min, 15–30 min, > 30 min
_____	cm	local excision < 3 cm, 3–5 cm
_____		split thickness skin graft
_____		fasciotomy (optional)
_____		leakage measurement
_____		leakage < 5% in first 5 minutes
_____		leakage > 15% in 60 minutes
_____		priming volume between 750 ml and 1000 ml, heparinization 20 mg/l
_____		final blood dilution ± 50% with an hematocrit of 25–30%
_____		perfusion fluid supplemented with bicarbonate
_____	ml	extracorporeal circulation > 40 ml per liter of perfused limb
_____	ml	how much overflow from body to extremity?
_____		rinsing out blood with 1 liter of low molecular weight dextran
_____		heparin neutralized with protamine sulphate
_____		postoperative anticoagulants (optional)
_____		blood count and protein dosage checked every day for 4–7 days
_____		grading system of tissue toxicity

SURGICAL QUALITY CONTROL IN THE EORTC TRIAL 18832/WHO TRIAL 15 (Perfusion and local excision versus local excision alone)

Since March 1, 1984, a randomized trial on prophylactic isolation perfusion for stage I high-risk (> 1.5 mm thickness) malignant melanoma of the limbs under auspices of the EORTC is going on. In June 1988, the Committee on Quality Control for the EORTC has selected this perfusion trial on melanoma as a surgical pilot study.

Surgery as a modality is considerably more difficult to quantify than radiotherapy and chemotherapy. While on a local level, it is relatively easy to determine that a certain surgeon obtains excellent results, such assurances are quite difficult on a multi-institutional level.

Although the protocol of the EORTC/WHO trial has been carefully outlined, deviations from it are bound to occur. An evaluation of the perfusion data from the DATA center reveals differences. The computer sheets of the period 1984 to 1987 showed intercenter discrepancies in the measured temperature of arterial blood and subcutaneous tissue. Although the protocol stipulates exactly at which temperature the cytostatic drug is to be injected, many centers made errors in this respect.

Apart from protocol misreadings of the temperatures to be used, typical operative errors can be recognized only by visiting the participating centers. At a meeting in September 1987, all trial participants agreed to on-site visits at the collaborating centers and, besides the site-visits, twice a year meetings with all the trial participants. One of the participating surgeons was chosen as responsible investigator.

The intention is that the visiting surgeon will contact the center at least 4 weeks in advance. Perfusion dates will be set by mutual agreement, preferably on two consecutive days. The center to be visited will receive a letter with specifications on the planned visit. These specifications include a complete checklist (Table 19-2) with possible shortcomings and problems in surgical technique. If errors in surgical technique are identified during on-site visits, the intention is to be constructive, educational, and corrective. This implies suggestions for improvements and lending a helping hand in surgical technique.

Between September 1988 and March 1991, eight centers were visited. Three other centers were contacted, but no suitable dates have yet been found (11 centers in Europe have introduced more than 10 patients in the perfusion trial). The operation (regional perfusion) was usually performed well and in accordance with the protocol. Nevertheless, several centers made certain errors that could easily have been avoided if the site visits had been started earlier. It was found that by jointly carrying out the procedure, together with the external reviewer, a number of errors could still be detected and corrected. Moreover, some rules formulated in the protocol were found to be misinterpreted, and the forms to be completed were not readily understood on some points. Various aspects were discussed at conclusion of the visit to the center, and a few days after the visit, the center was sent a report. In all cases communications were quite pleasant.

It is obvious that the frequency of errors could be reduced from 28 to 17 to 11 percent, respectively, during the period April 1984 to April 1987, April 1987 to April 1988, and since April 1988.

CONCLUSION

In our opinion, regional perfusion is justified for recurrent melanoma of the extremity. As Au and Goldman[53] stated, the disease has already demonstrated aggressive behavior in these cases and will progress unless its course can be modified. After regional perfusion, objective response rates of more than 80 percent are common in measurable disease. The 5-year survival rate is 29 to 80 percent for patients with local recurrence, satellitosis, and in-transit metastases with or without lymph node metastases. Even in the most advanced cases (those with in-transit and regional metastases) the 5-year survival is ± 30 percent, and the 10-year survival is ± 25 percent.

It is still unresolved whether mild hyperthermia (39–40°C) gives better results than normothermia. The role of true hyperthermia has to be explored further; the same holds true for the application of repeat perfusion schedules. It is unknown whether a combination of melphalan with different drugs might improve results. Preliminary results applying biological response modifiers (tumor necrosis factor, interferon-gamma) point in this respect to increased efficacy. An option for the future could be a combination of perfusion with infusion treatments or tourniquet infusions.

REFERENCES

1. Klopp C, Alford T, Bateman J, Berry G, and Winship T. Fractionated intra-arterial cancer chemotherapy with methyl bis-amine hydrochloride: A preliminary report. *Ann Surg* 132:811–832, 1950.
2. Creech O, Ryan R, and Krementz ET. Treatment of malignant melanoma by isolation perfusion technique. *JAMA* 169:339–343, 1959.
3. Stehlin J, Clark R, White EC, Smith JL, Griffin AC, Jess RH, and Healy JE. Regional chemotherapy for cancer: Experiences with 116 perfusions. *Ann Surg* 151:605–619, 1960.

4. Luck J. Action of P-di(2-chloroethyl)-amino-L-phenylalanine on Harding Passey mouse melanoma. *Science* 123:984–985, 1956.
5. Cavaliere R, Ciocatto E, Giovanella B, Heidelberger Ch, Johnson RO, Margottini M, Mondovi B, Moricca G, and Rossi-Fanelli A. Selective heat sensitivity of cancer cells: Biochemical and clinical studies. *Cancer* 20:1351–1381, 1967.
6. Aigner K, Hild P, Henneking K, Paul E, and Hundeiker M. Regional perfusion with cis-platinum and dacarbazine. *Recent Results Cancer Res* 86:239–245, 1983.
7. Franklin H, Schraffordt Koops H, Oldhoff J, Czarnetzki BM, Macher E, Kroon BBR, Welvaart K, Velden JW van der, Dijk E van, Esch EP van der, Oosterhuis JW, Huisman SJ, Hart AAM, and Rümke Ph. To perfuse or not to perfuse? A retrospective comparative study to evaluate the effect of adjuvant isolated regional perfusion in patients with stage I extremity melanoma with a thickness of 1.5 mm or greater. *J Clin Oncol* 6:705–708, 1988.
8. Edwards MJ, Soong S-J, Boddie AW, Balch CM, and McBride CM. Isolated limb perfusion for localized melanoma of the extremity. *Arch Surg* 125:317–321, 1990.
9. Illig L, and Aigner K. Therapie des malignen Melanoms unter besonderer Berücksichtigung der isolierten Extremitäten perfusion. *Dt Arztebl* 77:2911–2925, 1980.
10. Israels SP. Loco-regional drug delivery in cancer treatment, with special reference to isolation perfusion. In Veronesi U, *Drug Delivery in Cancer Treatment*. Berlin: Springer Verlag, 1987, 53–76.
11. Jönsson P, Hafström L, and Hugander A. Results of regional perfusion for primary and recurrent melanomas of the extremities. *Recent Results Cancer Res* 86:277–282, 1983.
12. Krementz ET, Ryan RF, Carter RD, Sutherland CM, and Reed RJ. Hyperthermic regional perfusion for melanomas of the limbs. In: Balch, Milton (ed.), *Cutaneous Melanoma*. Philadelphia: Lippincott, 1985, 172–195.
13. Kroon BBR. Regional isolation perfusion in melanoma of the limbs: Accomplishments, unsolved problems, future. *Eur J Surg Oncol* 14:101–110, 1988.
14. Lejeune FJ, Deloof T, Ewalenko P, Fruhling J, Jabri M, Mathieu M, Nogaret JM, and Verhest A. Objective regression of unexcised melanoma in-transit metastases after hyperthermic isolation perfusion of the limbs with melphalan. *Recent Results Cancer Res* 86:268–276, 1983.
15. Lejeune FJ. Is isolation perfusion with chemotherapy an improvement in the management of malignant melanoma? In: Kroon BBR, van Dongen J (eds.), *Oncologisch kabinet*. Antoni van Leeuwenhoek Huis, Nederlands Kanker Instituut, Amsterdam: 1987, 71–78.
16. Lejeune FJ, Liénard D, Douaihy ME, Seyedi JV, and Ewalenko P. Results of 206 isolated limb perfusions for malignant melanoma. *Eur J Surg Onc* 510–519, 1989.
17. Martijn H, Oldhoff J, and Schraffordt Koops H. Regional perfusion in the treatment of patients with a locally metastasized malignant melanoma of the limbs. *Eur J Cancer* 70:471–476, 1981.
18. Martin H, Oldhoff J, Schraffordt Koops H, and Oosterhuis JW. Hyperthermic regional perfusion with melphalan and a combination of melphalan and actinomycin-D in the treatment of locally metastasized malignant melanoma of the extremities. *J Surg Oncol* 20:9–13, 1982.
19. Martijn H, Schraffordt Koops H, Milton GW, Nap M, Oosterhuis JW, Shaw HM, and Oldhoff J. Comparison of two methods of treating primary malignant melanomas Clark IV and V, thickness 1.5 mm and greater, localized on the extremities. *Cancer* 57:1923–1930, 1986.
20. McBride C, Smith L, and Brown B. Primary malignant melanoma of the limbs: A reevaluation using microstaging techniques. *Cancer* 48:1463–1468, 1981.
21. Rochlin D, and Smart C. Treatment of malignant melanoma by regional perfusion. *Cancer* 18:1544–1550, 1964.
22. Schraffordt Koops H, Oldhoff J, Ploeg E van der, Vermey A, Eibergen R, and Beekhuis H. Some aspects of the treatment of primary malignant melanoma of the extremities by isolated regional perfusion. *Cancer* 39:27–33, 1977.
23. Schraffordt Koops H, Beekhuis H, Oldhoff J, Oosterhuis J, Ploeg E van der, and Vermey A. Local recurrence and survival in patients with (Clark's level IV/V and over 1.5 mm thickness) stage I malignant melanoma of the extremities after regional perfusion. *Cancer* 48:1952–1957, 1981.
24. Schraffordt Koops H, Kroon BBR, and Lejeune FJ. Isolated perfusion in the treatment of local recurrence, satellites and in-transit metastases of extremity melanomas. In: Rümke P, (ed.), Therapy of Advanced Melanoma. Basel, Switzerland: Karger, 10:67–78, 1990.
25. Storm FK, and Morton DL. Value of therapeutic hyperthermic limb perfusion in advanced recurrent melanoma of the lower extremity. *Am J Surg* 150:32–35, 1985.
26. Vaglini M, Belli F, Marolda R, Prada A, Santinami M, and Cascinelli N. Hyperthermic antiblastic perfusion with DTIC in stage IIIA-IIIAB melanoma of the extremities. *Eur J Surg Oncol* 13:127–129, 1987.
27. Vaglini M, Ammatuna M, Nava M, et al. Regional perfusion at high temperature in the treatment of stage IIA-IIIAB melanoma patients. *Tumori* 69:585–588, 1983.
28. Baas PC, Schraffordt Koops H, Hoekstra HJ, Oosterhuis JW, Weele LT van der, and Oldhoff J. Isolated regional perfusion in the treatment of local recurrence, satellitosis and in-transit metastases of extremity melanoma. *Reg Cancer Treat.* 1988;1:33–36.
29. Fontijne WPJ, Vries J de, Mook P, Elstrodt J, Oosterhuis JW, Schraffordt Koops H, Olhdoff J, and Wildevuur Ch. Improved tissue perfusion during pressure-regulated hyperthermic regional isolated perfusion in dogs. *J Surg Oncol* 26:69–76, 1984.
30. Schraffordt Koops H. Prevention of neural and muscular lesions during hyperthermic regional perfusion. *Surg Gynecol Obstet* 135:401–403, 1972.
31. Wieberdink J, Benckhuijsen C, Braat RP, Slooten EA van, and Olthuis GA. Dosimetry in isolation perfusion of the limbs by assessment of perfused tissue volume and grading of toxic reactions. *Eur J Cancer Clin Oncol* 18:905–910, 1982.
32. Benckhuijsen C, Kroon BBR, Geel AN van, and Wieberdink J. Regional perfusion treatment with melphalan for melanoma in a limb: An evaluation of drug kinetics. *Eur J Surg Oncol* 14:157–164, 1988.
33. Lejeune FJ, and Ghanem GE. A simple and accurate new method for cytostatic dosimetry in isolation perfusion of the limbs based on exchangeable blood volume determination. *Cancer Res* 47:639–643, 1987.
34. Kroon BBR, Geel AN van, Benckhuijsen C, and Wieberdink J. Normothermic isolation perfusion with melphalan for advanced melanoma of the limbs. *Anticancer Res* 7:441–442, 1987.
35. Shiu MH, Knapper WH, Fortner JG, Yeh S, Horowitz G, Schnog J, Guerra J, Gould-Rossbach P, and Ray C. Regional isolated limb perfusion of melanoma in-transit metastases using mechlorethamine, nitrogen mustard. *J Clin Oncol* 4:1819–1826, 1986.
36. Di Filippo F, Calabro A, Giannarelli D, Carlini S, Cavaliere F, Moscarelli F, and Cavaliere R. Prognostic variables in recurrent limb melanoma treated with hyperthermic antiblastic perfusion. *Cancer* 63:2551–2561, 1989.

37. Hartley JW, Fletcher WS. Improved survival of patients with stage II melanoma of the extremity using hyperthermic isolation perfusion with I-phenylalanine mustard. *J Surg Oncol* 36:170–174, 1987.
38. Stehlin JS, Greeff PJ, de Ipolyi PD, Giovanella BC, Klein G, McGaff CJ, Davis BR, Williams LJ, Natelson ET, and Anderson RF. Heat as an adjuvant in the treatment of advanced melanoma: An immune stimulant? *Houston Med J* 4:61–82, 1988.
39. Santinami B, Belli F, Cascinelli N, Rovini D, and Vaglini M. Seven years experience with hyperthermic perfusions in extracorporeal circulation for melanoma of the extremities. J Surg Oncol 42:201–208, 1989.
40. Friedman L, and McNeer G. Prognosis with local metastasis and recurrence in malignant melanoma. *Ann N Y Acad Sci* 100:123–130, 1963.
41. Stehlin JS, Smith JL, Jing B, and Sherrin D. Melanoma of the extremities complicated by in-transit metastases. *Surg Gynecol Obstet* 122:3–14, 1966.
42. McNeer G, and Carter J. Local failure in the treatment of melanoma. *Am J Roentgenol Radium Ther Nucl Med* 99:791–808, 1967.
43. Fortner JG, Strong EW, Mulcare RJ, Schottenfeld D, and Maclean BJ. The surgical treatment of recurrent melanoma. *Surg Clin North Am* 54:865–870, 1974.
44. Kroon BBR, Geel AN van, Franklin HR, Klaase JM, and Benckhuijsen C. Preliminary results of a double perfusion schedule with melphalan in measurable melanoma. In Jakesz R, and Rainer H (eds.), *Progress in Regional Cancer Therapy*. Berlin-Heidelberg: Springer Verlag, 1990, 192–194.
45. Karakousis CP, Kanter PM, Park HC, Sharma SD, Moore R, and Ewing JH. Tourniquet infusion versus hyperthermic perfusion. *Cancer* 49:850–858, 1982.
46. Zee J van der, Broekmeyer-Reurink MP, Berg AP van den, Geel AN van, Jansen RFM, Kroon BBR, Wijk J van, and Hagenbeek A. Temperature distribution and pH changes during hyperthermic regional isolation perfusion. *Eur J Cancer Clin Oncol* 25:1157–1163, 1989.
47. Kroon BBR. True hyperthermia in regional perfusion. Annual report. Amsterdam: The Netherlands Cancer Institute 1989, 109.
48. Jansen RFM, Geel AN van, Zee J van der, Hagenbeek A, and Levendag P. Intractible cutaneous non-Hodgkin's lymphoma of the lower limb. Complete remission after sequential regional isolated hyperthermic perfusion and perfusion with I-phenylalanine-mustard (Melphalan, L-PAM). *Cancer* 64:392–395, 1989.
49. Aigner K, Hild P, Breithaupt H, Hundeiker M, Schwemmle K, Henneking K, Illig L, Merker G, Paul E, Brodkorb J, and Jungbluth A. Isolated extremity perfusion with DTIC: An experimental and clinical study. *Anticancer Res* 3:87–94, 1983.
50. Cox KR. Survival after regional perfusion for limb melanoma. *Aust N Z J Surg* 45:32–36, 1975.
51. Coit D, Houghton A, Cordon-Cardo C, Shiu M, and Old L. Isolation limb perfusion with monoclonal antibody R24 in patients with malignant melanoma, meeting abstract. *Proc Ann Meet Am Soc Clin Oncol* 7:A962, 1988.
52. Lienard D, Ewalenko P, Delmotte J-J, Renard N, and Lejeune F. High doses of rTNFα in combination with IFN-gamma and melphalan in isolation perfusion of the limbs for melanoma and sarcoma. *J Clin Oncol* 10:52–60, 1992.
53. Au F, and Goldman L. Isolation perfusion limb melanoma: A critical assessment and literature review. In: Clark, Goldman, Mastrangelo. Human Malignant Melanoma. New York: Grune & Stratton, 1977, 295–308.

Chapter 20

ISOLATION PERFUSION OF THE LIMBS FOR IN TRANSIT MELANOMA METASTASES WITH CYTOKINES AND CHEMOTHERAPY

Ferdy J. Lejeune and Danielle Liénard

INTRODUCTION

In 1975, Carl Carswell, from the group of L. Old, at the Sloan Kettering Institute, discovered a soluble substance in the serum of animals treated either with BCG (Bacillus Calmette-Guerin) or endotoxin.[1] This substance, later identified as TNFα was able to produce hemorrhagic necrosis of the lesions leading to tumor regression in animal model. Later it was shown to be produced by activated macrophages and to consist of a peptide of 157 aminoacids. The cDNA for human TNFα was finally determined, rendering possible the production of recombinant (r) TNFα in escherichia Coli.[2]

rTNFα was found to be the first cytokine able to produce tumor regression comparable to the best chemotherapeutic agents.[3–5] However, TNFα is considered as one of the major mediators of septic shock.[6] TNFα induces a septic shock-like syndrome[7–8] which represents the major side effect of its administration, both in animals and in humans.

Phase I studies so far indicate that the maximal tolerated single (MTD) dose in humans is less or equal to 350 μg/m^2 intravenously.[8–9] Under these conditions, a negligible clinical response rate has been reported in all diseases including melanoma.[8–9] The beneficial antitumor effects of TNFα seem to be related to endothelial cell activation and vascular damage resulting in hemorrhagic necrosis, which starts within 1 to 4 hours after rTNFα administration, principally in tumors located on skin.[10] This might be due to the neovascular supply of superficial neoplastic nodules and/or to some specific property of the capillary bed of tumors in the skin. Another potential consequence of local administration of rTNFα is the lysis of the extracellular matrix resulting from the release of elastase by activated polymorphonuclear neutrophils as it was observed in our patients.[11] Neutrophils elastase is a major determinant of neutrophil-induced endothelial and tissue damage.

Since human tumor xenografts are sensitive to rTNFα and that its clinical use is limited by a low MTD, we decided to try the administration of the drug by Isolation Limb Perfusion for in transit melanoma metastases. Indeed this regional therapy using the chemotherapeutic agent melphalan alone is a well-established procedure for treating in transit metastases of melanoma with an overall complete response rate of 50 percent (cf. Chap. 19) resulting in a high-limb sparing. Therefore, the administration of effective doses, that is high doses of rTNFα, was decided in order to overcome not only the problem of side effects but also the lack of efficacy of systemic low-dose administration. As it will be seen, the pilot study with TNFα resolved the problem of systemic toxicity, but it was necessary to use rTNFα in combination therapy in order to achieve the very high-response rate that we finally obtained[12-13]

FEASIBILITY OF ADMINISTERING HIGH-DOSE (HD) rTNFα IN ISOLATED LIMB PERFUSION

Isolated Limb Perfusion (ILP) allows the delivery of a high dose of drug in a closed system with acceptable toxicity and minimal systemic side effects (cf. Chap. 19). With melphalan, the drug concentration reaches by 10- to 30-fold the concentration at the equilibrium obtained after systemic administration. The experience with intratumoral TNFα administration giving more tumor responses suggests that giving TNFα at high dose could be more efficient than the MTD. Therefore, the three patients in the pilot study received rTNFα only (Genentech, kindly given by Boehringer-Ingelheim, Germany) at doses of 2, 3, and 4 mg, respectively, in the arterial line of the circuit. The three patients (two females, one male) had regionally advanced melanoma (2 Stage IIIa, 1 Stage IIIab).[14]

The technique of isolation perfusion has been described elsewhere.[15] We used a membrane oxygenator (VPCML; Cobe Inc, Lakewood, CO) and silicone tubing. Priming consisted of 19 mL bicarbonate, 0.4 mL heparin, and 1 L Haemacel (Behringwerke, Marburg, Germany). It was supplemented either with 1 U of bank blood or autologous fresh blood. Perfusate flow was set as high as possible and was typically 700 mL/min for lower limb ILP. Potential leakage of the drugs was measured with radioiodinated human serum albumin (RIHSA; Institut de Radio-Eléments IRE, Fleurus, Belgium) injected into the circuit, and the radioactivity was assessed in the peripheral plasma at 5, 30, and 60 minutes. The arterial blood temperature of the perfused limb was maintained at 40°C during the whole ILP. Four thermistor probes were implanted in the subcutaneous tissues and into the muscles to monitor the tissue temperature, which ranged between 38°C and 40°C.

Side Effects

The first patient had been perfused previously two times for extensive in transit metastases of the lower limb; the first with melphalan alone, and the second with αMSH melphalan, with partial remission for the first, and no change in the second. The route had been the iliac vessel for the first two treatments, and the femoral for the third with TNFα. There were more than 40 tumor nodules and the overall leakage at 60 minutes was 34.4 percent due to the neovascularization of the previous operating site. The second patient had more than 100 nodules over the whole lower limb and was perfused by the iliac region. Leakage was minimal.

In those two patients, a profound circulatory shock developed, the first during perfusion because of leakage, and the second after releasing the tourniquet following extensive wash-out by 2 liters of fluid with the pump. In both cases, it responded well to fluid loading and dopamine. The third patient had 20 in transit metastases on the leg and knee. She received 4 mg of TNFα. She entered the prophylactic dopamine infusion protocole with fluid loading and had no systemic toxicity (see section on Prophylaxis of Septic Shock-like Syndrome). Prophylaxis of shock was given according to the protocol described in a separate paragraph. No septic shock-like syndrome was observed.

In addition to the hypotension problems, the two first patients—who did not receive prophylactic dopamine infusion nor indomethacine—experienced tachycardia and transient oliguria and WHO grade 3 renal toxicity for 29 days, respectively.

All three patients developed chills and temperature a few hours after the perfusion.

Tumor Response in the Pilot Study

The first patient experienced a complete response although a pigmentation remained on his leg. The complete softening of the nodules remained for 7 months, and then a relapse appeared which was treated with the combination therapy (see section on Efficacy of ILP with HD rTNFα, IFNγ, Melphalan on Unexcised in Transit Melanoma Metastases). The second patient presented a typical hemorrhagic necrosis of the in transit amelanotic metastases already 2 days after perfusion (Plate 55) but relapsed after 21 days. In the third patient however, only minor response was observed.

RATIONALE FOR USING A COMBINATION OF HD rTNFα, rIFNγ, AND MELPHALAN

It has been demonstrated that the number of the TNFα receptors on malignant cells increases when they are incubated with IFNγ.[16–17] In addition, a synergistic antiproliferative activity of rTNFα and IFNγ has been demonstrated in vitro and in vivo using human melanoma xenografts in nude mice.[18–19]

An enhancement of the cytolytic activity of rTNFα by hyperthermia (40°C) has been demonstrated in experimental tumors both in vitro and in vivo.[20] Cytotoxic activity of rTNFα is enhanced when chemotherapeutic drugs, especially alkylating agents, are added in vitro and in vivo.[21] Since melphalan is the first line ILP chemotherapy for the treatment of melanoma (see Chap. 19), we decided to combine rTNFα at high dose, rIFNγ at low dose and melphalan at the usual concentration for isolation perfusion of the limbs. Our protocol is presented in Fig. 20-1. IFNγ (Boehringer-Ingelheim, Germany) at the dosage of 0.2 mg is given subcutaneously on days -2 and -1. This dosage of IFNγ was chosen as it received an NCI clearance for biological response modifiers (BRM) protocols. The high dose of TNFα (Genentech, Boehringer-Ingelheim, Germany) of 4 mg for lower limb, was chosen because it was found to be tolerable in the pilot study and since it represents a 10-fold increase of the systemic dosage for MTD (maximum tolerated dose). For upper limb, the dosage was initially of 2 mg and was later increased to present dose of 3 mg.

Melphalan (Alkeran, Wellcome Foundation Beckenham, UK) dosage was calculated according to the liter-volume method,[15] 10 mg/l of perfused limb for lower and 13 mg/l for upper limb. Exchangeable limb blood volume (ELBV) was assessed with the hematocrit method and additional priming with Haemaccel solution was done in order to achieve a final concentration of 40 μg of melphalan per ml at the equilibrium for lower limb and of 20 μg for upper limb.[15]

rIFNγ and rTNFα were injected successively as a bolus in the arterial line. Melphalan was administered 30 minutes later. The whole perfusion lasted 90 minutes. At the end of the ILP, the limb was washed twice with 1 liter of Haemaccel (Travenol) and 1 liter of Macrodex® (Pharmacia, Sweden). Recently we replaced Haemaccel by plasmasteril.

PROPHYLAXIS OF SEPTIC SHOCK-LIKE SYNDROME

Since the pilot study[14] had shown in two patients a profound circulatory shock which responded well to fluid loading and dopamine, the patients included in the phase II study received a prophylactic treatment. It consisted in the use of continuous intravenous infusion of 2 μg/kg/min of dopamine, starting before the injection of rTNFα in the circuit and systematically during at least 48 hours postoperatively. Fluid loading was given before releasing the tourniquet after completion of the washout.[13] For achieving an optimal prophylaxis of shock, electrocardiogram, urine output, blood pressure, central venous pressure and pulmonary pressures, and arterial wedge pressure were recorded and monitored continuously by an arterial and a Swan-Ganz catheter from the beginning of the ILP until the second postoperative day.

Recently we added Indomethacine in order to reinforce the protection of the patient against side effects, as it had been shown in animal that Indomethacine can protect mice from a lethal shock from rTNFα.[5,22] We used indomethacin (Indocid®) at a fixed dosage of 50 mg for the first 4 hours with a pump intravenously, starting at the beginning of the ILP before injecting rTNFα. The last 20 hours to complete a full day, patients received 200 mg of

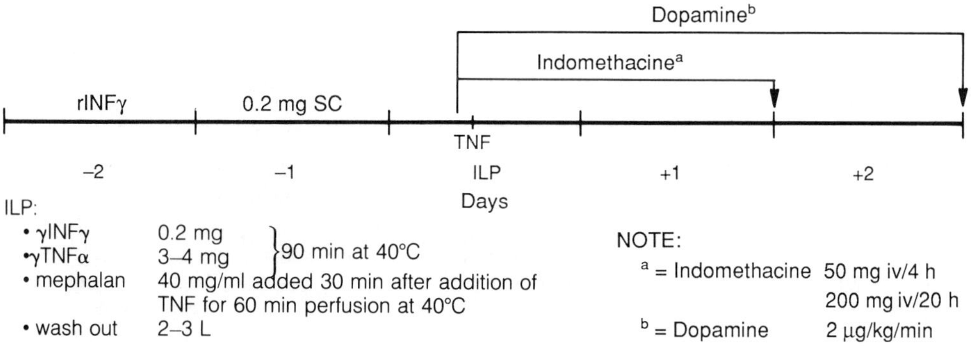

FIG. 20-1. Protocol for isolation perfusion of the limbs using TNFα, IFNγ, and melphalan.

indomethacin also with a pump. Indomethacin was not prolonged because it was not needed any longer (see section on Toxicity of ILP with rTNFα, rIFNγ, and Melphalan) and for avoiding the risk of gastric ulceration.

EFFICACY OF ILP WITH HD rTNFα, IFNγ, MELPHALAN ON UNEXCISED IN TRANSIT MELANOMA METASTASES

Forty-four consecutive melanoma patients entered the study. Their characteristics are listed in Table 20-1. Patients entered the phase II study from December 1988 in Brussels to March 1992 in Lausanne, after extended work-up and informed consent.

The 44 patients received 46 ILP, the majority being through the iliac vessels. There were 36 females and 8 males. The age ranged between 22 and 84, with a medium of 60. It should be stressed that we decided to treat old patients because of the well-known tolerance of elderly patients to TNF. All patients had in transit metastases (Stage IIIa). Thirteen had it associated to regional lymph node metastases and two had a Stage IV, that is advanced disease, because of liver metastases which were not diagnosed at the time of the work-up.

The majority of the patients (28 out of 44) had been previously treated. Twenty-eight had been perfused, three had received intra-arterial chemotherapy, and two had received the association of IFNα-2 and Interleukine-2. The tumor burden was considerable in 18 patients, that is from more than 10 to more than 100 nodules. The patients with a few nodules had been operated several times by local excision of in transit metastases with subsequent recurrences.

TABLE 20-1
TNF PERFUSION: MELANOMA

n = 44		→ 46	ILP:	Ax:	1
				Fem:	6
				Iliac:	39
36 F/81 M			Age:	60 (22–84)	
Stage:	IIIa:		29		
	IIab:		13		
	IV:		2		
Previous treatment: 28/44			ILP	Melphalan:	20
				TNF:	2
				TNF-Melphalan	1
			IA Cis DDP: 3		
			IV $IF\alpha_2$ + IL_2: 2		
Number of nodules:			**1 → 10:**	**26**	
			>10 → 50:	**11**	
			>50 → 100:	**3**	
			>100:	**4**	

Tumor Response

In all cases, an early and spectacular softening of the tumors was seen within the first 3 days after high dose of TNFα ILP, as the first sign of tumor response, an observation which was never made after chemotherapy alone. Objective regression rapidly appeared. Table 20-2 gives the account of the responses. There were 39 out of 44 complete responses (90.5%) and 5 partial remissions. There has been no failure after the triple drug regimen. Mean time to objective response was 9 days for CR and 16 days for PR. A striking observation is that most CR occurred with bulky tumors with numerous nodules and that the 5 PR were at least with 75 percent tumor shrinkage.

Median follow-up time has been 13 months and only 7 out of the 44 patients (16%) developed recurrence in the perfused limb. However, 17 out of the 44 developed distant metastases. This observation strongly suggests that a state of regional resistance of the tumor developed; it was dependent on the high dose of treatment received. An illustrative case is represented in Plate 56 where all the nodules disappeared, including those very close to the tourniquet; complete response duration was 8 months and at that time generalization together with recurrence in the perfused limb appeared but only at the root of the limb, that is, where perfusion had not been optimal. Plate 57 shows a female who developed distant metastases more than 2 years after the last perfusion, but never recurred in the perfused limb when she had more than 100 nodules. Figure 20-2 shows the disease-free interval and survival which are 60 and 74 percent at 2 years, respectively, a result which is unexpected if one considers the fact that most patients were recurring after previous therapy and had a heavy tumor burden.

Since the first aim of such a therapy is limb salvage from unnecessary amputation for such a poor prognosis population, it is of interest to know that 40 out of the 44 patients kept a functional limb. There have been four amputations: two for arterial

TABLE 20-2
OUTCOME OF TNF PERFUSION

Response:	39/44	CR	= 88.6%
	5/44	PR	= 11.4%
Follow-up time:		13 months (1–35)	
Recurrence:		7/44 (16%) (2 → 13 months)	
Distant Metastases:		17/44	
Limb Salvage:		40/44	2 arterial trombosis 1 recurrence < 1 toxicity due to hyperthermia

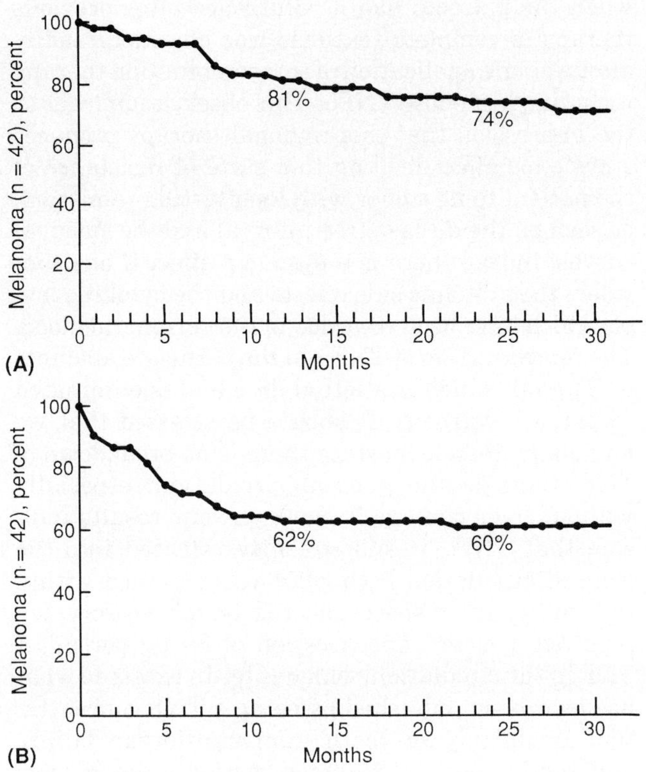

FIG. 20-2. Isolation perfusion TNF. A. Survival and B. disease free interval.

thrombosis, not related to TNF itself as it was associated to major vessel atheromatosis, one for heavy recurrence, and one for accidental burn caused by excessive hyperthermia.

TOXICITY OF ILP WITH HD rTNFα, rIFNγ, AND MELPHALAN

We analyzed systemic toxicity from a whole population of 60 patients because the same protocol was applied to soft tissue sarcoma and carcinoma patients.[12] In Table 20-3 it is obvious that chills and fever occurred in most patients with a lag period of 5 hours. It is of interest to note that this peak corresponds not to the TNFα level, but to Interleukine-6. Hypotension in the postoperative period was only severe in three patients who developed a multiorgan failure (MOF). It should be stressed that two out of the three patients were reperfused with TNFα because of partial remission or recurrence and had a significant systemic leakage. The third patient had an ulcerated and infected invasive carcinoma of the leg and developed, subsequently, a true septic shock from bacterial mobilization induced by the isolation perfusion. Since this case, we decided to exclude patients with ulcerated tumors unless they have been successfully treated to eliminate pathogens. The last patient died of septic shock, and one of the two other cases also died, not of the septic shock but from a

TABLE 20-3
SYSTEMIC TOXICITY (N = 60)

Chills, fever	mean 39.1°C	53/60	
	38°C to 40.9°C	lag period:	5 hours
Blood Pressure	Hypotension	7/60:	mild
		3/60:	MOF
Lungs	Hypoxia—ARDS	18/60	mod.→severe
		4/60:	MOF-
Kidneys	ARF	4/60:	2 grade 4
			1 grade 3
			1 grade 1
Liver	Bili	18/60	
	ENZ + bili	15/60:	4 grade 3
			2 grade 4

tension iatrogenic pneumothorax. Therefore, there has been only one lethal toxicity out of 60 perfusions.

Lung toxicity deserves some comments as it represents hypoxia and ARDS incipiens. Four patients had a MOF and 18 moderate to severe hypoxia which required intubation for a few days. It should be stressed that in some patients the x rays of the thorax showed diffused hyperdensity of both lungs accompanied with a drop of pO_2 and of saturation without any dyspnea which resolved spontaneously after 1 or 2 days.

Acute renal failure was found in four cases: there have been two grade IV, one grade III, and one grade I. It required dialysis for the two cases with grade IV and it was reversible except for one of them who died from a true septic shock (see above).

Bilirubine increase as seen in septicemia was encountered in 18 patients, but the association of increase of enzymes and hyperbilirubinemia was found in 18 patients, with four grade III and two grade IV liver failure. The two grade IV were associated with the MOF (see following).

Hematological toxicity was encountered in most patients with a drop of leukocytes and of platelets within the first 3 days with recovery by 30 days, but there has been one case of WHO grade IV for leukocytes and platelets. In that case, the cumulative systemic leakage during perfusion reached 31 percent, indicating that this toxicity can be attributed to melphalan.

Regional toxicity attributed to rTNFα was minimal, as the majority of the patients had only a grade II skin toxicity as we reported before.[12,13] Levels of TNFα and Interleukine-6 were recorded in about 20 patients. No correlation was found between the level of TNFα released from the perfused tissues after the perfusion and intense washout, indicating an individual sensitivity to the toxicity of cytokines.[23]

Although we felt that dopamine infusion and fluid loading were the major components of shock prophylaxis, we decided to add indomethacine in nine patients. Four experienced a cumulative leakage of more than 10 percent. In those patients there has been no haemodynamic, lung, or renal toxicity. In addition, no chills were observed, and the temperature ranged between 37.3 and 38.2°C. Of interest is the fact that the peripheral levels of TNFα and Interleukine-6 did not change as compared to those patients who did not receive indomethacine. Out of the nine patients, eight experienced a complete response and one a partial, indicating that protection against side effect offered by indomethacine does not compromise the antitumor activity of TNFα.

DISCUSSION AND CONCLUSION

Our work indicates that, by isolation perfusion of the limb, it is possible to deliver an effective high dosage of cytokine, achieving a very high response rate in human melanoma with acceptable toxicity. It is indeed the first evidence that the high efficacy of TNFα in animals can be confirmed in human with regional disease, when a high dosage of TNFα is administered together with IFNγ and melphalan. We strongly feel that the combination of chemotherapy to rTNFα is useful, as the cytokine alone resulted in higher recurrence rate when used alone in a pilot study. However, the necessity of using IFNγ, although supported by experimental data, has not been proven in patients. Therefore, we have decided to activate a phase II randomized trial, where in one arm IFNγ is omitted.

The mechanism whereby this treatment produces such a fast and effective tumor regression has been addressed, using morphology, immunohistology, angiography, and cytokine measurements.[12,13,23,24] We found that the prime cause of tumor destruction is the direct effect of TNFα, in addition to IFNγ, on the tumor endothelium. Within a few hours after the isolation perfusion with TNFα, there was an induction and an amplification of the expression of adhesion molecules, with resulting high recruitment of polymorphonuclear leukocytes (PMNs) which deeply and heavily invaded the metastatic nodules, a phenomenon accompanied with endothelial destruction. The latter effect was dramatically demonstrated by the angiographic disappearance of the tumor hypervascularization within 1 week after perfusion.[12] Thus, in melanoma metastatic nodule early softening and subsequent destruction in more than 90 percent of the cases seems to be related to a *primum movens* which is the destruction of the tumor microvascularization.

It is of importance to note that in most cases, whether the tumor burden was high or not, and even when the patients had a recurrence after previous therapy, a complete response was obtained readily after a single application of this combination therapy including high-dose TNFα. This observation leads to the impression that this regional therapy produces a systemic effect leading to a state of resistance of the patient to its tumor with long lasting remission, as seen on the disease-free interval and the survival curves. Indeed there is a systemic effect if one considers the systemic side effects and the cytokine levels which have been recorded in the peripheral blood. The concentration of TNFα in the perfusate amounts to 2 μg/ml, which is a lethal dose and is eliminated by intense washout. It should be stressed that we found a plateau level since there is no breakdown of TNFα outside the general circulation, especially without liver passage.[12] However, our results indicate that TNFα is subsequently released into the general circulation because it was retained within the intercellular space and the lymph vessels. We reported a mean concentration of 30 ng per ml of TNF in the circulation, which is far in excess to what has ever been published as being a TNF concentration accompanying death from multiorgan failure and septic shock.[23] Whereas, patients dying from septic shock present a TNFα concentration which does not reach the ng levels![25,26] Therefore, we question the concept of considering TNFα as being the main and/or the sole effector of septic shock toxicities. Indeed, it has been shown that endotoxin associated to TNFα dramatically increases toxicity in animals.[27] Therefore, our proposal is that TNFα being given at a high amount to patients suffering of cancer but not of septic disease do not have a significant level of endotoxin in the blood and, therefore, do not experience the high toxicity which has been reported in septicemia. At this point, we should stress the fact that we experienced one case of lethal shock because the patient had an infected tumor on the perfused limb, associated presumably to endotoxemia.

Since our first report on the successful use of rTNFα, IFNγ, and melphalan in isolation perfusion, Eggermont in Rotterdam and Schraffordt Koops in Groningen have used this protocol. The addition of their melanoma cases at the time of the writing of this chapter permits to add 8 more cases. The overall response rate from a total of 51 evaluable cases with in transit metastases is 46 complete responses (90.5%) and 5 partial responses (9.5%). Although in Brussels and Lausanne there has been 16 percent recurrences, 43 percent have been recorded in Rotterdam but it is too early to conclude, the overall local recurrence rate being 19 percent. At this time, metastases rate has been 18 out of 52, that is 36.5 percent.

The role of IFNγ is still questioned, as it may be that the upregulation of TNFα receptor may lead to more circulating soluble receptors. Therefore, we decided to design a randomized phase II study, where we compare the triple association to the association of TNFα with melphalan. This restricted trial is conducted by Lausanne, Rotterdam, and Groningen. The aim is to test whether the addition of IFNγ increases a response rate obtained with the association of high-dose rTNFα with melphalan.

In conclusion, these results demonstrate a rapid, impressive, and sustained response of in transit melanoma metastases to high-dose rTNFα when administered regionally in combination with IFNγ and chemotherapy. This triple drug regimen appears to be an attractive therapeutic approach in the treatment of regionally advanced melanoma, especially in case of melphalan failure. The limb sparing rate has been 48 out of a total of 52 cases treated in Brussels, Lausanne, Rotterdam, and Groningen, that is 92 percent with patients with a very large tumor burden.

Because of the unacceptable systemic toxicity of such a regimen, it should be limited to isolation perfusion of the limbs. Moreover, great care must be taken to avoid septic shock-like syndrome using fluid loading, dopamine, and indomethacine administration.

SUMMARY

Isolation perfusion of the limbs with high dose rTNFα (3 to 4 mg total dose) can be performed with acceptable toxicity, provided prophylaxis of septic shock-like syndrome is done. Prophylaxis of septic shock-like syndrome is effective with systemic administration of dopamine (2 μg/kg/min) starting with isolation perfusion—before rTNFα administration—and lasting at least 48 hours, fluid loading and indomethacine given systemically during 24 hours. High-dose rTNFα associated to rIFNγ and melphalan in isolation perfusion produced 90.5 percent complete remission of in transit metastasis of melanomas and 9.5 percent partial remissions with no failure. The necessity of using rIFNγ is currently studied in a randomized phase II trial.

REFERENCES

1. Carswell EA, Old JJ, Kassel RL, et al. An endotoxin induced serum factor that causes necrosis of tumors. *Proc Natl Acad Sci U S A* 72:3366–3370, 1975.
2. Aggarwal BB, Henzel WJ, Moffat B, Kohr WJ, and Harkins RN. Primary structure of human lymphotoxin derived from 1788 lymphoblastoid cell line. *J Biol Chem* 260:2334–2344, 1985b.
3. Haranaka K, Satomi N, Sukarai A. Antitumor activity of murine tumor necrosis factor against transplanted murine tumors and heterotransplanted human tumors in nude mice. *Int J Cancer* 34:263–267, 1984.
4. Balkwill FR, Ward BG, Fiers W. Effects of tumour necrosis factor on human tumour xenografts in nude mice. In (ed. by Ciba Foundation Symposium 131) *Tumour Necrosis Factor and Related Cytotoxins.* Chichester: J. Wiley & Sons, 1987, 154–169.
5. Fiers W, Brouckaert P, Goldberg AL, Kettelhut I, Suffys P, Tavernier J, Vanhaesebroeck B, and Van Roy F. Structure-function relationship of tumour necrosis factor and its mechanism of action. In (ed. by Ciba Foundation Symposium 131) *Tumour Necrosis Factor and Related Cytotoxins.* Chichester: J. Wiley & Sons, 1987, 109–123.
6. Tracey K, Beutler B, Lowry S, et al. Shock and tissue injury induced by recombinant human cachectin. *Science* 234:470–474, 1986.
7. Chapman PB, Lester TJ, Casper ES, et al. Clinical pharmacology of recombinant human tumor necrosis factor in patients with advanced cancer. *J Clin Oncol* 5:1942–1951, 1987.
8. Feinberg B, Kurzrock R, Talpaz M, et al. A phase I trial of intravenously administered recombinant tumor necrosis factor alpha in cancer patients. *J Clin Oncol* 6:1328–1334, 1988.
9. Spriggs DR, Sherman ML, Michie H, et al. Recombinant human tumor necrosis factor administered as a 24-hour intravenous infusion. A phase I and pharmacologic study. *J Natl Cancer Inst* 80:1039–1044, 1988.
10. Old, LJ. General discussion II. In: (ed. by Ciba Foundation Symposium 131), *Tumour Necrosis Factor and Related Cytotoxins.* New York: J. Wiley & Sons, 1987, 185–191.
11. Smedly LA, Tonnesen MG, Sandhaus RA, et al. Neutrophil-mediated injury to endothelial cells. Enhancement by endotoxin and essential role of neutrophil elastase. *J Clin Invest* 77:1233–1243, 1986.
12. Lienard D, LeJeune FJ, Delmotte JJ, Renard N, Ewalenko P. High-dose recombinant tumor necrosis factor-alpha in combination with interferon-gamma and melphalan in isolation perfusion of the limbs for melanoma and sarcoma. *J Clin Oncol* 10:52–60, 1992.
13. Lienard D, LeJeune FJ, Ewalenko P. In transit metastases of malignant melanoma treated by high dose rTNF-alpha in combination with interferon-gamma and melphalan in isolation perfusion. *World J Surg* 16:234–240, 1992.
14. Lienard D, LeJeune FJ, Ewalenko P, and Delmotte JJ. Isolation Perfusion (IP) with high dose Tumour Necrosis Factor (rTNF-alpha) and chemotherapy for Melanoma. In: Romagnani S, and Abbas AK (eds.) *Cytokines: Basic principles and clinical applications,* Vol. 68. Serono Symposia Publications. New York: Raven Press, 1990, 87–89.
15. LeJeune F, Ghanem G. A simple and accurate new method for cytostatics dosimetry in isolation perfusion of the limbs based on exchangeable blood volume determination. *Cancer Res* 47:639–643, 1987.
16. Tsujimoto M, Yip Y, Vilcek J. Interferon-gamma enhances the expression of cellular receptors for tumor necrosis factor. *J Immunol* 136:2441–2444, 1986.
17. Ruggiero V, Tavernier J, Fiers W, et al. Induction of the synthesis of tumor necrosis factor receptors by interferon-gamma. *J Immunol* 136:2445–2450, 1986.
18. Salmon SE, Young L, Scuderi P, Clark B. Antineoplastic effects of tumor necrosis factor alone and in combination with recombinant gamma-interferon on tumor biopsies in clonogenic assay. *J Clin Oncol* 5:1816–1821, 1987.
19. Marquet RL, Ijzermans JN, DeBruin RW, Fiers W, and Jeekel J. Anti-tumor activity of recombinant mouse tumor necrosis factor (TNF) on colon cancer in rats is promoted by rat recombinant gamma-interferon: Toxicity is reduced by indomethacin. *Int J Cancer* 40:550–553, 1987.
20. Watanabe N, Niitsu Y, Umeno H, et al. Synergistic cytotoxic and antitumor effects of recombinant human tumor necrosis factor and hyperthermia. *Cancer Res* 48:650–653, 1988.

21. Balkwill FR, and Moody EM. Positive interactions between human interferon and cyclophosphamide or Adriamycin in a human tumor model system. *Cancer Res.* 44:904–908, 1984.
22. Haranaka K, Nobuko S, Akiko S, and Haranaka R. Antitumour effects of tumour necrosis factor: Cytotoxic or necrotizing activity and its mechanism. In: (ed. by Ciba Foundation Symposium 131), *Tumour Necrosis Factor and Related Cytotoxins.* Chichester: J. Wiley & Sons, 1987, 140–153.
23. Gerain J, Lienard D, Ewalenko P, and LeJeune FJ. High serum levels of TNF-alpha after its administration for isolation perfusion of the limb. *Cytokine* vol 4, no 6 (Nov.), 1992.
24. Renard N, Lienard D, Robaye B, Van der Auwera P, LeJeune FJ. Morphological findings in melanoma, sarcoma and carcinoma metastases treated by high doses of rTNF combined with IFN and Melphalan. Correlation with in vitro studies on endothelial cells. *Cytokine* 3:520, 1991.
25. Retsas S, Leslie M, and Bottomley D. Intralesional tumor necrosis factor combined with interferon-gamma in metastatic melanoma. *Brit Med J* 298:1290–1291, 1989.
26. Fiers W, Brouckaert P, and Guisez Y. Recombinant interferon-gamma and its synergism with tumor necrosis factor in the human and mouse systems. In: Schellekens H, and Steward WE (eds.) *The Biology of the Interferon System.* Amsterdam: Elsevier Science, 1986, 241–248.
27. Soehnlen B, Liu R, and Salmon S. Recombinant TNF exhibit antitumor activity against clonogenic human tumor cells and synergism with gamma interferon. *Proc AACR* 26:303, 1985.

Chapter 21

PHYSIOLOGICAL AND PHARMACOKINETICS PARAMETERS IN ISOLATION PERFUSION OF THE LIMBS

D. Liénard, F. Lejeune, Ph. Autier, F. Sales, and G. Ghanem

INTRODUCTION

Isolation perfusion of the limbs is a therapeutic system aimed at increasing drug concentration into the limb while reducing systemic effects. This should result in an increased antitumor efficacy together with regional toxicity and a reduction of systemic side effects. It can be anticipated that all effects, beneficial and toxic, will depend on the *chemical structure of the drug* and of its pharmacokinetics, on the *perfusion conditions* such as temperature, pH, flow rate, oxygen tension and on the *patient's limb condition,* especially the vascular system.

In this chapter, we review the characteristics of different types of drugs, their dosimetry, pharmacokinetics, and toxicity studies which are by far the most useful parameters to optimize the use of isolation perfusion of the limbs.

DRUGS

Melphalan has been identified as one of the best agents to be used in isolation perfusion from the very beginning. Melphalan, a phenyl alanine mustard, is a bifunctional alkylating agent which binds loosely to plasma proteins via leucins, quickly penetrates tumor cells and readily alkylates with DNA and cross-link or strand DNA breakage.[1]

As listed in Table 21-1, other drugs have been also tried in isolation perfusion, either in association with melphalan or as single agent.

The association of melphalan with actinomycin D, a protein synthesis inhibitor, was used for a long time but seems not to bring more objective responses at the same time it seems to increase toxicity.[2]

DTIC, an imidazole carboxamide derivative, exhibiting some alkylating effects, was also tried in

TABLE 21-1
DRUGS USED IN ISOLATION PERFUSION OF THE LIMBS FOR MELANOMA IN TRANSIT MESTASTASES

DRUGS	PROPERTY	DOSE ILIAC	DOSE AXILLARY
Melphalan	Bifunctional alkylating agent	10 mg/l 40 μg/ml	13 mg/l 20 μg/ml
Actinomycin D	Antibiotic	0.014 mg/kg	0.010 mg/kg
DTIC	Alkylating agent	2.5 g/m²	1.5 g/m²
Cis-Platinum	Alkylating agent	3.2 mg/kg or 250 mg/m²	150 mg/m²
rTNFα + IFN-γ added to melphalan	Biological response modifiers	TNF-α 4 mg IFN-γ 0.2 mg	TNF-α 3 mg INF-γ 0.2 mg

isolation perfusion. As a single agent, it produces between 13 and 18 percent remission rate when systemically administered in disseminated melanoma. Although it requires a microsomal activation in the liver, it was used with some objective responses in isolation perfusion although the results reported appear inferior to the melphalan ones.[3]

Also cisplatinum, which is a very active alkylating agent, has been tried by several authors recently with and without hyperthermia. Response is certainly not higher than melphalan alone and the reported toxicity, specially neurotoxicity, seems to be higher.[4]

Recently, we designed and tried a combination regimen including melphalan with cytokines: rTNFα and IFN-γ. The rationale for such a combination is the following: there is a synergistic effect between chemotherapy and TNFα in human melanoma xenograft on the nude mouse; there is also a synergistic effect between TNFα and IFN-γ which also increases TNFα receptors.[5] This approach is reported in Chap. 20.

With the aim of melanoma targeting, an α-MSH-melphalan conjugate has been tried in isolation perfusion but is limited to perfusates with very low concentration of plasma protein because of its instability.[6]

Nowadays, melphalan is still the first choice drug with its 50 percent average complete remission rate on in transit metastases of melanoma.[7] (See Chap. 19.)

PHARMACOKINETICS OF MELPHALAN

As compared to intra-arterial infusion, continued drug delivery to the target tissue during isolated perfusion depends on drug penetration and stability of the drug in perfusate without any detoxification, metabolism, or clearance as normally occur in the liver and kidney following systemic administration.

Since isolation perfusion aims at delivering the highest tolerable dose, pharmacokinetics studies on the perfusate are useful in order to determine the disappearance curve of the drug in relation with its cytotoxic effects on the tumor cells, the toxic effects on normal tissues, and the interference of various parameters such as the volume of distribution, temperature, pH, and the injection mode. The latter was always bolus injection in the arterial line in the pharmacokinetics described in the following. However, the correlation of pharmacokinetics with drug effects in terms of tumor response and toxicity remains questionable (see following text). Figures 21-1 and 21-2 show typical biexponential disappearance curve of an iliac (Fig. 21-1) or axillary isolation perfusion (Fig. 22-2) with melphalan: α-curve with a half life of about 10 minutes is due to the drug distribution into the vascular compartment and in the extracorporeal circuit; β-curve results from drug hydrolysis and drug penetration in the tissues. It is difficult to assess the amount of melphalan taken up by the tissues but it can be indirectly measured since most of melphalan taken up by the tumor cells has

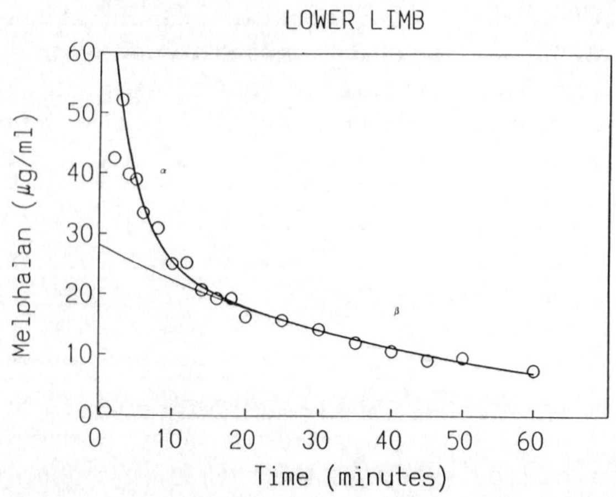

FIG. 21-1. Disappearance curve of melphalan concentration in lower limb isolation perfusion (iliac) after bolus injection in the arterial line of 40 μg/ml perfusate. Extrapolation at time 0 of β curve (see text).

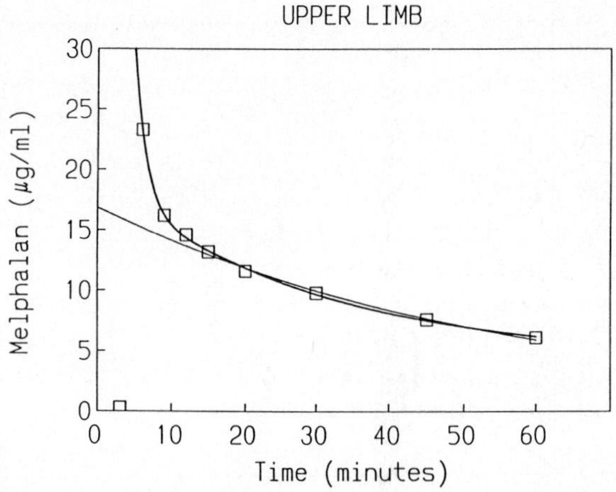

FIG. 21-2. *Same as Fig. 21-1 but for axillary isolation perfusion. Bolus injection of 20 μg/ml melphalan in the arterial line.*

reacted and is no longer detectable by high-performance liquid chromatography (HPLC), therefore, the amount of drug measured in the tissues[21] may reflect the intercellular melphalan.

The β-curve can also be used in order to calculate melphalan concentration at the equilibrium. This is done by extrapolation at time zero. This value is of great importance if one intends to check the efficacy of melphalan dosimetry as it will be shown in the following. This exponential curve seems to indicate that isolation perfusion behaves as a mammillary system where the vascular (intra- and extra-corporeal) system is sucked out by the perfused tissues. Out of 300 pharmacokinetics, we can identify a similar bi-exponential in more than 80 percent of the cases.

Instead of extrapolating at time 0, it is possible to take into account the whole pharmacodynamics. The easiest way is the measurement of the Area Under the Curve (AUC) of the drug. However, Benckhuijsen and colleagues[8] have used the steady state, considering that it represents the whole process, that is, blood distribution in the α and β phases.

More recently, Benckhuijsen and colleagues[9] suggested, thanks to a method for calculating tissue penetration, that one would be able to calculate the amount of melphalan taken by the isolated leg. The formula is based on the estimation of tissue water, where melphalan is dissolved. It was shown that the amount of drug uptaken by the normal tissue and presumably by the tumor is at least two to four fold lower than in the plasma. In addition, they found that the tissue levels were largely independent of the AUC^{60} of the plasma concentration. There was no significant difference in upper versus lower limb, when the doses of 13 and 10 mg/l limb were respectively applied.

Drug Assay in Perfusate

Drug assay in perfusate was performed by HPLC as previously described.[10] Briefly, perfusion blood samples were collected on ice and supernatants freezed at −20°C until assayed.

Sample extraction was carried out using Octadecylsilane 100 mg column (Bond Elut) previously washed with 2 ml of acetonitrile followed by 4 ml of water. One ml of each sample was pushed through the column, washed with 1 ml of water and eluted with 1 ml of acetonitrile/ammonium acetate 0,5M, pH:4.4 (1/1;v/v). 20 μl of the eluate were then chromatographed on an ODS C18 column (10 cm, 5 μm) under isocratic conditions (acetonitrile/ammonium acetate 30/70;v/v) over 10 minutes.

DOSIMETRY

Traditionally, the administration of cytostatic drug by systemic route was initially based on the body weight and is now based on the body surface. In contrast, in isolation perfusion, for decades, only the body weight has been used. The inaccuracy of this method seems to have been at least partly compensated by the magnitude of the total dose administrated. However, for accuracy of calculation of maximum tolerated dose of cytostatic during isolation perfusion of the isolated limb, a progress was needed. The first step was done by Wieberdink[11] who considered that the variable components of isolation perfusion were not the reservoir and the tubing but the volume of the perfused limb. Therefore, he designed a simple method based on the actual measurement of the whole limb volume by immersion. He found that the optimal dose was 10 mg of melphalan per tissue liter for lower limb and 13 mg/l for upper limb. Van Os and colleagues[12] further demonstrated that this method allowed to give to the individual patient a slightly higher dose of melphalan aiming at a higher antitumor effect, especially in the case of in transit metastases. Briele has proposed a method based on drug concentration versus time relationship[13] in the perfusate. More recently, a new method was designed for measuring the actual volume contained in the isolated limb.[10,14] It is based on the successive determinations of three hematocrits and is, therefore, named "the hematocrit method." The isolation perfusion system is seen as two compartments which are mixed during the perfusion. The first compartment is the pump with the oxygenator, the reservoir, and the tubing of which the volume is known since it corresponds to the priming. Its hematocrit will be very low if one unit of blood is added or equal to zero in case of no priming with blood is done. The second is the vascular compartment itself that is named exchangeable limb blood volume (ELBV) since there is no proof that the entire vascular tree is involved in the perfusion. This is the unknown volume but its hematocrit is known, equal to the patient's one. During perfusion, the two compartments will be mixed and will reach a resultant third hematocrit. Therefore, using three parameters and one unknown value, it is possible to calculate the exchangeable limb blood volume.

$$\mathrm{ELBV} = \left|\frac{\mathrm{Ha} - \mathrm{Hc}}{\mathrm{Hb} - \mathrm{Hc}}\right| \times \mathrm{Va}$$

where Ha is the hematocrit in the pump before circulation, Hb is the hematocrit of the patient at the moment of starting the isolation perfusion, Hc is the resulting hematocrit in the circuit after homogenization (at least 5 minutes after the start), and Va is the priming volume.

Then, the total volume is: ELBV + Va. Then, the total dose of melphalan to be given is calculated as follows: total volume × 40 μg melphalan for lower limb and total volume × 20 μg melphalan for upper limb.

The concentration of melphalan per ml was obtained from series of isolation perfusions where the dosage had been calculated by the Wieberdink method. In other terms, 10 mg/l with the Wieberdink method for lower limb equal 40 μg melphalan with the hematocrit method; for upper limb it is 13 μg and 20 μg, respectively.[10]

It has been proved that although the average total dose given to the patient is not very different when the three dosimetry methods are used, there are tremendous variations from patient to patient. It was actually demonstrated that no correlation exists between body weight and exchangeable blood volume or even with the volume of perfused limb.[14] Furthermore, the pharmacokinetics studies clearly demonstrated that the hematocrit method is the most accurate: there is an excellent correlation between the measured melphalan concentration and the calculated one. Figure 21-3 shows the results generated at Bordet, Brussels and Fig. 21-4 shows results from Antoni van Leeuwenhoekhuis, Amsterdam (Dr. B. Kroon) and from Royal Infirmary, Glasgow (Mr. McKay). In the latter, the hematocrit method was applied by the surgeon and the pharmacokinetics were done on samples sent to Brussels.

When the doses calculated with the Wieberdink method and the hematocrit method are compared, it is obvious that for individual patients, very little variation occurs with the Wieberdink method, while with the hematocrit method great differences are noted. This observation further demonstrates that the main variable in isolation perfusion is neither the full body weight nor the volume of the isolated limb but the volume of blood within the limb which

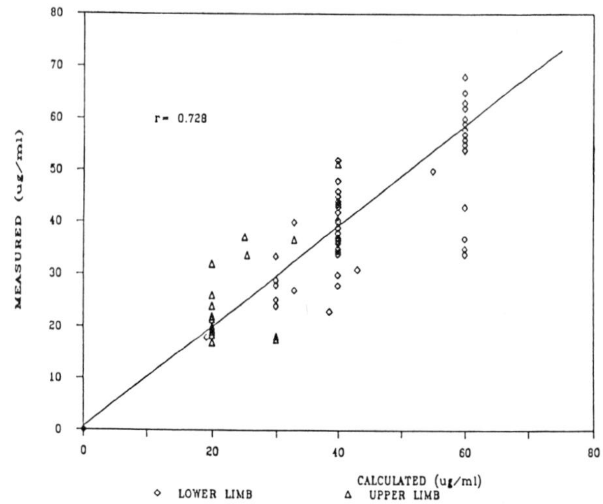

FIG. 21-3. Comparison between melphalan concentration at the equilibrium in the perfusate. Abcissa: calculated with the hematocrit method; Ordinate: measured by HPLC; n = *87 (Brussels cases).*

can be exchanged with the isolation perfusion system.

Using this hematocrit method, we found that we could even increase melphalan dosage in some patients as compared to the other methods.

Most protocols for isolation perfusion currently use Wieberdink method for calculation of drug dose which can be applied by any group. The hematocrit method requires the availability of a hematology laboratory during the procedure although hematocrits can be easily measured in the operating room with an adequate centrifuge. In the appendix, the methods for measuring the limb volume and the practical considerations for the hematocrit method are described.

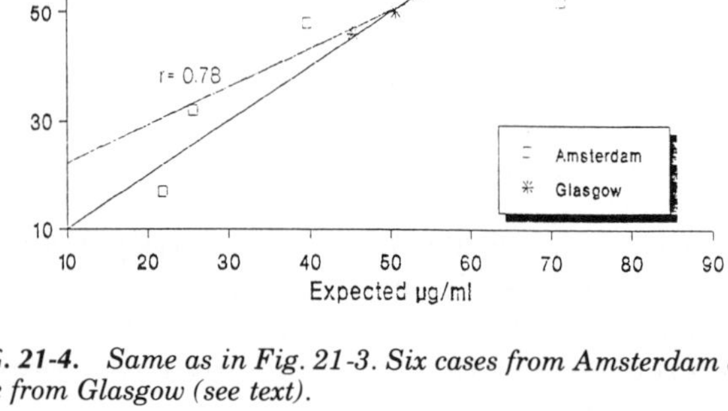

FIG. 21-4. Same as in Fig. 21-3. Six cases from Amsterdam and five from Glasgow (see text).

TOXICITY AND ISOLATION PERFUSION PARAMETERS

Systemic as well as regional toxicities should be separately considered.

Systemic Toxicity

The systemic toxicity will be mainly due to drug leakage during perfusion and leakage of unbound drug after it. Table 21-2 shows the differences in systemic and regional toxicities according to three commonly used drugs, that is, melphalan, *cis*-platinum, and rTNFα. It is clear that with all drugs, a systemic leakage during perfusion will produce systemic side effects, depending on the characteristics of the drug. All are able to induce hematological toxicity mainly thrombocytopenia and leucopenia. *Cis*-DDP is highly toxic for the kidneys as is TNFα in addition to its capacity to induce a septic shock-like syndrome.

After perfusion, the limb is thoroughly washed to remove unbound drug. One liter of Plasmalyte for wash is used following melphalan perfusion, 2 or 3 liters of Plasmalyte following TNFα perfusion. After melphalan isolation perfusion, washing usually does not release significant amounts of drugs because of its low level at the end of the procedure (see previous text). With *cis*-platinum however, consistent amounts of platinum are released by the perfused limb and recovered from the urine for 3 to 4 days after isolation perfusion.[15] Kidney toxicity should be prevented by hyperhydration during 72 hours. rTNFα levels have been measured in peripheral blood up to 24 hours after isolation perfusion and this commonly results chills and elevated temperature and in some cases a septic shock-like syndrome. (See Chap. 20.)

After most of the isolation perfusions, irrespective of the choice of drug, a significant drop in plasma total proteins is seen up to 3 days. It seems to be due to both a third compartment syndrome related to the capillary leak induced by the isolation perfusion at least in the limb and to hyperhydration. It is useful in some cases to administer up to 2 units of human albumin and 2 units of plasma proteins per day in order to counteract the hypoalbuminemia. An additional beneficial effect of this procedure is that most patients have only slight edema which does not require fasciotomy as used regularly by others (see Chap. 19).

Regional Toxicity

As indicated in Table 21-2, the most frequent regional toxicity include skin, muscles, nerves, and vessels in diminishing order.

Skin toxicity is the main criterion for assessing isolation perfusion regional toxicity and is well classified. Wieberdink has proposed a grading system[11] which is presented in Table 21-3. Grade 2 seems to correspond to the optimal isolation perfusion conditions since the erythema and the slight edema are well tolerated. Grade 3 with blistering corresponds to a more painful side effect on skin and soft tissues. In our opinion, this is unnecessary and does not necessarily result in a better tumor response. Grades 4 and 5 are not acceptable but can occur in case of excess of hyperthermia, excess of cytotoxic drug, and anoxemia.

We reviewed (Liénard et al, in preparation) 205 consecutive cases of adult isolation perfusion using mild hyperthermia and with melphalan in whom pharmacokinetics were done together with the measurement of volume parameters by the hematocrit method and limb volume. In order to evaluate the respective importance of various perfusion parameters they were compared as follows:

$$\begin{aligned}\text{Total dose} &= \text{dose} \times \text{volume}\\ &= \text{dose} \times (\text{priming} + \text{ELBV})\\ &= \text{dose} \times \text{priming} \times \left(1 + \frac{\text{Ha} - \text{Hc}}{\text{Hb} - \text{Hc}}\right)\end{aligned}$$

The dose was fixed by the operator. For the lower limb, the dose was either 40 μg/ml which correlates

TABLE 21-2
TOXICITY FROM ISOLATION PERFUSION

	SYSTEMIC TOXICITY				REGIONAL TOXICITY			
DRUG	RELEASED BY PERFUSED TISSUES AFTER ILP	SHOCK	RENAL	HEMATOLOGIC	MUSCLES	SKIN	NERVES	NORMAL VESSELS
Melphalan	−	−	−	+	+	+	+	−
Cis-platinum	+	−	+	+	+	+	++	+
rTNF-α	++	++	+	+	−	−	−	−[a]

[a] *Tumor vessels* are the target

TABLE 21-3
SKIN TOXICITY AFTER ISOLATION PERFUSION AFTER WIEBERDINK[15]

GRADE	
1 (mild)	No subjective or objective evidence of reaction
2 (moderate)	Slight erythema and/or edema
3 (high)	Considerable erythema and/or edema with some blistering; slightly disturbed motility permissible
4 (severe)	Extensive epidermolysis, superficial necrosis
5 (severe)	Obvious damage to the deep tissues, causing definite functional disturbances, threatening or manifest compartmental syndromes, necrosis requiring amputation

with Wieberdink's 10 mg/l of perfused limb or 60 μg/ml which was used sometimes for unresectable in transit metastases. For the upper limb, the dose was of 20 μg/ml. For the statistical analysis of toxicities, three kinds of data were considered: (1) the initial parameter based on hematocrit method of dosimetry; (2) the physiological parameters which may exert an influence on the effects of melphalan; (3) the pharmacokinetic parameters which result, in part, from the action of the dosimetry and which are potential predictors of melphalan toxicity. This analysis has considered these three sets of parameters separately.

Because of the small number of toxicities in Grades 1 and 4, the nonparametric Kruskall-Wallis test was used to compare between the four grades of toxicity. In all other univariate analyses, Student t-test or ANOVA F-test were applied.

Table 21-4 displays the univariate analysis of toxicity according to the initial parameters, the flow, and pharmacokinetics.

TABLE 21-4
TOXICITY ACCORDING TO INITIAL PARAMETERS OF ISOLATION PERFUSION

	p VALUE	
INITIAL PARAMETERS	LOWER LIMB	UPPER LIMB
Total dose (mg)	0.001	0.003
Total perfusate volume (ml)	0.45	0.18
Priming volume (ml)	0.65	0.03
Calculated concentration (μg/ml)	0.05	0.003
Flow (ml/min)	0.99	0.003
ELBV (ml)	0.60	0.91
PHARMACOKINETICS		
Peak concentration (μg/ml)	0.003	0.05
Concentration at equilibrum (μg/ml)	<0.0001	0.01
Area under the curve (mm^2)	<0.0001	0.003

For lower and upper limb, total dose and calculated concentration seem to be associated with toxicity together with the three parameters of pharmacokinetics. Flow played a major influence in upper limb but not in the lower limbs. This discrepancy may be due to the fact that the flow influences the AUC (Liénard et al., in preparation). A slow flow should result in a higher duration of contact of melphalan with the tissues.

In Table 21-5, the quantity of melphalan in the external circuit, that is, the priming volume, and in the limb vascular bed, that is, ELBV, are compared by univariate logistic regression. These data demonstrate that the extracorporeal quantity of melphalan is strongly associated with the toxicities. This finding points out the importance of standardizing and optimalizing the priming volume. This aim will not be easily achieved due to the great variety of oxygenators used around the world.

DRUG ADMINISTRATION AND ISOLATION LIMB PERFUSION PARAMETERS

Some practical considerations are of importance as they will determine the efficacy of isolation perfusion, and its toxicity since the drug delivery and metabolism can be altered.

Drug Injection into the Circuit

Melphalan may be given into the arterial line or into the venous reservoir. No comparative studies have been made to determine which method is more effective and less toxic. It has been suggested that bolus administration in the artery may cause severe arterial damage. We have never encountered this problem. The pharmacokinetics of melphalan injected either way is similar with a slight difference in that the initial peak can be higher when injected in the reservoir. Instead of bolus injection, fractionated injection can be used either three or four times during the 60 minutes.[16] The pharmacokinetics consists of several peaks but it seems that the area under the curves are not higher. There is no increased uptake of the drug into the tissue by fractionation.[17]

TABLE 21-5
TOXICITY ACCORDING TO THE DOSE OF MELPHALAN IN PRIMING VOLUME AND IN THE LIMBS

LOWER LIMB	$\chi 2$	p
Melphalan quantity in priming	9.5	<0.0001
Melphalan quantity in limb (ELBV)	1.4	>0.50
UPPER LIMB		
Melphalan quantity in priming	10.7	<0.0001
Melphalan quantity in limb (ELBV)	0.5	>0.50

Current protocol of the EORTC-WHO-NAPG recommends a bolus injection in the reservoir.[3]

Hyperthermia

It is widely recognized that in the past, due to the inefficient heating system, a hypothermia condition was applied with poor microhemodynamic and low-drug delivery into the tissues. Cavaliere and colleagues[18] showed that hyperthermia itself at a temperature around 42°C was able to induce tumor response. However, the regional toxicity was high and was followed by amputation in a few cases. Stehlin[19] proposed the use of mild hyperthermia, between 39°C and 40°C. These conditions have shown to produce an optimal microcirculation with maximal glucose and oxygen consumption in the tissues.[20] In addition, it seems that this temperature can potentiate the effect of melphalan[21] and also of rTNFα. Vaglini and colleagues have claimed that higher temperature results in higher response.[22] However, Kroon and colleagues[23] feel that there is no major difference in terms of efficacy and toxicity between mild hyperthermia and true normothermia which is between 37 and 37.5°C. Moreover, they reported (see Chap. 20) an increased toxicity with high antitumor effect when using "true" hyperthermia that is about 40°C. Since no randomized trial has been conducted so far due to the difficulty of the methodology of comparing slightly different temperatures with a lot of variations, it is difficult to arrive at any definite conclusion. However, it should be pointed out that true normothermia fits with blood temperature but not with tissue temperatures which are around 33 to 34 in the extremity skin. Therefore, most perfusionists nowadays use more or less hyperthermic conditions that are between 38°C and ≤40°C. Figure 21-5 illustrates a typical case treated according to the EORTC 18832 protocol (Figure 21-5).

Composition of the Perfusate

Diluted blood is mostly used because it facilitates the hemodynamics by significantly reducing the viscosity. The blood component can be either autologous blood or bank blood. It seems that this is not a major point although fresh blood will allow less hemolysis and, therefore, a better oxygen transport and also less error in hematocrit measurements. Proteins are important for drug transport and to minimize drug adsorption to the extracorporeal equipment. In review of isolation perfusion toxicity, no influence of whole problem content of perfusate was noted.

Sulfhydryl compounds such as glutathion can protect from alkylating toxicity.[24] This aspect is currently under investigation.

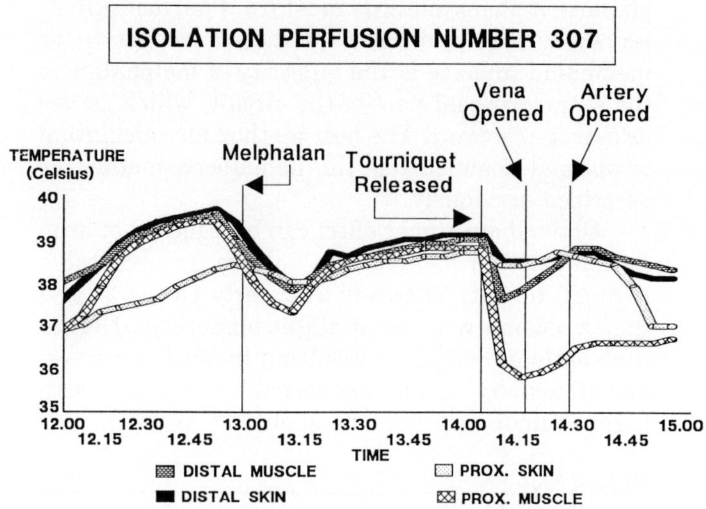

FIG. 21-5. Time course of tissue temperature measurements at four sites during and after iliac isolation perfusion. The first drop of temperature after melphalan administration is due to the reduction from 41°C to 38°C for 10 minutes. Second drop is due to the anoxemia during vessel repair. Proximal muscle seems less perfused in physiological conditions than during isolation perfusion.

Oxygenation

Adequate oxygenation depends on the flow. This was demonstrated by using partial pressure oxygen (pO_2) probes in the extremity tissues both in dogs[25] and in humans.[26] Since chemotherapy uptake by tumor cells is an active mechanism, it is of paramount importance that the tissues are not anoxic when the drugs reach them. Moreover, the pO_2 into the vessels and the surrounding tissues may be adequate, creating a higher uptake into the normal tissues, as compared to the tumor nodules. It has been also shown that drug delivery is optimal with an optimal flow. That is in contrast with the proposal made by Aigner of reducing drastically the pump flow when injecting the drugs. The pharmacokinetics of drugs in the perfusate seems to support this hypothesis but there is no proof that drug uptake by the tumor tissues in increased. Therefore, it seems that high flow is recommended because it permits an optimal microcirculation and an optimal drug delivery.

CONCLUSIONS

Although the pharmacokinetics of chemotherapeutics in isolation perfusion system are available, we still need information on the drug uptake by tumor tissues. This is a difficult problem since most available methods measure drug concentrations in the tissues but not necessarily uptake by the cells. It is hoped that new experimental models will address this question.

The single most efficacious drug used in isolation perfusion of the limbs for melanoma is melphalan—a phenylalanine mustard. Pharmacokinetics show that the most predictive criterion for melphalan toxicity is the quantity of melphalan in the extracorporeal part of the circuit, which serves as a drug reservoir. The best method for calculation of optimal dosimetry is the hematocrit method as described previously.

Optimal antitumor effect can be achieved at drug concentration which results only in an acceptable regional toxicity of Grade 2 or early Grade 3 (erythema, edema with no or slight blistering). Higher than optimal drug dose resulting in more severe regional toxicity is not necessarily associated with higher tumor response and should be avoided.

REFERENCES

1. Colvin M. The alkylating agent. In Chabner B. (ed.), *Pharmacologic Principles of Cancer Treatment.* Philadelphia: Saunders, 1982, 276–308.
2. Martijn H, Oldhjoff J, and Schraffordt Koops H. Hyperthermic regional perfusion with melphalan and a combination of melphalan and actinomycin D in the treatment of locally metastasized malignant melanomas of the extremities. *J Surg Oncol* 20:9–13, 1982.
3. Lejeune FJ and Vaglini M. Regional chemotherapy in melanoma, In: Cascinelli N, et al. (eds.), *Cutaneous Melanoma Biology and Management.* Milan: Masson, 1990, 233–239.
4. Hajarizadeh H, Mueller CR, Woltering EA, Small K, and Fletcher WS. Phase I-II trial of hyperthermic isolated limb perfusion with cisplatin in the treatment of high risk malignant melanoma of the extremities. *Melanoma Res* 1:55–61, 1991.
5. Liénard D, Ewalenko P, Delmotte J-J, Renard N, and LeJeune FJ. High doses of rTNFα in combination with IFN-gamma and melphalan in isolation perfusion of the limbs for melanoma and sarcoma. *J Clin Oncol* 10:52–60, 1992.
6. Ghanem G, Libert A, Arnould R, Vercammen-Grandjean A, and Lejeune FJ. Human melanoma targeting with α-MSH-melphalan conjugate. *Melanoma Res* 1:105–115, 1991.
7. Schraffordt Koops H, Kroon BB, and Lejeune FJ. Isolated regional perfusion in the treatment of local recurrence, satellites and in transit metastases of extremity melanomas. In: Rümcke P. (ed.) *Therapy of Advanced Melanoma, Pigment Cell Series,* Vol 10, Basel: Karger, 1990, 67–78.
8. Benckhuijsen C, Varossieau FJ, Hart AAM, Wieberdink J, and Noordhoek J. Pharmacokinetics of melphalan in isolated perfusion of the limbs. *J Pharmacol Exp Ther* 237:583–588, 1986.
9. Benckhuijsen C, Kroon BB, Van Geel AN, and Wieberdink J. Regional perfusion treatment with melphalan for melanoma in a limb: An evaluation of drug kinetics. *Eur J Surg Oncol* 14:157–163, 1988.
10. Lejeune FJ, and Ghanem GE. A simple and accurate new method for cytostatics dosimetry in isolation perfusion of the limbs based on exchangeable blood volume determination. *Cancer Res* 47:639–643, 1987.
11. Wieberdink J, Benckhuijsen C, Braat RP, Van Slooten EA, and Olthuis GA. Dosimetry in isolation perfusion of the limbs by assessment of perfused tissue volume and grading of toxic tissue reactions. *Eur J Cancer Clin Oncol* 18:905–910, 1982.
12. Van Os, Schraffordt Koops H, and Oldhoff J. Dosimetry of cytostatics in hyperthermic regional isolated perfusion. *Cancer* 55:698–701, 1985.
13. Briele HA, Djuric M, Jung DT, Mortell T, Patel MK, and Das Gupta TK. Pharmacokinetics of melphalan in clinical isolation perfusion of the extremities. *Cancer Res* 1885–1889, 1985.
14. Lejeune FJ, Ghanem G, Liénard D, and Ewalenko P. Assessment of the haematocrit method for dosimetry of cytostatics in isolation perfusion. *Reg Cancer Treat* 2:82–86, 1989.
15. Zwelling LA. Cisplatin and new platinum analogs. In: Pinedo HM and Chabner BA (eds.), *Cancer Chemotherapy/8, The EORTC Cancer Chemotherapy Annual.* Amsterdam: Elsevier, 1986, 97–116.
16. Krementz E and Saha S. Limb perfusion with melphalan for melanoma by increased dose and dilution compared to the standard technique—a pilot study. *Reg Cancer Treat* 2:233–237, 1989.
17. Scott RN, Blackie R, Byrne D, Kaye SB, MacKie RM, and McKay AJ. Tissue levels of melphalan achieved by isolated limb perfusion for malignant melanoma. ICRCT'89. Berchtesgaden, June 5–7, 1989, session MP9, pp 54.
18. Cavaliere R, Ciocatto E, Giovanella B, Heidelberger CH, Johnson RO, Margottini M, Mondovi B, Moricca G, and Rossifanelli A. Selective heat sensitivity of cancer cells: Biochemical and clinical studies. *Cancer* 20:1351–1381, 1967.
19. Stehlin JS, Giovanella BC, de Ipolyi PD, and Anderson RF. Results of eleven years' experience with heated perfusion for melanoma of the extremities. *Cancer Res* 39:2255–2257, 1979.
20. Vaupel P. Oxygen supply to malignant tumors. In: Peterson HI (ed.), *Tumor Blood Circulation: Angiogenesis, Vascular Morphology and Blood Flow of Experimental and Human Tumors.* Boca Raton, Fl: CRC Press, 1979, 144–168.
21. Natali, PG, Zupi G, Greco C, Cavaliere R, Giacomini P, and Ferrone S. Effect of hyperthermia and neoplastic drugs on cell survival and antigen-antigenic profile of two human melanoma cell lines. In: Hegermann, A/1170, Tom 15-SE: 12.1, 12.3, 246/9–246-18, Proc. Thirteenth International Congress Chemotherapy, Vienna: Springer-Verlag H. 1983.
22. Vaglini M, Belli F, Marolda R, Prada A, Santinami M, and Cascinelli N. Hyperthermiec antiblastic perfusion with DTIC in stage IIIa-IIIb melanoma of the extremities. *Eur J Sur Oncol* 13:127–129, 1987.
23. Kroon BB, Van Geel AN, Benckhiujsen C, and Wieberdink J. Normothermic isolation perfusion with melphalan for advanced melanoma of the limbs. *Anticancer Res* 7:441–442, 1987.
24. Calcutt, G and Conners TA. Tumor sulfhydryl levels and sensitivity to the nitrogen mustard merophan. *Biochem Pharmacol* 12:839–845, 1963.
25. Fontijne WPJ, de Vries J, Mook P, Elstrodt J, Oosterhuis JW, Schraffordt Koops H, Oldhoff J, and Wildevuur CH. Improved tissue perfusion during pressure-regulated hyperthermic regional isolated perfusion in dogs. *J Surg Oncol* 26:69–76, 1984.
26. Byrne DS, McKay AJ, Scott RN, Hughes J, Burnside G, and McKie RM. Assessment of regional perfusion for melanoma by preoperative transcutaneous oxygen tension (Ptc = 2) measurement. ICRCT'89 Berchtesgaden, June 5–7, 1989, session MP8, pp 53.

Chapter 22

ARTERIAL INFUSION TECHNIQUES FOR MALIGNANT MELANOMA

K.R. Aigner and H. Müller

INTRODUCTION

Approximately 15 to 20 percent of melanoma patients will eventually exhibit systemic metastasis. The treatment for metastatic melanoma in general remains unsatisfactory. Systemic chemotherapy, at the cost of moderate to high toxicity, results in low-partial response. One of the reasons for low incidence of response to systemic chemotherapy is low-level drug delivery to target tissue when the chemotherapeutic agent is administered intravenously. A higher systemic dose is precluded due to accompanying severe toxicity. Clinical studies of isolated perfusion for melanomas of the extremities have demonstrated that a higher drug dose can result in high rate of complete response and subsequent cure in selected cases.

The possibility of increase in the drug delivered to target tissue through intra-arterial administration have been evaluated for a wide variety of cancers. Drugs with short half-life such as 5 FU will have advantage of higher delivery at first passage. Also, manipulation of the blood flow rate to the target tissue can result in significant increase in drug delivery. Intra-arterial chemotherapies have been used for the treatment of melanoma. This chapter reviews the method, drug schedule, and toxicity of intra-arterial administration of chemotherapy for the treatment of melanoma.

INDICATIONS FOR INTRA-ARTERIAL INFUSION

Similar to isolated limb perfusion, intra-arterial chemotherapy for melanoma is suitable for metastasis localized to anatomic areas with defined dominant blood supply. However, unlike isolated perfusion system, intra-arterial chemotherapy is an open circuit. Therefore, after first pass effect and benefit of higher drug delivery following reduction of blood flow with intra-arterial balloon or external tourniquet compression, unbound drug will mix with systemic circulation with potential for the systemic toxicity. This excess drug escape to the systemic circulation can be reduced by chemofiltration of the venous blood. Intra-arterial chemotherapy may be instituted in partially open circuits like chest wall, shoulder, hip, inguinal region, accessible through subclavian or iliac artery. Simultaneous chemofiltration can be instituted to reduce the systemic leak of the drug and immediate and cumulative systemic toxicity with filtration catheter in subclavian or iliac vein.[1,2]

TECHNIQUE FOR THE CHEMOFILTRATION

A double lumen filtration catheter (PfM cologne, FRG) is inserted via the saphenous or the femoral vein and the tip is positioned under x ray control to the point where the maximum drug concentration is expected. The procedure is performed under systemic heparinization using local or general anesthesia. The filtration catheter is then connected to a chemoprocessor or a simple filtration unit consisting of three roller pumps, a filter, and scales. Filtrate container and substitution solution bags are both placed on the scales where an equilibrium is maintained throughout the procedure (Fig. 22-1). Dependency on the individual drug or drug combinations, intra-arterial infusion of chemotherapeutics is given over 30 to 60 minutes and chemofiltration is usually maintained for 60 to 90 minutes until the filtrate amounts to at least 10 liters.

Results

Melanoma data obtained so far shows that local response is improved in some cases, but nevertheless results were not striking, since impressive immediate tumor necroses as in isolated perfusion were not observed. However, systemic toxicity and side effects were lower, indicating a potential benefit of filtration.

In melanoma there is a need for prolongation of the local exposure time at higher drug concentrations in order to overcome the baseline level of chemoresistance, and achieve results similar to the isolation perfusion system. This can be attained either by blood-flow reduction, by temporary arterial blocking, or venous outflow occlusion.

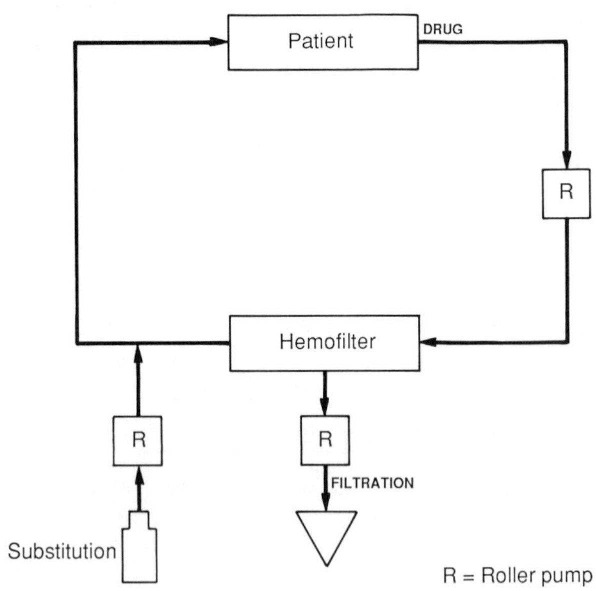

FIG. 22-1. Schematic illustration of chemofiltration.

CHEMOEMBOLIZATION

This method is suitable only for intra-arterial chemotherapy for liver metastasis especially from ocular melanoma. Chemoembolization combines temporary local ischemia and increase drug exposure, which results in an enhancement of cytotoxicity. Early experiences with Ethibloc®,[3] showed high morbidity and pain due to definitive blocking of capillary branches. Epidural anesthesia is mandatory when using Ethibloc®. Chemoembolization with Gel Foam® proved to be better in terms of morbidity and prevention of pain.

TECHNIQUE FOR CHEMOEMBOLIZATION

Vascular access may be achieved by means of an angiography catheter placed percutaneously through the femoral artery by the Seldinger technique with the tip of the catheter positioned into the common hepatic artery. Alternatively, surgical catheter placement may be performed with a routine technique using a port catheter (Jet Port II, PfM cologne, FRG) which tolerates high pressures in the port chamber as well as in the rigid polyurethane tube. The tip of the catheter is positioned and fixed in the gastroduodenal artery with its tip right at the origin from the common hepatic artery. The catheter is exited through the abdominal wall and connected to the port placed in a subcutaneous pouch on the fascia on the rectus abdominis muscle.

In order to keep side effects minimal, chemoembolization should be performed in three sittings on three consecutive days. For prophylaxis of pain just before each Gel Foam embolization, 3 to 5 ml of 0.5 percent Xylocaine is injected in 1 to 2 minutes through the arterial catheter.

In patients with average body weight of 70 kg, total doses of drugs for each cycle are calculated up to 20 mg of mitomycin C (MMC), 40 mg of melphalan (L-PAM) and 50 to 100 mg of Cisplatinin (CDDP). In case of extensive liver evolvement, MMC and L-PAM are reduced by 30 percent each. Daily doses do not exceed 10 mg of MMC, 20 mg of L-PAM, and 50 mg of CDDP. Combinations usually given are listed in Table 22-1. Embolisates consisting of 3 cm by 2 cm Gel Foam, 3 ml of 0.5 percent Xylocaine, and lyopholized drug injected over 3- to 5-minute period. This regimen is well tolerated by the patients. In general, epidural anesthesia is not necessary and remission induction usually can be seen in CT-scan a few days after the therapy showing hypodense metastases. Second look laparotomy, in case of marked response reveals tumor necrosis (Plates 58 and 59).

As mentioned previously, main indication for hepatic chemoembolization is metastases from ocu-

TABLE 22-1
DRUG DOSE AND SCHEDULE FOR HEPATIC CHEMOEMBOLIZATION

	MMC	L-PAM	CDDP	XYLOCAIN (1%)	GEL FOAM
Day 1	10 mg	20 mg		3 ml	3 cc
Day 2	10 mg		50 mg	3 ml	3 cc
Day 3		20 mg	50 mg	3 ml	3 cc

lar melanoma which has a tendency to metastasize predominantly to the liver. In most other anatomic areas of the body, however, chemoembolization cannot be applied due to excessive local ischemia. The appropriate technique to overcome this problem is reduction of the blood flow or complete blocking by means of tourniquet infusion.

TOURNIQUET INFUSION AND ARTERIAL BALLOON OCCLUSION

Both methods include temporary interruption of the arterial blood flow while the drug is injected into the main arterial vessel supplying a tumor-bearing limb or organ. The rationale are the local ischemia enhancing cytotoxicity of the drugs coupled with an increase in the local drug concentration resulting higher drug delivery due to low flow and low washout rate.

External Tourniquet Blocking

Although for advanced melanoma localized to the limb, isolation perfusion as described (see Chap. 19) is considered to be the treatment of choice, an effective alternative may be tourniquet infusion.[4–6] Duration of blocking can be chosen individually according to local tissue tolerance. This method is indicated for metastatic lesions in the limbs not reaching entirely up to the groin or axilla, since there must be some free space for the tourniquets such as inflatable cuffs or rubber bandages, placed as proximally as possible.

Arterial Balloon Catheter Occlusion

In contrast to the external tourniquet blocking method, this technique may be utilized for the lesions in the limb extending proximal to the inguinal ligament or the shoulder and also for lesion in the chest wall, pelvis, and lower abdominal area.

SUBCLAVIAN ARTERY INFUSION WITH BALLOON OCCLUSION

Presence of lesions in the axillary region and shoulder require placement of a balloon catheter into subclavian artery. Catheter is inserted by Sledinger technique from the groin and the tip is positioned distal to the origin of the vertebral artery to prevent infusion of the chemotherapeutic agents to the central nervous system. The balloon is then inflated and the blood flow through the subclavian artery is blocked. To verify correct positioning of the catheter, contrast imaging of all vascular branches is necessary (Plate 60). Homogeneous distribution of the drug to the target tissue is also checked by injection of blue dye through the catheter while the intra-arterial balloon is inflated (Plate 61). This procedure is considered mandatory to insure proper drug delivery to the target tissue since prior surgery and radiation therapy may alter the anatomic route of blood flow to the area of interest. Choice of the chemotherapeutics may be dictated by the protocol. We use single agent or combination of Melphalan, Cisplatinin, and Mitomycin C as described in the chemoembolization section (without Gel Foam). To avoid ischemic and vascular damage, occlusion time should not exceed 10 minutes. While catheter remains in place, it is connected to a perfusion pump with infusion of heparin at a rate of 20,000 unit per 24 hours. In responding patients where subsequent intra-arterial infusion for maintenance therapy is advisable, permanent port catheter may be implanted surgically. Through a supraclavicular incision, the subclavian artery is exposed, secured with a tape, and the tip of a jetport, all round catheter (PPM, cologne FRG) is inserted end-to-side in subclavian artery and fixed with a proline purse-string suture (Plate 62). The port is placed in a subcutaneous pouch on the pectoral muscle. This technique has been described. In order to achieve infusion in a more limited area, a pneumatic cuff is placed around the upper arm in order to stop the blood flow distally and preferentially infuse to the area supplied by axillary artery and to the chest wall.

ILIAC ARTERY BALLOON OCCLUSION

The technique for the iliac artery balloon occlusion for melanoma invading the groin or small pelvis is comparable to the subclavian access. Angiography catheters are introduced through the contralateral groin. The occlusion is achieved either in the common iliac artery or up in the aortic bifurcation. In case the diameter of the vessels is too large, one thin infusion catheter and one stronger blocking catheter are inserted simultaneously (Plate 63).

Depending on the location of the metastatic spread, blood flow to the distal limb can be blocked by means of a pneumatic cuff. Choice of drugs and their dosages are comparable to those for the subclavian infusion, however, they can be increased if the infused tissue volumes tend to be too large. As soon as the total doses reach or exceed systemically tolerable ranges, the addition of chemofiltration may be useful to prevent systemic toxicity.

DISCUSSION

Systemic chemotherapy for metastatic melanoma usually results in partial remission. Systemic toxicities limit use of higher dose of drug which would allow higher drug delivery to target tissue to improve response. Regional chemotherapy, as by administration of the drug by intra-arterial route, have several advantages. Tissue hypoxia, alteration of blood flow, drug exposure time, local hyperthermia, and so on, can all be utilized to improve drug delivery to tumor tissue to improve response. Intra-arterial administration of the drug for treatment of melanoma may be instituted using several different techniques such as chemoembolization, tourniquet infusion, or intra-arterial balloon occlusion. Each method has its own indication and advantages. Chemoembolization can only be used for melanoma in anatomic region which will tolerate embolization such as liver. Tourniquet infusion is applicable for lesions in the extremities not extending to inguinal region or shoulder area. For more proximal extremities lesions or lesions involving chest wall, gluteal region, and so forth, a balloon catheter occlusion chemoembolization technique is more applicable. This method can only be used for metastatic melanoma confined to an anatomic region which will tolerate embolism such as in liver. In the past decade, the techniques for chemoembolization were enveloped[3,7,8] and continuously improved by incorporation of results obtained from basic research.[9–11] To clinically exploit this concept of ischemia and prolonged drug exposure, it is important to optimize and standardize the method of chemoembolization as to make it easily feasible for the physicians and tolerable for the patients. Administration of total dose over 3 days is outlined in the protocol instead of single dose. Use of local anesthetics, and so on, decreased the morbidity significantly.

Intra-arterial administration with tourniquet infusion is an alternative to isolated perfusion. Similar to isolated perfusion, this method is suitable only for regional metastasis in the limb with disease limited below inguinal ligament or shoulder joint. However, this method may be utilized repeatedly without any antecedent surgical morbidity associated with isolation perfusion. The simplicity of the technique is its greatest advantage. This technique is also being improved continuously to achieve the best combination of occlusion time, extent of decrease of blood flow (complete vs. partial), and tissue tolerance.[4–6] Although it has been suggested that partial occlusion of blood flow may allow a more even distribution of the drug,[4] other investigators have showed fairly uniform drug distribution with both partial and complete occlusion.[6] We have shown that toxicity is not increased with 10 minutes occlusion compared to 5 minutes occlusion.[5] Yet, utilization of high-drug dose may necessitate reduction in occlusion time to avoid toxicity.

The technique of intra-arterial balloon occlusion can be utilized not only for melanoma confined to the extremities but also to disease extending more proximally to the chest wall and gluteal region and pelvis. In contrast to isolated perfusion, unbound drug administered by intra-arterial route will enter the systemic circulation and result in systemic toxicity. The possibility of these toxicity increase with utilization of higher drug dose. This systemic exposure to the drug can be effectively minimized by the use of the chemofiltration technique in conjunction with intra-arterial infusion.[3] Long-term control with improved survival as a result of intra-arterial infusion with blood-flow occlusion and reduction of systemic toxicity by concomitant use of hemefiltration needs to be studied in a prospective fashion.

REFERENCES

1. Aigner KR, Müller H, Walther H, and Link KH. Drug filtration in high dose regional chemotherapy. *Contr. Oncol.* Basel: Karger, 1988, 261–280.
2. Muchmore JH, Krementz ET, Carter RD, Meyer GM, Preslan JE, and George WJ. Management of advanced intra-abdominal malignancy using high-dose intra-arterial chemotherapy with concomitant hemofiltration. *Reg. Cancer Treat.* Vol. 3. Heidelberg: Springer, 1990, 211–216.
3. Schultheis KH. Chemoembolisation: A new treatment for malignant tumors and metastases. *Rec. Res. Cancer Res. 86,* Heidelberg: Springer, 1983, 46–47.
4. Jönsson PE, Ingrar C, and Stridbeck H. Tourniquet infusion chemotherapy in extremities with DTIC in therapy resistant melanoma on the extremities: A pilot study. *Rec. Res. Cancer Res.* Heidelberg: Springer, 1983, 13–217.
5. Karakousis CP, Rao V, Holtermann OA, Kauter PM, and Holyoke ED. Tourniquet infusion chemotherapy in extremities with malignant lesions. *Surg Gynecol Obstet* 149:481–487, 1979.
6. Karakousis CP, Kanter PM, Lopez RE, Moore R, and Holyoke ED. Modes of regional chemotherapy. *J Surg Res* 26:134–138, 1979.
7. Kato T, Nemoto R, Hisashi M, and Takahashi M. Arterial chemoembolization with mitmycin C microcapsules in the treatment of primary or secondary carcinoma of the kidney, liver, bone and intrapelvic organs. *Cancer* 49:674–680, 1981.
8. Wallace S, Chuang VP. The radiological diagnosis and management of hepatic metastases. *Radiology* 22:56–64, 1982.
9. Link KH, Aigner KR, Kuehn W, Schwemmle K, and Kern DH. Prospective correlative chemosensitivity testing in high-dose intraarterial chemotherapy for liver metastases. *Cancer Res* 46:4837–4840, 1986.
10. Link KH, Staib L, and Beger HG. Influence of exposure concentration and exposure time c x t on toxicity of cytostatic drugs to HT29 human colorectal carcinoma cells. Characterization of drugs for (regional) chemotherapy. *Reg. Cancer Treat.* Vol. 2. Heidelberg: Springer, 1989, 189–198.
11. Storm FK, Kaiser LR, and Goodnight JE. Thermochemotherapy for melanoma metastases in liver. *Cancer* 49:1243–1248, 1982.

Chapter 23

SURGICAL MANAGEMENT OF BRAIN METASTASES

Per-Ebbe Jönsson, Larsolof Hafström, and Lars-Göran Strömblad

INTRODUCTION

Today more malignant melanomas are diagnosed each year; however, there is no comparable rise in mortality, which means that the primaries are diagnosed at an earlier stage. Metastases to the brain occur in up to 30 percent of patients with systemic cancer and malignant melanoma represents the third most common cause of such spread.[1] Most statistical data on brain metastases are uncertain, as they are based on a selected clinical and autopsy patient series of limited size. An estimation is that 75 percent of all diagnosed brain metastases in autopsy series are symptomatic in the clinical situation.[2,3] Brain metastases of melanoma are the consequence of a hematogenous dissemination of melanoma cells distributed in the brain, well-correlated to the relative brain weight and blood flow distribution patterns.[1,4] In malignant melanoma, independent of the metastatic sites, treatment modalities such as chemotherapy and immunotherapy have not been shown to improve the survival rate.[5] It is, however, possible that the use of those treatments may produce a relative increase of symptomatic brain metastases. Today the role of neurosurgery in melanoma brain tumors is well-established as the only possibility for a curative treatment and long term survival.

GENERAL CONSIDERATIONS

Our Own Patient Series

We have recently reviewed our experience of neurosurgery for brain metastases of malignant melanoma with the aim of evaluating survival time and quality of life after surgical resection alone and to define which patients could benefit from such treatment.[6] All together 40 patients (26 men and 14 women in the age range 23–75 years with a median age of 53 years) have been treated during the period from 1968 to 1984.

In all cases the brain metastases were histologically proven to be malignant melanoma. In 28 patients (70 percent), primary malignant melanoma was diagnosed and the median time interval from this diagnosis to the development of brain metastasis was four years. Five patients had a longer interval of more than 10 years. Twenty-four patients (60 percent) developed extracerebral manifestations of melanoma before the brain metastases were diagnosed. Seventeen of those 24 patients were successfully treated by surgical resection of lymph node metastases and subcutaneous disease and, in one patient, a partial lung resection. The brain metastases were symptomatic in all but two patients at the time of diagnosis and neurosurgery. The two asymptomatic patients were diagnosed for other reasons in the routine work-up by computer tomography.

Our preoperative work-up included carotid angiography and brain scan until 1978, when the computer tomography technique was introduced. Thereafter, computer tomography was the only diagnostic method used in all patients. At the time for neurosurgery, eight of our 40 patients had multiple brain metastases, five of those had a single metastasis diagnosed preoperatively by the CT-scan.

The localization of all metastases considered for neurosurgery was supratentorial. Dominating sites were the parietal lobes without any preference for either hemisphere.

The hospital mortality (within 30 days) was 7/40 patients (17.5 percent) of whom two patients died from postoperative complications, such as intracerebral hematoma and septicemia, and the remaining five from progressive melanoma disease because of multiplicity. All together eight complications were registered. Five were minor without influence on the hospital stay.

Survival Data

The survival data is illustrated in Fig. 23-1 and Fig. 23-2. Five out of 40 patients are still alive, without signs of metastatic melanoma, 3.5, 5, 11, and 14 years after the surgery. The overall median survival time is 8 months. Six patients have survived more than 5 years, that is a 5-year survival of 15 percent. We performed an analysis of the survival data regarding different factors such as single versus multiple metastases, extracranial versus no extracranial metastases, unknown primary versus known primary tumor, and longtime interval between primary tumor and brain metastases versus short interval (Fig. 23-2). The significance of the different comparisons is evident from the figures. Of interest is that successfully treated extracerebral metastases prior to brain metastases did not affect the survival.

Surgery was judged as macroscopically radical in 31 patients and recurrent brain disease developed in 28 patients. A second craniotomy was performed in four of those after 11, 24, 24, and 56 months, and two patients survived another 2 years, and one is still alive 12 months after the secondary neurosurgery.

Quality of Life and Symptom Relief

Quality of life was estimated both from the chart showing the relief of symptoms as well as according to the more well-established Karnofsky index. There was a shift of Karnofsky index preoperatively compared to one month postoperatively (Fig. 23-3). In the majority of patients (71 percent) the Karnofsky index exceeded 50 until one month or less before death. This was well-related to the improvement of neurological symptoms and remained so during the mean time of 12 months in patients who could leave the hospital. Median duration time of the improvement was 5 months compared with a median survival time of 6 months in the overall series. The same improvement was seen in those few patients who were operated on a second time.

Protocol

The marked propensity of metastatic tumor to produce extensive edema in the surrounding brain pa-

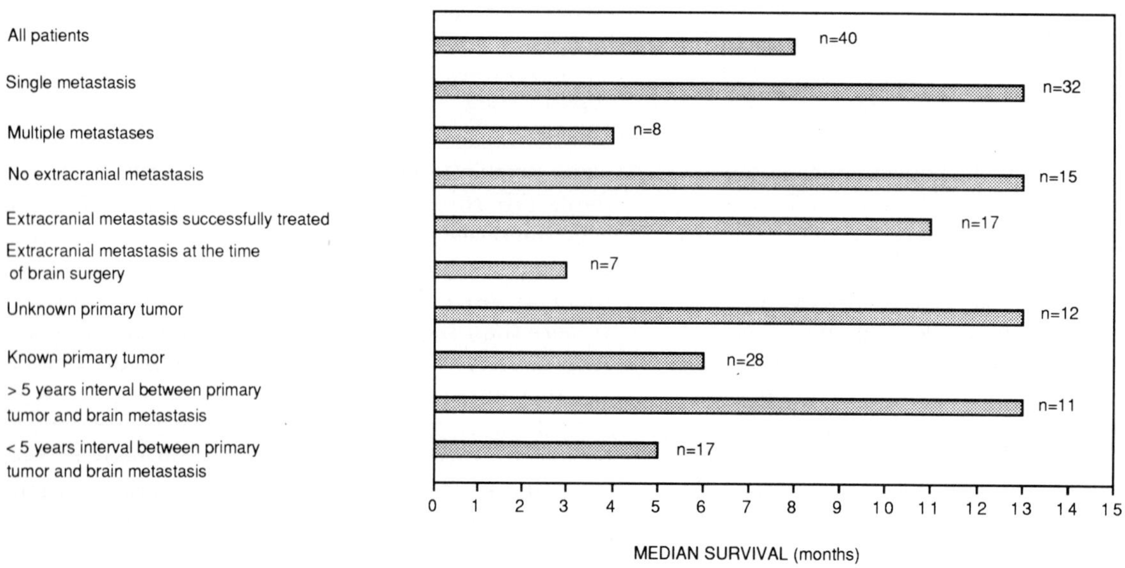

FIG. 23-1. Median survival time for all patients in various subgroups of patients after resection of malignant melanoma metastases to the brain.

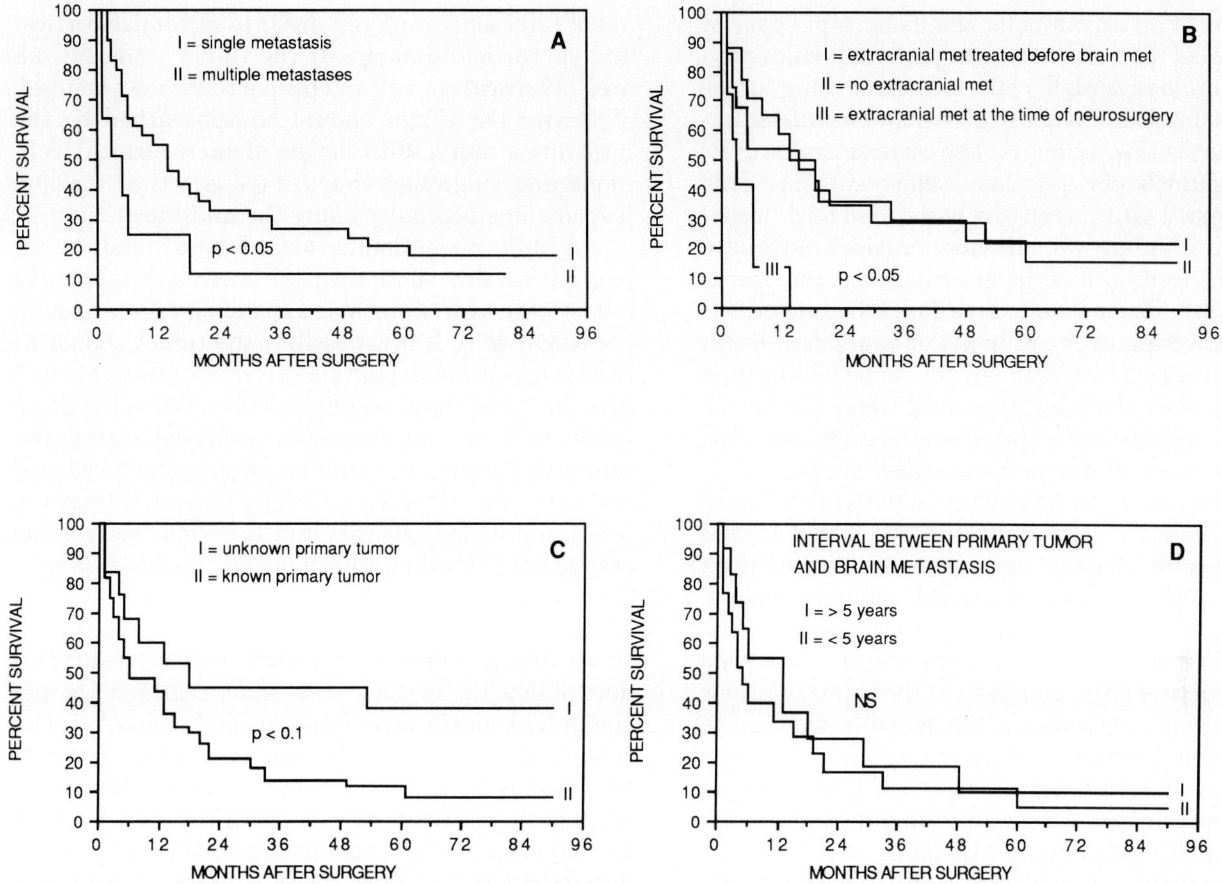

FIG. 23-2. Life table comparing various subgroups of patients treated by surgery for malignant melanoma metastases to the brain. A. Single versus multiple metastases; B. Presence of extracranial metastases before brain metastases versus no extracranial metastases; C. Unknown primary tumor versus known primary tumor; D. Long interval between primary tumor in brain metastases versus short interval.

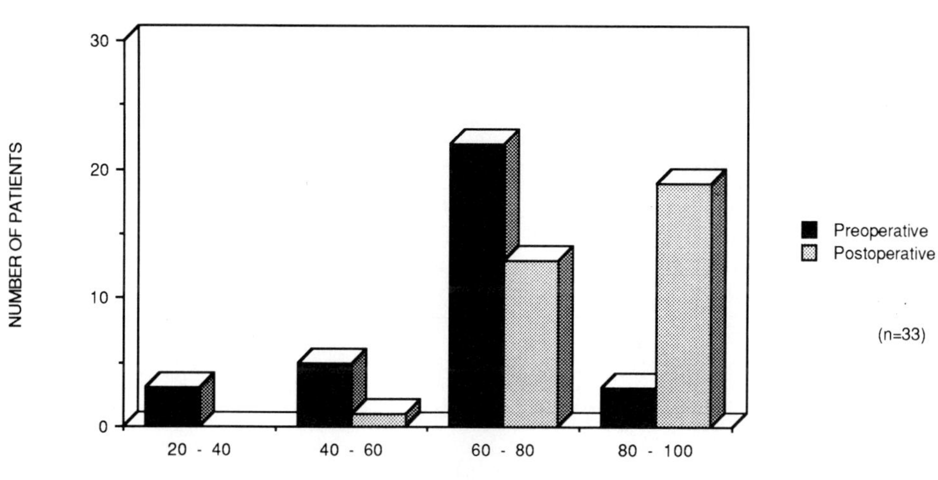

FIG. 23-3. Quality of life as estimated by Karnofsky index before (.) and 30 days after (−) surgery on malignant melanoma metastases to the brain (n = 33). Patient deceased within 30 days after surgery have been excluded (n = 7).

renchyma often accounts for the usual rapid pace of neurological deterioration in patients. High-dose corticosteroids are highly effective in reducing tumor induced edema and usually give notable clinical improvement within 12 hours. The corticosteroid treatment should begin 3–5 days before surgery. This time interval will usually be associated with maximal clinical improvement and provides adequate treatment to minimize edema caused by the operative trauma. The most effective dose schedule is dexamethason 8 mg every 12 hours or equivalent doses of an analogue. The treatment should be maintained 3–5 days after the operation, and when the tumor has been successfully extirpated, the corticosteroids can be tapered off during a two-week period.

In the preoperative staging of patients who are potential candidates for neurosurgery, it is of utmost importance to identify those who can benefit from surgery. This assessment should not only include what has already been mentioned concerning the extent of the systemic disease, the length of the time interval between the diagnosis of the primary tumor and the brain metastases, the possible damage to other organ systems from prior treatment, and the likelihood of occult brain metastases but also an evaluation of cardiopulmonary function and the patient's nutritional state. The coagulation parameters must strictly be observed, especially in patients who might previously have been treated by chemotherapy.

Prior to the operation a computer tomography is carried out in order to facilitate the planning of the scalp incision and bone flap. Brain metastasis represents growth of tumor emboli trapped at a site of arterial narrowing, often at a cortical-white matter junction. Most are, therefore, adjacent to the brain surface. About 25 percent of brain metastases will reach the cortical surface and are thus easily found. Others should be intraoperatively localized with the aid of ultrasonography in order to minimize cortical and subcortical damage. If the tumor underlies an area of critical cortex, an oblique route may be used, otherwise the tumor should be approached by the most direct route. With the use of microsurgical technique and magnified vision a transcortical incision is made longitudinally along the midline of a gyrus.

A blunt dissection is carried out around the tumor with a fine suction tip. It is advisable to leave a very thin rim of normal-appearing tissue around the tumor wall. If it is possible, the tumor should be removed as an intact single specimen, since this will give the lowest local recurrence rate. When handling larger tumors that cannot be removed intact, the center of the tumor should be progressively reduced and then the periphery carefully dissected from the brain and folded inwards and removed. Meticulous care should be taken to remove all visible tumor.

Discussion

In the literature there are several reports of survival data following various treatment regimens in patients with brain metastases of melanoma.[7–12] The results of neurosurgery for metastatic melanoma to the brain without radiotherapy as an additive treatment postoperatively are shown in Table 23-1. Those are papers published during the 1980s, and we have extracted patients from more comprehensive series of patients where several treatment modalities have been used. Most of those studies are retrospectively evaluated, so it is very important to be aware of the shortcomings from those. There is no complete information from the others; however, the results are mostly comparable, and it is interesting to find out that there is longterm survival without symptoms in about 10–15 percent for at least three years. In some papers a comparison between the surgically treated patients and patients treated by radiotherapy with or without drugs was done. In the analyses

TABLE 23-1
RESULTS OF SURGICAL RESECTION FOR METASTATIC MELANOMA WITHOUT POSTOPERATIVE RADIOTHERAPY

AUTHORS	NUMBER OF PATIENTS n	POSTOPERATIVE COMPLICATIONS %	HOSPITAL MORTALITY (30 DAYS) %	RELIEF OF SYMPTOMS %	SURVIVAL MEDIAN (MONTHS)	SURVIVAL 2 YEARS	SURVIVAL 3 YEARS
Fell 1980	13	—[a]	5,4	87	3.5	0	—
Madajewicz 1984	11	22	22	—	6.5	10	10
Wornom 1986	17	22	11	77	8.0	16	13
Neuss 1987	18	—	0	—	5.0	16	—
Mendez 1988	12	—	0	—	5.5	25	—
Guazzo 1989	31	24	0	64	—	25	10
Our own series 1990	40	20	17.5	71	8	—	15

[a]— means not mentioned.

by Fell et al.,[7] 42 patients underwent neurosurgery with supplementary radiotherapy in 19 and they were compared in a nonrandomized manner to 38 patients who were untreated or treated by radiotherapy and/or chemotherapy. The median survival time was 1.5 months in the nonsurgical group and 5 months in the surgically treated patient group. The overall median survival in other series of patients are comparable to ours and underline that neurosurgery is indicated in patients with solitary brain metastases and no sign of extracerebral disease. Previous extracranial metastases that have been successfully treated do not interfere with this statement.

Chemotherapy and radiotherapy alone or in combination do not give results comparable to surgery. In one report here the response to chemotherapy was only 10 percent in patients with brain tumor from malignant melanoma.[7] Radiotherapy alone had a response rate of 37–100 percent, with a median survival time of three months or less. It is difficult to compare the effect on neurological symptoms achieved by systemic treatment and radiotherapy versus the effect achieved by surgery because of different use of high dose cortical steroid therapy, which interferes with the evaluation. Thus, the results of neurosurgery are superior to those reported after radiotherapy and chemotherapy. The quality of life is of utmost importance when palliation is discussed. There is one more study where a comparison of the Karnofsky index before and after surgery was performed and this found a shorter survival time in patients with severe preoperative neurological deficits and a Karnofsky index less than 50.[13]

The use of surgery in combination with chemotherapy or radiotherapy has to be evaluated prospectively in a randomized way to establish the optimal treatment. Recently a randomized trial of surgery in treatment of single metastases to the brain alone or followed by radiotherapy was published.[14] That study included 25 patients for surgery and 23 patients for radiation. However, there were only two melanomas in the first group and one in the second. The dominating primary tumor in this study was lung cancer in 18 of the first group and 19 patients of the second group. However, the results are very interesting because they showed that a patient with a solitary brain metastasis removed by surgery and treated by radiotherapy lived longer and had fewer recurrences in the brain and a better quality of life than similar patients treated with radiotherapy alone.

Overall brain metastasis in metastatic cancer is a common problem, especially in patient with malignant melanoma. In most cases it is difficult to immediately limit the neurological disability therapeutically. However, usually the quality of life and duration of survival is improved. With careful selection criteria, it is possible to offer neurosurgery to approximately 5–10 percent of patients with brain metastasis from malignant melanoma. The ideal patient has only a single lesion with minimal neurologic impairment. The results are often bad in patients with severe neurological deficits preoperatively. We have found both in our earlier evaluation as well as in our recent update that carefully selected patients will benefit from neurosurgery and some will gain a longterm survival (30 percent) up to 3–5 years or more.[6,15] The use of surgery in combination with radiotherapy compared to surgery alone is not evaluated in brain metastases from malignant melanoma.

CONCLUSION

The indication for neurosurgery is a single metastasis with restricted neurological deficits and no evidence of extracranial disease at the same time. Refinement in surgical technique, improvements in preoperative localization, and the use of steroids have gradually led to a change in surgical approach to metastasis. It is also possible to do smaller incisions today by use of a microtechnique and magnified vision in conjunction with excellent preoperative localization.

REFERENCES

1. Wright DC. Surgical treatment of brain metastases. In: Rosenberg SA (ed.) *Surgical Treatment of Metastatic Cancer.* Philadelphia: I.B. Lippincott, 1987, 165–222.
2. Amer MH, Al-Sarraf M, Baker LH, and Vaitkevicius VK. Malignant melanoma and central nervous system metastases. Incidence, diagnosis, treatment and survival. *Cancer* 42:660–668, 1978.
3. Bullard DE, Cox EB, and Seigler HF. Central nervous system metastases in malignant melanoma. *Neurosurgery* 8:26–30, 1981.
4. Kindt GW. The pattern of location of cerebral metastatic tumors. *J Neurosurg* 21:54–57, 1964.
5. Feun LG, Gutterman J, Burgess MA, et al. The natural history of resectable metastatic melanoma. *Cancer* 50:1656–1663, 1982.
6. Oredsson S, Ingvar C, Strömblad L-G, and Jönsson P-E. Palliative surgery for brain metastases of malignant melanoma. *Eur J Surg Oncol* 16:451–456, 1990.
7. Fell DA, Leavens ME, and McBride CM. Surgical versus nonsurgical management of metastatic melanoma of the brain. *Neurosurgery* 3:238–242, 1980.
8. Madajewicz S, Karakousis C, West CR, Caracandas I, and Avellanosa AM. Malignant melanoma brain metastases; review of Roswell Park Memorial Institute experience. *Cancer* 53:2550–2552, 1984.
9. Wornam IL, Soomg SL, Vrist MM, Smith IW, McElvein R, and Balch CM. Surgery as palliative treatment for distant metastases of melanoma. *Ann Surg* 204:181–185, 1986.
10. Neuss M, Konig A, and Herrman H-D. Intracranial melanoma metastases: Surgical treatment and follow-up of 18 patients. *Anticancer Research* 7:445–446, 1987.

11. Mendez IM, and Del Maestro RF. Cerebral metastases from malignant melanoma. *Can J Neurol Sci* 15:119–123, 1988.
12. Guazzo EP, Atkinson RL, Weidmann M, and Effeney DJ. Management of solitary melanoma metastasis to the brain. *Aust N Z J Surg* 59:321–324, 1989.
13. Sundaresan N, and Galicich JH. Surgical treatment of brain metastases; Clinical and computerized tomography evaluation of the results of treatment. *Cancer* 55:1382–1386, 1985.
14. Patchell RA, Tibbs PA, Walsh JW, et al. A randomized trial of surgery in the treatment of single metastases to the brain. *N Engl J Med* 8:494–500, 1990.
15. Hafström L, Jönsson P-E, and Strömblad L-G. Intracranial metastases of malignant melanoma treated by surgery. *Cancer* 46:2088–2090, 1980.

Chapter 24

SURGICAL MANAGEMENT OF PULMONARY METASTASES

D. Liénard and P. Rocmans

The lungs are the most common site for metastatic melanoma[1] excluding the skin and lymph nodes. Lung metastases have been found in 70 to 78 percent of cases in autopsy series.[2] In contrast, Das Gupta[2] found the lungs to be the only site for metastatic disease, on clinical ground, in 7 percent of stage III patients.

It seems that an aggressive surgical approach may save some patients with pulmonary metastases from melanoma. It is known that this approach provides consistent five-year survival in sarcoma and carcinoma patients.[3,4] As the melanoma metastatic pattern involves multiple organs, it is commonly believed that surgical removal of metastases does not offer survival benefit. However, a number of reports do suggest that selected patients can benefit from surgical resection of metastases[5] with prolonged survival.

BORDET EXPERIENCE BETWEEN 1980 AND 1990

Eight patients treated in our Institute had lung metastases resected by wedge, segmental excisions, or

TABLE 24-1
REMOVAL OF MELANOMA LUNG METASTASES: CLINICAL PARAMETER OF PRESENT SERIES

CASE	PREOPERATIVE THERAPY	THORACOTOMY RESECTION	N METASTASES RESECTED	LYMPH NODE METASTASES	ADJUVANT TREATMENT	OTHER SITES OF METASTASES	STATUS
1	CisDDP + VDS + DTIC	Sternotomy Segmentectomy	2 bilateral	Mediastinal	—	8 mos brain	Died 9 mos
2	—	Lateral Wedge	3 ipsilateral	None	—	9 mos brain	Died 12 mos
3	—	Sternotomy Wedge	1	Incomplete dissection	Radiotherapy Chemotherapy	59 mos brain and liver	Died 72 mos
4	Tamoxifen	Sternotomy Wedge	6 bilateral	None	—	Brain, lung and pharynx	Died 40 mos
5	—	Sternotomy Wedge	2 ipsilateral	None	—	Neurofibrosarcoma arm	Died 22 mos
6	—	Lateral Wedge	2 ipsilateral	None	—	Lymph node, skin, liver, heart	Died 22 mos
7	—	Lateral Pneumectomy	1	Hilar and mediastinal	Gangliosides	Liver and stomach	Died 3 mos
8	—	Lateral Wedge	2 ipsilateral	None	Gangliosides	—	Alive 5 mos

pneumectomy at the Department for Thoracic Surgery, Hôpital Erasme, ULB, Brussels. This was associated with node dissection in three cases: number 1 and 3 for proven mediastinal metastases and number 7 for hilar and mediastinal nodes. Major patient characteristics are depicted in Table 24-1. Mean number of resected nodules was 2.4 per patient (range 1 to 6). Our median survival reached 22 months and the overall five-year survival rate reaches 25 percent in the series of UCLA[6] and 36 percent in the series reported by Cahan.[5] In contrast, in most of the other series, the five-year survival approached 0 percent and no long-term survivor was observed, and the median survival varied between 7 and 24 months.[6,7] Three out of eight patients in our series survived longer than two years (range 3 to 92 months). No patient except one recurred in the lung. The recurrence of this patient was observed after 36 months and in a different site from the previous nodules. This is especially interesting as more than half of the failures occurred in the lung within 12 months in other series.[3] The most common site for further distant metastases in our series was the central nervous system in four out of eight cases. This has been reported by Dalbäck et al.[8] in 50 percent of their patients.

DETECTION AND TECHNICAL WORK-UP

Most melanoma metastases are routinely detected on chest radiographs and are confirmed by conventional tomography and more recently by computed tomography (CT). Chang[9] in 1979 demonstrated that CT with 13 mm thick, contiguous slices is more sensitive than conventional tomography for detecting small pulmonary nodules. This has been widely confirmed recently.[10,11] Karp[12] demonstrated that CT is also mandatory to detect enlarged mediastinal lymph nodes preoperatively, especially to exclude from thoracotomy patients with massively nonresectable invaded lymph nodes.

PATIENTS SELECTION

Several criteria for lung metastases resection have been established over the years[13,14] and include:

- complete resection of the primary tumor,
- good medical status of the patients (PS 0-1 ECOG),[15]
- surgical resectability of lung metastases as to their number and distribution,
- no evidence of other unresectable metastatic sites.

Joseph et al.[16] emphasized the need to measure the tumor doubling time (TDT) of lung metastases for osteosarcomas. TDT is a good and accurate indicator of long-term survivors after surgical removal of lung metastases in sarcoma and carcinoma. It seems that this concept can be applied to malignant melanoma. According to the work of Wong[6] in 1988, patients with TDT longer than 40 days appear to benefit most likely from lung metastasectomy. However, in most other series, this criterion has not been included.

Long-term survivors reported in the literature by Cahan,[5] MacCormack and Martini[17] had solitary metastases. However, in experience of the others, as by Thayer[18] and our own, long-term survivors among patients with multiple metastases were observed (Table 24-2). It should also be pointed out that for Pogrebniak et al.[11] the number of diagnosed nodules on preoperative tomograms did not correlate with the survival rate. Therefore, patients with bilateral, multiple nodules should not be excluded from surgery even if their long-term survival appears to be poorer.

TABLE 24-2
LUNG MELANOMA METASTASES RESECTION—THERAPEUTICAL RESULTS

AUTHOR	YEAR	NUMBER	MEDIAN SURVIVAL	RANGE
Cahan	1972	29		10/29 2 years 6/29 2–5 years
Merlier	1978	9	12 months	(3–27 months)
Mathisen	1979	23	12 months	(3–25 months)
Dahlbäck	1980	8	7 months	(2–32 months)
Feun	1982	26	16 months	
Thayer	1984	18	16.5 months	(1–172 months)
Wornom	1986	17	9 months	
Pogrebniak	1988	31	22 months	(max. 120 months)
Wong	1988	47	19 months	
Karp	1990	29	11 months	
Liénard	1991	8	22 months	(3–72 months)

SURGICAL TECHNIQUES

Resectability

Patients selected for surgery are expected to have a *complete* resection (no residue, free margins) of all detectable metastases. Computed tomography with contiguous thin slices added to AP and profile chest film is mandatory to assess the topography and resectability of metastatic nodules as follows:

- detection of nodules down to 3 mm diameter,
- assessment of resectability (contact with bronchus and vascular branches, "free" access, preservation of function),
- topography of hilar and mediastinal lymph nodes to be explored by thoracotomy or initial mediastinoscopy.

Our data stress two prognostic factors specific of melanoma, not recognized in the classical approach of lung metastases from other primary tumors, especially osteosarcoma.[19]

1. All pulmonary metastases are usually detected preoperatively by X ray and CT scan.
2. High frequency of lymph node metastases to the mediastinum. The resectability of such deposit must be assessed, by methods including cervical mediastinoscopy.

Surgical Approach

Median sternotomy is mandatory for bilateral dissemination or if radical mediastinal dissection is expected for enlarged lymph nodes associated with left lung metastases. Lateral thoracotomy is advised for unilateral left lung metastases with disease-free mediastinum and for all unilateral right lung disseminations (even with enlarged mediastinal lymph nodes). Large size metastases of lower lobes are poorly dissected by median sternotomy and require lateral thoracotomy for excision.

A double-lumen endotracheal tube is routinely used to explore the lung visually and by palpation during inflation and complete deflation. All nodules detected on X ray and CT scan are identified as the first step of exploratory thoracotomy. All visible and palpable nodules are resected to assess their quality

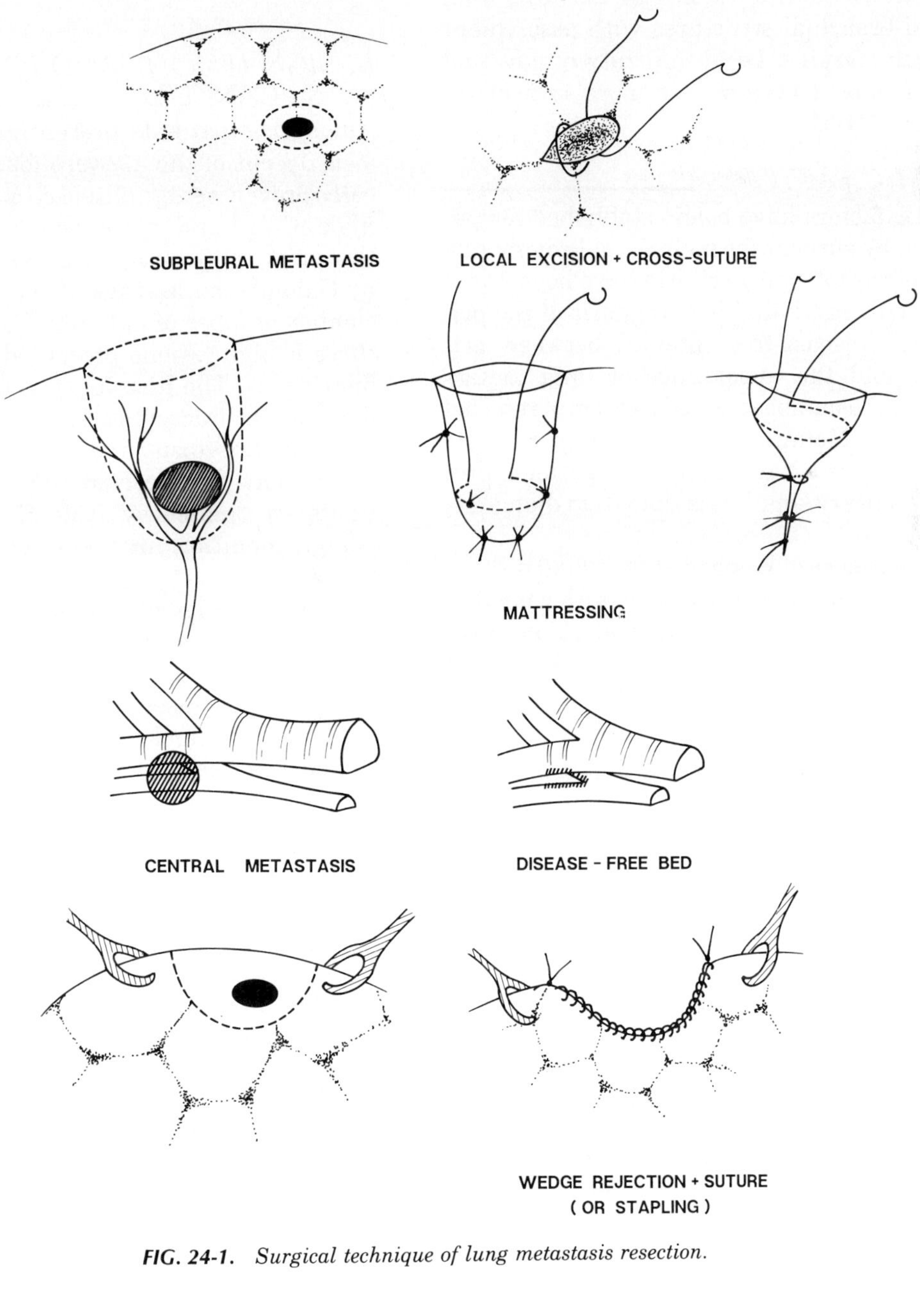

FIG. 24-1. Surgical technique of lung metastasis resection.

of fibrosis or necrosis, subpleural lymph node, primary lung cancer, or others. Normal and enlarged lymph nodes are collected. Positive lymph nodes detected by frozen sections necessitate radical dissection of hilum and/or mediastinum to assure tumor for status of the mediastinum.

Technique of Resection

All nodules are resected with a 2 to 5 mm margin of disease-free tissue, assessed if necessary by frozen section. Subpleural nodules are excised; the resection bed is treated by cautery and mattressed with silk suture. Nodules in the edge of the lung need wedge resection with local mattress suture or stapling. Deep nodules are funnel-excised with cautery and the local excision cone is mattressed with deep to surface stitches. Central nodules are dissected from vascular and bronchial structures with assessment of disease-free margins. Local infiltration may lead to segmentectomy, lobectomy, or more radical resections (Table 24-3).

PROGNOSTIC FACTORS

No prognostic factors have been established for patients treated by surgery for melanoma lung metastases. None of the following criteria have been found to correlate with survival: histoprognosis of the primary tumor,[11] disease-free interval between primary tumor and the appearance of lung metastases,[4,11,18] and the number and the location of resected metastases.[8,11,18] Mountain et al.[3] showed in their study of 60 patients a trend in favor of patients presenting with solitary small (less than 3 cm diameter) metastases.

In the experience of Wong et al.[6] residual disease after thoracotomy had a bad prognosis with a median survival of six months and no survival at the fifth-year. Patients with complete resection had 40 months median survival time and 25 percent five-year survival. In other series[7,11] there was no difference between patients who had incomplete resection as compared to apparently complete resection.

Involvement of the hilar lymph nodes is rarely observed among the five-year survivors, as noted in the study of Cahan.[5] In our experience, among three patients with metastatic mediastinal lymph nodes, one with residual mediastinal melanoma survived five years after surgery and adjuvant radio-chemotherapy, while two others died after three and nine months from disseminated melanoma (Table 24-1).

Adjuvant treatment—immuno- or chemotherapy pre- or post-operatively did not improve survival in the studies reported by Mountain et al.,[3] and Wong et al.,[6] especially in patients treated with incomplete resections.

TABLE 24-3
RESECTION OF MELANOMA LUNG METASTASES

RESECTION	CAHAN 1972	DÄHLBACK 1980	THAYER 1984	LIENARD 1991
SOLITARY	18	4	10	2
Wedge	2	2	2	1
Segmental	5		2	0
Lobectomy	8	2	6	0
Pneumonectomy	3			1
Lymph node +	5			2
MULTIPLE	11	4	8	6
Wedge	6	3	3	4
Segmental	3		2	2
Lobectomy	1	1		0
Pneumonectomy	1		3	0
Lymph node +	4			1
Lymph nodes	9/29			

BENIGN LESIONS AND PRIMARY LUNG CANCERS

Among the patients presenting with a solitary lesion, 16 out of the 49 were found to have histologically proven benign disease in the series of Pogrebniak et al.[11] and in the one of Juttner et al.[20] with two cases, confirming the previous observation made by Cahan[5] and Mathisen[7] ten years before, with a smaller number of patients (Table 24-4). Clinically, these benign lesions presented as classical solitary metastases. The histologies included granulmatous disease, anthracocylicotic nodules, lymphoid aggregates, histiocytosis, and nonspecific pneumonitis.

It may be expected that some melanoma patients are treated by systemic chemotherapy for a benign condition mistaken for a solitary lung metastasis.

In the series of Pogrebniak et al.,[11] one out of the 16 patients with solitary nodules and five of the 18 from the Cahan series[5] had primary lung cancer and not metastases from melanoma. Most of these patients were smokers and did not show any typical radiological feature for a primary lung carcinoma.

CONCLUSIONS

In conclusion, reaction of pulmonary metastases from melanoma may benefit a small number of patients with the following criteria:

- All the extrapulmonary sites should be controlled either by surgery or by any other treatment.
- In case of a solitary lesion it is mandatory to insure that the lesion is not a benign lesion or a primary lung tumor.
- Presence of a small number (not exceeding 4) of lung metastases.
- All the lesions should be resectable.

TABLE 24-4
LUNG NODULES IN MELANOMA—NATURE AND DISTRIBUTION

	NON SURGICAL		SURGICAL						
AUTHOR	WEBB	CHEN	CAHAN	MERLIER	MATHISEN	DÄHLBACK	POGREBNIAK	JUTTNER	LIÉNARD
Year	1977	1981	1972	1978	1979	1980	1988	1986	1991
N cases	65	130	29	14	33	8	49	2	8
Lung metastases									
Multiple	49	54	11	5	9	4	23		6
Solitary	14	26	18	9	8	4	10		2
Lymph nodes	28 (43%)	9 (6%)	9 (30%)				3		3
Pleural effusion	10	3							
Bony	6	1							
Extrapleural		1							
Combined		36							
Separate lung primary			5				1	1	
Benign tumor					10		16	1	
Pulmonary disorder									

In case of associated lymph node involvement, a complete clearance should be possible.
The patient should be in good medical condition.

It should be stressed that a definite proof of the value of the above mentioned criteria is presently lacking in the literature.

REFERENCES

1. Patel JK, Kidolkar MS, Pickren JW, and Moore RH. Metastatic pattern of malignant melanoma, a study of 216 autopsy cases. *AM J Surg* 135:807, 1978.
2. Das Gupta T, and Brasfield R. Metastatic melanoma: A clinicopathological study. *Cancer* 17:1323–1339, 1964.
3. Mountain CF, McMurtrey MJ, and Hermes KE. Surgery for pulmonary metastasis: A 20-year experience. *Ann Thorac Surg* 38:323–330, 1984.
4. Takita H, Edgerton F, Karakousis C, Douglass HO et al. Surgical management of metastases to the lung. *Surg Gynecol Obstet* 152:191–194, 1981.
5. Cahan WG. Excision of melanoma metastases to the lung: Problems in diagnosis and management. *Ann Surg* 178:703–709, 1973.
6. Wong JH, Euhus DM, and Morton DL. Surgical resection for metastatic melanoma to the lung. *Arch Surg* 123:1091–1095, 1988.
7. Mathisen DJ, Flye MW, and Peabody J. The role of thoracotomy in the management of pulmonary metastases from malignant melanoma. *Ann Thorac Surg* 27:295–299, 1979.
8. Dahlbäck O, Hafström L, Jönsson PE, and Sundqvist K. Lung resection for metastatic melanoma. *Clin Oncol* 6:15–20, 1980.
9. Chang AE, Schaner EG, Conkle DM, Flye MW et al. Evaluation of computed tomography in the detection of pulmonary metastases. A prospective study. *Cancer* 43:913–916, 1979.
10. Pass HI, Dwyer A, Hakuch R et al. Detection of pulmonary metastases in patients with osteogenic and soft tissue sarcomas: The superiority of CT scans compared with conventional linear tomograms using dynamic analyses. *J Clin Oncol* 3:1261, 1985.
11. Pogrebniak HW, Stovroff M, Roth JA, and Pass HI. Resection of pulmonary metastases from malignant melanoma: Results of a 16-year experience. *Ann Thorac Surg* 46:20–23, 1988.
12. Karp NS, Boyd A, DePan JH, Harris MN, and Roses DF. Thoracotomy for metastatic malignant melanoma of the lung. *Surgery* 107:256–261, 1990.
13. Van Dongen JA, and Van Slooten EA. The surgical treatment of pulmonary metastases. *Cancer Treat Rev* 5:29–48, 1978.
14. Ramming KP. Surgery of pulmonary metastases. *Surg Clin North Am* 60:815–824, 1980.
15. Oken MM, Creech H, and Tormey DC. Toxicity and response criteria of the ECOG. *Am J Clin Oncol* 5:649–655, 1982.
16. Joseph WL, Morton DL, and Adkins PC. Prognostic significance of tumor doubling time in evaluating operability in pulmonary metastatic disease. *J Thorac Cardiovasc Surg* 61:23–32, 1971.
17. McCormack PM, and Martini NM. The changing role of surgery for pulmonary metastases. *Ann Thorac Surg* 28:139–145, 1979.
18. Thayer JO, and Overholt RH. Metastatic melanoma to the lung: Long-term results of surgical excision. *Am J Surg* 149:588–562, 1985.
19. Kern KA, Pass HI, and Roth JA. Surgical treatment of pulmonary metastases. In: Rosenberg SA (ed.), *Surgical Treatment of Metastatic Cancer*. Philadelphia: J.B. Lippincott, 1987, 69–100.
20. Juttner FM, Smolle J, Popper H, and Schneider G. Pitfalls in the diagnosis of pulmonary metastases in melanoma. *Dermatologica* 172:113–115, 1986.

Chapter 25

SURGICAL MANAGEMENT OF DISTANT METASTASES: GI TRACT

J. C. Pector

INTRODUCTION

Metastatic spread from a tumor originating outside the peritoneal cavity rarely involves the gastrointestinal (GI) tract. However, in approximately 60 percent of patients who die from malignant melanoma, the autopsy reveals metastases in the GI tract.[1] On the other hand, GI tract metastatic melanomas are generally clinically undetectable in the early stages.[2] It has been estimated that, with the use of radiologic and endoscopic techniques, between 1 and 4 percent of all patients with malignant melanoma can be diagnosed before death as having GI metastases.[3] In a retrospective series of 2500 patients with melanoma reported by Reintgen et al.,[4] only 110 patients (4.4 percent) had been identified to have premortem GI metastatic disease.

The difference may be due to the fact that GI metastases normally occur in the course of the disease when other organ systems, such as brain and lungs, are already involved. In such cases, the clinical symptoms of these organs usually predominate and the digestive symptoms tend to be nonspecific.

There are isolated reports of malignant melanomas as primary tumors in the GI area. However, the possibility of these tumors being merely a secondary manifestation of a cutaneous or intraocular melanoma must always be considered. It is not unusual for a patient with metastatic malignant melanoma to first present with signs and symptoms due to a metastatic lesion rather than those due to the primary lesion. Usually, a careful search in such patients will reveal the site of the primary tumor. The great majority of patients with metastatic malignant melanoma to the GI tract have had a previous history of a primary skin melanoma or have shown evidence of metastatic lesion elsewhere before the manifestations of GI tract involvement have been apparent. The occurrence of GI metastases does not show a good correlation with either the histologic type of primary tumor or its location. Usually, the invasion depth of the cutaneous melanomas with GI metastases exceeds Clark level III, but not always.[5]

In this study, special attention will be made to melanoma involvement of each part of the digestive system, its clinical manifestations, and the role of surgical treatment.

ESOPHAGUS

Melanoma involving the esophagus can be metastatic or primary since melanoblasts have been identified in esophageal epithelium.[6] According to Allen and Spitz,[7] the main criteria to assess the primary nature of the disease is the presence of junctional change of the overlying epithelium.

TABLE 25-1
INCIDENCE OF METASTATIC MELANOMA IN THE GI TRACT (AUTOPSY SERIES)

REFERENCE	DAS GUPTA AND BRASFIELD[10]	MOSIMANN ET AL.[45]	EINHORN ET AL.[47]	PATEL ET AL.[48]
PERIOD	1935–60	1972–80	1967–73	1959–74
PAT. NO.	125	22	96	216
	(%)	(%)	(%)	(%)
Esophagus	4	0	3	9
Stomach	26	14	7	23
Liver	68	68	76	58
Gall bladder	15	27	4	9
Biliary tract	6		0	0
Pancreas	53	45	38	38
Spleen	36	0	43	31
Small bowel	58	27	26	36
Colon	22	18	14	28
Rectum	5	0	0	0
Anus	1	0	0	0

Primary melanoma of the esophagus accounts for only .1 percent of primary esophageal malignant neoplasms.[8] A series of more than a hundred cases have been reported.[9] Although metastatic melanoma of the esophagus is present in up to 4 percent of an autopsy series,[10] only few cases have been clinically detected.[11–14]

Dysphagia is a common symptom. Radiology and endoscopy show a polypoid lesion, which is difficult to differentiate from other lobulated masses.

The outlook of primary and metastatic malignant melanoma of the esophagus is generally poor, with survival in most cases of less than a year from diagnosis. However, in selected patients, surgical resection may provide a satisfactory palliation.[14]

STOMACH

Although malignant melanoma of the stomach is almost invariably a metastatic tumor, a possibly primary origin, from Meissner's plexus of the gastric submucosa, has been postulated, but not substantiated.[15]

In a review of the literature, Lee[16] reported an incidence of 7 to 26 percent gastric metastases in autopsy series of patients with malignant melanoma. Clinically, however, the gastric metastases are seldom diagnosed. Booth[17] reported that 51 cases were in the literature until 1964. In the retrospective series of 2500 melanomas, Reintgen et al.[4] found only eight cases. In addition, gastric invasion is most often associated with the invasion of other organs.[17] Isolated gastric metastases were exceptionally reported.[18,19]

Symptoms of gastric involvement by malignant melanoma usually include nausea and vomiting, abdominal discomfort, pain imitating peptic ulcer disease, and weight loss. The intramural nodule is the most common melanoma lesion in the stomach and is usually multiple. Growth of the tumor results in intraluminal polypoid masses. Ulceration may occur, giving the tumor the classic "bull's eye" or target radiographic appearance.[20]

Surgery for symptomatic lesions can improve the quality of life and even extend life expectancy.

Laser photocoagulation can successfully manage bleeding from unresected lesions.[21]

GALLBLADDER AND BILIARY TRACT

Metastatic melanoma of the gallbladder is rare: Shimkin et al.[22] reported an incidence of 14 percent in an autopsy series; Das Gupta and Brasfield[10] found metastatic lesions in the mucosa of the gallbladder in only 7 out of 125 patients dying from disseminated malignant melanoma. However, melanoma is the most common metastatic lesion of the gallbladder, comprising 50 to 66 percent of all gallbladder metastases.[23]

Henriques[24] first reported a case of gallbladder metastasis associated with acute cholecystitis. Thereafter, only few cases of gallbladder metastases have been documented in living melanoma patients.[25,26] Ultrasonography and CT Scan can allow early recognition of asymptomatic lesions. Surgical removal is a worthwhile palliative procedure.

Jaundice in patients with known malignant melanoma is most always caused by metastases in the liver; more rarely, there is compression of the main bile duct due to lymph node metastasis. Exceptionally, obstructive jaundice may be the consequence of an intraductal melanoma metastasis. Only six such cases were in the Anglo-Saxon literature until 1990.[27–31] An additional case was recently treated in our institution (see Plate 65).

Because of the rarity of this occurrence, the appropriate treatment of melanoma metastatic to the bile duct remains undefined. Patients with diffuse involvement of multiple organ systems should be treated by implantation of a bilio-duodenal endoprosthesis, or palliative cholecystojejunostomy or choledochojejunostomy. Selected patients may benefit from resection "for cure"; however, strong evidence is lacking to support an aggressive approach, especially if it involves a high-risk procedure such as pancreatoduodenectomy.[31]

PANCREAS

Pancreatic involvement is frequent in patients who die from malignant melanoma. Metastatic deposits were found in the pancreas in 32 to 53 percent of the patients in different autopsy series.[16] However, be-

TABLE 25-2
INCIDENCE OF METASTATIC MELANOMA IN THE GI TRACT (CLINICAL SERIES)

REFERENCE	*REINTGEN ET AL.*[4]	*KLAASE ET AL.*[46]	*GARRAMONE ET AL.*[49]	*JORGE ET AL.*[36]	*GUTMAN ET AL.*[44]
PERIOD	*1972–83*	*1981–87*	*1975–88*	*1973–82*	*1973–84*
PAT. NO.	*110/2500*	*30/835*	*13/450*	*15/320*	*11/348*
Esophagus	1	0	0	0	1
Stomach	8	0	7	1	1
Duodenum	0	0	2	5	0
Gall bladder	0	0	1	0	0
Biliary tract	0	1	0	0	0
Small bowel	38	17	6	10	6
Colon	16	4	2	2	2
Anus	0	0	0	1	3

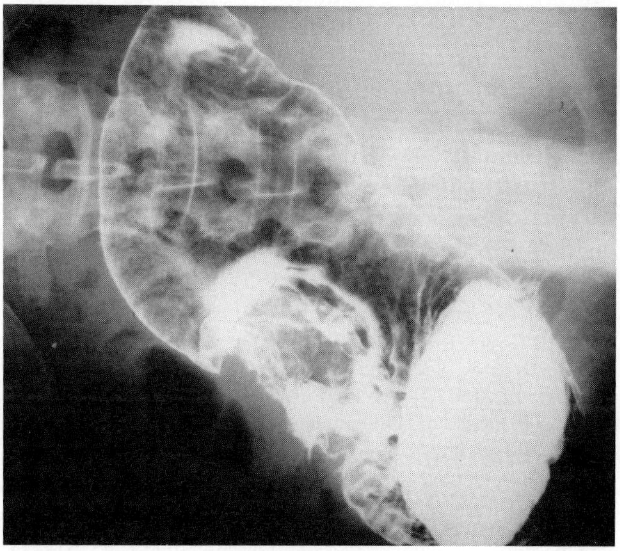

FIG. 25-1. *Gastric metastasis of malignant melanoma in a patient who underwent, 1 year before, a left axillary dissection followed by chemotherapy with dacarbazine for a lymph node metastasis. An enlarged subtotal gastrectomy was performed. More than 10 years after surgery, the patient was in good health and apparently free of disease.*

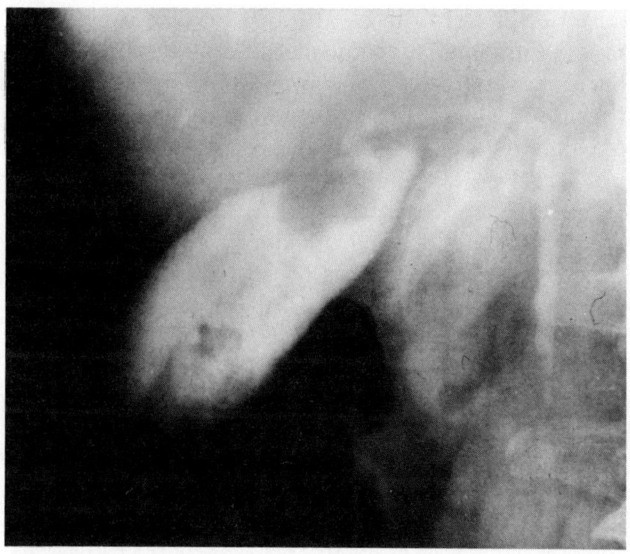

FIG. 25-2. *Cholecystogram showing a polypoid lesion into the gallbladder of a 59-year-old female. The lesion was discovered during the course of routine follow-up, 6 years after the excision of a primary malignant melanoma of the lower limb and 4 years after groin dissection for regional lymph node metastases.*

cause of the lack of any evidence of pancreatic dysfunction, its clinical diagnosis has been extremely rare.

SMALL BOWEL

The small bowel is the most common site for alimentary tract metastases from malignant melanoma. Involvement of the small bowel is found at autopsy in 58 percent of patients with malignant melanoma.[1]

Melanoma is responsible for 50 to 70 percent of the metastatic lesions to the small bowel.[32] In the series of 110 melanoma patients with symptomatic GI metastatic disease reported by Reintgen et al.,[4] the small bowel was involved in 35 percent of the cases.

Metastases usually implant in the submucosa and develop polypoid lesions, which act frequently as leading points for intussusception and resultant bowel obstruction.[33] Ulceration leads to chronic GI bleeding.

The predominate complaints in patients with symptomatic small bowel melanoma involvement are abdominal pain, chronic GI bleeding, obstruction, and weight loss.[34] Even though it is frequently negative, small bowel enteroclysis is the radiographic procedure of choice in these patients. Treatment includes bowel resection or intestinal by-pass. Several authors[35,36] have reported prolonged survival times after resection of solitary as well as multiple small bowel metastatic lesions.

COLON, RECTUM

Reviewing autopsies of 125 patients who died from melanoma, Das Gupta and Brasfield[1] found that 22 percent had colonic metastases. Among patients with symptomatic GI metastases from malignant melanoma, colonic involvement is unusual.[37] However, Willbanks and Fogelman[38] reported colonic metastases in 10 of 18 patients with symptomatic melanoma involvement of the GI tract. Malignant melanoma of the rectal ampulla was described as primary occurrence in rare instances.[39]

Initial signs and symptoms in patients with metastatic melanoma of the colon usually suggest obstruction, gastrointestinal blood loss, or a palpable mass. Work-up for colonic metastases should include barium enema and colonoscopy with biopsy. Surgical therapy includes resection of the affected segment of colon.

ANUS

Anal melanomas are considered primary tumors arising from melanocytes in the anal canal.[40] They represent 1 to 3 percent of all melanomas[41] and 1 percent of all anal tumors.[42]

Presenting complaints are bleeding, perception of a mass, change in bowel habits, pain or pruritus.[43,44] These signs are often mistakenly attributed to benign conditions or other tumors.

Diagnosis of anal melanoma is based on history, digital examination, proctoscopic evaluation, and biopsy. Diagnosis is usually delayed so that 38 to 62 percent of patients already have lymph node involvement at the time of diagnosis.[43]

Treatment for potential cure includes local excision and abdominoperineal resection. Although not proven by controlled studies, no significant difference in survival was found when patients treated by abdominoperineal resection were compared with those treated by local excision.[43] In the same way, the beneficial role of groin dissection has not been established.

CONCLUSIONS

Despite the high frequency of metastatic melanoma in the GI tract, it rarely causes symptoms. The clinician should be alerted by nonspecific symptoms such as anorexia, nausea and vomiting, weight loss, distention, diarrhea, melena, and anemia in any patient with a previous history of malignant melanoma. The use of aggressive radiologic and endoscopic procedure is justified in the attempt to diagnose and stage patients with melanoma.

TABLE 25-3
MALIGNANT MELANOMA METASTATIC TO THE GI TRACT REVIEW OF LITERATURE BY SITES

SITE	REFERENCE
Esophagus	Eng et al.[14]
Stomach	Booth[17]
Gall bladder	Murphy et al.[25]
Biliary tract	Kohler et al.[30]
Small bowel	Fraser-Moodie et al.[35]
Colon	Alexander et al.[39]
Anus	Cooper et al.[43]

Although most patients with GI involvement present with metastases elsewhere, it is not necessarily at an end stage, and most authors agree that surgery is usually useful.[36,45,46] Moreover, no effective chemotherapy is available as alternative treatment. The quality of life of these patients improves considerably after palliative surgery. The immediate, life-threatening complications, as well as pain and discomfort, are alleviated. This allows for further treatment when indicated. In some instances, survival after resection of a solitary intestinal metastasis can be very long.

REFERENCES

1. Das Gupta T, and Brasfield R. Metastatic melanoma of the gastrointestinal tract. *Arch Surg* 88:969–973, 1964.
2. Sacre R, and Lejeune FJ. Pattern of metastases distribution in 173 stage I or II melanoma patients. *Anticancer Res* 2:47–52, 1982.
3. Backman H. Metastasis of malignant melanoma in the gastrointestinal tract. *Geriatrics* 24:112–120, 1969.
4. Reintgen DS, Thompson W, Garbutt J, and Seigler HF. Radiologic, endoscopic, and surgical considerations of melanoma metastatic to the gastrointestinal tract. *Surgery* 95:635–639, 1984.
5. Geboes K, De Jaeger E, Rutgeerts P, and Vantrappen G. Symptomatic gastrointestinal metastases from malignant melanoma. *J Clin Gastroenterol* 10:64–70, 1988.
6. Raven RW, and Dawson I. Malignant melanoma of the oesophagus. *Br J Surg* 51:551–555, 1964.
7. Allen AC, and Spitz S. Malignant melanoma: A clinicopathological analysis of the criteria for diagnosis and prognosis. *Cancer* 6:1–45, 1953.
8. Turnbull AD, Rosen P, Goodner JT, and Beattie EJ. Primary malignant tumors of the esophagus other than typical epidermoid carcinoma. *Ann Thorac Surg* 15:463–473, 1973.
9. Chalkiadakis G, Wihlm JM, Morand G, Weill-Bousson M, and Witz JP. Primary malignant melanoma of the esophagus. *Ann Thorac Surg* 39:472–475, 1985.
10. Das Gupta T, and Brasfield R. Metastatic melanoma; a clinicopathological study. *Cancer* 17:1323–1339, 1964.
11. Butler ML, Van Heertum RL, and Teplick SK. Metastatic malignant melanoma of the esophagus: A case report. *Gastroenterology* 69:1334–1337, 1975.
12. Wood CB, and Wood RAB. Metastatic malignant melanoma of the esophagus. *Am J Dig Dis* 20:786–789, 1975.

13. Nelson RS, and Lanza F. Malignant melanoma metastatic to the upper gastrointestinal tract. *Gastrointest Endosc* 24:156–158, 1978.
14. Eng J, Pradhan GN, Sabarnathan S, and Mearns AJ. Malignant melanoma metastatic to the esophagus. *Ann Thorac Surg* 48:287–288, 1989.
15. Chandler AB, and Jones GF. Malignant melanoma of gastrointestinal tract. *Am Surg* 17:719–721, 1951.
16. Lee YN. Malignant melanoma: Pattern of metastasis. *CA Cancer J Clin* 30:137–142, 1980.
17. Booth JB. Malignant melanoma of the stomach: Report of a case presenting as an acute perforation and review of the literature. *Br J Surg* 52:262–270, 1965.
18. Calkins WG, and Hoppel CL. Malignant melanoma of the stomach. *Am J Gastroenterol* 43:150–154, 1965.
19. Pector JC, Crokaert F, Lejeune F, and Gerard A. Prolonged survival after resection of a malignant melanoma metastatic to the stomach. *Cancer* 61:2134–2135, 1988.
20. Potchen EJ, Khung CL, and Yatsuhashi M. X-ray diagnosis of gastric melanoma. *N Engl J Med* 271:133–136, 1964.
21. Colombel JF, Cortot A, Deloziere V, Houcke M, Hervouet P, Mosquet L, Brunetaud JM, and Paris JC. Métastase gastrique d'un mélanome malin de la choroïde. *Gastroentérol Clin Biol* 8:754–757, 1984.
22. Shimkin P, Soloway M, and Jaffee E. Metastatic melanoma of the gallbladder. *Am J Roetgenol* 116:393–395, 1972.
23. McFadden PM, Drementz ET, McKinnon WMP, Pararo LL, and Ryan RF. Metastatic melanoma of the gallbladder. *Cancer* 44:1802–1808, 1979.
24. Henriques CQ. A case of secondary melanoma of the gallbladder presenting as acute cholecystitis. *Br J Surg* 42:663–665, 1955.
25. Murphy MN, Lorimer SM, and Glennon PE. Metastatic melanoma of the gallbladder: A case report and review of the literature. *J Surg Oncol* 34:68–72, 1987.
26. Velchik MG. Acute gangrenous cholecystitis due to metastatic melanoma detected by cholescintigraphy. *Clin Nucl Med* 14:327–329, 1989.
27. Bowdler DA, and Leach RD. Metastatic intrabiliary melanoma. *Clin Oncol* 8:251–255, 1982.
28. McArthur MS, and Teergarden DK. Metastatic melanoma presenting as obstructive jaundice with hematobilia. *Am J Surg* 145:830–832, 1983.
29. O'Connel JB, Whittemore DM, Russel JC, Ellis WA, and Becker DR. Malignant melanoma metastatic to the cystic and common bile ducts. *Cancer* 53:184–186, 1984.
30. Kohler B, and Riemann JF. Obstructive jaundice due to an intraductal melanoma metastasis. *Endoscopy* 19:79–80, 1987.
31. England MD, and Sarr MG. Metastatic melanoma: An unusual cause of obstructive jaundice. *Surgery* 107:595–596, 1990.
32. Macbeth WA, Gwynne JF, and Jamieson MG. Metastatic melanoma in the small bowel. *Aust N Z J Surg* 38:309–315, 1969.
33. Kruse J, and Heath R. Melanoma metastatic to the gastrointestinal tract. *Am Fam Physician* 41:165–168, 1990.
34. Goodman PL, and Karakousis CP. Symptomatic gastrointestinal metastases from malignant melanoma. *Cancer* 48:1058–1059, 1981.
35. Fraser-Moodie A, Hughes RG, Jones SM, Shorey BA, and Snape L. Malignant melanoma metastases to the alimentary tract. *Gut* 17:206–209, 1976.
36. Jorge E, Harvey HA, Simmonds MA, Lipton A, and Joehl RJ. Symptomatic malignant melanoma of the gastrointestinal tract: Operative treatment and survival. *Ann Surg* 199:328–331, 1984.
37. McClenathan JH. Metastatic melanoma involving the colon. *Dis Colon Rectum* 32:70–72, 1989.
38. Willbanks OL, and Fogelman MJ. Gastrointestinal melanosarcoma. *Am J Surg* 120:602–606, 1970.
39. Alexander RM, and Cone LA. Malignant melanoma of the rectal ampulla: Report of a case and review of the literature. *Dis Colon Rectum* 20:53–55, 1977.
40. Morson BC, and Volkstadt H. Malignant melanoma of the anal canal. *J Clin Pathol* 16:126–132, 1963.
41. Mason JK, and Helwig EB. Ano-rectal melanoma. *Cancer* 19:39–50, 1966.
42. Oropeza R. Melanoma of special sites. In: Andrade R, Gumport SL, Popkin GL, and Rees TD (Eds.), *Cancer of the Skin*. Philadelphia: WB Saunders, 1976, 987–992.
43. Cooper PH, Mills SE, and Allen MS. Malignant melanoma of the anus. Report of 12 patients and analysis of 255 additional cases. *Dis Colon Rectum* 25:693–703, 1982.
44. Gutman M, Klausner JM, Inbar M, Chaitchik S, and Rozin RR. Surgical approach to malignant melanoma in the gastrointestinal tract. *J Surg Oncol* 36:17–20, 1987.
45. Mosimann F, Fontolliet C, Genton A, Gertsch P, and Pettavel J. Resection of metastases to the alimentary tract from malignant melanoma. *Int Surg* 67:257–260, 1982.
46. Klaase JM, and Kroon BBR. Surgery for melanoma metastatic to the gastrointestinal tract. *Br J Surg* 77:60–61, 1990.
47. Einhorn LH, Burgess MA, Vallegos C, Bodey GP, Gutterman JU, Mavligit G, Hersh EM, Luce JK, Frey E, Freireich EJ, and Gottlieb JA. Prognostic correlations and response to treatment in advanced metastatic malignant melanoma. *Cancer Res* 34:1995–2004, 1974.
48. Patel JK, Didolkar MS, Pickren JW, and Moore RH. Metastatic pattern of malignant melanoma: A study of 216 autopsy cases. *Am J Surg* 135:807–810, 1978.
49. Garramone RR, and Crombie HD. Gastrointestinal complications of metastatic malignant melanoma. *Conn Med* 54:130–132, 1990.

Chapter 26

ADJUVANT TREATMENT OF MELANOMA

U. R. Kleeberg

INTRODUCTION

The high rate of malignancy, the variable course of disease, and the marked resistance to therapy of metastatic melanoma represent a major challenge to the physician and scientist.

Occasional spontaneous remissions in melanoma,[1,2] the absence of a primary tumor in approximately 3 percent, the development of asymmetrical vitiligo in approximately 11 percent of patients[3] and the observation of halo-nevi with dense mononuclear cell infiltrates[4–6] as a result of unexplained destruction of the normal melanocytes, the coexistence of tumor progression and regression in up to 40 percent of primary melanomas,[3,7] especially of the superficial-spreading type[8] and finally, phases of clinical latency with involution of metastases,[9–12] which are occasionally observed in the same patient alongside fulminant courses of the disease,[13] point to the fact that "biological factors" play a role in melanoma and can influence the proliferation of the tumor.

Meanwhile it has become clear that both, lymphokines as mediators of the immune surveillance as well as "oncokines" aborted natural growth factors produced by the tumor, may influence its growth in an endocrine, paracrine, or autocrine fashion. Any form of regional (for example, radiotherapy) or systemic (for example, immune- or chemotherapy) treatment may induce production of such factors as well as expression of their receptors on the tumor cell membrane, thus turning any nonspecific intervention into a specific growth promoting or inhibiting stimulus. In view of the autonomous course of melanoma progression, every new treatment modality requires particularly critical evaluation before its clinical introduction.[14]

In the treatment of melanoma, it is remarkable that a large number of "standardized" therapeutical recommendations for adjuvant surgical, radiotherapeutic, local or systemic treatments have had to be revoked after sober examination in a controlled prospective way. As a lesson from medical history, the prospectively randomized multicentric study of the EORTC-Melanoma Cooperative Group (MCG), the intention of which was to examine the value of adjuvant BCG skin scarifications started in 1969 and terminated in 1974, should be noted at this point.[15,16]

Impressed by enthusiastic case reports and self-consciously articulated, unicentric empiricism, based on retrospective, "historical" comparisons of different patient collectives,[17,18] it was criticized as being "unethical" to withhold active nonspecific immunization with bacille Calmette-Guérin (BCG) from a melanoma patient. It then took another 10 years before, in 1982, first the WHO Melanoma Group (trial No. 6),[19] followed by the Piedmont Oncology Group,[20] and EORTC-MCG[21] were able to show that adjuvant BCG therapy is ineffective in melanoma patients. The natural course of disease in melanoma can be correlated with a series of clinical, cytologic, and immunohistochemically defined prognostic factors. Only with these criteria as a basis can the value of a treatment modality be judged conclusively. Using melanoma as an example, several generally applicable maxims for oncology can also be impressively supported.

Prerequisites for a scientifically sound proof of efficacy are the initial definition and careful documentation of proliferation rate and parameters of the tumor—biology, type, and location of metastases and stratification according to the previously mentioned prognostic criteria, as well as an external quality control ("extramural review") and "clinical audit"—which, as a rule, can only be realized in multicentric studies.[22,23]

BASIC PRINCIPLES OF ADJUVANT IMMUNOTHERAPY

Great importance is placed on the immune system in protecting the patient against the development of malignant tumors. It is often reasoned that stimulation of the immune response to tumor-associated antigens should therefore inhibit the proliferation of malignant growth and be able to destroy tumor cells, especially in minimal residual disease.

These postulations are derived from epidemiological, clinical, and experimental observations, which show that chemical carcinogens, particularly RNA viruses, X-, and UV-rays can induce malignant growth and concomitant reactions of the immune system:[24] Activation of oncogenes is followed by synthesis of aberrant proteins that, after being incorporated into the cell wall, become an obvious signal to be recognized by the immune surveillance. These proteins become antigens if they react with factors of the immune defense, or immunogens if they can provoke an immune response.

As we know, for example, from the post partum trophoblastic choriocarcinoma and from experiments on the nude mice, immunogenic tumors can be eliminated using immunological intervention. These successes and observations of spontaneous tumor remissions, however, are set against the backdrop of the majority of "hard" tumors in which no relevant immune reaction could be reproducibly defined, let alone therapeutically used.

In the facultatively immunogenic melanoma, we know of specific responses on the part of the host organism directed against particular tumor stem cell lines. Proof of a cellular defense reaction to autologous[25] and allogenic[26] melanoma cells, and the observation of humoral antibodies against membrane antigens early on and against cytoplasmic antigens late in the course of the disease,[27] and antigen evolution, in which a particular tumor cell population can change its antigenic phenotype[28–31] speak for the fact that these host factors are of an immunological nature. However, they seem to be blocked, or to remain ineffective, in the physiological control of tumor growth. As much as the histological evidence of infiltration of lymphocytes and macrophages in or around the tumor correlates with a better prognosis in some patients[5,32] and worse in others,[33] in the long run the host organism is not able to stand up against the widely proliferating tumor.

Melanoma cells are characterized by the varying expression of constitutional, differentiation, proliferation, and sporadically some telltale "tumor-associated antigens" (TAA), which together define a highly variable tumor cell phenotype.[34–38]

Melanoma cells can reproduce billionfold from one single atypical clone growing into a highly heterogenous of variants. Early in the course there may be such an occasional variant caught by the (augmented) immune surveillance, but later there is an ever rising number of clones evading the supervision of the most sophisticated defense mechanisms. It is difficult to imagine how, in such a situation, a specific or nonspecific stimulation of humoral and/or cell-mediated components of the natural immune system could successfully intervene in advanced tumor cell growth. Only if it were possible to permanently express a considerably larger number of TAA on the melanoma cells in vivo, as has been achieved in cell cultures using recombinant interferon,[39] and then to locate these antigens, for instance with selective monoclonal antibodies (mAbs), and damage the cells through co-transported cytostatics (immunotoxins, "drug targeting"), could specific "immunotherapy" become a reality.

First attempts to make tumor cells visible through a coupling of mAbs with fluoresceins, peroxidase, and radioisotopes in histological sections, cytological preparations, or in vivo ("tumor imaging") have been published.[40–44]

The specificity and selectivity of these mAbs, however, are not yet sufficient. Cross-reactions with endothelial and nerve cells, macrophages, and so on, make clinical application more difficult.[42] Without any doubt, however, monoclonal antibodies have brought us to the verge of a new development.

The unrealistic hopes, favored by a broad lay public, of curing cancer patients through "natural methods" that stimulate the immune system can in part be traced back to medical successes in eradicating smallpox, polio, diphtheria, and so on. Apart from the fact that every infectious agent involves an exogenous antigen that is foreign to the host, the control of these epidemics was not achieved through "immuno*therapy*," but through "immuno*prophylactics*," in which the host was sensitized with the immunogen *before* exposure to the pathogenic virus. Experimental oncology also knows of this phenomenon, whereby experimental animals reject genetically identical tumor transplants and become resistant to tumor growth if they have *previously* been immunized with a small amount of the tumor antigen.[16] Up to now, however, it has not been possible to obtain cross-reacting immunogenic tumor cell extracts as a human immunoprophylactic, so that this principle has been currently ruled out in the treatment of human tumors.

In a majority of malignant diseases, and especially melanoma, even after radical removal of the primary tumor and clearance of the regional lymph node drainage areas, systemic occult micrometastases remain, to which patients may succumb after a phase of clinical latency, the so-called disease-free interval.

Supported by cell-kinetic data from the 1960s,[45] attempts were made to further reduce the suspected minimal residual tumor mass through pre-, peri-, or post-operative systemic cytostatic therapy, and one hoped that the physiological immune defense could then finally conquer the remaining tumor cells. It, therefore, seemed reasonable through additional stimulation and/or augmentation of the immune system by means of active, passive, specific, and nonspecific measures to destroy any tumor cell remaining in immunological hideouts.

Finally, one hoped to equalize a possibly disadvantageous, cytostatic-induced immunosuppression with a combination of chemo- and immunotherapy, and to potentiate the cytotoxic effect by mobilizing all available defense mechanisms. There has been no lack of attempts to influence the fate of melanoma patients with the aid of adjuvant specific or nonspecific immunotherapy.

Unfortunately, all efforts so far have not produced tangible results, whereby it remains open whether or not adjuvant therapy is falsely conceived, incorrectly practiced, or whether the available treatment modalities are still simply too weak for the highly therapy-resistant melanoma.

The results of latest studies with monoclonal antibodies directed against various antigen structures of the tumor cell membrane allow the assumption that the tumor-phenotype constantly alters, regulating its antigenic structures as a result of the conflict with the host organism and possibly also through therapeutical intervention.[39,28,29] In human melanoma approximately 70 different antigens expressed by the tumor cells have been defined by mAbs. Only in rare instances have tumor antigens been found on malignant cells but not on any normal cells of the same or other lineages. As far as we can tell now, there are quantitative, and only rarely relevant qualitative, differences in the phenotypic expression of proliferating benign versus malignant cells.[16] As a result of the permanent selective pressure, tumor cell clones proliferate that evade the physiological defense mechanisms thus obtaining decisive growth advantages. The metastases that ultimately kill the host have undergone a long development of constant mutation and selection and are hardly vulnerable to any conventional stimulation or augmentation of the "immune defense."

The results of representative studies on adjuvant immuno-, chemo-, and combination therapy, as well as secondary adjuvant indicator therapy are presented in the following.

TREATMENT OPTIONS IN ADJUVANT IMMUNOTHERAPY

Supported by experimental and morphological studies, as well as clinical observation, regarding the significance of "host" factors for the growth of melanoma, the following treatment options have been evaluated.

Active, Nonspecific Immunotherapy

This therapy is understood as the direct stimulation of a generalized immune response leading to a nonspecific rejection of tumor cells. This has been attempted with different antigens, such as the microorganisms bacille Calmette-Guérin (BCG), *Corynebacterium parvum* (*C. parvum*), vaccinia virus, or their components as well as through methanol extractable residues (MER) from BCG or picibanil from *Streptococcus hemolyticus* A, and so on. Based on erroneous veterinary observations in the south of France that the most frequent malignant growth in white horses, the melanoma, is less common in tuberculosis-infested horses living wild in the Camargue as compared with the tuberculosis-free farm livestock, the first clinical experiments were already carried out in the late 1960s.

In animal and human experiments, it could be shown that BCG vaccination can induce hyperplasia of the reticulohistiocytic system (RHS) with activation of macrophages.[46–49]

In 1978 it became known that the efficacy of these immunomodulators is dependent on the concentration of such membrane components as trehalose dimycolate or muramyl dipeptide, which were isolated from MER of wild and attenuated (BCG) bacteria, similarly from *C. parvum* and Nocardia rubra.[50,51] With the assumption that any relevant effect of the human immune response could be expected predominantly in minimal residual disease, a large number of clinical studies with intracutaneous,[19,52] peroral,[53] parenteral,[54] intralymphatic,[55] and intralesional[48,49,56] administration of the mentioned bacteria and their extracts, as well as of viruses[57,58] were initiated. How little is known about the interaction between the immunosurveillance of the host and the immunogenicity of the tumor is revealed by the results of a series of controlled clinical studies: Besides a questionable benefit, one and the same BCG therapy can bring a definite disadvantage to the patient resulting in unrestrained stimulation of tumor growth.[30,59–63,64]

Other immunomodulators were used besides those mentioned, such as smallpox viruses,[65] levamisol,[16,66] transfer factor,[67–69] thymosin,[70] isoprinosine,[16] alpha-, beta-, and gamma-interferons,[16] tumor cells, and so on, but only a few produced a scientifically sound conclusion.[50,55,71] Out of some 30 adjuvant treatment trials, both in patients with stage I and stage II melanoma, a selection of representative, controlled study protocols will be discussed.

BCG—Bacille Calmette-Guérin

Between 1970 and 1980, the WHO "International Melanoma Working Group" adjuvantly treated, in a randomized phase III protocol, 761 patients with prognostically unfavorable stage I (only trunk) or stage II (trunk and limb) melanomas over 2 years with BCG, 75 mg per scarification, initially weekly, then monthly and/or DTIC (200 mg/m^2 i.v., d1-5, 6 times monthly).[19] The survival times and disease-free intervals of the patients, who have now been followed over 10 years since surgery, and who were stratified according to prognostic criteria and allocated to different treatment groups or a control arm, do not differ significantly from one another, both regarding disease-free and overall survival. A discrete trend in favor of the DTIC and/or BCG treated patients could be seen so that a few questions remained open that were to be clarified in two follow-up studies by the EORTC-Melanoma Cooperative Group.

The first, a postoperative phase III study with BCG in prognostically unfavorable melanomas initiated by the EORTC-MCG in 1974 and discontinued in 1975[15] produced just as little support for an improvement of the disease-free interval or survival rates[72] as a similar ECOG study concluded in 1976.[71] In the WHO study those patients had a better prognosis who converted on BCG from an initially negative or weak to a strong reaction—in contrast with the results from the EORTC-trial[15] showing that the degree of a patient's immune reaction to BCG administered systemically was of paramount importance in determining the likelihood of survival: The more intense the reaction to BCG and (independent from the level of invasion) the higher the Breslow's tumor thickness, the shorter was the disease-free and total survival.

Production procedures, quality, quantity of the bacteria, as well as way and site of administration, appeared to be of importance for the effect of BCG: BCG-RIV from Bilthoven consists exclusively of live bacteria, whereas BCG-Pasteur from Paris contains large amounts of dead bacteria and soluble proteins. Humoral antibodies against Tbc-bacteria and delayed-type immune reactions were virtually only observed in patients immunized with the French vaccine.[73] On the other hand, specific cellular immune reactions could be better induced with the Dutch BCG.[72]

For this reason, the EORTC-MCG began a second prospective controlled study in 1978 for patients with prognostically unfavorable stage I melanomas (Breslow > 1,5 mm) with randomization either into a therapy arm with BCG Pasteur (n = 119) or BCG-RIV (n = 118) over 3 years, respectively, or into a placebo controlled arm (n = 117). Survival time and disease-free intervals (DFI) observed at 7 years was identical in the groups.[21] The preliminary results are depicted on Fig. 26-1. The effect of an adjuvant, 2-year BCG treatment on a possible inhibition of micrometastases were also tested in stage II melanoma with regional lymph node metastasis: Compared to a control group with surgery only, more favorable[74] (historical control), identical,[52,71] and worse courses,[63] with a possible "enhancement" of tumor growth were documented.

Corynebacterium Parvum

After Halpern[75] demonstrated immunostimulation through heat-inactivated corynebacteria in 1966 with a better immunotherapeutical efficacy as compared to BCG in human melanoma xenotransplants,[76] *C. parvum* was introduced into experimental medicine.

In a nonrandomized study, 34 patients with stage I melanomas received *C. parvum* s.c. (4 mg/m^2 weekly 6 times, then monthly 6 times, then every 6 months up to the fifth postoperative year), without identifiable advantage over a historical comparative population.[77]

Nor in stage II was it possible to significantly influence survival times in 30 patients with *C. parvum* (4 mg s.c. over 5 days, then weekly over 3 years).[78] In contrast, in patients with a prognostically unfavorable stage I melanoma (depth of penetration > 3 mm), an extension of the free interval occurred in a randomized, although too small group, with 23 treated against 26 control patients. In the remaining 175 patients with less than 3 mm thick melanomas, both therapy arms had identical disease-free survival times (DFS) of 83 percent after 3 years observation.[79]

A prospective and randomized comparison of *C. parvum* (5 mg/m^2 s.c.) with BCG (3 × 10^8 live bacteria per scarification) given over 2 years did not yield any significant difference in the 5-year survival rates in 68 stage I patients but possible difference in DFS of 48 stage II patients treated with *C. parvum*.[80] It remained open whether extending the DFS resulted in improved cure rates. Negative results have been obtained in a randomized study with *C. parvum* following surgery for 115 stage II patients, increasing the likelihood that nonspecific adjuvant immunotherapy will not improve the prognosis of high risk stage I or II melanoma patients.

Active Specific Immunotherapy

This therapy is understood as the attempt to induce an "autoimmune reaction" against tumor-associated antigens. For this purpose, autologous or heterolo-

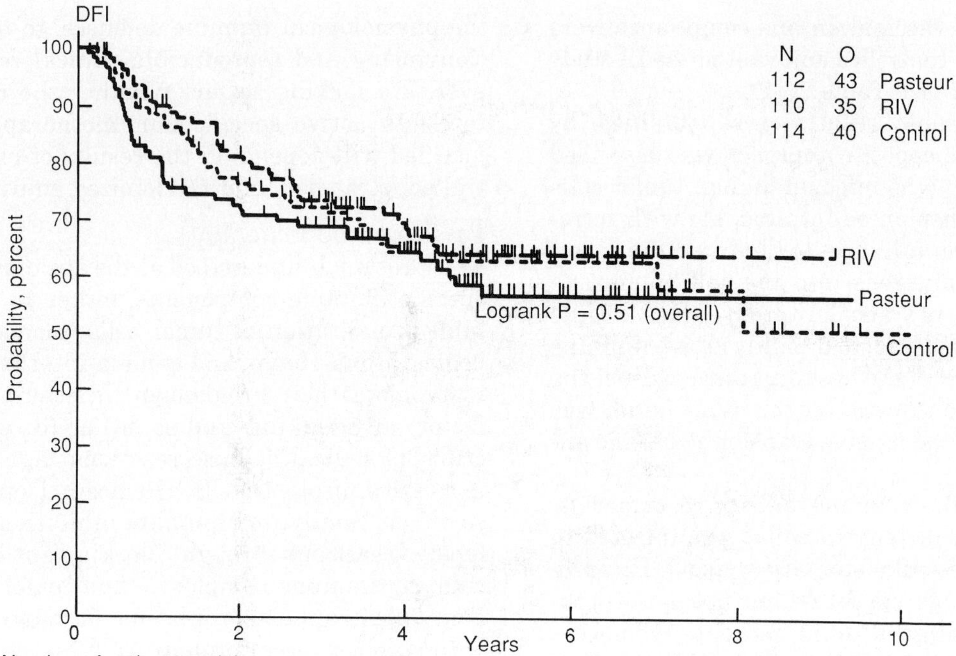

Number of patients at risk:

0	2	4	6	8	
112	75	50	17	3	Pasteur
110	81	52	20	2	RIV
114	78	48	22	7	Control

FIG. 26-1. *Adjuvant BCG-treatment in melanoma patients (for explanation see text).*

gous melanoma cells were obtained and following devitalization by chemical, thermal, or radiogenic means reinjected either in toto or as a membrane mixture. The basis of these experiments were experiences from transplantation immunology and evidence of differences in HLA-A, B, and DR, constitutive or differentiation antigens between tumor cells and their normal precursors.

Whereas it was possible in animal experiments to trigger a rejection reaction of the transplanted melanoma through prior immunization of the host, initial clinical experiments produced negative or contradictory results.[3,63,81–83] In some cases even insufficiently inactivated melanoma cells started growing in HLA-compatible donors or an enhancement of tumor growth was observed resulting in reduction of survival rates in treated patients as compared with a historical control.[84,85]

Livingstone et al.[86] treated 20 patients with radio-inactivated allogen (SK-MEL 13-) melanoma cells, injected intradermally at the site where an inflammatory reaction had been triggered with BCG scarification 2 to 3 weeks earlier. All patients developed antibodies against the HLA alloantigen of the transferred melanoma parent cell line, but only one against melanoma-associated and neuroectodermal antigens. A clinical effect was not observed.[87]

Other vaccinations with melanoma-associated antigens were used, for example, a vaccinia melanoma cell lysate given to 80 stage II patients in a phase II adjuvant study: Overall survival of 39 patients at a 2-year follow-up period was 75 percent, compared to 57 percent in a historical control group.[88]

In another adjuvant study, vaccination with the sialo-ganglioside GM2 in cyclophosphamide pretreated stage II patients seemed to delay recurrences.[89] The EORTC-MCG initiated a similar approach, starting off with a pilot study vaccinating patients in stage II and III with high risk of recurrence following curative surgery with native gangliosides first followed by liposomal preparations, then additional aluminum as adjuvants. Out of 32 evaluable patients, 17 presented a significant increase in antibody titer, mostly of the IgG isotype. The disease-free intervals for the patients who showed an antibody response to the treatment were significantly higher ($p < 0.001$) than those of the nonresponding group.[147]An innovative idea was presented by Wallack in 1979.[58,90] Based on the observation that the virus capsid partly consists of virus-specific proteins synthesized by the host cell, and partly of lipid components from its plasma membrane, he infected melanoma parent cell lines with smallpox viruses. After passage through the tumor, cell antigens common to both, the virus-capsid and the cell membrane occurred as well as a virus-related alteration of the surface structure of the infected melanoma cells. A mixture of smallpox-infected allogenic melanoma cells, the so-called "vaccinia-oncolysate" was then injected intradermally into patients with stage II melanoma. Seven of 19 patients immunized, remained free of disease for 6 to 24 months. Because tolerability of the vaccination and compliance were good, a prospective controlled adjuvant phase III study has been initiated (see Table 26-1).

Similar favorable results were obtained by Hersey et al.[91] The opposite approach was described by Iglehart et al.[57] who infected human tumor cells that had been transplanted into rodents with retroviruses and thus simultaneously induced the incorporation of viral antigens into the cell membrane and the expression of transplantation antigens. This resulted, on the one hand, in a highly active immune reaction on the part of the host organism against the tumor cells, whose growth, on the other hand, was inhibited through the passive transfer of specific antiviral antisera.[92]

To increase the immunogenicity of tumor-associated antigens, melanoma cells were infected in vitro with VSV (vesicular stomatitis virus). This produced antibodies against HLA- but not against tumor-associated antigens in 11 patients who were vaccinated with cell-free lysates fromVSV-infected autologous and allogenic melanoma cell cultures.[86]

At least in theory, the combination of various options of active and passive immunotherapy should allow control of a progressing tumor which has evaded the physiological immune defenses, to be regained. Convincing and reproducible clinical results, however, are lacking so far. Whether the renewed interest in active specific immunotherapy is indeed justified will depend on the results of properly controlled, stratified, and randomized adjuvant trials.

Passive Immunotherapy

This therapy is understood as the attempt to transfer specific immune components, either to directly inhibit proliferation of tumor cells (monoclonal antibodies, alpha-, beta-, and gamma-interferons) and/or to promote their breakdown (interferons, transfer factor, interleukins, and so on) or to indirectly recruit "biological defense reactions" against the tumor (Levamisole, DNCB, Thymosin, Isoprinosin and so on) or, finally, to eliminate inhibition of host defensive reactions through "blocking antibodies," circulating immune complexes, and "exfoliated" antigens (plasmapheresis, plasma immune absorption with staphylococcal protein A).[16]

Adoptive Immunotherapy

This therapy is used to describe the use of individual factors or the administration of whole, as a rule heterologous immune mixtures, such as fresh cells, im-

TABLE 26-1

RANDOMIZED PHASE III TRIALS FOR PATIENTS WITH HIGH RISK MELANOMA WHO ARE CLINICALLY DISEASE-FREE FOLLOWING CURATIVE SURGERY (PDQ—TRIAL RETRIEVAL 1992)

LEAD ORGANIZATION (PROTOCOL NUMBER) STUDY COORDINATOR	TITLE OBJECTIVES
Canadian Clinical Trials Group (Can-NCIC-ME7) J.C. Quirt: Princess Margaret Hospital, Toronto, Canada	Comparison of Levamisole versus rIfn gamma in high risk stage I/II patients
US Natl. Cancer Institute (NCI-89-C-168) J.W. Smith II: NCI Nat. Institutes of Health, Frederick Md.	Levamisole alone or in combination with rIfn gamma in high risk stage II A-B/II patients
Mt. Sinai Med. Center Miami (NCI-V88-0479) M.K. Wallack: Mt. Sinai Med. Center, Miami Beach, Fla.	Double-blind study of Vaccinia Oncolysate versus Vaccinia alone in high risk stage II patients
MGH Cancer Center (MGH-M1/SEG-Int/MEl 3044504) H.C. Hoover Jr: MGH, Boston, Mass.	BCG-tumor vaccination with versus without cyclophosphamide versus surgery alone in clinical stage II/III patients
Eastern Coop. Oncol. Group (ECOG-EST-1684) J.M. Kirkwood: Pittsburgh Cancer Institute, Pittsburgh, Pa.	rIfn alpha 2 versus no adjuvant therapy in high risk stage I/II patients
EORTC-Mel. Coop. Group AIO German Cancer Society (EORTC-MCG 18871) U.R. Kleeberg: Haem.-Onkol. Praxis Altona, Hamburg, Germany	rIfn alpha 2 versus rIfn gamma versus Iscador versus no adjuvant therapy in stage I (>3 mm) and II B patients
EORTC-Mel. Coop. Group WHO Mel. Group NAPG/SWOG/CNCIC (EORTC-MCG 18832) F. Lejeune: Inst. J. Bordet, Free University, Bruxelles, Belgium	Isolation perfusion with L-PAM plus hyperthermia in melanoma of the extremities versus surgery alone +/− reg. lymphadenectomy in stage I (> 1,5 mm) patients
North Centr. Can. Treat. Group (NCCTG 89705) R.J. Dalton: Duluth Clinic, Duluth, Minn.	Double-blind study of Megestrol vs. placebo in high risk stage I/II patients

munized T lymphocytes, hyperimmunoglobulin, transfer factor, thymus extracts, and so on, under the partly vague, partly refuted impression that it would serve to correct the immune deficiency that inhibits the recovery of the tumor patient. More recent experiments with tumor infiltrating lymphocytes have emerged as the possibly only clinically relevant approach. None of these treatment modalities have been tested in adjuvant phase III trials.

Levamisole

After it was found that the antihelmintic Levamisole promotes cell mediated immunity in animals[93] and man,[94] several animal experiments showed that tumor growth could be inhibited and survival times lengthened in certain species,[95,96] whereas in others Levamisole was ineffective.[97] In melanoma patients, Levamisole improved specific humoral and cellular immunity directed at the tumor,[98] and favorable results in bronchial carcinoma,[99,100] mammary carcinoma,[101] and colorectal cancer,[148,149] were obtained in initial clinical studies.

With the hypothesis that patients with minimal residual tumor mass[102] ought to profit from treatment with Levamisole, especially when simultaneously subjected to effective "cytoreductive" therapy, a series of adjuvant mono- and combined chemo-immunotherapeutical studies were carried out. In a prospective randomized placebo-controlled double-blind study, the action of Levamisole was tested in an adjuvant setting in 203 patients with primary and regional metastatic melanomas.[103] In stage I a trend resulted in favor of Levamisole regarding the disease-free intervals ($p = 0{,}07$) but, as a whole, this form of immunotherapy had no effect on survival time and rates over a total observation period of up to $5^1/_2$ years. The EORTC-Melanoma Coop. Group (Protocol No. 18781) carried out a prospective, randomized, double-blind phase III trial of DTIC versus Levamisol versus placebo in stage I high-risk patients (Breslow > 1,5 mm) after surgical removal of primary melanoma of the skin: No significant difference in time to progression, disease-free, and overall survival could be observed in 325 patients over a mean observation period of 5 years.[104] The combination of Levamisole with cytostatic therapy, tested by SWOG[105] on 280 patients with metastatic melanomas, who received either BCNU, hydroxyurea, or DTIC with or without Levamisole, did not lead to improved rates of objective remission either. Due to a trend towards shortening of survival time in the Levamisole group, the suspicion was even expressed that this immunotherapy may have been disadvantageous (see Fig. 26-2).

Transfer Factor

The transfer factor (TF) was first described by Lawrence[69] as a dialysable leukocyte extract with

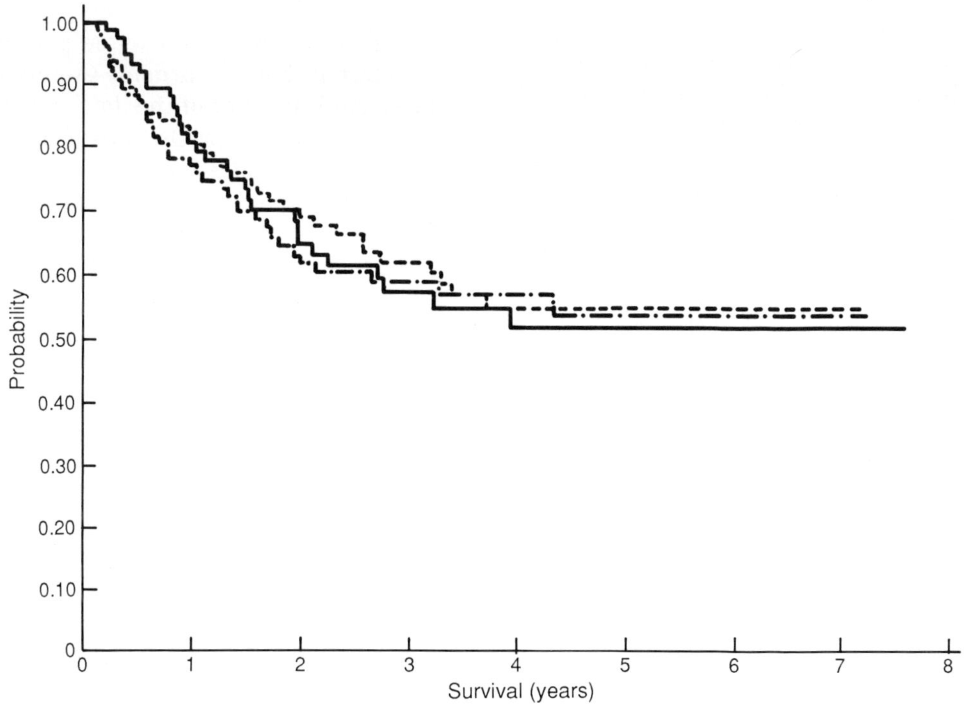

Number patients at risk:

78	55	36	27	16	10	6	2	0
102	78	57	39	25	16	4	1	0
96	66	46	33	21	14	11	3	0

FIG. 26-2. *Adjuvant treatment with DTIC (——), Levamisole (---), placebo (—·—·—) in 376 patients with a stage I melanoma, Breslow > 1,5 mm, EORTC-Melanoma Coop. Group (Macher et al.[104]).*

which a previously actively induced delayed-type immune reaction could passively be transferred from one organism to the other. In addition, later investigations demonstrated a nonspecific stimulatory action on cell-mediated immunity.[67]

It, therefore, seemed obvious to also test TF in the adjuvant immunotherapy of different types of malignant diseases.[106] The free intervals of 96 stage I melanoma patients treated with TF s.c. were investigated in a larger, nonrandomized, uncontrolled study. After a mean observation period of 30 months, only nine patients showed progression.[107]

The latest randomized, controlled study on melanoma published on this subject describes 36 stage II patients who after curative resection of lymph node metastases were treated with TF (1 unit = extract from 1 × 10^9 leukocytes i.m., 6 times weekly, then monthly) over 2 years or until further progression. The mean disease-free intervals, 12 months in the 18 treated and 10 months in the untreated patients, were not statistically significantly different from one another.[68] Despite a trend in favor of the TF patients, further investigations with TF are only meaningful if the active ingredient of this cell mixture, a supposed lymphokine, can be successfully isolated, standardized, and applied under controlled conditions.

Interferons

The reason to use interferons as antiproliferative agents in melanoma stems from the initial work of Ratner et al.[108] showing the inhibition of growth in mouse melanoma and a whole variety of immunoregulatory effects on the host immune surveillance[88,109] and on the antigen expression of melanoma cells.[39,110]

Phase I and II evaluations of the interferons in metastatic melanoma yielded objective response rates between 10 to 20 percent depending on total tumor burden, site of disease, and to a minor degree on the doses applied[16] without, however, altering the course of advanced disease to any substantial degree. In view of their differing biological effects and because of the greater susceptibility of microscopic disease to immune manipulation in experimental systems, the early application of recombinant interferon alpha and gamma (rIfn alpha + gamma) in an adjuvant setting appeared of particular interest. Various adjuvant trials in stage I, II, and III melanoma patients have been initiated, puzzling the oncologist with contradictory results. Only few of them are worth mentioning: The only recognized method that avoids almost all bias is the random allocation of the treatments with sophisticated prerandomization stratification. The only criterion of success is a significant increase in overall survival. Up to 1991, the answer remains open (for current interferon trials see Table 26-1). A definitive answer is expected from the ongoing international trial of the EORTC-Melanoma Cooperative Group, started in 1987, comparing rIfn alpha with rIfn gamma with Iscador M versus a control group in melanoma patients immediately following curative resection of either high risk primary stage I (Breslow's > 3 mm) or regional lymph node metastasis (stage IIb).

Diverse Adjuvant Immunological Therapy Trials

An active specific immunotherapy with the Newcastle disease virus-oncolysate from autologous melanoma cells was tested in phase II study on 32 stage II and III patients after curative resection of their metastasis. Only four of the patients treated experienced progression within the following 3 years.[111]

In a randomized, prospective-controlled study, stage II melanoma patients were treated postoperatively either with BCG (49 patients) or with BCG and a tumor cell vaccine (52 patients) and compared with a control group of 48 patients who had only received surgery.[112]

After a mean observation time of 62 months, the relapse rate were identical in all three groups, although the survival times of those treated with BCG were slightly more favorable, with a mean of 14,4 months, compared to 5,2 months in the control group and 6,8 months in the tumor vaccine group.

In a prospectively controlled trial, an adjuvant passive immunotherapy with thymostimulin (TP1) was given postoperatively to 26 stage I (tumor thickness > 1,25 mm) and 11 stage II patients.[113] After 1 year, the DFS of the treated patients appeared to be better in both treatment groups as compared to the control. In light of the data, which are available now from well-controlled prospectively randomized multicentric studies, recruiting enough evaluable cases for proper statistical evaluation, the results obtained with active-nonspecific or passive adjuvant immunotherapy presented here must be judged with great caution. Many problems arise from biased patient selections, ill-defined clinical and microstages, unequal distribution of relevant prognostic factors, mixing of historical and prospective control populations, and, last but not least, uncritical final evaluation. The only valid parameters in this adjuvant setting are disease-free and total survival.

And another word of caution: Also unfavorable clinical courses have been observed under immunological manipulation with possible tumor enhancement.[30,59–64,84,114,115] Therefore, great care is recommended in view of our still insufficient knowledge of the mechanisms of action of the various biomodulators and immunotherapy in general.

ADJUVANT CYTOSTATIC THERAPY

The number of effective cytostatics and their combinations in the treatment of metastatic melanoma is small and their duration of action limited. At the end of the 1960s, 20 to 30 percent remissions were reported on chemotherapy with 5-(3,3-dimethyl-1-triazeno)-imidazole-4-carboxamide (DTIC), and this substance was used in adjuvant treatment protocols (as a rule at a dosage of 200 to 250 mg/m^2 i.v. d1-5 every 4 weeks for 6 times).

In 1974 the WHO Melanoma Group[19] and in 1976 the EORTC-Melanoma Cooperative Group (MCG)[104] initiated adjuvant treatment studies with DTIC in high risk stage I and II melanoma patients. Both were conducted as prospective, randomized studies and, with 761 (WHO) and 325 (EORTC) evaluable patients, the numbers were sufficient to permit stratification according to the different prognostic criteria. After 5 years' observation time, there were no statistically significant differences found, neither with regard to disease-free interval nor survival times between DTIC and control groups. However, a trend in favor of adjuvant DTIC therapy occurred in the WHO study in patients with stage II melanomas of the extremities with up to three positive lymph nodes ($p = 0{,}01$) and those with stage I trunk disease ($p = 0{,}06$).

This trend is confirmed by Wood et al.[116,17] who described an improvement in survival time in 70 stage I and II patients (Breslow > 1,5 mm) in a controlled, randomized study. In 25 stage II patients with more than five positive lymph nodes, no improvement in survival times could be achieved with DTIC[74] and the "Central Oncology Group"[118] found, if anything, an unfavorable effect in 81 stage I, II, and III patients treated with DTIC as compared to 84 controls after a mean observation period of 2.5 years.

Even raising the DTIC dosage from 4,5 mg/kg/day i.v. × 10 for 4 courses to twice this amount made no difference to the disadvantageous results, so that the authors advise against adjuvant monotherapy with DTIC. Apart from the well known and regularly encountered side-effects of the highly emetic DTIC such as anorexia, nausea, and vomiting, potentially serious complications may occur such as the veno-occlusive syndrome leading to acute liver dystrophy and intrahepatic thrombosis.[119,120]

Twelve months of polychemotherapy with BHD: BCNU, Hydroxyurea, DTIC was also unsuccessful in 60 stage I (Clark III-V) patients as compared to 63 postoperatively untreated controls in a prospectively randomized study conducted by the "Southwest Oncology Group" (SWOG).[121]

In stage II disease, six courses of adjuvant BHD polychemotherapy following curative resection of regional lymph node metastases yielded a significant advantage in disease-free interval for the 33 treated versus 29 untreated patients without any effect however on overall survival.[122]

For the time being an end ought, therefore, to be put to the attempts at trying to favorably influence the fate of melanoma patients using an adjuvant cytostatic mono- or polychemotherapy. The positive results initially described in patients who were compared with a historical collective[17,123,124] as control could not be confirmed in the prospectively randomized studies or were contradictory. Also apart from being of doubtful value, DTIC treatment may be detrimental in a small, and highly unpleasant in a large group of patients reducing their lifetime without tumor symptoms and treatment toxicity.[125]

For a subpopulation of patients, regional extremity perfusion may be an answer. A first study, lacking proper stratifications and quality controls, yielded favorable results[126] but was discontinued prematurely. This technique also may cause some toxicity and late functional restrictions.[127]

Again, we will have to wait for the results of a properly stratified and prospectively randomized trial such as listed on Table 26-2, before such an approach can be adopted as a new adjuvant treatment strategy. A large international trial inaugurated in 1983 by the EORTC-MCG in cooperation with the WHO Melanoma Group and the North American Perfusion Group (NAPG) so far recruited some 800 patients with melanoma of the extremities, receiving isolation perfusion with L-PAM in hyperthermia compared to a control group.

Adjuvant Trials with Biological Response Modifiers (BRM)

Among various hypothetical approaches based primarily on in vitro data, adjuvant treatment with Retinoids merits mentioning: These natural and synthetic analogues of Vitamin A inhibit growth and induce differentiation in many human malignancies. In vitro experiments also demonstrated that Retinoids may have synergistic activity in combination with other BRMs, hormones, and irradiation.[128]

To test this possibility, adjuvant therapy with 13-Cis-Retinoid acid was given to 18 patients with high risk stage I and II melanoma and compared with 19 concomitant controls. At a median observation time of 18 months, no difference in DFS was observed.[129]

ADJUVANT COMBINED CYTOSTATIC AND IMMUNOTHERAPY

A multitude of observations that suggest an influence of the immune system on the course of disease, as well as both animal experiments and clinical studies with DTIC (from which immunosensitization in the form of antigen modulation of the tumor cell[130] without identifiable immunosuppression[26,131,132] was

TABLE 26-2
ADJUVANT TREATMENT OPTIONS TESTED IN CONTROLLED OR RANDOMIZED TRIALS FOR PATIENTS WITH STAGE I/II MELANOMA OF POOR PROGNOSIS

TREATMENT OPTIONS	DRUGS	NUMBER OF TRIALS
Monochemotherapy versus control	DTIC	8
	MeCCNU	2
Monochemo- versus +/−	DTIC sh BCG	7
Immunotherapy	DTIC +/− BCG	2
	DTIC +/− MER	1
	DTIC / *C. parvum*	1
	DTIC +/− *C. parvum*	1
	Ac + D +/− BCG	1
Mono- versus polychemotherapy	MeCCNU +/− VCR	1
	DTIC / BHD	1
Poly- versus polychemotherapy	5 versus 6 rugs	1
Polychemotherapy versus control	DTIC + CPA	1
	BHD	3
	6 drugs	1
Polychemo- versus Immunotherapy	BHD +/− BCG	1
Immunotherapy versus control/placebo	BCG	5
	MER	3
	C. parvum	3
	Levamisole	3
	Transfer factor	2
	Isoprinosine	1
	Retinoids	1
	Melanoma cells	2
Immuno- versus Immunotherapy	BCG / *C. parvum*	2
Immunochemotherapy	BHD +/− BCG	1
	DTIC +/− BCG	2
	DTIC +/− *C. parvum*	2
	DTIC +/− MER	1
	DTIC + CPA + *C. parvum*	1
	DTIC + BCG + Mel. cells	1
	Polychemo + Isoprinosine	1

Adapted from Lejeune and Kleeberg 1986

shown) have formed the rationale for a combination of various immunomodulators with DTIC.

After it initially appeared as if it would be possible to raise the efficacy of DTIC through BCG or *C. parvum* in palliative therapy of metastatic melanoma, this principle was also applied to the adjuvant treatment of stage I and II melanoma patients. At first, studies with or without historical comparative collectives appeared to confirm this thesis. Between 1972 and 1975, Serrou et al.[98] treated 35 stage I and II patients with the combination of BCG (75 mg per scarification) and vincristine (1 mg/m^2 i.v. days 1 and 2), DTIC (200 mg/m^2 i.v. days 3 and 4), and CCNU (50 mg/m^2 per os, days 5 and 6) every 6 weeks over 2 years. Their disease-free survival times were significantly longer ($p = 0.001$) than those of patients who had only received surgery in the same institutions between 1962 and 1972. Growing skepticism vis-à-vis the methodical problems of uncontrolled studies, small case numbers and short observation periods soon led to the merging of different research groups (EORTC-MCG, WHO Melanoma Group, Oncofrance in Europe and ECOG, SWOG, etc. in the United States) and the beginning of cooperative multicentric studies.

BCG-Combinations

In a first controlled prospective study by Wood et al.,[116] 70 patients (Clark III-V, Breslow > 1,5 mm) were allocated after surgery either to a DTIC (see previous discussion), a BCG, or DTIC and BCG group. Whereas 6 out of 20 patients on DTIC and 5 of 28 on BCG experienced progression within 1 year, all 22 treated with the combination remained free of disease.

In a Canadian randomized study[133] with 57 stage I and 37 stage II melanoma patients, either operated on only or treated with DTIC and BCG over 6 or 24 months, a trend emerged in favor of the combination in stage II patients. With the same DTIC and BCG protocol, 181 stage I and II patients were prospectively given adjuvant treatment in the controlled previous WHO study reported[19] no significant difference in regard to survival times after more than 5 years' observation in comparison with the 185 patients who only received surgery. However, a favorable trend was again described in stage II patients with up to three positive lymph nodes.

A third similar study[124] with 75 stage I and II patients who were allocated to a treatment with DTIC, BCG, or the combination, showed a trend towards improvement of disease-free interval after a period of 18 months observation. However, this effect also documented in the WHO study was lost later after 30 and 60 months. The SWOG performed a randomized study giving a 1 year adjuvant chemotherapy with BCNU, Hydrea, and DTIC (BHD) with or without BCG in stage II and III patients with high risk of recurrence. The addition of BCG here appeared to shorten the DFS from 99 to 60 weeks.[134]

The results of the Oncofrance Melanoma Study[135] in which BCG was compared to BCG and DTIC in 278 prospectively randomized patients between 1975 and 1980, no significant difference was shown in DFS after an observation period of 8 years. Similar result was observed when the 6-month DTIC therapy (150 mg/m^2 i.v. d 2-5 every 4 weeks) was intensified with CCNU (60 mg/m^2 per os d2 + 8 every 8 weeks) and Etoposide (60 mg/m^2 i.v. d1 every 4 weeks). After further tumor progression, on the other hand, the survival time of men in the combined polychemotherapy arm was less favorable, so that a possible negative effect of adjuvant chemotherapy was considered.

Two other French trials with a combination of Velbe, Thiotepa, Rufocromomycin, Methotrexate, Procarbazine plus "when possible" preoperative intraarterial DTIC and Vincristine in 62 stage I patients versus 55 controls, and 33 male patients receiving in addition *C. parvum* without proper controls, and different treatments for female patients, are confusing and hard to interpret.[136]

Combinations with Corynebacterium Parvum

Whereas a favorable effect on survival time and cure rates through "immunoprophylaxis" and adjuvant immunotherapy[137] can be noted in animal experiments, corresponding trials in man remain disappointing: In a controlled, prospectively randomized study, 117 stage I and II patients received either *C. parvum* with or without DTIC and cyclophosphamide (both in the dosage of 600 mg/m^2 i.v. every 3 weeks, 9 times) adjuvantly after curative surgery. In neither group was it possible to achieve an improvement of disease-free intervals and survival times.[79,138]

Combinations with MER-BCG

Seventy stage I and II patients were prospectively randomized into one of two treatment groups by the "Piedmont Oncology Group"[20]: 19 stage I and 14 stage II patients received DTIC cytostatic therapy (300 mg/m^2 d 1-5 every 5 weeks for 2 years) and 19 stage I and II patients were administered DTIC in combination with MER (methanol extracted residue of BCG, 4 × 100 μg s.c. every 5 weeks for 1 year). After a mean observation period of nearly 5 years, there was no statistically significant difference between the two groups with only a trend towards longer disease-free intervals in the stage II group treated with the combination.

Summarizing these combined immuno- and chemotherapy trials, it must be stated that it has not been possible to improve the fate of melanoma patients in the prognostically unfavorable stages I and II in a significant way. Trends that favor one or other modality proved to be either transitory or only of little clinical importance.

The question that had previously been left open in studies with historical comparative collectives[18,48] or small case numbers[136,139] as to the value of adjuvant chemotherapy, active nonspecific immunotherapy, or a combined chemo-immunotherapy in melanoma stages I and II does not lead to great optimism. At the same time, it must still be taken into account that our inability to recognize all of the many prognostic factors and to stratify the studies accordingly can conceal individual advantages of the one or other treatment modality.

SECONDARY ADJUVANT INDICATOR THERAPY

Due to the minimal efficacy of cytostatics in both adjuvant and palliative treatment of melanoma with objective remission rates up to a maximum of 25 percent, possibilities for prior testing of tumor sensitivity to various cytostatics are being sought in different ways. Testing melanoma stem cells in tissue cultures or in xenotransplanted nude mice is of limited relevance for predicting clinical response. We were, therefore, posed with the question of whether the decision to suggest adjuvant cytostatic therapy to individual patients with particularly unfavorable stages II and III or following curative resection of solitary (pulmonary) metastasis could not be based on the prior response of the tumor to cytostatic treatment with the same agents.[140–142]

This founded the concept of the *indicator therapy,* a secondary adjuvant treatment in which only those patients were further treated with the same protocol, in whom it had been possible to achieve a preoperative objective remission. Through such "in vivo testing," it should be possible to spare the large majority, approximately 80 percent of patients, an ineffective adjuvant cytostatic therapy.

In an EORTC-MCG pilot study (No. 18782), after cytologically securing the tentative clinical diagnosis of metastatic disease, we observed the effect of two chemotherapy courses.[140] Only in those patients attaining partial or complete remission was the same cytostatic protocol continued after *curative tumor resection* as a *secondary adjuvant therapy.* Our own initial results in 24 patients show that such a procedure was technically feasible. No complications were noted with regards to operability or wound healing following prior treatment with Cisplatinum, Dacarbazine, and Vindesine. Only in eight of these patients was treatment continued, as indicator therapy for another four, that is, a total of six courses. After a 5 year observation period, half of these patients are still alive and free of disease. It is up to a prospective controlled study, of course, to prove whether such indicator therapy improves cure rates rather than lengthening the disease-free interval only at the expense of the patients' time without symptoms and toxicity.

CONCLUSIONS

The development of adjuvant medical treatment modalities in patients with clinical stage I and II melanoma of poor prognosis is characterized by early optimism and sobering corrections later on. Most if not all of the positive results showing an increase in disease-free or overall survival initially, had to be revoked after results of prospectively controlled and randomized trials became available. It is interesting to observe how many favorable studies in accordance with the biostatistic "law of the first cases" presented partly as preliminary results on renowned conferences "got lost," were abandoned, or couldn't be verified or reproduced.

Cancer medicine has learned that enthusiastic reports and consciously articulated, unicentric empirism, usually based on retrospective "historical" comparisons of different patient collectives, leads to erronous therapeutical recommendations. The number of false "standard treatments" is legion in oncology in general and expressively in melanoma.

Adjuvant immunotherapy, in particular, has to be viewed with great caution since "restoration of the immune-defense," specific or nonspecific immunization, and activation or unbalanced stimulation of parts of the immune surveillance may result in its blockade or even uncontrolled enhancement of tumor growth.

So far none of the many options of systemic treatment with cytostatic agents, biological response modifiers and/or any active or passive immunotherapy have improved the cure rates. The only acceptable criterion in adjuvant trials is the disease-free overall survival. The only recognized method to avoid treatment biases is the prospectively planned random allocation of patient populations following sophisticated stratification according to well-defined risk factors. It remains open, whether or not adjuvant therapy is falsely conceived, incorrectly practiced, or whether the available treatment modalities are simply not effective enough to treat this heterogenous and highly resistant disease.

To overcome the autistic-undisciplined thinking in medicine, as wisely defined by E. Bleuler in 1919,[143] remains the dominant task of the true scientist.

REFERENCES

1. Everson TC and Cole WH. Spontaneous regression of cancer. Philadelphia: Saunders, 1966.
2. Nathanson L. Spontaneous regression of malignant melanoma: A review of literature on incidence, chemical features and possible mechanisms. *J Natl Cancer Inst Monogr* 44:67–76. 1976.
3. Peter HH. The immunology of malignant melanoma and possible immunotherapeutic approaches. *Pigment Cell Res* 6:65–92, 1983.
4. Baldwin RW and Pimm MV. Tumor immunotherapy—experience, evaluation, and clinical prospects. In: Flad HD, Herfarth Ch, and Betzler M (eds.), *Immunodiagnosis and Immunotherapy of Malignant Tumors.* Berlin, Heidelberg, New York: Springer, 1979, 195–205.
5. Cochran AJ. Histology of "borderline" and atypical cutaneous malignant melanoma. *Pigment Cell Res* 6:36–64, 1983.
6. Lewis MG and Copeman PW. Halo-naevus. A frustrated malignant melanoma. *Br Med J* II:47, 1972.
7. Lévine A. On the histological diagnosis and prognosis of malignant melanoma. *J Clin Pathol* 33:101–124, 1980.
8. Césarini JP and Roubin R. Host reaction against tumor aggression in cutaneous primary human malignant melanoma of the superficial spreading type: Macroscopic, microscopic, and ultrastructural features. *Behring Inst Mitt* 56:65–73, 1975.
9. Bodurtha AJ. Spontaneous regression of malignant melanoma. In: Clark WH, Goldmann LJ, and Mastrangelo MJ (eds.), *Human Malignant Melanoma.* Clinical Oncology Monographs. New York, San Francisco, London: Grune & Stratton, 1979, 227–241.
10. Braun-Falco O. Spontanregression des malignen Melanoms. *Dtsch Med Wochenschr* 105:714, 1980.
11. Feun LG, Gutterman J, Burgess MA, et al. The natural history of resectable metastatic melanoma (Stage IVa Melanoma). *Cancer* 50:1656–1663, 1982.
12. Manelis G, Shasha SM, Manelis J, Suprun H, and Robison E. Spontaneous regression of malignant melanoma. *Oncology* 35:83–86, 1978.
13. Voigt H and Kleeberg UR. Herausforderung Melanom. *Hamburger Ärzteblatt* 2:41–45, 1983.
14. Kleeberg UR. Maligne Hauttumoren: Medikamentöse Therapiemöglichkeiten aus der Sicht des internistischen Onkologen. *MMW* 126:1044–1047, 1984.
15. Cochran AJ, Buyse ME, Lejeune FJ et al. EORTC-Malignant Melanoma Coop. Group: Adjuvant reactivity predicts survival in patients with "high-risk" primary melanoma treated with systemic BCG. *Int J Cancer* 28:543–550, 1981.
16. Kleeberg UR and Voigt H. Experimentelle Therapieansätze. In: Voigt H and Kleeberg UR (eds.), *Malignes Melanom.* Berlin: Springer Verlag, 1986, 127–171.
17. Gutterman JU, Mavligit GM, Gottlieb JA, Burgess MA, McBride CM, Einhorn L, Freireich EJ, and Hersh EM. Chemoimmunotherapy of disseminated malignant melanoma with DTIC and BCG. *N Engl J Med* 291:592–597, 1974.
18. Gutterman JU, McBride CM, Freireich EJ, Mavligit GM, Frei E, and Hersh EM. Active immunotherapy with BCG for recurrent malignant melanoma. *Lancet* I:1208–1212, 1973.
19. Veronesi U, Adamus J, Aubert C (WHO-Melanoma Study Group), et al. A randomized trial of adjuvant chemotherapy and immunotherapy in cutaneous melanoma. *N Engl J Med* 307:913–916, 1982.
20. Sterchi JM, Bradley Wells H, Case LD, Spurr CL, White DR, Richards F, Muss HB, Jackson DV, Stuart JJ, and Cooper MR for the Piedmont Oncology Group. A randomized trial of adjuvant chemotherapy and immunotherapy in stage I and stage II-melanoma. An interim report. *Cancer* 55:707–712, 1985.
21. Czarnetzki B for the EORTC-Malignant Melanoma Coop. Group. Trial No. 18781. A controlled trial on long term immunotherapy comparing two BCG preparations for stage I high risk malignant melanoma. To be published in *Melanoma Research,* 1992.
22. Kleeberg UR, Erdmann H, and Richter-von Arnauld HP. *Vademecum der Zytostatikatherapie.* Freiburg: Kehrer, 1982.
23. Rümke Ph: The EORTC Malignant Melanoma Cooperative Group. In: *Decimo corso di aggiornamento in oncologia medica.* Rome, 5.–9.11.1984, 664–674.
24. Rajewsky M. Molecular and cellular mechanisms of chemical cancerogenesis. EORTC Melanoma Coop. Group, Macher Z (ed.), Meetin, Münster 28.4.1984.
25. Currie GA, Lejeune F, and Hamilton-Fairley G. Immunization with irradiated tumor cells and specific lymphocyte cytotoxicity in malignant melanoma. *BMJ* 2:305–309, 1971.
26. Hellström J, Hellström KE, and Sjögren HO. Demonstration of cell-mediated immunity in human neoplasms of various histological types. *Int J Cancer* 1:1–7, 1971.
27. Lewis MG. Immunology and immunotherapy of malignant melanoma. In: Milton GW (ed.), Malignant Melanoma of

the Skin and Mucous Membrane. Edinburgh: Churchill Livingstone, 1977, 102–151.

28. Engel E, Kleeberg UR, Dietel M, Bröcker EB, and Carrel S. Alteration of melanoma cell phenotype following in vitro culturing and exposure to cytostatic agents. *Anticancer Res* 9:873–878, 1989.
29. Herlyn M, Menrad A, and Koprowski H. Structure, function and clinical significance of human tumor antigens. *J Natl Cancer Inst* 82:1883–1889, 1990.
30. Meyskens FL Jr, Loescher L, Serokman R, and Moon TE. Potential uses of biological response modifiers (BRM) in the adjuvant treatment of melanoma and results form a trial of BCG +/− Vitamin A. In: Salmon SE and Jones SE (eds.), *Adjuv Ther Cancer* 4:583–589, 1984.
31. Schlom J, Greiner J, Horan-Hand P, Colcher D, Inghirami G, Weeks M, Pestka S, Fisher PB, Toivanen A, Granberg J, and Nordman E. Lymphocyte subpopulations in patients with breast cancer after postoperative radiotherapy. *Cancer* 54:2919–2923, 1984.
32. Hansen MG and McCarten AB. Tumor thickness and lymphocytic infiltration in malignant melanoma of the head and neck. *Am J Surg* 138:557–561, 1974.
33. Bröcker EB, Brüggen J, Suter L, Sorg C, and Macher E. Immunologische Aspekte maligner melanome. In: Voigt H und Kleeberg UR (eds.), *Malignes Melanom.* Berlin: Springer Verlag, 1986, 203–226.
34. Herlyn M and Koprowski H. Melanoma antigens: Immunological and biological characterization and clinical significance. *Ann Rev Immunol* 6:283–308, 1988.
35. Holzmann B, Bröcker EB, Lehmann JM et al. Tumor progression in human malignant melanoma: Five stages defined by their antigenic phenotypes. *Int J Cancer* 39:466–471, 1987.
36. Lehmann JM, Holzmann B, Rothbächer U, Riethmüller G, and Johnson JP. Schrittweise Expression von Melanomassoziierten Antigenen während der Tumorprogression. *Onkologie* 12:273–276, 1989.
37. Ruiter DJ, Dingjan GM, Steijlen PM, et al. Monoclonal antibodies selected to discriminate between malignant melanomas and nevocellular nevi. *J Invest Dermatol* 85:4–8, 1985.
38. Suter L, Brüggen J, Bröcker EB et al. Tumor-associated antigen expressed in melanoma cells with lower malignant potential. *Int J Cancer* 35:787–791, 1985.
39. Carrel S, Schmidt-Kessen A, and Giuffrè L. Recombinant interferon-gamma can induce the expression of HLA-DR and -DC on DR-negative melanoma cells and enhance the expression of HLA-ABC and tumor associated antigens. *Eur J Immunol* 15:118–124, 1985.
40. Brüggen J and Sorg C. Detection of phenotypic differences on human malignant melanoma lines and their variant sublines with monoclonal antibodies. *Cancer Immunol Immunother* 15:200–205, 1983.
41. Brüggen J, Bröcker EB, Suter L, Bedmann K, and Sorg C. The expression of tumor-associated antigens in primary and metastatic human malignant melanoma. *Behring Inst Mitt* 74:19–22, 1984.
42. Kleeberg UR, Loycke A, Meier T, Bröcker EB, Lejeune F, and Carrel S. Sensitivity, selectivity and specificity of monoclonal antibodies directed at tumor associated antigens from metastatic melanoma. *Eur J Cancer Clin Oncol* 24 [Suppl 2]:47–50, 1988.
43. Oldham RK, Thurman GB, Talmage JE, Stevenson HC, and Foon KA. Lymphokines, monoclonal antibodies, and other biological response modifiers in the treatment of cancer. *Cancer* 54:2795–2806, 1984.
44. Suter L, Bröcker EB, Brüggen J, Ruiter DJ, and Sorg C. Heterogeneity of primary and metastatic human malignant melanoma as detected with monoclonal antibodies in cryostat sections of biopsies. *Cancer Immunol Immunother* 16:53–58, 1983.
45. De Vita VT. Cell kinetics and the chemotherapy of cancer. *Cancer Chemother Rep* 2:23–33, 1971.
46. Alexander P. Activated macrophages and the anti-tumor action of BCG. *Monogr Natl Cancer Inst* 39:127–133, 1973.
47. Jones PDE and Castro JE. Immunological mechanisms in metastatic spread and the antimetastatic effects of corynebacterium parvum. *Br J Cancer* 35:519–621, 1977.
48. Morton DK, Eilber FR, Malmgren RA, and Wood WC. Regression of cutaneous lesions of malignant melanoma after intralesional BCG-injections. *Surgery* 68:158–164,1970.
49. Morton DK. Immunologic and immunotherapeutic studies: Human melanomas. In: Immunologic Aspects of Neoplasia: A Rational Basis for Immunotherapy. *Am Int Med* 74:591–595, 1971.
50. Bekierkunst W. Immunotherapy of cancer with nonliving BCG and fractions derived from Mycobacteria. *Infect Immun* 74:1044–1050, 1974.
51. Ribi E, Milnar KC, Gragner DL et al. Components of BCG cell walls. *Ann NY Acad Sci* 277:228–238, 1976.
52. Silver HKB, van Hazel EMA, Reynolds PM, Lemish WM, and Holman CDJ. Adjuvant BCG-Immunotherapy for stage I and II malignant melanoma. *Can Med Assoc J* 128:1291–1298, 1983.
53. Varella AD, Bandiera DC, de Amorim AR, Calvis LA, Santos JO, Escaleira N, and Centil F. Treatment of disseminated malignant melanoma with high dose oral BCG. *Cancer* 48:1353–1362, 1981.
54. Cascinelli N, Bajetta E, Vaglini M, Buzzoni R, and Nava M. Present status and future perspectives of adjuvant treatment of cutaneous malignant melanoma. *Pigment Cell Res* 6:187–198, 1983.
55. Orefice S, Vaglini M, and Rovini D. Intralymphatic administration of BCG in stage I melanoma of lower extremities. Proc. Int. Symp. New trends in diagnosis, prognosis, treatment of malignant melanoma. Peter H (ed.), Hannover. 1980, 15.
56. Nathanson L, Schoenfeld D, Regelson W, Colsky J, and Mittelman A. Prospective comparison of intralesional and multipuncture BCG in recurrent intradermal melanoma. *Cancer* 43:1630–1635, 1979.
57. Iglehart JD, Ward EC, Zitiert IN: Immunotherapy of melanoma. In: Seigler HF (ed.), *Clinical Management of Melanoma. Developments in Oncology.* Den Haag: *J Natl Cancer Inst* Martinus Nijhoff, 1982, 503–513.
58. Wallack MK, McNally KR, Leftheriotis E, Seigler G, Balch C, Wanebo H, Bartolucci AA, and Bash JA. A southeastern cancer study group phase I/II trial with vaccinia melanoma oncolysates. *Cancer* 57:649–655, 1986.
59. Colmerauer ME, Koziol JA, and Pilch YH. Enhancement of metastasis development by BCG-immunotherapy. *J Surg Oncol* 15:235–241, 1980.
60. Costanzi JJ. Chemotherapy and BCG in the treatment of disseminated malignant melanoma. In: Terry WD, Windhorst D (eds.), *Immunotherapy of Cancer: Present Status of Trials in Man.* New York: Raven Press, 1978, 87–93.
61. Ishibashi T, Yamada H, Harada S, Takamoto M, and Sugiyama K. Inhibition and promotion of tumor growth by BCG. Evidence for stimulation of humoral enhancing factors by BCG. *Int J Cancer* 21:67–71, 1978.
62. Levy NL, Mahaley MS, and Day ED. Serum-mediated blocking of cell-mediated antitumor immunity in a melanoma patient: Association with BCG immunotherapy and clinical deterioration. *Int J Cancer* 10:244–248, 1972.

63. McIllmurray MB, Ambleton MJ, Reeves WG, Langsam M, and Deane M. Controlled trial of active immunotherapy in management of stage II B malignant melanoma. *Br J Med* 2:540–542, 1977.
64. Piessens WF, Lachapelle FL, Legros N, and Heuson JC. Facilitation of rat mammary tumor growth by BCG. *Nature* 228:1210–1211, 1970.
65. Hunter-Craig J, Newton KA, Westbury G, and Lacey BW. Use of vaccinia virus in the treatment of metastatic malignant melanoma. *Br J Med* 2:512–515, 1970.
66. Lejeune F, Macher E, Kleeberg UR, Rümke Ph, Prade M, Thomas D, and Suciu S. An assessment of DTIC versus levamisole or placebo in the treatment of high risk stage I patients after surgical removal of a primary melanoma of the skin. A phase III adjuvant study (EORTC No. 18761). *Eur J Cancer Clin Oncol* 24 [Suppl 2]:81–90, 1988.
67. Bloom BR. Does transfer factor act specifically or as an immunologic adjuvant? *N Engl J Med* 288:908–909, 1973.
68. Bukowski RM, Deodhar S, Hewlett JS, and Greenstreet R. Randomized controlled trial of transfer factor in stage II malignant melanoma. *Cancer* 51:269–272, 1983.
69. Lawrence HS. The transfer of generalized cutaneous hypersensitivity of the delayed tuberculin type in man by means of constituents of disrupted leukocytes. *J Clin Invest* 33:951–952, 1954.
70. Berengo MG, Barbara C, De Matteis A, Meregalli M, and Zina G. In vitro effects of a calf thymus extract in one hundred melanoma patients and preliminary results in vivo. In: Ainti F, Wigzell H (eds.), *Thymus, Thymic Hormones and T-Lymphocytes.* London: Academic Press, 1980, 313–322.
71. Pinsky CM, Hirshaut Y, Wanebo HJ, Fortner JG, Miké V, Schottenfeld D, and Oettgen H. Randomized trial of BCG (percutaneous administration) as surgical adjuvant immunotherapy for patients with stage-II melanoma. *Ann NY Acad Sci* 277:187–193, 1976.
72. Rümke Ph. Malignant melanoma. In: Pinedo HM and Chabner BA (eds.), *The EORTC Cancer Chemother. Annual 6.* Amsterdam: Elsevier, 1984, 427–435.
73. Ikonopisov R. Delayed hypersensitivity in the comparison of BCG-strains in immunotherapy of malignant melanoma in man. *Proc Int Symp New Trends in Diagn Progn Treatment of Malignant Melanoma*, Hannover, 1980, p 10.
74. Gutterman JU, Richman SP, McBride CM, Burgess MA, Bartold SW, Kennedy A, Gehan EA, Mavligit GM, and Hersh EM. Immunotherapy for recurrent malignant melanoma: Efficacy of BCG in prolonging the postoperative disease-free interval and survival. *Recent Results Cancer Res* 68:359–362, 1979.
75. Halpern BV, Biozzi G, Stiffel C, et al. Inhibition of tumor growth by administration of killed C. parvum. *Nature* 212:853–854, 1966.
76. Garrett AJ, Reeson DE, Osborn TW, et al. Effects of BCG and C. parvum treatment on human melanoma xenografts. *Dev Biol Stand* 38:363–369, 1978.
77. Murray JL, Ishmael DR, Bottomby RH, Grozea PN, and Lee ET. Inefficacy of s.c. Corynebacterium parvum in stage I malignant melanoma: Preliminary results of a single-institution pilot study. *Cancer Treat Rep* 67:191–192, 1983.
78. Hilal EY, Pinsky CM, Hirshaut Y, Wanebo HJ, Hansen IA, Braun DW, Fortner JG, and Oettgen HF. Surgical adjuvant therapy of malignant melanoma with Corynebacterium parvum. *Cancer* 48:245–251, 1981.
79. Balch CM, Smalley RV, Bartolucci A, Burns D, Presant CA, Durant JR, the Southeastern Cancer Study Group. A randomized prospective clinical trial of adjuvant C. parvum immunotherapy in 260 patients with clinically localized melanoma (stage I): Prognostic factors analysis and preliminary results of immunotherapy. *Cancer* 49:1079–1084, 1982.
80. Lipton A, Harvey HA, Lawrence B, Gottlieb R, Kukrika M, Dixon R, Graham W, Miller S, Heckard R, Schelzel D, and White DS. Corynebacterium parvum versus BCG adjuvant immunotherapy in human malignant melanoma. *Cancer* 51:57–60, 1983.
81. Bluming AZ, Vogel CL, Ziegler JL, and Kiryabwire JWM. Delayed cutaneous sensitivity reactions to extracts of autologous malignant melanoma: A second look. *J Natl Cancer Inst* 48:17–24, 1972.
82. Ikonopisov RL. Autoimmunization with irradiated tumor cells in human malignant melanoma. *Br Med J* 2:752–54, 1970.
83. Tritsch H. Dermale Reaktionen auf Melanom-Autohomogenate. *Hautarzt* 21:258–265, 1970.
84. Hedley DW, McElwain TJ, and Currie GA. Specific active immunotherapy does not prolong survival in surgically treated patients with stage II-B malignant melanoma and may promote early recurrence. *Br J Cancer* 37:491–496, 1978.
85. Shibata HR, Jerry LM, Lewis MG, Mansell PW, Capek A, and Marquis G. Immunotherapy of human malignant melanoma with irradiated tumor cells, oral BCG, and Levamisole. *Ann NY Acad Sci* 277:355–366, 1976.
86. Livingston PO, Takeyama H, Pollack MS, Houghton AN, Albino A, Pinsky CM, Oettgen HF, and Old LJ. Serological responses of melanoma patients to vaccines derived from allogeneic cultured melanoma cells. *Int J Cancer* 31:567–576, 1983.
87. Rümke Ph. Malignant Melanoma. In: Pinedo HM (ed.), *The EORTC Cancer Chemother. Annual 3.* Amsterdam: Excerpta Medica, 1981, 397–408.
88. Hersey P, MacDonald M, Hall C, Spurling A, Edwards A, Coates A, and McCarthy W. Immunological effects of recombinant interferon alpha 2a in patients with disseminated melanoma. *Cancer* 57:1666–1674, 1986.
89. Livingston PO, Natoli EJ, Calves MJ, Stocker E, Oettgen HF, et al. Vaccines containing purified GM_2 ganglioside elicit GM_2 antibodies in melanoma patients. *Proc Natl Acad Sci USA* 84:2911–2913, 1987.
90. Wallack MK, Mayer M, Bourgoin A, and Leftheriotos E. The use of vaccinia oncolysates in the treatment of recurrent stage II malignant melanoma. *Medical Oncology: Abstracts of the 5th Annual Meeting of the Medical Oncology Society.* 1.–3. December 1979, Nizza.
91. Hersey P, Edwards A, Coates A. Shaw L, and McCarthy W. Evidence that treatment with vaccinia melanoma cell lysates (VMCL) may improve survival of patients with stage II melanoma. *Cancer Immunol Immunother* 25:257–262, 1987.
92. Seigler HF, Shingleton WW, Metzgar RS, Buckley CE, Bergoc PM, Miller DS, Fetter BF, and Phaup MB. Nonspecific and specific immunotherapy in patients with melanoma. *Surgery* 72:162–174, 1972.
93. Renoux G and Renoux M. Action immunostimulante des dérivés du phenylimidothiazide sur les cellules spléniques formatrice d'anticorps. *CR Acad Sci (D) (Paris)* 274:756–757, 1972.
94. Tripodi D, Parks LC, and Brugmans J. Drug-induced restoration of cutaneous delayed hypersensitivity in anergic patients with cancer. *N Engl J Med* 289:354–357, 1973.
95. Renoux G and Renoux M. Levamisole inhibits and cures a solid malignant tumor and its pulmonary metastases in mice. *Nature* 240:217–218, 1972.
96. Sadowski MJ and Rapp F. Inhibition by Levamisole of me-

tastases by cells transformed by herpes simplex virus type I. *Proc Soc Assoc Biol Med* 149:219–222, 1975.
97. Potter CW, Carr I, Jennings R, et al. Levamisole inactive in treatment of four animal tumors. *Nature* 249:567–569, 1974.
98. Serrou B, Pujol H, Dorras J, and Gauci L. Results of a nonrandomized trial in malignant melanoma patients (Clark's stage III-V) treated by post-surgical chemoimmunotherapy. *Recent Results Cancer Res* 68:363–366, 1979.
99. Amery WK. A placebo controlled Levamisole study in resectable lung cancer. In: Terry WD and Windhorst D (eds.), *Immunotherapy of Cancer: Present Status of Trials in Man.* New York: Raven Press, 1978, 191–202.
100. Amery WK. Four year results from double-blind study of adjuvant Levamisole treatment in resectable lung cancer. In: Terry WP and Rosenberg SA (eds.), *Immunotherapy of Human Cancer.* New York: Excerpta Medica, 1982, 123–133.
101. Rojas AL, Michrewitz F, Feuerstein IN, Glait H, and Olivar AJ. Levamisole in advanced human breast cancer. *Cancer* 1:211–215, 1976.
102. Chirigos MA, Pearson IW, and Pryor J. Augmentation of chemotherapeutically induced remission of a murine leukemia by a chemical immunoadjuvant. *Cancer Res* 33:2615–2618, 1973.
103. Spitler LE and Sagebiel R. A randomized trial of Levamisole vs. placebo as adjuvant therapy in malignant melanoma. *N Engl J Med* 303:1143–1147, 1980.
104. Lejeune F, Macher E, Kleeberg UR, Rümke P, Prade M, Thomas D, and Suciu S for the EORTC-Malignant Melanoma Coop. Group. A randomized study on DTIC, Levamisole and placebo as adjuvant treatment of high risk stage I primary melanoma. *Eur J Cancer Clin Oncol* 24:581–590, 1988.
105. Costanzi JJ, Fletcher WS, Balcerzak SP, Taylor S, Eyre HJ, O'Bryan RM, Al-Sarraf M, and Frank J. Combination chemotherapy plus Levamisole in the treatment of disseminated malignant melanoma. *Cancer* 53:833–836, 1984.
106. Lo Buglio AF and Neidhardt IA. A review of transfer factor immunotherapy in cancer. *Cancer* 34:1563–1570, 1974.
107. Blume MR, Rosenbaum EH, Cohen RJ, Gershow J, Glassberg AA, and Shepley E. Adjuvant immunotherapy of high risk stage I melanoma with transfer factor. *Cancer* 47:882–888, 1981.
108. Ratner L, Nordlund JJ, and Lengyel P. Interferon as an inhibitor of cell growth: Studies with mouse melanoma cells. *Proc Soc Exp Biol Med* 163:267–272, 1980.
109. Kirchner H. Das Interferonsystem unter besonderer Berüksichtigung des gamma Interferons. *Dtsch Med Wschr* 111:64–70, 1986.
110. Liao SK, Kwong PC, Khosravi M, and Dent PB. Enhanced expression of melanoma-associated antigens and beta-2-microglobulin on cultured human melanoma cells by interferon. *JNCI* 68:19–25, 1982.
111. Cassel WA, Murray DR, and Phillips HS. A phase-II-study on the postsurgical management of phase-II malignant melanoma with a Newcastle disease virus oncolysate. *Cancer* 52:856–860, 1983.
112. Morton DL, Eilber FR, Weisenburger TH, and Lin PY. Multimodality therapy of malignant melanoma. In: Salmon SE and Jones SE (eds.), *Adjuv Ther Cancer III.* New York: Grune and Stratton, 1981, 241–251.
113. Azizi E, Brenner HJ, and Shoman J. Postsurgical adjuvant treatment of malignant melanoma patients by the thymic factor Thymostimulin. *Arzneimittelforsch-ung* 34:1043–1046, 1984.
114. Gershon RK and Metzler CM. Regulation of the immune response. In: Towney JJ and Good RA (eds.), *The Immunopathology of Lymphoreticular Neoplasms.* New York: Plenum Press, 1979, 23–51.
115. Patt YZ, Hersh EM, Schafer LA, Smith TL, Burgess MA, Gutterman JU, Goldstein AL, and Mavligit GM. The need for immune evaluation prior to Thymosin-containing chemoimmunotherapy for melanoma. *Cancer Immunol Immunpathol* 7:131–136, 1979.
116. Wood WC, Cosimi AB, Carey RW, and Kaufman SD. Randomized trial of adjuvant therapy for high risk primary malignant melanoma. *Surgery* 83:677–681, 1978.
117. Wood WC, Cosimi AB, Carey RW, and Kaufman SD. Adjuvant chemotherapy in stage I and II-melanoma. In: Terry WD and Rosenberg SA (eds.), *Immunotherapy of human cancer.* New York: Excerpta Medica, 1982, 265–270.
118. Hill GJ, Krementz ET, and Hill HZ. DTIC and combination therapy for melanoma. *Cancer* 53:1299–1305, 1984.
119. Runne U and Pullmann H. Adjuvant Dacarbazine in cutaneous melanoma. (Letter to the editor). *N Engl J Med* 308:777, 1983.
120. Voigt H, Kleeberg UR, and Caselitz J. Pathogenetische and präventiv-diagnostische Hinweise zu Dacarbazin-induzierten Todesfällen. *Tumor Diagn Ther* 3:150–155, 1982.
121. Tranum BL, Dixon D, Quagliana J, et al. for the SWOG. Lack of benefit of adjunctive chemotherapy in stage I malignant melanoma. *Cancer Treat Rep* 71:643–644, 1987.
122. Czarnetzki BM, Aragon V, Bröcker EB, Krieg V, Bünte H, and Macher E. Adjuvante Polychemotherapie zusätzlich zur radikalen operativen Behandlung regionaler Lymphknotenmetastasen beim malignen Melanom. *Dtsch Med Wochenschr* 111:732–736, 1986.
123. Gutterman JU, Mavligit GM, Reed RC, and Hersh EM. Immunotherapy of human cancer. *Semin Oncol* 1:409–423, 1974.
124. Kaufman SD, Cosimi AB, Wood WC, and Carey RW. Adjuvant therapy in malignant melanoma: A trial of immunotherapy, chemotherapy, and combined treatment. *Recent Results Cancer Res* 68:380–386, 1979.
125. Gelber RD and Goldhirsch A. A new endpoint for the assessment of adjuvant therapy in postmenopausal women with operable breast cancer. *J Clin Oncol* 4:1772–1779, 1986.
126. Ghussen F, Nagel K, Groth W, Müller JM, and Stützer H. A prospective randomized study of regional extremity perfusion in patients with malignant melanoma. *Ann Surg* 200:764–768, 1984.
127. van Geel AN, van Wijk J, and Wieberdink J. Functional morbidity after regional isolated perfusion of the limb for melanoma. *Cancer* 63:1092–1096, 1989.
128. Lippman SM, Kessler JF, and Meyskens FL Jr. Retinoids as preventive and therapeutic anticancer agents. *Cancer Treatm Reports* 71:391–405, 1987.
129. Legha SS, Papadoupoulos N, Pickett S, Plager C, Dimery JW, Benjamin RS, and Itri L. Adjuvant therapy for high risk local and regional melanoma using 13-cis Retinoic acid. *Adjuvant Ther of Cancer* 4:577–582, 1984.
130. Bonmassar E, Bonmassar A, Vadlamudi S, and Goldin A. Antigenic changes of L-1210 leukemia in mice treated with DTIC. *Cancer Res* 32:1446–1450, 1972.
131. Herbst WP. Malignant melanoma of the choroid with extensive metastases treated by removing secreting tissue of the testicles. *JAMA* 122:597, 1943.
132. Luce JK, Thurman WG, Isaacs BL, and Talley RW. Clinical trials with the antitumor agent DTIC. *Cancer Chemother Rep* 54:119–124, 1970.
133. Quirt JC, et al. Randomized controlled trial of adjuvant

chemoimmunotherapy with DTIC and BCG after complete excision of primary melanoma with poor prognosis or melanoma metastases. *Can Med Assoc J* 128:929–931, 1983.

134. Quagliana J, Tranum B, Neidhardt J, and Gagliano R for the SWOG. Adjuvant chemotherapy with BCNU, Hydrea and DTIC (BHD) with or without immunotherapy (BCG) in high risk melanoma patients. *Proc ASCO* 21:399 (C-316), 1980.
135. Misset IL, Delgado M, Mathé G, et al. Eight year update of the Oncofrance Melanoma adjuvant trial. In: Salmon SE and Jones SE (eds.), *Adjuv Ther Cancer* 4:557–566, 1984.
136. Jacquillat C, Banzet P, Civatte J, et al. Adjuvant chemotherapy and chemoimmunotherapy in the management of primary malignant melanoma of level III, IV and V. *Recent Results Cancer Res* 68:346–358, 1979.
137. Milas L, Gutterman JU, and Basic I, et al. Immunoprophylaxis and immunotherapy for a murine fibrosarcoma with C. granulosum and C. parvum. *Int J Cancer* 14:493, 1974.
138. Balch CM, Murray DR, Presant CA, Bartolucci A, the Southeastern Cancer Study Group. A randomized evaluation of adjunctive chemoimmunotherapy versus immunotherapy in patients with resected metastatic melanoma. *Int J Radiat Oncol Biol Phys* [Suppl 1] 7:38, 1981.
139. Seigler HF. Immunotherapy of melanoma. In: Seigler HF (ed.), *Clinical Management of Melanoma.* Developments in Oncology 5. Den Haag: Martinus Nijhoff, 1982, 503–513.
140. Kleeberg UR, Voigt H, and Erdmann H. Die Zytodiagnostik von Melanommetastasen und ihre Bedeutung für die Wahl der Therapie. *Tumor Diagn Ther* 5:49–54, 1984.
141. Kleeberg UR. Selective adjuvant chemotherapy in stage II-melanoma. Pilot-study of the EORTC Malignant Melanoma Coop. Group. Hamburg, Protocol No. 18782, 1978.
142. Kleeberg UR and Voigt H. Indicative chemotherapy in melanoma: A new concept in stage II, III and IV? *Verh Dtsch Krebs Ges* 5:135, 1984.
143. Bleuler E. *Das autistisch-undisziplinierte Denken in der Medizin and seine Überwindung.* Berlin: Springer Verlag, 1919.
144. Lejeune F. Phase III adjuvant studies in operable malignant melanoma (Review). *Anticancer Res* 7:701–706, 1987.
145. Lipson RL, Baldes EJ, and Olsen AN. The use of a derivative of hematoporphyrine in tumor detection. *J Natl Cancer Inst* 26:1–8, 1961.
146. Paterson AHG, Willans DJ, Jerry LM, Hanson J, and McPherson TA. Adjuvant BCG in malignant melanoma stage I. *Adj Ther of Cancer* 4:567–575, 1984.
147. Portoukalian J, Carrel S, Dové Jean-François, and Rümke Ph, on behalf of the EORTC Melanoma Coop. Group. Humoral immune response in disease-free advanced melanoma patients after vaccination with melanoma-associated gangliosides. *Int J Cancer* 49:893–899, 1991.
148. Moertel CG, Fleming TR, MacDonald JS, et al., for the ECOG, NCCTG and SWOG. Levamisole and Fluorouracil for adjuvant therapy of resected colon carcinoma. *N Engl J Med* 322:352–358, 1990.
149. Krook JE, Moertel CG, Gunderson LL, et al., for the NCCTG. Effective surgical adjuvant therapy for high-risk rectal carcinoma. *N Engl J Med* 324:709–715, 1991.

Chapter 27

SYSTEMIC CHEMOTHERAPY: NEW STRATEGIES

Alan Coates and Philip Rümke

Disseminated melanoma is virtually always a lethal disease. Most patients die within a few years after the first hematogenous metastases have been diagnosed. The survival duration can, however, vary considerably. In some patients with soft tissue metastases, particularly with skin metastases only, it may take a long time before visceral metastases become manifest. These patients live longer with their disease than those in whom dissemination occurs first at visceral sites. Exact figures are not known, but it can be stated that the great majority die within 5 years of the first manifestation of metastatic disease, and probably half of them do not live longer than 2 years.

GENERAL EXPECTATION FROM SYSTEMIC CHEMOTHERAPY

Numerous trials have been carried out with single agents or with combinations of cytotoxic drugs.[1–5] None of these have resulted in the achievement of a standard therapy. Although, very rarely, chemotherapy has possibly cured a patient, in clinical practice chemotherapy aims to palliate, not to cure. The result of a trial is generally expressed in the response rate percentage. This figure comprises the fraction of patients that experience a complete regression of all metastases for at least 1 month plus the fraction in whom the total tumor burden has regressed by at least 50 percent for a minimum of 1 month. Too often this figure is interpreted as the proportion of the patient population that has benefited from the chemotherapy. In view of the fact that the majority of the responses last only some weeks or, at most, a few months, and that chemotherapy, due to serious side effects, nearly always impairs the quality of life, it is clear that the proportion of patients who really benefit from the therapy is much lower than the response rate percentage. When confronted with the toxic side effects of chemotherapy and knowing that the treatment will have little chance to be curative, many patients may only accept treatment if there is a reasonable chance for a remission of—say—at least 6 months. Such clinically meaningful remissions, being partial or complete, probably occur in fewer than one quarter of the conventionally cited responses.

The response rate to the most effective and most used single agent, that is, dacarbazine (DTIC), is around 23 percent. Trials of combinations of cytotoxic drugs, seldom show better results than with dacarbazine alone. And if they do, the remissions are generally of short duration and toxicity is considerable, so that the real clinical benefit remains as low as with monotherapy with dacarbazine. It is for these reasons that, in spite of many efforts in the past decades, no standard systemic therapy for metastatic melanoma has yet emerged. What has been learned, however, is that certain categories of patients will have a higher chance to respond than others. Generally, it can be stated that patients who have metastases involving soft-tissue sites (that is, skin and lymph nodes) rather than visceral organs, who have a relatively small total tumor burden, who are young and have a good performance status, and who have not previously failed to respond to other chemotherapy, have a better chance of responding to the therapy. These factors are, therefore, relevant to the decision whether or not to treat in the individual case, as well as for the design of trial protocols. An example of a good reason for abstention from chemotherapy is the presence of brain metastases.

Since most drugs do not pass the blood-brain barrier, brain metastases are rarely affected by the drugs. For this reason most oncologists will give priority to surgery or to radiotherapy if brain metastases have to be treated. In study protocols, patients with brain metastases are therefore often excluded.

It should be clear from this introduction that good medical practice for the individual patient may well imply not to treat at all, or at least not to attempt systemic chemotherapy with all its disabling toxic side effects.

CURATIVE POTENTIAL OF SYSTEMIC CHEMOTHERAPY

In exceptional cases, cure has been achieved, but almost exclusively in patients with soft-tissue metastases only. Hill et al.[6] reviewed the results of three phase III studies with dacarbazine given alone or in combination with other cytostatic agents. Of 580 patients, 26 (4.5 percent) achieved a complete remission, and six of these 26 were still in complete remission 30 to 259 weeks after the complete response was induced. It was concluded that only 1 percent had long-sustained remissions and that relapses are rare in those who remain in complete remission for 2 years or more. Remarkably, these possible cures were only achieved with dacarbazine (± other drugs), and in patients with soft-tissue metastases only, whereas with other cytostatic agents no long-sustained remissions were reported. Recently, Ahmann et al.[7] reported only 10 complete remissions in 503 patients treated with a variety of investigative cytotoxic regimens. Three patients survived disease-free for more than 5 years, confirming that durable responses to chemotherapy are infrequent, possibly in the order of less than 1 percent.

The question arises whether these long lasting remissions are not occurring spontaneously rather than being induced by chemotherapy. However, spontaneous regression of metastases occurs even more seldom. It has been estimated that .25 percent of patients with metastatic disease show this phenomenon and that 40 percent of these patients develop no recurrence.[8] In our own experience, it is highly unlikely that the long lasting remissions after chemotherapy were coincidental. In a pilot study conducted by one of us (P. Rümke, unpublished), five patients have possibly been cured by the combination of dacarbazine with the topical application of the hapten dinitrochlorobenzene (DNCB). In 45 patients, all selected on the basis that they had cutaneous metastases (while half of them had also some metastases elsewhere), 3 percent DNCB in acetone was used topically and repeatedly to induce severe eczematous delayed-type skin reactivity in the skin metastases. This procedure itself did not result in complete remissions, but when dacarbazine was subsequently administered, 10 patients experienced a complete remission. Most remarkably, five of these 10 patients are still, 6 to 13 years later, in complete remission and are therefore likely to be cured. Two of these five had, in addition to the cutaneous metastases, also lung metastases. It has to be mentioned that four of these five patients had received six or more dacarbazine cycles after achieving a complete remission. The same was the case with the long-surviving patients in the study of Hill et al.[6] In seven of the eight patients with sustained remission, dacarbazine had been administered for at least 6 months after the complete remission was achieved. Unfortunately, no studies have ever addressed the question of the value of maintenance therapy with dacarbazine after a complete remission has been achieved with the drug, so that it remains uncertain whether maintenance therapy with dacarbazine should indeed be given to prolong disease-free survival in complete responders.

INCONSISTENCY OF PUBLISHED CHEMOTHERAPY TRIAL RESULTS

Often new regimes, which seemed encouraging, are less effective in confirmatory trials than in the original publication. An example is the combination of bleomycin, vincristine (Oncovin), CCNU (lomustine), and dacarbazine, called the BOLD regime. Initially, in 1980 and 1983, response rates of 40, 46, and 30 percent were reported. York et al.[9] however, found 22 percent in 46 patients, with the Prudence Foundation[10] only 4 percent in 51 patients.

There are several reasons for such differences. Patient selection is an important one. Obviously, the more patients entered who have had no prior chemotherapy and who have soft tissue metastases only or a low tumor burden, the better the results will be. Another important bias comprises the diagnostic criteria. The aforementioned study of York et al.[9] exemplifies the importance of rigorous diagnostic restaging at 4 weeks after the second cycle of chemotherapy. Clinically silent metastases in originally negative sites were found in 12 patients. Had these extensive (and expensive) scannings not been repeated, the response rate would have been twice as high. Particularly in patients with metastatic melanoma, silent sites of metastases can regularly be found, a fact which is often neglected in the designs of the study protocols! The duration of treatment necessary to fulfill evaluation by criteria may also vary. In most studies at least two courses of chemotherapy are required to evaluate whether the therapy had an effect. Patients, who received only one course because progressive illness may have precluded a second course, would then be nonevaluable. It is evident that if these patients are excluded the outcome of the study is favorably influenced. Yet another point of misinterpretation is that if a partial remission makes it possible to surgically remove the last remaining metastases, and the patient remains thereafter disease-free for a period of time, according to standard terminology this patient cannot be called a complete responder. This rule is sometimes disregarded. A misleading point concerns the reported difference in the duration of survival between responders and nonresponders. The difference may suggest a prolongation of life due to the response. However, since patients with a low tumor burden (that is, patients in whom dissemination occurred relatively recently) have a better chance to respond than those with a larger tumor burden (that is, patients at a later stage of their disease). It can even be anticipated that responding patients ought to live longer on the average than nonresponders. This has indeed been found. For example, one study of high-dose melphalan and autologous bone-marrow transplantation has reported a response rate of 12/28 (43 percent). The median survival of the responders was 9 months and of nonresponders 4 months—a difference that was statistically significant. However, when calculated from the time of the first recorded evidence of distant metastases, there was no significant difference in survival between responders and nonresponders.[11]

EFFECTIVENESS OF ADJUVANT CHEMOTHERAPY

In most tumor types, therapies which prove to be effective in the adjuvant setting also have objective tumor response rates of 50 percent or above when used for measurable metastatic disease. This rate of response cannot usually be achieved in metastatic melanoma at present. It is, therefore, not surprising that adjuvant trials of cytotoxic therapy in melanoma have been negative.[12,13] Theoretically, biological response modifiers might be effective against the smaller tumor loads that might be expected after surgical resection of a primary melanoma, even though they were unable to cope with the large number of tumor cells in patients with overt metastases. In practice, adjuvant therapy has been unimpressive. Lejeune[14] reviewed 21 randomized trials involving 2850 patients with stage I melanoma. None of the systemic therapies tested, including cytotoxic chemotherapy, immunotherapy, and combined chemoimmunotherapy, proved effective. Similar results were reported in the 15 studies involving 1972 patients with stage II melanoma.[14] (See also Chap. 26.)

CURRENT RECOMMENDATION

The older literature has been extensively reviewed,[1–5] and we will therefore focus on recent reports of what can be achieved now and on the reasonable prospects for the immediate future. A summary of response rates reported in some recent publications is provided in Table 27-1, but these are not intended to guide selection of routine treatment for patients, since the therapies listed vary widely in toxicity and many are completely unsuitable for use outside specialized centers. (See Chap. 28.)

Combination chemotherapy has yet to demonstrate superiority over the standard single agents in a prospective controlled trial in metastatic melanoma. Cisplatin, as a single agent, has modest reported activity in melanoma[15,16] but Glover et al.[17] reported a higher response rate using the combination of cisplatin with the organic thiophosphate WR-2721, which protects normal tissues against cisplatin toxicity. Thirty-six patients were treated at cisplatin doses varying from 60 to 150 mg/M^2 and partial responses were observed in 19, for a response rate of 53 percent (95 percent confidence limits (c.l.) 36–70 percent). The combination was well tolerated, and responses included cases with liver metastases, which are notoriously difficult to treat, as well as the more readily responsive nodal, subcutaneous, and lung metastases. This result is interesting and is being tested in further studies.

Cisplatin is an important component of the combination chemotherapy regiments used for many tumor types, but in melanoma earlier combinations of cisplatin with vinblastine and bleomycin yielded widely varying response rates.[18,19] Several early studies[16,20,21] used the combination of cisplatin and dacarbazine. Goodnight et al.[16] reported a study of 11 patients treated with cisplatin 15 mg/M^2 daily for 4 days and dacarbazine 200 mg/M^2 daily for 5 days each 4 weeks. Only one partial response was observed, giving an overall response rate of 9 percent (95 percent c.l. 2–41 percent).

Friedman et al.[20] treated 18 patients with cisplatin 75 mg/M^2 and dacarbazine 600 mg/M^2 each 4 weeks, with dose escalation as tolerated in subsequent cycles. In their study, two complete and four partial responses were observed, for an overall response rate of 33 percent (95 percent c.l. 13–59 percent).

Recent trials of the combination of dacarbazine and cisplatin, sometimes also including a vinca alkaloid, include that of the Southwest Oncology Group[22] who used full doses of each agent. Dacarbazine 750 mg/M^2 and cisplatin 100 mg/M^2 were given each 3 weeks. All 30 patients entered were evaluated, with two complete and nine partial responses,

TABLE 27-1
CHEMOTHERAPY RESPONSE RATES[1]

DRUGS USED	FIRST AUTHOR	NO. OF PATIENTS	% RESP.	95% C.L.	REF.
STANDARD AGENTS					
Dacarbazine	Various	978	22	19–25	1–5
Nitrosoureas	Various	693	14	12–17	1–5
COMBINATION CHEMOTHERAPY					
Cisplatin, WR-2721	Glover	36	53	36–70	17
Cisplatin, dacarbazine	Various	84	29	19–40	16,20,22,23
Cisplatin, vindesine, dacarbazine	Verschraegen	105	21	14–30	24
Pool of above studies cisplatin, dacarbazine	Various	189	24	14–30	
Fotemustine	Jacquillat	169	22	16–29	27
HIGH DOSE ALKYLATING AGENTS					
Melphalan	Cornbleet	28	39	22–60	11
Melphalan	Lazarus	20	60	36–81	30
Thio-tepa	Wolff	71	41	29–53	31
Cyclophosphamide, cisplatin, carmustine	Antman	20	55	32–77	32
TAMOXIFEN (TAM) COMBINATIONS					
Dacarbazine, TAM	Cocconi	60	28	17–42	34
Dacarbazine, cisplatin, carmustine, TAM	McClay	59	49	36–63	3

[1]Complete plus partial responses as a percentage of all entered patients. Confidence limits by Fisher's exact method, or Wilson's approximation for $N > 180$.

giving an overall response rate of 37 percent (95 percent c.l. 20–56 percent). Median response duration was a respectable 31 weeks, but responses were seen almost exclusively in soft tissue, nodal, and lung metastases. As in other studies, patients with liver or brain metastases had shorter survival. Toxicity was considerable, with "severe" renal toxicity in 13 percent, neurological in 10 percent, and hematological in 33 percent.

Lower doses of the same agents were tested by Oratz et al.[23] Dacarbazine 350 mg/M^2 daily for 2 days was combined with cisplatin 20 mg/M^2 daily for 3 days. All patients were evaluated, with one complete and five partial responses, for a somewhat low overall response rate of 24 percent (95 percent c.l. 9–45 percent). Toxicity was, however, correspondingly less severe, with no severe renal or neurological toxicity, and only 8 percent severe hematological toxicity. Verschraegen et al.[24] described an EORTC study of dacarbazine 450 mg/M^2, cisplatin 50 mg/M^2, and vindesine 3 mg/M^2 repeated at days 1 and 8 of each 4 week course in 105 patients. Responses were evaluated by extramural review according to strict EORTC guidelines, and included four complete and 18 partial among 92 evaluable patients, giving an overall response rate of 24 percent of evaluable and 21 percent of all entered patients (95 percent c.l. 14–30 percent).

Overall, response rates were higher in the studies using higher doses, though the confidence intervals overlap. Pooling the five studies, nine complete and 37 partial responses were seen among 189 patients, for a response rate of 24 percent (95 percent c.l. 19–31 percent).

The nitrosoureas lomustine (CCNU), carmustine (BCNU), and semustine (methyl-CCNU) are regarded as standard active agents in melanoma.[2] In a comparative trial, the Eastern Cooperative Oncology Group found that semustine and dacarbazine gave equal response rates, and that the combination of the two agents was more toxic but no more efficacious.[25] Newer nitrosoureas have, therefore, been studied in phase II trials. Khayat et al.[26] reported a study of the nitrosourea fotemustine (S 10036) in 33 patients with disseminated melanoma. Eight partial responses were seen among 30 evaluable patients (27 percent, 95 percent c.l. 12–46 percent), including two responses among seven patients with cerebral metastases. Jacquillat et al.[27] recently extended these results, reporting three complete and 34 partial responses among 169 entered (152 evaluated) patients, a response rate of 24 percent of evaluable and 22 percent (95 percent c.l. 16–29 percent) of all entered patients. Responses were again reported in cerebral and visceral metastases. Hepatic intra-arterial fotemustine was also effective, producing two complete and six partial responses among 17 treated patients.[28] The combination of fotemustine and dacarbazine was reported by Avril et al.[29] to produce four complete and eight partial responses among 36 evaluable of 40 patients entered, an overall response rate of 33 percent of evaluable and 30 percent (95 percent c.l. 17–47 percent) of all entered patients. This agent deserves study in a phase III setting.

ROLE OF AUTOLOGOUS BONE MARROW TRANSPLANT

Conventional doses of alkylating agents are almost completely inactive in melanoma, but resistance can be overcome, at a price, by the use of higher doses. Cornbleet et al.[11] first used high-dose melphalan in 28 patients. They received doses varying from 140 to 260 mg/M^2, followed by autologous bone marrow transplantation. Most of the patients also received cyclophosphamide, prior to the melphalan, to reduce bone marrow suppression. Two complete and nine partial responses were observed, for a response rate of 39 percent (95 percent c.l. 22–60 percent), and despite the logistic complexity and need for prolonged supportive therapy, seven patients were retreated. Only one of the five early deaths was due to toxicity.

A similar trial was later reported by Lazarus et al.[30] who treated 20 patients with melphalan doses ranging from 180 to 225 mg/M^2. They observed six complete and six partial responses for a response rate of 60 percent (95 percent c.l. 36–81 percent), but reported three toxic deaths. The North American Bone Marrow Transplantation Group[31] used Thiotepa 180 to 1575 mg/M^2 over 3 days followed by autologous bone marrow transplantation in 71 patients with metastatic melanoma. Fifteen patients died early without tumor progression, four achieved complete and 25 partial responses for a response rate of 53 percent of evaluable and 41 percent (95 percent c.l. 29–53 percent) of all treated patients. As in other high dose studies, hemorrhage into cerebral metastases was a major problem, with major bleeds in three of 31 patients with cerebral metastases.

One further study of high-dose therapy deserves mention, if only because of its extreme approach. Antman et al.[32] used a combination of cyclophosphamide 5620 mg/M^2 cisplatin 165 mg/M^2 and carmustine (BCNU) 600 mg/M^2 with autologous bone marrow transplantation. Seventeen of 20 patients were evaluable, with one complete and 10 partial responses, giving a response rate of 65 percent of the evaluable and 55 percent (95 percent c.l. 32–77 percent) of all treated patients. Again cerebral bleeding was a problem, occurring in two (10 percent) of the patients.

Despite the relatively high response rates, such treatments are unlikely to become standard. They serve mainly to emphasize that melanoma is not altogether resistant to alkylating agents. Perhaps more easily manageable protocols can be devised with the availability of colony stimulating factors.

ROLE OF HORMONAL THERAPY

A number of observations support the belief that melanoma cell growth may be influenced by hormones.[33] The prognosis is worse in men than in women, and the doubling time of lung metastases is shorter in men than in women; exacerbations as well as remissions of metastatic melanoma have been seen during pregnancy, and estrogen and progesterone receptors were found in the metastases of some patients. For these reasons, hormonal therapies have been tried, but generally without success.

The only hormonal drug still in use is tamoxifen. Although it was disappointing as a single agent,[2,3,5] tamoxifen has recently produced promising results in combination with cytotoxic agents. Phase II studies of tamoxifen with cisplatin, dacarbazine, and carmustine show a cumulative response rate of 49 percent,[3,5] while a controlled trial by the GOIRC[34] showed the combination of dacarbazine and tamoxifen to be superior to dacarbazine alone.

DRUG RESISTANCE

Tumor cells protect themselves from potentially toxic substances by a variety of mechanisms and correspondingly show resistance to many anticancer drugs. Overcoming such resistance is an important goal of cancer therapy. One mechanism of resistance with potential application in the treatment of melanoma is the glutathione system. Glutathione is the major intracellular nonprotein sulfhydryl molecule. In mammalian cells, most glutathione is present as the reduced form (GSH), in dynamic equilibrium with lesser concentrations of the disulfide (GSSG). GSH concentration is determined by the rate of synthesis, involving gamma-glutamyl-cysteine synthetase and GSH synthetase, the rate of oxidation, either nonenzymatic or mediated by glutathione peroxidase to GSSG, and reduction via glutathione reductase.

High glutathione levels may be in part responsible for the resistance of various cell lines to alkylating agents,[35] as well as providing protection against endogenous reactive oxygen intermediates.[35] Glutathione-S-transferase (GST) enhances binding of GSH to toxic compounds and may thus be important in determining the resistance of melanoma cells to alkylating agents. Direct binding of reactive substances to GST or peroxidation by GST may also be involved.[36]

Manipulation of GSH levels in tumor cells was studied by Russo et al., who found that artificially elevated GSH levels conferred protection of normal fibroblasts against melphalan, cisplatin, and bleomycin, while the same pretreatment did not alter glutathione levels in a lung tumor line.[37]

Depletion of GSH using buthionine sulfoximine has been studied in several models. Exposure of human ovarian cancer cell lines to .5 mM buthionine sulfoximine for 20 to 28 hours reduced glutathione to 10 to 20 percent of control levels, and increased the toxicity of melphalan approximately two-fold.[38] Similar potentiation was observed with murine leukemia cells. The effect of this level of glutathione depletion on cisplatin toxicity was much less marked,[38] suggesting differences in the intracellular interaction of GSH with cisplatin as compared to the alkylating agents.

Similar potentiation of the cytotoxic effect of melphalan against a human ovarian carcinoma cell line both in vitro and in a nude mouse model has been described by Ozols et al.,[39] but pretreatment of normal bone marrow cells with buthionine sulfoximine had little potentiating effect on the toxicity observed in a colony forming unit assay.[39] This may indicate that the impact of alteration of GSH levels might be predominantly seen in tumor cells and thus confer a therapeutic advantage.

Inhibition of GST by ethacrynic acid or piriprost was found by Tew et al.[40] to increase the sensitivity of a human colon cancer cell line to the alkylating agent chlorambucil. Ethacrynic acid, an older diuretic, is available for clinical use and is being tested in a phase I–II clinical trial in combination with intravenous melphalan in the Sydney Melanoma Unit.

Buthionine sulfoximine, used as a means of reducing glutathione, may have antimelanoma activity in its own right. Kable et al.[41] studied the effects of buthionine sulfoximine on cell lines in vitro and found a direct cytotoxic effect unrelated to GSH depletion.

CONCLUSION

Chemotherapy for malignant melanoma remains largely unsatisfactory. There is an urgent need for new approaches. Among these, combined chemohormonal therapy, analogues of current effective agents, rational design of drugs exploiting the melanin synthetic pathway, treatments aimed at reducing drug resistance, and newer biological agents are perhaps the most promising. High dose alkylating agents, although unsuitable as routine treatment, show a degree of activity that suggests that resistance to these agents is relative and thus encourages approaches aimed at overcoming drug resistance.

Meanwhile, routine adjuvant systemic therapy is premature outside clinical trials. Asymptomatic patients with metastatic disease may be observed without specific therapy, unless patient anxiety prohibits this approach. The remote chance of a prolonged complete response is compelling for some patients, but the major aim of treatment is palliation. If treatment is given, it should, whenever possible, be in a formal clinical trial. Off study, single agent dacarbazine or lomustine are reasonable, perhaps with tamoxifen in female patients. The duration of therapy and any decision to use second line agents must always be governed by the primary aim of improving quality of life for the patient.

REFERENCES

1. Luce JK. Chemotherapy of melanoma. *Semin Oncol* 2:179–185, 1975.
2. Coates AS and Durant JR. Chemotherapy for metastatic melanoma. In: Balch CM, and Milton GW (eds.), *Cutaneous Melanoma. Clinical Management and Treatment Results World Wide.* Philadelphia: Lippincott, 275–282, 1985.
3. McClay EF, Mastrangelo MJ. Systemic chemotherapy for metastatic melanoma. *Semin Oncol* 15:569–577, 1988.
4. Legha SS: Current therapy for malignant melanoma. *Seminars in Oncology* 16:34–44, 1989.
5. Kleeberg UR, Rümke Ph, Kirkwood JM. Systemic chemotherapy of advanced melanoma. In: Ph. Rümke (ed), *Therapy of Advanced Melanoma* (Pigment Cell, Vol. 10, series ed. R.M. MacKie). Basel, Switzerland: Karger, 1990, 91–104.
6. Hill GJ, II, Krementz ET, Hill HZ. Dimethyl triazeno imidazole carboxamide and combination therapy for melanoma. IV. Late results after complete response to chemotherapy (Central Oncology Group protocols 7130, 7131, and 7131A). *Cancer* 53:1299–1305, 1984.
7. Ahmann DL, Creagan ET, Hahn RH et al. Complete responses and long-term survivals after systemic chemotherapy for patients with advanced malignant melanoma. *Cancer* 63:224–227, 1989.
8. Nathanson L. Spontaneous regression of malignant melanoma: A review of the literature on incidence, clinical features and possible mechanisms. *Natl Cancer Monogr* 44:67–77, 1976.
9. York RM, Foltz AT. Bleomycin, vincristine, lomustine, and DTIC chemotherapy for metastatic melanoma. *Cancer* 61:2183–2186, 1988.
10. The Prudente Foundation Melanoma Study Group. Chemotherapy of disseminated melanoma with bleomycin, vincristine, CCNU, and DTIC (BOLD regimen). *Cancer* 63:1676–1680, 1989.
11. Cornbleet MA, McElwain TJ, Kumar PJ, et al. Treatment of advanced malignant melanoma with high-dose melphalan and autologous bone marrow transplantation. *Br J Cancer* 48:329–334, 1983.
12. Veronesi U, Adamus J, Aubert C, et al. A randomized trial of adjuvant chemotherapy and immunotherapy in cutaneous melanoma. *N Engl J Med* 307:913–916, 1982.
13. Lejeune F, Macher E, Kleeberg U, et al. An assessment of DTIC versus levamisole or placebo in the treatment of high risk stage I patients after surgical removal of a primary melanoma of the skin. *Eur J Cancer Clin Oncol* 24:S81–S90, 1988.
14. Lejeune FJ. Phase III adjuvant studies in operable malignant melanoma (review). *Anticancer Res* 7:701–705, 1987.
15. Al-Sarraf M, Fletcher W, Oishi N, et al. Cisplatin hydration with and without mannitol diuresis in refractory disseminated malignant melanoma: A Southwest Oncology Group study. *Cancer Treat Rep* 66:31–35, 1982.

16. Goodnight JE, Moseley HS, Eilber FR, et al. Cis-dichlorodiammine-platinum II alone and combined with DTIC for treatment of disseminated malignant melanoma. *Cancer Treat Rep* 63:2005–2007, 1979.
17. Glover D, Glick J, Weiler C, et al. WR-2721 and high dose cisplatin: An active combination in the treatment of metastatic melanoma. *J Clin Oncol* 5:574–578, 1987.
18. Nathanson L, Kaufman SD and Carey RW. Vinblastine, infusion bleomycin and cis-dichlorodiammine-platinum chemotherapy in metastatic melanoma. *Cancer* 48:1290–1294, 1981.
19. York RM, Lawson DH, and McKay J. Treatment of metastatic malignant melanoma with vinblastine, bleomycin by infusion and cisplatin. *Cancer* 52:2220–2222, 1983.
20. Friedman MA, Kaufman DA, Williams JE, et al. Combined DTIC and cis-dichlorodiammineplatinum(II) therapy for patients with disseminated malignant melanoma: A Northern California Oncology Group study. *Cancer Treat Rep* 63:493–495, 1979.
21. Karakousis CP, Getaz EP, Bjornsson S, et al. Cis-diamminedichloroplatinum(II) and DTIC in malignant melanoma. *Cancer Treat Rep* 63:2009–2010, 1979.
22. Fletcher WS, Green S, Fletcher JR, et al. Evaluation of cisplatinum and DTIC combination chemotherapy in disseminated melanoma. *Am J Clin Oncol* 11:589–593, 1988.
23. Oratz R, Speyer JL, Green M, et al. Treatment of metastatic malignant melanoma with dacarbazine and cisplatin. *Cancer Treat Rep* 71:877–878, 1987.
24. Verschraegen CF, Kleeberg UR, Mulder J, et al. Combination of cisplatin, vindesine and dacarbazine in advanced malignant melanoma. A Phase II study of the EORTC Malignant Melanoma Cooperative Group. *Cancer* 62:1061–1065, 1988.
25. Costanza ME, Nathanson L, Schoenfeld D, et al. Results with methyl-CCNA and DTIC in metastatic melanoma. *Cancer* 40:1010–1015, 1977.
26. Khayat D, Bizzari JP, Frenay M, et al. Interim report of phase II study of new nitrosourea S 10036 in disseminated malignant melanoma. *J Natl Cancer Inst* 80:1407–1408, 1988.
27. Jacquillat CL, Khayat D, Banzet P, et al. Final report of the phase II study of the nitrosourea fotemustine (S 10036) in 153 patients with disseminated malignant melanoma including brain metastases. *Cancer* 66:1873–1878, 1990.
28. Khayat D, Cour V, Aigner C, et al. Malignant melanomas—hepatic intra-arterial chemotherapy (HIAC). *Pathol Biol* 38:872–875, 1990.
29. Avril M-F, Bonneterre J, Delaunay M, et al. Combination chemotherapy of dacarbazine and fotemustine in disseminated malignant melanoma: Experience of the French Study Group. *Cancer Chemother Pharamcol* 27:81–84, 1990.
30. Lazarus HM, Herzig RH, Wolff SN, et al. Treatment of metastatic malignant melanoma with intensive melphalan and autologous bone marrow transplantation. *Cancer Treat Rep* 69:473–477, 1985.
31. Wolff SN, Herzig RH, Fay JW, et al. High-dose thiotepa with autologous bone marrow transplantation for metastatic malignant melanoma: Results of phase I and II studies of the North American Bone Marrow Transplantation Group. *J Clin Oncol* 7:245–249, 1989.
32. Antman K, Eder JP, Elias A, et al. High-dose combination alkylating agent preparative regimen with autologous bone marrow support: The Dana-Farber Cancer Institute/Beth Israel Hospital experience. *Cancer Treat Rep* 71:119–125, 1987.
33. Colbourn DS, Nathanson L, Belilos E. Pregnancy and malignant melanoma. *Seminars in Oncology* 16:377–387, 1989.
34. Cocconi G, Bella M, Calabresi F, et al. DTIC vs DTIC plus tamoxifen in metastatic malignant melanoma (meeting abstract). *Proc Am Soc Clin Oncol* 9:A1076, 279, 1990.
35. Arrick B, and Nathan CF. Glutathione metabolism as a determinant of therapeutic efficacy: A review. *Cancer Res* 44:4224–4232, 1984.
36. Wang AL, and Tew KD. Increased glutathioneS-transferase activity in a cell line with acquired resistance to nitrogen mustards. *Cancer Treat Rep* 69:677–682, 1985.
37. Russo A, DeGraff W, Friedman N, et al. Selective modulation of glutathione levels in human normal versus tumor cells and subsequent differential response to chemotherapy drugs. *Cancer Res* 46:2845–2848, 1986.
38. Andrews PA, Murphy MP, and Howell SB. Differential sensitization of human ovarian carcinoma and mouse L1210 cells to cisplatin and melphalan by glutathione depletion. *Mol Pharmacol* 30:643–650, 1986.
39. Ozols RF, Louie KG, Plowman J, et al. Enhanced melphalan cytotoxicity in human ovarian cancer in vitro and in tumor bearing nude mice by buthionine sulfoximine depletion of glutathione. *Biochem Pharmacol* 36:147–153, 1987.
40. Tew K, Bomber AM, and Hoffman SJ. Ethacrynic acid and piriprost as enhancers of cytotoxicity in drug resistant and sensitive cell lines. *Cancer Res* 48:3622–3625, 1988.
41. Kable EPW, Favier D, and Parsons PG. Sensitivity of human melanoma cells to L-DOPA and D,L-buthionine sulfoximine. *Cancer Res* 49:2327–2331, 1989.

Chapter 28

CONTROLLED STUDIES IN CHEMOTHERAPY FOR ADVANCED MELANOMA

Michael J. Mastrangelo

INTRODUCTION

Although the incidence of cutaneous melanoma is rapidly increasing, effective lay and professional education has resulted in earlier diagnosis at a time when modest surgery can be curative. Nonetheless, significant numbers of patients continue to present with, or to develop, metastatic disease. The successful treatment of these patients represents a difficult challenge. For an exhaustively detailed analysis of the chemotherapy of melanoma, the reader is referred to a recent review.[1] This chapter will consider the results of traditional phase II and III chemotherapy trials wherein melanoma-bearing patients served as their own controls and objective tumor regression was the measure of outcome. As background, the results of conventional dose, single agent chemotherapy trials will be briefly presented. Emphasis is placed on promising new combination and high-dose chemotherapy regimens.

CONVENTIONAL DOSE, SINGLE AGENT CHEMOTHERAPY

Of the single agents subjected to phase II testing at conventional doses, DTIC (dimethyl triazeno imidazole carboxamide, dacarbazine) remains the most effective with an overall objective response rate of 20 percent.[2] Although complete responses are rare, the cost/benefit ratio is favorable in that significant organ toxicity is infrequent. A nitrosourea is a common choice as second-line single agent chemotherapy. Reported objective response rates with nitrosoureas are as follows: carmustine (BCNU), 22/122 (18 percent); lomustine (CCNU), 35/270 (13 percent); semustine (methyl-CCNU), 54/347 (16 percent).[1,3] Bonafide, but infrequent, objective remissions can also be achieved with the vinca alkaloids (111/739, 15 percent), cisplatin (17/114, 15 percent) and alpha interferon (43/379, 11 percent).[1] With all of these agents, subcutaneous, lymph node, and pulmonary metastases are most likely to respond.

Central nervous system metastases remain a major clinical problem. They rarely respond to systemic chemotherapy even with lipid soluble agents. New hope in this regard is offered by fotemustine, a new 2-chloroethyl-nitrosourea in which 1-amino-ethyl phosphonic acid is grafted onto a nitrosourea molecule to facilitate cell penetration using active amino acid transport and to achieve better passage through the blood-brain barrier.[4] Although the overall objective response rate achieved with fotemustine (3 complete and 34 partial remissions among 153 evaluable patients) is within the range of responses seen with DTIC, the 9 partial responses in 36 patients with cerebral metastases suggest a markedly improved level of central nervous system activity.[5]

COMBINATION CHEMOTHERAPY REGIMENS

Of the several dozen combination chemotherapy regimens subjected to phase II and III clinical trials, a majority contain DTIC as the most active single agent. These are summarized in Table 28-1. Of the two drug regimens, only the combination with alpha interferon seems more effective than DTIC alone. However, in a randomized trial of modest size, an advantage for the combination over either agent alone could not be confirmed.[7–14] Also of interest is the four-drug combination of DTIC + BCNU + cisplatin + tamoxifen with a complete response rate of 11 percent and an overall response rate of 46 percent. This regimen was designed by Del Prete et al.,[22] who reported four complete and seven partial responses among 20 evaluable patients. Regressions were durable and included metastases in visceral sites. The Jefferson Medical College Group[23] confirmed these results but were concerned when six of 20 patients developed deep venous thrombosis. In an effort to eliminate this complication, tamoxifen was dropped from the regimen in a subsequent phase II trial.[18] Although thromboembolic events were eliminated, only one complete and one partial response were noted among 20 patients. With reintroduction of tamoxifen, the higher objective response rate was restored.[24] The Jefferson Medical College Group has

TABLE 28-1
COMBINATION CHEMOTHERAPY REGIMENS CONTAINING DACARBAZINE (DTIC)

REGIMENS	EVALUABLE PATIENTS	CR[a]	PR	CR + PR	RESPONSE RATE (%)	REFERENCES
DTIC + VA	223	10	30	40	18	1
DTIC + NU	343	25	46	71	21	1,6
DTIC + DDP	98	4	18	22	22	1
DTIC + Procarb	94	2	12	14	15	1
DTIC + CTX	111	6	10	16	14	1
DTIC + Act-D	131	16	10	26	20	1
DTIC + Anth	46	0	9	9	20	1
DTIC + HU	28	0	5	5	19	1
DTIC + Cyclo	17	1	2	3	18	1
DTIC + IFN	251	26	44	70	28	7–14
Totals	1342	90	186	276	20	
DTIC + VA + Bleo	31	5	5	10	32	15
DTIC + VA + Anth	18	1	6	7	39	1
DTIC + VA + CTX	110	5	25	30	27	1
DTIC + VA + NU	1114	66	185	251	23	1
DTIC + VA + DDP	255	18	63	81	32	1,16,17
DTIC + NU + Act-D	91	11	13	24	26	1
DTIC + NU + HU	331	21	57	78	24	1
DTIC + DDP + Procarb	13	0	2	2	15	1
DTIC + DDP + NU	20	1	1	2	10	18
DTIC + DDP + TAM	21	2	1	3	14	19
Totals	2004	130	358	488	24	
DTIC + NU + VA + HU	89	10	17	27	30	1
DTIC + NU + VA + Bleo	296	27	61	88	30	1,20
DTIC + NU + VA + Procarb	25	2	4	6	24	1
DTIC + NU + VA + ACT-D	57	5	9	14	25	1
DTIC + NU + VA + Chl	121	12	15	27	22	1
DTIC + NU + Bleo + VP-16	27	2	6	8	30	21
DTIC + NU + DDP + TAM	141	16	49	65	46	18,22–27
Totals	756	74	161	235	31	

VA, vinca alkaloid; NU, nitrosourea; DDP, cisplatin; CTX, cyclophosphamide; Act-D, dactinomycin; Anth, adriamycin or epirubicin; HU, hydroxyurea; Cyclo, cyclocytidine; IFN, Interferon alpha; Procarb, procarbazine; Chl, chlorpromazine; TAM, tamoxifen; Bleo, bleomycin; VP-16, etoposide; CR, complete response; PR, partial response.

[a]This category may be under-represented in that all responses not specifically designated complete were included as partial remissions.

Revised and reprinted with permission from Reference 1.

reported a total of 81 evaluable patients treated with DTIC + BCNU + cisplatin + tamoxifen at several dosage schedules.[25] There have been 11 complete and 24 partial responses for an overall response rate of 43 percent (95 percent confidence interval: 32–55 percent). Several of the complete responders have continued in unmaintained remission for greater than 5 years. It may now be possible to speak of cures in about 5 percent of patients with metastatic melanoma.

The role of tamoxifen in producing this high rate of tumor regression in this traditionally chemotherapy resistant tumor seems critical but is as yet unexplained. DeGregorio and co-workers, as well as other investigators, have demonstrated in vitro that tamoxifen can enhance the cytotoxicity of chemotherapeutic agents.[28,29] This phenomenon is noted at concentration $> 2\ \mu M$ and is associated with a steep dose-response curve. The doses of tamoxifen originally employed in this regimen (20–40 mg/d) do not routinely achieve this minimum plasma concentration. In an effort to explore a possible dose-response effect, the Jefferson Medical College Group treated 15 evaluable patients with a brief, intense course of tamoxifen (160 mg/dx7d) just prior to initiating chemotherapy.[25] The 47 percent response rate was similar to that seen with conventional doses of tamoxifen; however, there was a higher proportion of complete responses in the high-dose group (27 percent vs. 9 percent). Peak plasma concentrations of tamoxifen and the active N-desmethyl metabolite were each approximately 1–2 μM, levels at which reversal of drug resistance has been demonstrated in vitro.

There are clinical and in vitro data that provide some insight about the drug or drugs in which tamoxifen may be interacting. The work of Cocconi et al.[30] suggest that tamoxifen (20 mg/m^2/d) enhances the antitumor effect of DTIC. These investigators noted four complete and 13 partial remissions in 52 patients treated with the combination but only three complete and two partial remissions among 60 patients treated with DTIC alone ($p = 0.03$). In vitro data implicate cisplatin as a possible target for tamoxifen interaction.[31] However, in the Jefferson Medical College Group's short-course, high-dose tamoxifen trial[25] hematologic toxicity, but not neurologic or renal toxicity, was significantly increased suggesting that BCNU is the major interactive partner in that DTIC and cisplatin have minimal marrow toxicity. This conclusion is supported by the work of Buzaid, et al.[19] These investigators noted just three responses in 21 evaluable patients when BCNU was dropped from the regimen even though the dose of cisplatin was doubled.

Table 28-2 lists several non-DTIC containing regimens that are of potential clinical utility. The 38 percent response rate reported for cisplatin + ifosfamide includes 5/58 complete responses (32–34). The combination of nitrosourea + vinca alkaloid + procarbazine is likewise of interest because of the 12 percent complete response rate (14/115).[1,35] Although a 48 percent response rate has been reported with nitrosourea + cisplatin + bleomycin,[36] the number of evaluable patients is small and no complete responses were noted. Unfortunately, these three regimens all share one or more drugs in common with the seemingly more active combination of DTIC + BCNU + cisplatin and tamoxifen.

Based upon preclinical data several investigators have combined IL-2 with one or more chemotherapeutic agents.[37] The reported trials are modest in size. The addition of IL-2 (with or without LAK cells) to DTIC is no better than DTIC alone. A 40 percent response rate (three complete and five partial responses) was seen in 20 patients treated with IL-2 + cisplatin. Of greatest interest are the results of Richards, et al.[38] who integrated IL-2 and alpha interferon between courses of DTIC + BCNU + cisplatin + tamoxifen and achieved a 100 percent objective response rate in a series of just seven patients. Confirmation in a larger series is required.

DOSE INTENSIFICATION

Hematologic toxicity is dose limiting for most chemotherapeutic agents when administered systemically. This toxicity can be circumvented by autologous bone marrow or peripheral blood stem cell rescue. The critical question in patients with melanoma is whether increasing the doses of marginally effective

TABLE 28-2
COMBINATION CHEMOTHERAPY REGIMENS EXCLUSIVE OF DACARBAZINE (DTIC)

REGIMEN	EVALUABLE PATIENTS	CR	PR	RESPONSE RATE (%)	REFERENCES
DDP + Ifosfamide	58	5	17	38	32–34
NU + VA + Procarbazine	115	14	16	26	1,35
NU + DDP + Bleo	25	0	12	48	36

DDP, cisplatin; VA, vinca alkaloid; NU, nitrosourea; Bleo, bleomycin drugs will yield a clinically significant increment in therapeutic outcome. Several groups have explored systemic dose intensification with hematologic rescue (Table 28-3). The alkylating agents have been most extensively studied in this fashion. The overall response rates range from 20 to 100 percent with a mean of 53 percent. Complete responses are rare (12 percent) as are remissions of greater than 1 year's duration. Toxicity is substantial. Over time deaths due to sepsis have become far less frequent and will be further reduced with the use of hematopoietic growth factors. However, nonhematologic toxicity remains a serious obstacle to further dose escalation. Enrollment of patients earlier in the course of their disease and perhaps retreatment may improve therapeutic efficacy.

At conventional doses (≤ 100 mg/m^2), cisplatin is only minimally active (15 percent response rate) against melanoma. However, the lack of substantial hematologic toxicity makes cisplatin a suitable candidate for systemic dose escalation trials in patients with advanced melanoma. The results of such trials are summarized in Table 28-4. The mean complete (6 percent) and overall (32 percent) response rates are not impressive. Most investigators administered cisplatin in divided doses. On such schedules, aggregate doses of 200 mg/m^2 produced only modest success.[51,53,54] However, using cisplatin at 150 mg/m^2 as a single 30-minute infusion every 3 to 4 weeks (with WR-2721), Glover et al.[52] reported six remissions among nine patients. In a series of 36 patients so treated, she noted five complete and 15 partial remissions (53 percent). When compared with response rates noted at lower doses, the median duration of remission was doubled to 6 months (personal communication, October 18, 1990). These data suggest that brief but intense exposure to cisplatin is more effective than exposure to a higher total dose

TABLE 28-3
SYSTEMIC HIGH-DOSE CHEMOTHERAPY WITH AUTOLOGOUS BONE MARROW RESCUE

		RESPONSE			
		FREQUENCY			DURATION (MOS)
INVESTIGATORS	DRUG (DOSE)	CR/PR	# PTS	RR (%)	MEDIAN (RANGE)
Lazarus et al.[39]	MEL (180–225 mg/m^2)	6/6	20	60	CR = 6 (4–14) PR = 3 (2–5)
McElwain et al.[40]	MEL (140 mg/m^2)	1/3	8	50	CR = 4 PR = 2 (2–3)
McElwain et al.[41]	MEL (140 mg/m^2)	2/10	20	60	CR = 5,7 PR = 5 (4–11)[a]
Phillips et al.[42]	NU (1200 mg/m^2)	4/7	29	38	CR = 12 (3–29+) CR + P = 5.7 (1.5 − 29+)
Thomas et al.[43]	MEL (35–90 mg/m^2) NU (400–800 mg/m^2)	1/5	8	75	CR = 10.5+ PR = 2.5 (1–5)
Ciobanu et al.[44]	NU (1050 mg/m^2) DDP (200 mg/m^2)	1/2	7	43	CR = 3 PR = 1+,5
Slease et al.[45]	CTX (160–200 mg/kg) NU (600–900 mg/m^2)	0/2	6	33	PR = 2,3
Eder et al.[46]	CTX (6 g/m^2) TPA (180–900 mg/m^2)	0/2	4	50	PR = ?
Wolff et al.[47]	TPA (180–1575 mg/m^2)	4/25	51	57	3(1–31+)
Shea et al.[48]	CTX (1500–7500 mg/m^2) DDP (75–180 mg/m^2) NU (150–750 mg/m^2) ± MEL	1/10	19	58	4.7 (1–23)
Thatcher, et al.[49]	DTIC + MEL (Various) DTIC + IFO (Various)	5/11 0/2	27 10	59 20	— —
Moormeier, et al.[50b]	CTX (7.5 g/m^2) TPA (675 mg/m^2) NU (150–750 mg/m^2)	0/3	3	100	PR = ?
	Totals	25/88	212	53	

CR, complete response; PR, partial response; # Pts, number of evaluable patients; RR, combined response rate; DTIC, dacarbazine; NU, carmustine; MEL, melphalan; DDP, cisplatin; CTX, cyclophosphamide; TPA, thiotepa; IFO, Ifosfamide; [a], survival; [b], stem cell rescue.
Reprinted with permission from Reference 37.

TABLE 28-4
HIGH-DOSE CISPLATIN IN THE TREATMENT OF METASTATIC MELANOMA

INVESTIGATORS	REGIMEN	CR/PR	EVALUABLE PATIENTS	RESPONSE RATE (%)
Mortimer et al.[51]	DDP: 40 mg/m²/dx5	1/1	14	14
	100 mg/m²,d1 + 8	1/5	23	26
Glover et al.[52]	WR-2721:740–910 mg/m²			
	Plus			
	DDP: <100 mg/m²	0	3	0
	120 mg/m²	11	25	44
	135 mg/m²	6	13	46
	150 mg/m²	6	9	67
		(2/21)	(51)	(45)
Murren et al.[53]	DDP: 100 mg/m²,d1 + 8	0/0	8	0
	DTIC: 300 mg/m²,d1,2,8,9			
	DDP: 50 mg/m²,d1 + 8	3/4	14	50
	DTIC: 350 mg/m² × 3d			
Luger et al.[54]	DDP: 40 mg/m²/dx5d	1/7	28	29
	DTIC: 500 mg/m²/dx2d			
Buzaid et al.[19]	DDP: 50 mg/m²,d1–3	1/1	21	10
	DTIC: 350 mg/m²,d1–3			
	TAM: 20 mg daily			
	Totals	9/39	149	32

DDP, cisplatin; DTIC, dacarbazine; TAM, tamoxifen; WR-2721, S-2-(3-aminopropylamino) ethyl phosphorothioic acid; CR, complete response; PR, partial response.
Reprinted with permission from Reference 37.

over a longer period of time. This concept is supported by two studies in which dose intensification at the tumor site was achieved with regional angioocclusive techniques. Bland et al.[55] reported a 67 percent partial regression rate in 15 patients with locally recurrent or in transit melanoma of an extremity treated with intra-arterial cisplatin and temporary total outflow occlusion (pneumatic tourniquet). Thirty patients with hepatic metastases from ocular melanoma were treated by Mavligit et al.[56] with hepatic arterial chemoembolization using a mixture of cisplatin and polyvinyl sponge. One complete and 13 partial (46 percent) regressions were noted in a group of patients where objective remissions are rarely seen.

CONCLUSION

The medical management of patients with metastatic melanoma remains a formidable task. However, recent developments in chemotherapy justify cautious optimism. Fotemustine appears to have bonafide activity against brain metastases and is deserving of further study. Although most combination drug regimens have not yielded a sufficient increment in response rates to justify the added toxicity, the combination of DTIC + BCNU + cisplatin + tamoxifen is an exception. Remissions are frequent, include visceral sites, and are durable. Further exploration of the possible chemopotentiating effects of tamoxifen may not only improve this regimen but also provide insights applicable in the treatment of other tumors. Also of interest is bolus high-dose cisplatin (150 mg/m²) + WR-2721. These two regimens warrant comparative testing for efficacy and toxicity in a randomized prospective phase III trial. Pending the results of such a trial and with a consideration of the restricted availability of WR-2721, the Jefferson Medical College Group recommends DTIC + BCNU + cisplatin + tamoxifen as first line chemotherapy for patients with surgically incurable melanoma, exclusive of central nervous system metastasis.

REFERENCES

1. Mastrangelo MJ, Bellet RE, Kane MJ, and Berd D. Melanoma. In: Perry MC (ed.), *Chemotherapy Source Book.* Baltimore: Williams and Wilkins, 1992, 866–907.
2. Comis RL. DTIC (NSC-45388) in malignant melanoma: A perspective. *Cancer Treat Rep* 60:165–176, 1976.
3. Ahmann DL. Nitrosoureas in the management of disseminated malignant melanoma. *Cancer Treat Rep* 60:747–751, 1976.
4. Khayat D, Lokiec F, Bizzari J-P, Weil M, Meeus L, Sellami M, Rouesse J, Banzet P, and Jacquillat C. A phase I clinical study of the new amino acid-linked nitrosourea, S10036, administered on a weekly schedule. *Cancer Res* 47:6782–6785, 1987.
5. Jacquillat C, Khayat D, Banzet P, Weil M, Fumoleau P, Avril M-F, Namer M, Bonneterre J, Kerbrat P, Bonerandi JJ, Bugat R, Montcuquet P, Cupissol D, Lauvin, R, Vilmer C, Prache C, and Bizzari, JP. Final report of the French multicenter phase II study of the nitrosourea fotemustine in 153 evaluable patients with disseminated malignant mel-

anoma including patients with cerebral metastases. *Cancer* 66:1873–1878, 1990.

6. Avril MF, Bonneterre J, Delaunay M, Grosshans E, Fumoleau P, Israel L, Bugat R, Namer M, Cupissol D, Kerbrat P, Montcuquet P, Arcaute V, and Bizzari J-P. Combination chemotherapy of dacarbazine and fotemustine in disseminated malignant melanoma. Experience of the French Study Group. *Cancer Chemother Pharmacol* 27:81–84, 1990.
7. McLeod GRC, Thomson DB, and Hersey P. Recombinant interferon alpha-2a in advanced malignant melanoma. A phase I-II study in combination with DTIC. *Int J Cancer Suppl* 1:31–35, 1987.
8. Vorobiof DA, Falkson G, and Voges CW. DTIC versus DTIC and recombinant interferon alpha 2b in the treatment of patients with advanced malignant melanoma. *Proc Am Soc Clin Oncol* 8:284, 1989.
9. Bajetta E, Negretti E, Giannotti B, Brogelli L, Brunetti I, Sertoli MR, Bernengo MG, Sofra MC, Maifredi G, Zumiani G, Comella G, Buzzoni R, and Cascineli N. Phase II study of interferon alpha-2a and dacarbazine in metastatic melanoma. *Proc Am Soc Clin Oncol* 8:286, 1989.
10. Kerr R, Pippen P, Mennel R, and Jones S. Treatment of metastatic malignant melanoma with a combination of interferon alpha-2a and dacarbazine. *Proc Am Soc Clin Oncol* 8:288, 1989.
11. Mulder NH, Schraffordt Koops H, Sleijfer DTh, de Vries EGE, and Willemse PHB. Dacarbazine and α interferon for disseminated malignant melanoma. *Proc Am Soc Clin Oncol* 9:279, 1990.
12. Mickiewicz E, Estevez R, Rao F, Brier S, Balbiani L, Cabalar E, Cazap E, Cassini J, Gerchunoff M, Temperley G, and Caparros C. Interferon alpha 2b alone or in combination with DTIC in metastatic melanoma. Copiled data. *Proc Am Soc Clin Oncol* 9:281, 1990.
13. Breier S, Pensel R, Roffe C, Giangiacomo G, and Traine G. High dose DTIC with recombinant human interferon alpha 2b for the treatment of metastatic malignant melanoma. *Proc Am Soc Clin Oncol* 9:281, 1990.
14. Kirkwood JM, Ernstoff MS, Guiliano A, Gams R, Robinson WA, Costanzi J, Pouillart P, Speyer J, Grimm M, and Spiegel R. Interferon α-2a and dacarbazine in melanoma. *J Natl Cancer Inst* 82:1062–1063, 1990.
15. Mulder NH, Sleijfer D Th, De Vries EGE, Schraffordt Koops H, Samson MJ, and Willemse PHB. Phase II study of bleomycin, dacarbazine (DTIC) and vindesin in disseminated malignant melanoma. *J Cancer Res Clin Oncol* 115:93–95, 1989.
16. Legha SS, Ring S, Papadopoulos N, Plager C, Chawla S, and Benjamin R. A prospective evaluation of a triple-drug regimen containing cisplatin, vinblastine and dacarbazine (CVD) for metastatic melanoma. *Cancer* 64:2024–2029, 1989.
17. Pectasides D, Yianniotis H, Alevizakos N, Bafaloukos D, Barbounis V, Varthalitis J, Dinitriadis M, and Athanassiou A. Treatment of metastatic malignant melanoma with dacarbazine,vindesine and cisplatin. *Br J Cancer* 60:627–629, 1989.
18. McClay EF, Mastrangelo MJ, Sprandio JD, Belet RE, and Berd D. The importance of tamoxifen to a cisplatin—containing regimen in the treatment of metastatic melanoma. *Cancer* 63:1292–1295, 1989.
19. Buzaid AC, Murren J, and Durivage HJ. High-dose cisplatin with DTIC and tamoxifen in treatment of metastatic melanoma. *Cancer* 68:1238–1241, 1991.
20. Ceschia T, Cartei G, Clocchiatti L, Fasola G, Sibau A, Contessi E, Morandini G, and Galletti D. BELD polychemotherapy in advanced melanoma. *Proc Second Int Conf Melanoma.* Venice, Italy: 16–19 October 1989, 412.
21. Caparrotti G, Silvestro L, Bruni GS, Villari P, Lacava VFA, and Pergola M. DTIC, CCNU, Bleomycin and VP-16 in metastatic melanoma. *Proc Second Int Conf Melanoma.* Venice, Italy; 16–19 October 1989. 387.
22. Del Prete SA, Maurer LH, O'Donnell J, Forcier RJ, and LeMabre P. Combination chemotherapy with cisplatin, carmustine, dacarbazine and tamoxifen in metastatic melanoma. *Cancer Treat Rep* 68:1403–1405, 1984.
23. McClay E, Mastrangelo MJ, Bellet RE, and Berd D. Combination chemo/hormonal therapy in the treatment of malignant melanoma. *Cancer Treat Rep* 71:465–469, 1987.
24. McClay EF, Mastrangelo MJ, Bellet RE, and Berd D. Effective combination chemo/hormonal therapy for malignant melanoma: Experience with three consecutive trials. *Int J Cancer* 50:553–556, 1992.
25. Berd D, McLaughlin CJ, Hart E, Wiebe VJ, Mastrangelo MJ, Bellet RE, and DeGregorio WW. Short course, high-dose tamoxifen with cytotoxic chemotherapy for metastatic melanoma. *Proc Am Soc Clin Oncol* 10:291, 1991.
26. Adlaka A, Robinson WA, Gonzalez R, Lamb MR, and Ferguson J. Combination chemotherapy and tamoxifen in the treatment of disseminated malignant melanoma. *Proc Second Int Conf Melanoma.* Venice, Italy; 16–19 October, 1989, 401.
27. Richards JM, Mehta N, Ramming K, and Skosey P. Sequential chemoimmunotherapy in the treatment of metastatic melanoma. *J Clin Oncol* 10:1338–1343, 1992.
28. Ramu A, Glaubiger D, and Fuks Z. Reversal of acquired resistance to doxorubicin in P388 murine leukemia cells by tamoxifen and other triparanol analogues. *Cancer Res* 44:4392–4395, 1984.
29. DeGregorio MW, Ford JM, Benz EC, and Wiebe VJ. Toremifene: Pharmacologic and pharmacokinetic basis of reversing multidrug resistance. *J Clin Oncol* 7:1359–1364, 1989.
30. Cocconi G, Bella M, Calabresi F, Tonato M, Canaletti R, Boni C, Buzzi F, Ceci G, Corgna E, Lottici R, Papadia F, Sofra M, and Bacchi M. DTIC vs DTIC plus tamoxifen in metastatic malignant melanoma. *Proc Am Soc Clin Oncol* 9:278, 1990.
31. Hofmann J, Doppler W, Jakob A, Maly K, Posch L, Uberall F, and Grunicke HH. Enhancement of the anti-proliferative effective of cis-diamminedichloroplatinum (II) and nitrogen mustard by inhibitors of protein kinase C. *Int J Cancer* 42:382–388, 1988.
32. Verweij J, Planting AS Th, Gaast AvD, and Stoter G. Phase II study of cisplatin plus 24-hr. infusion of ifosfamide in advanced malignant melanoma. *Ann Oncol* 1:77–78, 1990.
33. Becher R, Seeber S, and Schmidt CG. Combination chemotherapy with ifosfamide and cis-dichlorodiammineplatinum (II) in advanced malignant melanoma. *J Cancer Res Clin Oncol* 97:301–306, 1980.
34. Berdel WE, Fink U, Emmerich B, Maubach PA, Busch U, Remy W, and Rastetter J. Chemotherapie maligner melanome mit cis-diaminodichloroplatinum und ifosfamid. *Dtsch Med Wschr* 107:26–28, 1982.
35. Evans BD, Hardy J, Thompson PT, Davis A, and Harvey VJ. A phase II study of combination chemotherapy with procarbazine, vincristine, and CCNU (POC) in patients with metastatic melanoma. *Proc Am Soc Clin Oncol* 9:276, 1990.
36. Cohen SM, Ohnuma T, Ambinder EP, and Holland JF. Lomustine, bleomycin and cisplatin in patients with metastatic malignant melanoma. *Cancer Treat Rep* 70:688–689, 1986.
37. Mastrangelo MJ, Bellet RE, and Berd D. Aggressive chemotherapy for melanoma. *PPO Updates* 5:1–11, 1991.
38. Richards JM, Ramming K, Bitran JD, Doane LL, and Priest ER. Combination of chemotherapy and biological therapy for the treatment of melanoma. *Clin Res* 38:844A, 1990.

39. Lazarus HM, Herzig RH, Wolff SN, Phillips GL, Spitzer TR, Fay JW, and Herzig GP. Treatment of metastatic malignant melanoma with intensive melphalan and autologous bone marrow transplantation. *Cancer Treat Rep* 69:473–477, 1985.
40. McElwain TJ, Hedley DW, Burton G, Clink HM, Gordon MY, Jarman M, Juttner CA, Millar JL, Milsted RAV, Prentice G, Smith IE, Spence D, and Woods M. Marrow autotransplantation accelerates hematological recovery in patients with malignant melanoma treated with high-dose melphalan. *Br J Cancer* 40:72–80, 1979.
41. McElwain TJ, Hedley DW, Gordon MY, Jarman M, Millar JL, and Pritchard J. High dose melphalan and non-cryopreserved autologous bone marrow treatment of malignant melanoma and neuroblastoma. *Exp Hematol* 7(Suppl 5):360–371, 1979.
42. Phillips GL, Fay JW, Herzig GP, Herzig RH, Weiner RS, Wolff SN, Lazarus HM, Karanes C, Ross WE, Kramer BS, and Southeastern Cancer Study Group. Intensive 1,3-bis (2-chloroethyl)1-nitrosourea (BCNU), NSC #4366650 and cryopreserved autologous marrow transplantation for refractory cancer. A phase I-II study. *Cancer* 52:1792–1802, 1983.
43. Thomas MR, Robinson WA, Hartmann D, Glode LM, Koppler H, and Morton NJ. Treatment of advanced malignant melanoma with high dose chemotherapy and autologous bone marrow transplantation. Preliminary results. *Am J Clin Oncol* 5:611–622, 1982.
44. Ciobanu N, Dutcher J, Gucalp R, Sparano J, Goldman M, Adinolfi C, Fitzgerald E, and Wiernik PH. High dose chemotherapy with autologous bone marrow transplantation (ABMT) for malignant melanoma after failure of interleukin-2 (IL2) and lymphokine activated killer (LAK) cells. *Proc Am Soc Clin Oncol* 8:281, 1989.
45. Slease RB, Benear JB, Selby GB, Reitz CL, Hughes WL, Watkins CL, and Epstein RB. High dose combination alkylating agent therapy with autologous bone marrow rescue for refractory solid tumors. *J Clin Oncol* 6:1314–1320, 1988.
46. Eder JP, Antman K, Elias A, Shea TC, Teicher B, Henner WD, Schryber SM, Holden S, Finberg R, Critchlow J, Flaherty M, Mich R, Schipper L, and Frei E III. Cyclophosphamide and thiotepa with autologous bone marrow transplantation in patients with solid tumors. *J Natl Cancer Inst* 80:1221–1226, 1988.
47. Wolff SN, Herzig RH, Fay JW, LaMaistre CF, Frei-Lahr D, Lowder J, Bolwell B, Giannone L, and Herzig GP. High-dose thiotepa with autologous bone marrow transplantation for metastatic malignant melanoma: Results of phase I-II studies of the North American Bone Marrow Transplantation Group. *J Clin Oncol* 7:245–249, 1989.
48. Shea TC, Antman KH, Eder PJ, Elias A, Peters WP, Schryber S, Henner WD, Schoenfeld DA, Schnipper L, and Frei E III. Malignant melanoma. Treatment with high-dose combination alkylating agent chemotherapy and autologous bone marrow support. *Arch Dermatol* 124:878–884, 1988.
49. Thatcher N, Lind M, Morgenstern G, Carr T, Chadwick G, Jones R, and Craig P. High-dose double alkylating agent chemotherapy with DTIC, melphalan or ifosfamide and marrow rescue for metastatic malignant melanoma. *Cancer* 63:1296–1302, 1989.
50. Moormeier JA, Willams SF Kaminer LS, Garner M, and Bitran J. High-dose tri-alkylator chemotherapy with autologous stem cell rescue in patients with refractory malignancies. *J Natl Cancer Inst* 82:29–34, 1990.
51. Mortimer JE, Schulman S, MacDonald JS, Kopecky K, and Goodman G. High-dose cisplatin in disseminated melanoma: A comparison of two schedules. *Cancer Chemother Pharmacol* 25:373–376, 1990.
52. Glover D, Glick J, Weiler C, Fox K, Grabelsky S, and Guerry D. High dose cis-platinum (DDP) and WR-2721 (WR) in metastatic melanoma. *Proc Am Soc Clin Oncol* 7:247, 1988.
53. Murren JR, DeRosa W, Durivage HJ, Davis C, Makuch R, and Portlock CS. High-dose cisplatin plus DTIC in the treatment of metastatic melanoma. *Cancer* 67:1514–1517, 1991.
54. Luger SM, Kirkwood JM, Ernstoff MS, and Vlock DR. High-dose cisplatin and dacarbazine in the treatment of metastatic melanoma. *J Natl Cancer Inst* 82:1934–1937, 1990.
55. Bland KI, Kimura AK, Brenner DE, Basinger MA, Hirsch M, Hawkins IF Jr, Pierson KK, and Copeland EM III. A phase II study of the efficacy of diammine-dichloroplatinum (cisplatin) for the control of locally recurrent and intransit malignant melanoma of the extremities using tourniquet outflow-occlusion techniques. *Ann Surg* 209:73–80, 1989.
56. Mavligit GM, Charnsangavej C, Carrasco CH, Patt YZ, Benjamin RS, and Wallace S. Regression of ocular melanoma metastatic to the liver after hepatic arterial chemoembolization with cisplatin and polyvinyl sponge. *JAMA* 260:974–976, 1988.

Chapter 29

IMMUNOTHERAPY OF MELANOMA

L.M. Jost and J.M. Kirkwood

Malignant melanoma might be predicted to interact with, and to respond to, the immune system of the host in which it arises, given its ontogeny from the neural crest and biologic features partially resembling those of immunocompetent cells. One of the highest rates of spontaneous regression among all tumors has been observed for melanoma and has been estimated to be approximately 0.22 percent; as many as 40 percent of those patients who exhibit spontaneous regression may have a cure without relapse of the malignant melanoma until death from other reasons.[1,2] Since malignant melanoma is one of the tumors most resistant to standard modalities of radiation and chemotherapy after failure of surgery, melanoma was an early obvious target for immunotherapeutic trials. We shall review both historic and current efforts to modulate the immune response to melanoma, encompassing both nonspecific and specific agents and methods.

NONSPECIFIC IMMUNOTHERAPY

Immunostimulants Derived from Bacteria

Prior to the availability of purified and recombinant cytokines, immunomodulation was attempted by administration of a range of bacterial agents, extracts, or toxins. Early trials were based on anecdotal reports of tumor regression after recovery from severe bacterial infections and corroborative animal data suggesting a protective effect of tuberculosis upon development of melanoma in wild white horses. Numerous trials have been reported using either *Corynebacterium parvum* (CP),[3–5] Coley's toxin,[6] bacillus Calmette-Guerin (BCG)[7–10] or Picibanil,[11] often administered in conjunction with chemotherapy or following surgery for melanoma. Despite earlier claims[12] there remains no compelling evidence for meaningful antitumor activity in terms of tumor regression, disease-free and overall survival with these agents administered by various systemic routes at a range of dosages. In contrast, tumor regression has been seen more frequently after intratumoral injection of these agents: BCG induced tumor regression in 10 of 22 patients treated with intralesional injections while only 2 of 22 responded after systemic treatment with scarification.[13] Similar results have been reported for regional and systemic use of CP.[14] Conclusive studies were finally performed by the SWOG and the WHO: The SWOG trial compared BCNU + Hydroxyurea + DTIC (BHD), BHD + BCG, and DTIC + BCG in 269 patients randomized to one of these arms.[15] The study failed to detect statistically significant differences among the three arms. The WHO trial examined 761 patients with melanoma stage I or II, who were treated either with DTIC alone, DTIC + BCG, BCG alone, or were left untreated in a control arm.[16] No statistically significant overall survival differences were identified among the groups despite relapse-free and overall survival differences seen in a subset of patients who initially had a negative BCG skin reaction (that is, had neither undergone BCG-vaccination nor experienced tuberculosis before study entry).[17] The first exposure to an antigen usually elicits a more complex, broader reaction of the immune system than does a subsequent exposure where the antigen is more quickly eliminated by a limited specific recall reaction. This observation favors the hypothesis that secondary immunologic stimuli may not be of the proper quality and magnitude to effectively activate the components of the immune system that are essential to induce tumor regression.

Picibanil, a pulverized product of heat-killed and penicillin G-treated Streptococcus pyogenes, has lately been reintroduced for in vitro and in vivo use in animal and human pilot studies. The role of picibanil as an immunomodulator for treatment of melanoma is currently under study (phase IB-II), because of its wide-ranging ability to induce or enhance activity of TNF,[18] IL-2 + LAK[19], IL-2 + TIL[20] in vivo and to augment CTL and NK/LAK activity[21,22] in vitro.

Chemically Defined Immunostimulatory Drugs

LEVAMISOLE

The immunostimulatory properties of the antihelmintic agent Levamisole were detected in animals[23] and humans[24] leading to pilot and then randomized, placebo-controlled studies. One major trial in 203 patients[25] showed no significant difference in survival between the groups despite a trend for longer disease-free survival in stage I patients treated with Levamisole ($p = 0.07$). Further studies,[26] including one using a combination with BHD chemotherapy,[27] gave largely negative results. Recently, the National Cancer Institute of Canada Clinical Trials Group completed a phase III trial studying 543 patients with completely resected malignant melanoma of poor prognosis, defined by Clark level ≥ III or lymph node metastasis. The four arms compared Levamisole 2.5 mg/kg on 2 days/week for 3 years, BCG 4 weekly doses of 40 mg followed by 1 monthly dose for 3 years, and Levamisole alternating with BCG to a control group. After a median follow-up of 8.5 years, a trend to prolonged median disease-free survival (66 versus 55 months, $p = 0.067$), and a significant prolongation of the median overall survival (74 versus 62 months, $p = 0.027$) has been documented for the Levamisole group in comparison to the controls.[28] The benefit was seen after 3 years and the recurrence rate was reduced by 29 percent for the Levamisole group ($p = 0.08$) and 6 percent for the BCG + Levamisole group ($p = 0.73$), but increased by 3 percent for the BCG group ($p = 0.87$). Gastrointestinal and mucocutaneous side effects as well as reversible leukopenia prompted an early discontinuation of Levamisole in 55 of 135 patients with only 47 patients receiving the full 3-year course of Levamisole therapy. Despite these side effects, the results justify further studies testing different treatment schedules, comparing Levamisole with other adjuvant treatment modalities, and evaluating the combination with chemotherapy in analogy to the encouraging findings in patients with colon cancer.[29]

CIMETIDINE/COUMARIN

Based on the stimulatory activity of coumarin upon macrophages and the stimulatory effects of cimetidine upon T-helper cells coupled with inhibitory effects on T-suppressor cells, the drug combination was tested in a nonrandomized fashion in patients with advanced malignant melanoma. Significant tumor regressions have been achieved in occasional patients,[30] but no randomized trial has yet been performed to establish any benefit of the combination over its components or over no treatment.

Recombinant Biological Response Modifiers

INTERFERONS

The interferons (IFN) consist of a large group of antigenically and genetically distinct species and subspecies with differing immunomodulatory and directly cytostatic and cytotoxic antitumor activities. They are produced by many cell types upon stimulation with viruses, nucleic acids, inflammatory mediators, and other cytokines. IFN-alpha, IFN-beta, and IFN-gamma entered widespread testing once they could be produced by means of recombinant DNA-technology. Their antiproliferative activity has been related to their ability to inhibit protein synthesis, following binding to specific membrane receptors.[31,32] Beyond their antiproliferative activity, the IFNs are able to induce changes in the expression of the major histocompatibility (MHC) class I and class II antigens, tumor-associated antigens (TAA),[33,34] and receptors for melanocyte stimulating hormone (MSH) by melanoma cells. Changes in MHC- and TAA-expression may lead to enhanced immunogenicity and altered susceptibility to cell-mediated cytotoxicity, whereas increased expression of MSH-receptors may enhance differentiative effects of MSH, that is, enhanced tyrosinase production and melanization.[35] Of equal or greater importance, the antitumor actions of the IFNs have been suggested to arise from immunomodulatory effects. NK-cell activation has been related to the antitumor effects of IFNs in experimental animals.[36] However, studies performed in humans, including melanoma patients, have not yet consistently correlated immune and antitumor responses.

The clinical toxicity of IFN is well characterized[37,38] and consists mainly of a flu-like syndrome of fever, chills, headache, malaise, myalgias, and arthralgias. Cardiovascular, renal, and neurologic toxicities are less frequent and may be most problematic among elderly patients. Hematologic toxicity is generally not dose-limiting, and commonly includes leukopenia and thrombocytopenia without evidence for bone marrow hypocellularity; the toxicity is correlated with dosage, schedule, and route of administration. Hepatotoxicity reflected in elevated transaminases has generally been well tolerated and is quickly reversible upon withdrawal of the IFNs. Rarely, cholostasis has been observed and this potentially life-threatening toxicity may be correlated with antecedent liver pathology or failure to monitor and modify treatment according to toxicity.

Therapy of advanced disease: The results of protocols using recombinant IFN, administered generally s.c. or i.m., are summarized in Table 29-1. An average response rate of approximately 15 percent for IFN-alpha and IFN-beta[39–49] is notable, while phase I studies suggest a lower response rate with

TABLE 29-1
INTERFERON-ALPHA/-BETA THERAPY OF MALIGNANT MELANOMA

YEAR	REFERENCE	NUMBER OF PATIENTS ENTERED	EVALUABLE	PATIENTS WITH CR	PR	PERCENT RESPONSE RATE ENTERED	EVALUABLE	IFN TYPE	ROUTE	DOSE MU/m²	SCHEDULE d/w
84	Creagan et al.[39]	30	30	1	5	20	20	a-2a	im	12	3d/w*12
84	Creagan et al.[40]	31	31	3	4	23	23	a-2a	im	50	3d/w*12
86	Coates et al.[41]	16	15	0	0	0	0	a-2a	iv	20	5d/2w
85	Hersey et al.[42]	20	18	1	1	10	11	a-2a	im	50	3d/w
87	Legha et al.[43]	35	31	0	3	9	10	a-2a	im	3-36	7d/w
		31	31	0	2	6	6	a-2a	im	3-36	3d/w
87	Elsasser et al.[44]	21	21	3	0	14	14	a-2a	im	18	7d/2*10 →3d/w
87	Steiner et al.[45]	12	12	1	0	8	8	a-2a	im	18	7d/w
85	Kirkwood et al.[46]	23	23	3	2	22	22	a-2b	im/iv	10-100	7d/w*4
86	Dorval et al.[47]	22	22	2	4	27	27	a-2b	sc	10	3d/w
86	Robinson et al.[48]	51	40	4	6	20	25	a-2b	sc/iv	30	3d/w*12
89	Sertoli et al.[49]	21	21	0	3	14	14	a-2b	im	10	3d/w
87	Sarna et al.[184]	19	17	0	0	0	0	B-Ser	iv	12	5d/w
	Total	332	312	18	30	14.5	15.4				

CR: complete response, d/w: treatment days per week, IFN: interferon, MU: mega unit ($1*10^6$ cetus units), PR: partial response, Pts: patients

IFN-gamma.[50–52] Unfortunately, no optimal dosage or treatment schedule can presently be established for treatment of melanoma patients. Patients with minimal disease appear to respond better, in keeping with earlier findings with cytotoxic drugs and other biomodulators. Responses are seen at all sites, but appear to be most frequent in subcutaneous and lymph node metastases[53] and lung disease.

Therapies utilizing combinations of IFNs of different subclasses administered concurrently have been associated with increased toxicity without substantial synergistic antitumor effects in melanoma patients.[54,55] Trials of sequenced delivery of interferons gamma and alpha-2, reported to achieve improved therapeutic and immunomodulatory activity in renal cell carcinoma,[56] have not yet been tested in melanoma patients.

Preliminary studies combining IFN with IL-2 have resulted in minimally improved response rates.[57–66] The combination with chemotherapy given in standard doses has not consistently yielded significantly improved response rates, when judged on the basis of reports in limited numbers of patients.[67–70] The concept of combining IFN with low-dose cyclophosphamide chemotherapy given as another immunomodulator, hypothesized to prevent the emergence of suppressor activity, has shown no benefit in an initial report,[35] and further evaluation of the concept is required.

Intra- or perilesional application of IFN has proven to be of approximately equal systemic efficacy as the s.c. administration with an overall response rate of 18 percent including those occurring at sites distant from the injections.[71]

Therapy of micrometastic disease: Adjuvant IFN therapy for patients with poor prognostic factors is based on the negative correlation between the tumor mass and the likelihood of a response. A number of studies addressing these questions have been completed (but the results are not yet published). Further large phase III studies are under way, and may lead to more clinically significant results for melanoma patients (see Chap. 26).

TUMOR NECROSIS FACTOR (TNF)

Tumor necrosis factor is a 17-kDa protein with a variety of effects that is secreted by activated T cells and monocytes. TNF is a potent endogenous pyrogen and mediates endotoxic shock and cachexia. TNF is also involved in the regulation of hematopoiesis. Its antitumor activity includes direct cytostatic antitumor effects, indirect immunomodulatory, and procoagulant effects. The induction of hemorrhagic necrosis within tumor nodules may be mediated by TNF effects upon endothelial cells, leading to enhanced platelet aggregation and activation of the coagulation system. Many tumor cells express high affinity receptors for TNF, which have been shown to be down-regulated in vitro by treatment with the protein synthesis inhibitor cycloheximide, and upregulated by IFN-gamma. These modulations lead to altered tumor cell sensitivity to direct cytotoxicity by TNF.[72] Unfortunately, the in vitro susceptibility of tumor cells cannot be predicted accurately by the presence or absence of these TNF receptors, which appears to be a characteristic of a given tumor cell clone.[73] The direct effects on the tumor cells may be cell cycle specific causing arrest in G_2 with following cell lysis during mitosis.[74] The form of cell death induced by TNF has been described as apoptic as opposed to necrotic, due to the DNA fragmentation induced early in the process of cell destruction.[75] In human tumor colony assays, 25 percent of 28 tested melanoma cell lines were sensitive to TNF with an ID_{50} of < 100 U/ml,[76] a level clearly attainable by direct parenteral administration of TNF, or by indirect induction of TNF as a secondary cytokine of several immunotherapy protocols with other immunostimulants, such as BCG, Picibanil, and IL-2.

Indirect or immunomodulatory effects of TNF include the release of interleukin-1, granulocyte-macrophage colony-stimulating factor,[77] and interferons. Augmentation of macrophage,[78] natural killer cell,[79] and granulocyte[80] tumoricidal activity have been documented, along with expression of activation markers including HLA-DR and interleukin-2 receptors on T-lymphocytes,[81] and induction of MHC class I antigens,[82] as well as several adhesion molecules on both endothelial and tumor cells. TNF also stimulates fibroblast proliferation.[83] In addition to its function in these positive loops in the immunoregulatory network, TNF also induces negative feedback mechanisms in lymphoid and macrophage populations with the production of inhibitory substances like prostaglandin E_2[84] within days after their initial activation.

Despite the encouraging data obtained in vitro and in animals and theoretically beneficial effects on the immune system, the clinical results obtained to date in phase I and II studies using a variety of schedules of systemic TNF therapy have been disappointing, with response rates of 0 to 5 percent. Significant toxicity has included fever, rigors, a flu-like syndrome, headache, hyper- and hypotension, nausea, vomiting, diarrhea, phlebitis, and all kinds of organ dysfunction. TNF does not seem to have achieved sufficient impact against cancer to date to argue for systemic monotherapy. To date, only preliminary trials using regionally administered TNF have been undertaken in bladder cancer[85] (intravesically), and peritoneal carcinomatosis (i.p.),[86] and in extremity melanoma using isolation-perfusion technique,[87] (see Chap. 20 for update results).

INTERLEUKIN-2

Interleukin-2, a glycoprotein with a molecular weight of approximately 15,000, is produced by activated lymphocytes. This hormone-like growth factor for NK- and antigen-primed T-cells enhances the cytotoxic activity of NK-cells, monocytes, and cytotoxic T-cells. It broadly activates a population of cytotoxic lymphocytes called LAK cells and induces the release of many secondary cytokines including IL-1, IL-2, TNF, and the interferons among others. In contrast to the interferons and TNF, there seems to be minimal direct cytostatic/cytotoxic effect on most tumor cell lines mediated by IL-2, although functional IL-2 receptors have been found on tumors of several different histotypes.[88] Effects of IL-2 upon tumor cells may include alterations in the expression of adhesion and MHC molecules, as well as tumor associated antigens, but these effects have not been adequately studied to date.

The toxicity of IL-2 is well-characterized,[89,90] and includes fever, rigors, malaise, skin rashes, pruritus, stomatitis, nausea, and occasional vomiting and diarrhea. Dyspnea, tachycardia, and arrhythmias have been correlated with significant capillary leak syndrome, with dose-dependent hypotension and weight gain due to extravasation of the plasma volume. Hematologic toxicity predictably includes lymphopenia and eosinophilia, which are reversible on withdrawal of the agent. Hepatotoxicity, renal toxicity, and altered mental function are common but also rapidly reversible after cessation of IL-2 treatment. Remarkably, patients receiving IL-2 are more susceptible to bacterial infections, chiefly manifested as intravenous line infections and septicemias; this has been correlated to granulocyte dysfunction during IL-2 infusion.[91] Bullous skin eruptions[92] and a toxic shock-like syndrome found in association with IL-2 may be due to the synergism of IL-2 with bacterial exotoxins or allergic reactions to antibiotics given to prevent infections. The MTD of IL-2 depends on the schedule and route of administration used and is below 12 MU/m^2/d (Cetus units) for i.v. bolus therapy according to the schedule used by Rosenberg's group for their initial studies and 3.75 MU/m^2/d for five-day continuous infusion.

Based on animal studies indicating a synergistic antitumor effect of IL-2 administered with adoptive transfer of lymphokine-activated killer (LAK) cells,[93–95] few trials using IL-2 alone were performed initially. Additional data have been gathered from studies using IL-2 alone, compared to IL-2 + LAK cells in one of the study arms however (see Table 29-2). The response rate noted from these studies of IL-2 was 19 percent[96–104] and may not be much different from the 15 percent (0–27 percent) reported for several interferon trials. Randomized comparisons between IFN and IL-2 have not yet been performed.

As for the interferons, the optimal dose and schedule for IL-2 as a monotherapy has not been well characterized. Administration by continuous infusion seems to be less effective,[105] and the optimal

TABLE 29-2
CLINICAL RESULTS OBTAINED WITH IL-2 MONOTHERAPY

YEAR	REFERENCE	NUMBER OF PATIENTS ENROLLED/	EVALUABLE	PATIENTS WITH CR	PR	PERCENT RESPONSE RATE ENROLLED/	EVALUABLE	SCHEDULE (i.v.)
89	Rosenberg et al.[96]	60*	42	0	10	?	24	Bolus
90	Parkinson et al.[97]	?	46	2	8	?	22	Bolus
86	Atkins et al.[98]	3	3	0	0	0	0	Bolus
88	Thompson et al.[99]	15	15	0	0	0	0	Bolus or Cont.
88	Sosman et al.[100]	7	7	0	0	0	0	Bolus or Cont.
90	Richards et al.[101]	?	33	0	3	?	9	Continuous
88	Kohler et al.[102]	3	3	0	0	0	0	Continuous
88	Paciucci et al.[103]	3	3	0	3	100	100	Continuous
87	Creekmore et al.[104]	3	3	0	1	33	33	Continuous
	Total	?	160	2 (1.3%)	28 (17.5%)	?	18.8%	

*Including some patients treated in adjuvant setting
Cont.: 24-h intravenous continuous infusion, CR: complete response, IL-2: interleukin-2, PR: partial response, Pts: patients

schedule is likely to consist of moderate doses given repeatedly over short periods of time with intervals between therapy cycles that are long enough to avoid activation of long-lasting negative feedback mechanisms and a decline in the patient's performance status. The clinical studies performed to date have documented modulation of multiple components of the immune system during IL-2 treatment. None of many parameters such as degree of rebound lymphocytosis, NK- and LAK-activity of PBL, rise in serum levels of TNF-alpha, interferon-gamma, or soluble IL-2 receptor has correlated reproducibly in a statistically significant manner with tumor response. In one study that has not been confirmed to date, the expression of tumor cell DR-antigen in metastatic melanoma was associated with tumor response.[106]

Combination therapy of IL-2 (see Table 29-3) with alpha-interferon may result in somewhat augmented antitumor effects,[58–66] but to date these do not meaningfully exceed the results of IL-2 or IFN alone. For other current trials, including those combining IL-2 with IL-4 or IL-7, it is too early to report reliable results. Their immunologic data will have to be carefully analyzed in order not to overlook potential positive and negative interactions, through which we may improve our understanding of the regulation of the immune network in cancer patients. Combinations of IL-2 with chemotherapy[107–116] have given some responses (see Table 29-4), but further evaluation in randomized tests against chemotherapy alone will be required before definitive conclusions can be drawn.

Adoptive Cellular Immunotherapy

IL-2/LAK STUDIES

Technical and biological aspects: As previously mentioned, most trials including IL-2 also used the ex vivo generation of LAK cells derived from PBL harvested by leukapheresis, usually after pretreatment

TABLE 29-3
CLINICAL RESULTS OF IL-2 AND OTHER BIOMODULATORS

YEAR	REFERENCE	NUMBER OF PATIENTS ENROLLED/	EVALUABLE	PATIENTS WITH CR	PR	PERCENT RESPONSE RATE ENROLLED/	EVALUABLE	SECOND BIOMODULATOR
89	Budd et al.[58]	6	6	0	1	17	17	IFN-alpha
89	Rosenberg et al.[59]	41	39	3	10	32	33	IFN-alpha
89	Lee et al.[60]	16	16	1	3	25	25	IFN-alpha
90	Sznol et al.[61]	7	7	0	0	0	0	IFN-alpha
90	Bukowski et al.[62]	3	3	0	0	0	0	IFN-alpha
90	Whitehead et al.[63]	14	14	0	0	0	0	IFN-alpha
90	Goey et al.[64]	47	35	0	10	21	29	IFN-alpha
88	Krigel et al.[65]	3	3	0	1	33	33	IFN-beta
90	Redman et al.[66]	1	1	0	0	0	0	IFN-gamma
	Total	138	124	4	25	21.0	23.4	

Cont.: 24-h intravenous continuous infusion, CR: complete response, IL-2: interleukin-2, IFN: interferon, PR: partial response, Pts: patients

TABLE 29-4
CLINICAL RESULTS OBTAINED WITH IL-2 AND CHEMOTHERAPY

YEAR	REFERENCE	NUMBER OF PATIENTS ENROLLED/EVALUABLE		PATIENTS WITH CR	PATIENTS WITH PR	PERCENT RESPONSE RATE ENROLLED/EVALUABLE		SECOND AGENT
88	Mitchell et al.[107]	27	24	1	5	25	27	CTX low dose
89	Lindemann et al.[108]	18	18	0	2	11	11	CTX low dose
89	Stoter et al.[109,110]	29	24	1	4	17	21	DTIC
89	Flaherty et al.[111]	32	29	1	6	22	24	DTIC hosp.
90	Flaherty et al.[112,113]	25	24	2	7	36	38	DTIC outpat.
90	Atkins et al.[114,115]	20	20	3	5	40	40	cisDDP
91	Redman et al.[116]	13	13	1	4	38	38	DTIC/cisDDP
	Total	164	152	9	33	25.6	27.6	

CTX: cyclophosphamide, DDP: Cisplatin, DTIC: Dacarbazine, CR: complete response, hosp.: IL-2 given in inpatient setting, IL-2: interleukin-2, outpat.: IL-2 given in a outpatient setting, PR: partial response, Pts: patients

of the patient with IL-2. This preparatory therapy with IL-2 leads to a rebound lymphocytosis and an increase of circulating LAK cell precursors. After cultivation and activation of isolated PBMNC for 3 to 4 days in medium containing high doses of IL-2 (1000 Cetus U/ml), these cells acquire significantly enhanced LAK activity. These cells, in numbers ranging from 1×10^{10} to 1×10^{11}, are adoptively retransfused into the patient. Adoptive therapy with LAK cells has not resulted in the appearance of qualitatively different side effects than those incurred by high doses of IL-2 alone. However, enhancement of these adverse effects as seen in higher systemic doses of IL-2 was noted. Studies with intravenously administered labeled LAK cells indicate that these cells are initially detained in the circulation of the lung and may then redistribute to lymphatic organs after 24 to 48 hours. Convincing enrichment of ex vivo generated LAK cells within the tumor has only rarely been reported. A four-fold (range 1–10) enrichment of frozen/thawed unstimulated PBL at the site of subcutaneous metastases has been observed when compared to the surrounding normal skin.[117] The latter ratio may reflect an enrichment of PBL localization within the tumor or may be due in part to the presence of more intravascular lymphocytes in vascularized tumors. One may conclude that, after systemic administration, only a very small fraction of LAK cells really gains access to tumor cells in metastatic foci.

Results of IL-2/LAK phase I-II trials: The mean response rate for IL-2/LAK therapy of patients with advanced melanoma appears to be around 17 percent (see Table 29-5) if IL-2 is given as bolus injec-

TABLE 29-5
CLINICAL RESULTS OBTAINED WITH IL-2 AND LAK THERAPY

YEAR	REFERENCE	NUMBER OF PATIENTS ENROLLED/EVALUABLE		PATIENTS WITH CR	PATIENTS WITH PR	PERCENT RESPONSE RATE ENROLLED/EVALUABLE		SCHEDULE (i.v.)
NCI, intramural								
89	Rosenberg et al.[96]	66*	48	4	6	?	21	Bolus
Other centers								
89	Dutcher et al.[118]	36	32	1	5	17	19	Bolus
89	Cascinelli et al.[119]	15	14	0	0	0	0	Bolus
89	Stahel et al.[120]	7	7	0	1	14	14	Bolus
88	Rayner et al.[122]	?	42	0	6	?	14	Hybrid
90	Gaynor et al.[90]	30	30	0	1	3	3	Continuous
90	Richards et al.[101]	?	35	0	2	?	6	Continuous
89	West et al.[121]	?	22	0	8	?	36	Continuous
88	Paciucci et al.[103]	?	3	0	1	?	33	Continuous
88	Schoof et al.[185]	?	9	1	4	?	56	Low Dose
	Total	?	242	6 (2.5%)	34 (14.0%)	?	16.5%	

*Including some patients treated in adjuvant setting
CR: complete response, IL-2: interleukin-2, LAK: lymphokine-activated killer cells, PR: partial response, Pts: patients

tions.[96,118–120] Slightly lower response rates have been noted when IL-2 is given as a continuous infusion[90,101,103,121] (13 percent) or in hybrid schedules[122] (14 percent). Overall, these results suggest that the LAK cells do not increase the response rate above that which can be achieved with IL-2 (or IFN alone) in melanoma patients. Furthermore, as is true for IL-2 alone, no parameter predictive for tumor regression has been characterized convincingly so far for IL-2/LAK therapy. A moderate positive correlation ($r = 0.623$) of the amount of GM2-ganglioside expressed by tumor cells with their LAK susceptibility in vitro[123] has yet to be confirmed in vivo.

ADHERENT LAK CELLS (A-LAK OR A-NK)

Given the lack of any superiority of IL-2/LAK over IL-2 alone in melanoma patients, it has to be considered that classic bulk LAK cultures consist of a phenotypically heterogeneous cell population, most of which cells may be irrelevant with respect to the cytotoxic response against the tumor. Worse yet, the bulk LAK populations may contain counter-regulatory populations including suppressor and suppressor-inducer cells, which may interfere with the antitumor responses in vivo. One way to get around this problem is to isolate and expand only pure NK/LAK cells. After initial elimination of monocytes, adherence of LAK cells after 24 hours of stimulation with IL-2 affords a new method to purify so-called adherent LAK (A-LAK/A-NK) cells. Such cultures exhibit considerable enrichment for NK-/LAK cells, with only occasional outgrowth of $CD3^{+}CD4^{+/-}CD8^{-/+}$ cells. Enhanced NK-/LAK-activity on a per cell basis has been shown, and the first clinical trial of A-LAK/A-NK cells has recently been completed from the Pittsburgh Cancer Institute. For melanoma and renal cell cancer patients, these clinical studies have not given results that are qualitatively significantly different from those of classic IL-2/LAK protocols[124] but revealed unexpected difficulties with the growth of sufficient A-LAK cells to fully test the limits of these effector cells in patients with melanoma or renal cell carcinoma.

TUMOR INFILTRATING LYMPHOCYTES (TIL)

Based on the limited response rates obtained in human IL-2/LAK studies, the phenotypic and functional heterogeneity of bulk LAK cell cultures derived from PBL, and the widely recognized lack of correlation between the in vitro generated NK-/LAK-activity with tumor regression, the possibility that lymphocytes resident in tumor tissue might afford a more active and specific effector population was explored. In animal models, preliminary studies suggested that TIL were 50 to 100 times more potent in mediating regression of freshly established lung metastases than LAK cells.[125] This observation was attributed to the priming to the tumor that TIL may have experienced prior to their in vitro expansion.

An initial report of Rosenberg et al.[126] showed a 55 percent response rate in 20 melanoma patients, including some with earlier unsuccessful LAK-therapy. But this concept of enhanced specificity and antitumor efficacy of the TIL effector cells is subject to qualification, in that selection of patients is implicit in this methodology: 20 further patients were biopsied for TIL culture establishment during the above-cited study, but became ineligible for the investigational treatment mainly because of rapid disease progression ($N = 7$) or inadequate TIL growth ($N = 10$). The complexity of the TIL culture technique and functional suppression noted in most freshly isolated TIL[127] explains these difficulties. The response rate calculated, based on "intent to treat" analysis, was actually only 28 percent (confidence interval 15–44 percent),[128] a result not statistically different from IL-2/LAK studies. A report of Kradin et al. showed PR in 3/13 (23 percent) of melanoma patients,[129] while Oldham et al. documented 1 CR and 3 PR (20 percent) among 20 melanoma patients,[130] further suggesting that the lower overall response rate may be valid. The last report of the NCI group[131] described 67 melanoma patients, of whom 55 were treated and evaluable. The response rate among those was 40 percent, corresponding to 33 percent of the enrolled patients (see Table 29-6). This report has, for the first time, correlated the lytic activity of the cultured TIL effectors against autologous tumor with the clinical response ($p < .002$).

The complexity and costs of the IL-2/TIL therapy, as well as the notable absence of an enhanced fraction of complete responses achieved with this investigational approach, must temper the initial high expectations.

Why are the TIL in human trials not convincingly more effective than LAK cells? Key questions in this regard relate to the tumor access of TIL cells after retransfusion. It is unclear whether retransfused TIL are able to reach tumor deposits in relevant numbers after systemic administration. Studies designed to answer this question using TIL marked with ^{111}Indium[117,132] or by means of gene transfer[133] show that TIL persist in circulation for 3 to 8 weeks and can be recovered from tumor biopsies in three of five patients. The enrichment ratio between subcutaneous melanoma metastases and surrounding normal skin was 12-fold (range 2–40), a result only three-fold higher than that of unstimulated labeled PBL (ratio = 4, range 1–10). Thus, at least a small fraction of adoptively transfused TIL may reinfiltrate residual tumor masses, achieving this end

TABLE 29-6
CLINICAL RESULTS OBTAINED WITH IL-2 AND TIL THERAPY

YEAR	REFERENCE	NUMBER OF PATIENTS ENROLLED/EVALUABLE		PATIENTS WITH CR	PATIENTS WITH PR	PERCENT RESPONSE RATE ENROLLED/EVALUABLE	
89	Kradin et al.[129]	?	13	—	3	?	23
90	Oldham et al.[130]	?	20	1	3	?	20
91	Aebersold et al.[131]	67	55	2	20	33	40
	Total	?	88	3 (3.4%)	26 (29.6%)	?	33.0%

CR: complete response, IL-2: interleukin-2, PR: partial response, Pts: patients, TIL: tumor infiltrating lymphocytes

better than LAK cells. But the number of TIL found in the tumor was still very low and never reached the effector-to-target ratios known to be required for demonstration of in vitro cytotoxicity in conventional assays. TIL-associated tumor regression may, therefore, not be mediated by a direct tumor cell lysis mechanism, in which the in vitro expanded TIL are cytotoxic to tumor cells in situ, but rather by cytokines secondarily released by IL-2 expanded TIL, such as IFN-gamma or TNF. Which cell subpopulation contributes the most to tumor regression and whether the "right" lymphocytes are being optimally expanded and transfused is not yet known. The correlation of cytotoxicity against autologous tumor with clinical response seems to confirm the importance of tumor-specific cytotoxic $CD8^+$ T-cells as a main effector population. But partial[126] and complete responses[134] after retransfusion of TIL consisting almost exclusively of $CD4^+$ lymphocytes also have been reported. It could, therefore, be that tumor-specific $CD4^+$ T-helper cells are even more important than tumor-specific cytotoxic $CD8^+$ T-cells. Most of the protocols used so far utilized very high doses of interleukin-2 for in vitro TIL expansion. This favors the outgrowth of NK-/LAK cells and other non MHC-restricted effector (T-)cells. Therefore, clinical results similar to those of LAK studies should not have come as a surprise. Furthermore, it seems likely that high dose IL-2 stimulation protocols can expand irrelevant lymphocytes, perhaps originating from contamination of the tumor specimen with blood. This may frequently happen because the desired TIL may show inhibited proliferative, cytotoxic, and secretory functions, as mentioned before. The use of IL-4 or other newer cytokines or counter-regulatory measures may help to circumvent this problem.[135] Last, but not least, it has been suggested by cloning assays that tumor-specific suppressor cells may be part of the initially isolated TIL-population, and that proliferation of these cells may effectively abrogate the generation or function of tumor-specific cytotoxic T-cells.[136,137] Therefore, the relative failure of TIL to effectively induce tumor regression may be attributed to

1. insufficient numbers of effector cells within the tumor,
2. harvest and propagation of the "wrong" lymphocyte subpopulations for adoptive transfer,
3. inhibition of growth and function of retransfused TIL in the tumor microenvironment,
4. tumor cell heterogeneity of providing a reservoir enabling the outgrowth of subclones resistant to TIL[138]; this phenomenon may be more likely after adoptive transfusion of mono- or oligoclonal TIL.

To improve the clinical results, methods for generating specific TIL of greater cytotoxic or helper potential are needed. This may be possible by use of methods to eliminate irrelevant or suppressor cells or the genetic alteration of TIL, in order to make them resistant to inhibitory influences or also more stable producers of effector cytokines. This would provide the locally missing help for delivery of the cytotoxic potential of the cells already in place and for further recruiting of fresh PBL. The random introduction of the TNF gene into the genome of TIL to be retransfused is currently in testing, and whether it achieves these goals will soon be known. Finally, new designs for the concomitant application of drugs and cytokines may circumvent the stimulation of a broad variety of negative feedbacks within the immune system, which may often limit the therapeutic benefit of TIL and other highly potent stimuli of the patient's immune system.

SPECIFIC CYTOTOXIC T-CELLS DERIVED FROM TUMOR- OR VACCINE-DRAINING LYMPH NODE LYMPHOCYTES

Another source of specifically cytotoxic T-cells potentially active against the autologous tumor may be the regional tumor draining lymph nodes or lymph nodes obtained after vaccination with autologous tumor cells.[139] Their superiority over specific CTL inducible from peripheral blood lymphocytes has yet to be confirmed in vitro and pilot clinical studies designed to evaluate the optimal timing of immunization and harvest, adjuvant agents, and type of immunogen are now appropriate.

SPECIFIC IMMUNOTHERAPY

Active Immunization

In contrast to the nonspecific immune stimulation discussed earlier, the use of viable, autologous, or allogeneic tumor cells, or tumor-derived products such as shed antigens, cell or membrane extracts for immunization elicits a response specifically targeted against the tumor (see Tables 29-7 and 29-8). To promote an effective humoral and cellular immune response, the immunogenicity of the specific antigens used may require potentiation either by combination with an adjuvant, enzymatic treatment, coupling with haptens, or admixture with viruses.

SHED ANTIGENS

By using a polyvalent vaccine derived from supernatants of pooled melanoma cell cultures, 1 of 13 patients was reported to respond.[140] Further studies with the same vaccine in 63 stage II melanoma patients in an adjuvant setting[141,142] showed a longer survival among those 25 patients in whom a cellular and antibody response was detectable. The four melanoma cell lines used for production of the vaccine were initially reported to be of allogeneic origin, but it has been detected that one of the lines included in this "polyvalent vaccine" is an xenogeneic hamster melanoma line. This leaves open the question whether allogeneic human melanoma specificities, or possibly more immunogenic xenogenic specificities, might have been responsible for effects obtained with this polyvalent "human" MAA vaccine. Unfortunately, data that will resolve this problem are not yet available, although larger scale testing of this polyvalent antigen is in progress.

PURIFIED TAA OR GANGLIOSIDES

In a multicenter three-arm study comparing immuno-, chemo-, and combination therapy in stage III melanoma patients, Hollinshead et al.[143] reported an unparalleled rate of clinical response with 8 of 23 patients responding after vaccination with purified TAA from sonicated allogeneic melanoma cell membranes and 11 of 16 patients reported responding with vaccination plus dacarbazine (DTIC) chemotherapy. In contrast, only 2 of 17 patients treated with DTIC alone responded. Livingston et al. reported the development of significant, but short-lived, anti-GM2 IgM-antibody titers in 17 of 31 stage III melanoma patients after immunization with either purified GM2-ganglioside or whole cells with high expression of GM2.[144] Nevertheless, the 17 patients with an increase in anti-GM2 titers were more likely to be disease-free after 15 months than the 14 others (14 of 17 versus 5 of 14). This encouraging serological correlate bears out earlier suggestions that IgM response to melanoma may be associated with improved prognosis[145] but is to be contrasted with one report in which IgG alloantibody was associated with relapse of melanoma.[146] (See also Chap. 26.)

MECHANICAL ALLOGENEIC WHOLE MELANOMA CELL LYSATES

Such cell lysates in combination with *detox* as an adjuvant lead to two CR, three PR, and three minor

TABLE 29-7
THERAPY OF ADVANCED MELANOMA WITH ACTIVE IMMUNIZATION

YEAR	REFERENCE	NUMBER OF PATIENTS	CR	PR	VACCINE TYPE USED	ADJUVANT
82	Hollinshead[143]	39	6	13	TAA from allogeneic sonicated melanoma cell membranes	FcA
86	Bystryn[140]	13	1	0	Shed antigens from pooled allo-/xenogeneic cell lines	None
88	Bystryn[186]	19	1	1	Shed antigens from pooled allo-/xenogeneic cell lines	None
88	Mitchell[147]	17	2	3	Mechanical lysates of two allogeneic melanoma lines	DETOX
90	Mitchell[148]	25	1	3	Mechanical lysates of two allogeneic melanoma lines	DETOX
89	Morton[152]	15	1	3	Three pooled irradiated allogeneic melanoma lines	BCG
90	Berd[153]	40	4	1	Autologous irradiated tumor cells	BCG
	Total	168	16	24	(=23.8% Response rate)	

BCG: bacille Calmette-Guerin, CR: complete response, FcA: Freund's complete adjuvant, PR: partial response, Pts: patients, TAA: tumor-associated antigen

TABLE 29-8
ADJUVANT ACTIVE IMMUNIZATION

YEAR	REFERENCE	NUMBER OF PATIENTS/ CHARACTERISTICS	VACCINE/ADJUVANT	CLINICAL OUTCOME	CONTROL GROUP
79	Seigler et al.[151]	719 Clark III-IV	Allogeneic cells/BCG	"Encouraging survival curves"	None
81	Jones et al.[145]	40 stage II	Allogeneic cells/BCG	Enhanced DFS in patients with IgM response	Immunologic nonresponders
87	Wallack et al.[150]	39 stage II	Allogeneic cells VMO	Enhanced DFS (p = 0.04)	Matched patients
89	Bystryn et al.[141]	63 stage II	Shed antigens/alum	Two years longer DFS in patients with strong DTH response	Immunologic nonresponders

BCG: bacille Calmette-Guerin, DFS: disease-free survival, DTH: delayed hypersensitivity reaction, IgM: immunoglobulin type M

responses in 17 patients. All of the responders showed increased peripheral blood CTL-precursor levels.[147] In the following phase II trial, one CR, three PR, two mixed, one minor response, and disease stabilization in one patient was achieved in patients showing evidence for both humoral and cellular immune responses.[148]

VMO-LYSATES OF AUTOLOGOUS MELANOMA CELLS

Wallack et al. showed the feasibility of using autologous melanoma cells after infection and production of a lysate with vaccinia virus (vaccinia melanoma oncolysates, VMO) in patients with advanced melanoma and preliminary evidence for clinical usefulness.[149] The SEG conducted a nonrandomized study involving 39 stage II patients, suggesting a prolonged disease-free survival of patients with adjuvant VMO-treatment compared to matched controls treated with either BCG or *Corynebacterium parvum,* and showed a correlation between serologic and clinical response.[150]

VIABLE IRRADIATED TUMOR CELLS

Seigler et al.[151] studied the survival of 719 patients with various stages of disease after vaccination with neuraminidase-treated, irradiated viable allogeneic melanoma cells. These authors claim encouraging survival results even for poor risk patients with advanced disease, but have never conducted a randomized controlled trial to verify the benefit. In the absence of a comparison with a retrospective control group carefully matched for important risk factors, it has been difficult to draw conclusions about the impact of this therapy despite large series of patients. Jones et al.[145] treated 40 stage II melanoma patients with a vaccine consisting of pooled allogeneic melanoma cells admixed with BCG and observed improved disease-free survival in 14 subjects who exhibited an immunologic response with an increasing IgM titer against an oncofetal antigen, compared to vaccinated subjects without immunologic response or untreated patients without spontaneously elevated IgM titer. Morton et al.[152] used a new, more immunogenic version of the same vaccine in 15 patients with advanced melanoma and obtained a 21 percent response rate, including one CR.

Berd et al.[153] have reported therapy of advanced melanoma with irradiated autologous tumor cells admixed with BCG after pretreatment of the patients with cyclophosphamide. The authors have found four CR and one PR in a group of 40 evaluable patients. Thus, there is considerable evidence for a therapeutic potential of tumor immunization in the adjuvant setting, and even for long-lasting complete responses to immunization with autologous, HLA-matched or -unmatched allogeneic viable melanoma cells, or membrane extracts in advanced disease.

Immunization combined with concomitant and sequential application of cytokines may be predicted to improve both immunologic and clinical responses. Experimental studies in mice show that the immunogenicity of tumor cells can be drastically enhanced by transfection of the tumor cells with cytokine genes, for example, IL-2 genes.[154,155] Genetically nonresponsive strains of mice can be shown to give immune response to proteins only when immunized with use of IL-2 as an adjuvant.[156] Further improvement may result from the combination of cellular adoptive immunotherapy with in vitro expansion of lymphocytes harvested after successful immunization. Studies testing this approach are underway.

Passive Specific Immunotherapy

Passive immunotherapy involves the administration of antibodies (generally monoclonal, mAbs) against melanoma-associated antigens (MAA) that are common to melanoma of different individuals. These MAA are of several biochemical categories and may be located on cell surface and intracellularly: gangliosides include GD3 and GD2 on the cell surface; melanotransferrin (p97) and melanoma chondroitin sulfated proteoglycans (mCSP) are cell surface and cytoplasmic antigens. They can be demonstrated to mediate growth inhibition by blocking of critical growth factor receptors, complement-dependent cytotoxicity (CDC), antibody-dependent cellular cytotoxicity (ADCC), which may occur through arming of macrophages or NK cells. Activation of an idiotype-anti-idiotype network[157] may achieve sustained host immunity against tumor cells by circumventing tolerance.[158,159]

Initial phase I studies with mouse mAbs administered systemically to cancer patients have demonstrated localization to tumor and induction of inflammatory responses in the tumor with modest toxicity. Clinical responses to this type of therapy have been limited,[160–163] a fact that may be attributed to a lack of definitive information on the mechanism of antitumor activity operative in vivo and a lack of knowledge about the optimal dose, route, or schedule of therapy. It may also be limited by a deficiency of CDC and ADCC mediated by the particular mAb in patients with advanced cancer.

More recent studies (see Table 29-9) using mAbs capable of potent activation of CDC (complement dependent cytotoxicity) and/or ADCC (R24 mAb against GD3,[164,165] 3F8 against GD2,[166] or Me36.1 against GD2/GD3[159] have shown an average response rate of 19 percent with one CR of 13 subjects treated with Me36.1. Coupling of mAbs to radioisotopes[167–169] may result in higher response rates and more precise delivery of radiotherapy. But this has yet to be proven, and problems with tumor specificity may be of even greater concern for this modality than for unlabeled mAbs. Coupling mAbs to toxins such as Ricin-A chains has been tested clinically in lymphoma patients; a phase I study of this approach[170] resulted in one CR, five mixed responses, and five patients with stable disease. A phase II study[171] involving 51 melanoma patients of whom 43 were evaluable has shown three PR (7 percent). A new generation of immunotoxins with blocked Ricin toxin may bear further promise.

MAbs have generally been produced in rodent hybridoma systems, where problems arise with clinical use in human subjects due to induction of host immune responses against rodent antibodies which may a) neutralize the primary mAb and accelerate its clearance, b) form immune complexes that may potentially cause immunosuppression or even enhanced tumor growth as well as nephropathy and serum sickness, and c) produce anaphylactic reactions after repeated administration (reviewed Wong et al.[172]). These problems certainly have limited the clinical application of mAbs in the previously-cited studies. Efforts to produce human monoclonal antibodies (h-mAbs) in sufficient quantities for clinical studies have proven to be difficult and resulted mostly in mAbs of the IgM classes, lacking the potential to

TABLE 29-9
PASSIVE IMMUNOTHERAPY WITH MONOCLONAL ANTIBODIES

YEAR	REFERENCE	NUMBER OF PATIENTS EVALUABLE	PATIENTS WITH CR	PATIENTS WITH PR	RESPONSE RATE (%)	MONOCLONAL ANTIBODY NAME	MONOCLONAL ANTIBODY CLASS	MONOCLONAL ANTIBODY SPECIES	TARGET (MAA)	COMBINATION OR LIGAND
Systemic										
88	Vadham-Raj et al.[165]	21	0	4	19	R24	IgG3	murine	GD3	—
88	Dippold et al.[164]	5	0	2	40	R24	IgG3	murine	GD3	—
87	Cheung et al.[166]	9	0	2	22	3F8	IgG3	murine	GD3	—
88	Lichtin et al.[159]	13	1	0	8	Me36.1	IgG2a	murine	GD2/GD3	
	Subtotal	48	1	8	18.8%					
Intralesional										
89	Irie et al.[176]	2	1	0	50	L55	IgM	human	GM2	—
86	Irie et al.[175]	8	0	4	50	L72	IgM	human	GD2	—
Combined with Cytokines										Cytokine
90	Bajorin et al.[179]	16	0	1	6	R24	IgG3	murine	GD3	IL-2
90	Caulfield et al.[178]	15	0	0	0	R24	IgG3	murine	GD3	alpha-IFN
Radiolabeled mAbs and Immunotoxins										
85	Larson et al.[168]	6	0	1	17	48-7	Fab	murine	HMW	^{131}I
87	Spitler et al.[170]	22	1	0	5	?	IgG2a	murine	mCSP?	Ricin-A
88	Spitler et al.[171]	43	0	3	7	?	IgG2a	murine	mCSP?	Ricin-A
90	Oratz et al.[187]	20	0	4	20	?	IgG2a	murine	mCSP?	Ricin-A
	Total	180	3	21	13.3%					

CR: complete response, GD/GMx: gangliosides, HMW: hgh molecular weight antigen, IL-2: interleukin-2, INF: interferon, MAA: melanoma associated antigen, mCSP: melanoma chondroitin sulfated proteoglycans, PR: partial response, Pts: patients

stimulate ADCC.[173,174] A first clinical trial injecting the L72 h-mAb against GD2 intralesionally showed tumor regressions in four of eight patients[175] and that of L55 against GM2 in one of two patients.[176] Studies testing other h-mAbs are underway. Recent developments in molecular technology allowed the construction of chimeric and hyperchimeric mAbs[177] with hypervariable regions of murine origin combined with the other parts of the immunoglobulin molecule derived from the human amino acid sequence. These may eliminate most of the problems evoked by purely murine mAbs and offer the possibility of switching a primary IgM to a more active IgG3 h-mAb. The impact of these techniques on the treatment of melanoma patients has yet to be studied. It is likely that they may permit prolonged treatment with reduced risk of anaphylactic reactions and development of neutralizing human anti-mouse antibodies (HAMA).

Combinations of mAbs with cytokines are promising, given the ability of cytokines to augment the numbers and activity of effector cells (ADCC) and the potential of interferons and other cytokines to modulate cell surface antigen expression on effector and target cells. A recently published phase I trial combining IFN-alpha and R24 mAb at low doses showed moderate toxicity, not much different from that to be expected with IFN-alpha alone. Only one transient minor response was noted among 15 patients,[178] but one must consider our lack of information regarding optimal doses/routes/schedules of R24 alone, or in combined modality trials, in assessing therapeutic outcome. In addition to the potential therapeutic synergism between IFNs (or other cytokines) and mAbs, there is also the possibility of interference, for example, by earlier and stronger induction of HAMA. This is likely for the combination of mAb with IL-2, which has resulted in one PR and two minor responses among 20 patients.[179] We will probably have to wait for human or humanized mAbs to be able to reasonably explore the potential of mAbs in combination with cytokines, which may increase not only the level of ADCC but also the efficiency of mAb targeting by increasing the permeability of the capillaries and postcapillary venules. Concomitant alteration of other factors, such as tissue pressure that may physiologically impede mAb delivery to tumor sites, may further improve the results.

The combination of cellular immunotherapy with mAbs has also been attempted in several ways. Hetero-cross-linked antibodies (hcl-Abs) have been constructed, which possess a binding site directed against a tumor-associated antigen on one side and one directed against Fc-gamma-receptors on the other side. Their Fc-receptor binding site allows such hcl-Abs to bind to large granular lymphocytes that affect ADCC. The TAA-specific part of the hcl-Abs serve the nonspecific killer cells as artificial receptors and convert them to effector cells specific for the TAA recognized by the hcl-Ab. Using this method, peripheral blood mononuclear cells (PBMNC) show substantially increased specific tumor cell lysis in vitro and inhibition of tumor growth in animal systems.[180] LAK cells may also be "armed" in this manner, but the benefit may be smaller, since these cells may localize less to the tumor than hcl-Ab-coated T-lymphocytes. The same may be true if tumor cells are to be precoated in vivo by injection of conventional mAbs in order to make them easier targets before LAK cells are to be adoptively transfused. Increased tumor destruction may be less impressive than in vitro, due to the fact that not the cells expanded in vitro but those recruited de novo from PBMNC may be the truly effective cell population in vivo.

POSSIBLE REASONS FOR FAILURE OF MODERN POTENT IMMUNOTHERAPY

Even though developments in biotechnology have provided us with formidable tools for immunotherapy and will allow further progress, limitations that may explain the suboptimal results in trials to date must be considered.

First of all, the principles of homeostasis apply to the immune system as to most other dynamic biological systems that are vital to life. It is inevitable that after an immunologic stimulus, negative feedback mechanisms are activated to bring the immune system back towards its resting steady state. The stronger the perturbing stimuli are, the stronger the negative feedback mechanisms are likely to be, balancing the perturbation. In the case of malignancy and some infections, the down-regulation of an immune response can take place long before the adverse antigenic stimulus (organism or tumor) is eliminated. Clearly, increased doses and repetitive or continuous exposure to the maximal stimuli may not give superior results over moderate stimuli. A better understanding of the regulatory network and the influence of dose and treatment schedule eliciting immune responses in individual patients will allow us to improve the efficacy of future immunotherapy.

Despite actual and future improvements, the heterogeneity of the expression of tumor-associated and MHC antigens, as well as adhesion molecules, make the tumor cells heterogeneous in regard to susceptibility to immunologic therapies and will always provide a basis for selection of resistant clones in vivo as has already been documented[138,181] and is reflected in the mixed responses frequently observed with immunotherapy.

Furthermore, poor vascularization and the presence of substances like fibrinogen[182] and tumor-associated haptoglobin,[183] which can obscure tumor from immune effector cells, may prevent both recognition and effector function by the immune system. Carefully designed and rationally developed combinations of immunologic modalities and drugs, as well as radiotherapy, may overcome some of these limitations.

CONCLUSION

Immunotherapy has found its place in the armamentarium employed against malignant melanoma. After results from a myriad of studies with agents like *Corynebacterium parvum* and BCG during the "pre-cytokine" era, monotherapy with interferons has achieved a consistent track record of objective responses in 15 to 20 percent of patients, and has been accompanied by tolerable side effects. Interleukin-2 monotherapy has achieved comparable response rates of approximately 20 percent, at a cost of toxicity that has mandated high-level support when IL-2 is given as maximally tolerable bolus i.v. injections, the route of administration that has appeared most active. In contrast to animal studies, the usefulness of adoptive cellular therapy with in vitro generated LAK cells for melanoma patients remains unproven, and the enormous costs of this modality have no clinical justification to date in routine practice. Studies using tumor infiltrating lymphocytes are at least as costly and have been grounded in conceptual framework that differs from the concept of massive nonspecific stimulation and favors the generation of autologous tumor-specific, MHC-restricted T-killer lymphocytes and, even more important for the future, autologous tumor-specific $CD4^+$ T-helper cells, which may be more likely to overcome the well-recognized general and local immunosuppression in tumor patients. Genetic alteration of the adoptively transfused TIL and the use of rationally designed combinations of multiple cytokines will certainly further improve the response rate of 25 to 50 percent. Passive specific immunotherapy with murine mAbs has consistently shown an ability to achieve responses, but to the present time these have not exceeded 20 percent. The possibility of producing humanized murine or purely human mAb against melanoma-associated antigens may elevate this form of therapy, avoiding the induction of neutralizing antibodies. Active specific immunotherapy has also shown successes but is earlier in standardization and broader scale application for therapy of melanoma. By introducing more efficient adjuvants, combinations with cytokines during immunization, or by genetic alteration of the tumor cells to be used as immunogen or vaccine, significant improvements may be anticipated in this area. A better understanding of the immunoregulatory network may enable us to adapt therapy to the immunologic reactions seen in individual patients and may allow us to circumvent negative feedback loops, which presently may damp the successful application of immunotherapy for cancer. Future studies will also have to address the question of whether it is just one subset of melanoma patients who are likely to respond to any kind of immunotherapy or whether each form of immunotherapy has its own subset of responders. If so, this would greatly enhance the total number of patients likely to benefit from immunotherapy, assuming we will be able to select the appropriate form of immunostimulation in advance.

REFERENCES

1. Everson TC. The spontaneous regression of cancer. *Prog Clin Cancer* 3:79, 1967.
2. Nathanson L. Spontaneous regression of malignant melanoma: A review of the literature on incidence, clinical features, and possible mechanisms. *J Natl Cancer Inst Monogr* 44:67–76, 1976.
3. Reed RC, Gutterman JU, Mavligit GM, Burgess MA, and Hersh EM. Corynebacterium parvum: Preliminary report of a phase I clinical and immunological study in cancer patients. In: Halpern B (ed). *Corynebacterium Parvum.* New York: Plenum Press, 1975, 349–366.
4. Karakousis CP, Didolkar MS, and Han T. Chemoimmunotherapy (DTIC and Corynebacterium parvum) for disseminated malignant melanoma. Letter to Editors. *Cancer Treat Rep* 65(9–10):925–926, 1981.
5. Robidoux A, Gutterman JU, Bodey GP, and Hersh EM. Actinomycin-D plus 5-(3,3-dimethyl-1-triazeno)-imidazole-4-carboxamide (DTIC) with or without intravenous Corynebacterium parvum in metastatic malignant melanoma. *Cancer* 49:2246–2251, 1982.
6. Morton DL. Adjuvant immunotherapy of malignant melanoma: Results of a randomized trial in patients with LN metastasis. In: Terry WD, and Rosenberg SA (eds.), *Immunotherapy of Human Cancer.* New York: Elsevier, 1982, 245–249.
7. Gutterman JU, Mavligit GM, and Gottlieb JA. Chemoimmunotherapy of disseminated malignant melanoma with dimethyl triazano imidazole carboxamide (DTIC) and bacillus Calmette Guerin (BCG). *N Engl J Med* 291:592–597, 1974.
8. Eilber FR, Morton DL, Holmes EC, Sparks FC, and Ramming KP. Adjuvant immunotherapy with BCG in treatment of regional lymph node metastases from malignant melanoma. *N Engl J Med* 294(5):237–240, 1976.
9. Pinsky CM, Hirshaut Y, Wanebo HJ, Fortner JG, Mike V, Schottenfield D, and Oettgen HF. Randomized trial of bacillus Calmette-Guerin (percutaneous administration) as surgical adjuvant immunotherapy for patients with stage-II melanoma. *Ann N Y Acad Sci* 49(6):1079–1084, 1982.
10. Lipton A, Harvey HA, Lawrence B, Gottlieb R, Kukrika M, Dixon R, Graham W, Miller S, Heckard R, Schelzel D, and White DS. Corynebacterium parvum versus BCG ad-

juvant immunotherapy in human malignant melanoma. *Cancer* 51(1):57–60, 1983.

11. Chiba M, Jimboco K, Kizukuri K, and Homma K. Chemoimmunotherapy for disseminated malignant melanoma with DTIC, ACNU, VCR and OK 432. *J Dermatol* 9:23, 1982.
12. Israel L. Report on 414 cases of human tumors treated with Corynebacterium parvum. In Halper B (ed.), *Corynebacterium parvum*. New York: Plenum Press, 1975, 389–401.
13. Nathanson L, Schoenfeld D, Regelson W, Colsky J, and Mittelman A. Prospective comparison of intralesional and multipuncture BCG in recurrent intradermal melanoma. *Cancer* 43:1630–1635, 1979.
14. Cunningham-Rundles WF, Hirshaut Y, Pinsky CM, and Oettgen HF. Phase I trial of intralesional C. parvum. *Clin Res* 377:1975.
15. Costanzi JJ. Chemotherapy and BCG in the treatment of disseminated malignant melanoma. In: Terry WD, and Windhorst D (eds.), *Immunotherapy of Cancer: Present Status of Trials in Man*. New York: Raven Press, 1978, 87–93.
16. Veronesi U, Adamus J, Aubert C, Bajetta E, Beretta G, Bonadonna G, Bufalino R, Cascinelli N, Cocconi G, Durand J, De Marsillac J, Ikonopisov RL, Kiss B, Lejeune F, MacKie R, Madej G, Mulder H, Mechl Z, Milton GW, Morabito A, Peter H, Priario J, Paul E, Rumke P, Sertoli R, and Tomin R. A randomized trial of adjuvant chemotherapy and immunotherapy in cutaneous melanoma. *N Engl J Med* 307(15):913–916, 1982.
17. Cascinelli N, Rumke P, MacKie R, Morabito A, and Bufalino R. The significance of conversion of skin reactivity to efficacy of bacillus Calmette-Guerin (BCG) vaccinations given immediately after radical surgery in stage II melanoma patients. *Cancer Immunol Immunother* 28(4):282–286, 1989.
18. Inagawa H, Oshima H, Soma G-I, and Mizuno D. TNF induces endogenous TNF in vivo: The basis of EET therapy is a combination of rTNF together with endogenous TNF. *J Biol Response Modif* 7:596–607, 1988.
19. Nio Y, Zighelboim J, Berek JS, and Bonavida B. Sensitivity of ovarian tumor cells to effector cells generated by various biological response modifiers. *Nat Immun Cell Growth Regul* 9:283–296, 1990.
20. Lafreniere R, Borkenhagen K, Bryant LD, Ng S, and Hayton S. Synergistic actions of picibanil (OK-432) on recombinant interleukin-2 induction of tumor-infiltrating lymphocyte expansion, cytotoxicity, and phenotypic differentiation. *J Biol Response Modif* 9:53-60, 1990.
21. Uchida A, and Micksche M. In vitro augmentation of natural killing potential by OK-432. *Int J Immunopharmac* 3:365–375, 1981.
22. Hoshino T, and Uchida A. OK-432 (picibanil): Property, action and clinical effectiveness. In: Hoshino T and Uchida A (eds.), *Clinical and Experimental Studies in Immunotherapy. Proceedings of an International Congress of Chemotherapy, Vienna, September 1983*. Amsterdam: Excerpta Medica, 1984, 1–19.
23. Renoux G, and Renoux M. Levamisole inhibits and cures a solid malignant tumor and its pulmonary metastases in mice. *Nature* 240:217–218, 1972.
24. Serrou B, Pujiol H, Dorras J, and Ganci L. Results of a nonrandomized trial in malignant melanoma patients (Clark's stage III-V) treated by post-surgical chemoimmunotherapy. *Rec Res Cancer Res* 68:363–366, 1979.
25. Spitler LE, and Sagebiel R. An randomized trial of levamisole versus placebo as adjuvant therapy in malignant melanoma. *N Engl J Med* 303(20):1143–1147, 1980.
26. Lejeune F, Macher E, Kleeberg UR, Rümke P, Prade M, Thomas D, and Suciu S, for the EORTC Malignant Melanoma Cooperative Group. A randomized study on DTIC, levamisole and placebo as adjuvant treatment of high risk stage-I primary melanoma. *Eur J Cancer Clin Oncol* 24:S81–S90, 1988.
27. Costanzi JJ, Fletcher WS, Balcerzak P, Taylor S, Eyre HJ, O'Bryan RM, Al-Sarraf M, and Frank J. Combination chemotherapy plus levamisol in the treatment of disseminated malignant melanoma. *Cancer* 53:833–836, 1984.
28. Quirt IC, Shelley WE, Pater JL, Bodurtha AJ, McCulloch PB, McPherson TA, Paterson AHG, Prentice R, Silver HKB, Willan AR, Wilson K, and Zee B. Improved survival in patients with poor prognosis malignant melanoma treated with adjuvant levamisole: A phase III study by the National Cancer Institute of Canada Clinical Trials Group. *J Clin Oncol* 9:729–735, 1991.
29. Moertel CG, Fleming TR, Macdonald JS, Haller DG, Laurie JA, Goodman PJ, Ungerleider JS, Emerson WA, Tormey DC, Glick JH, Veeder MH, and Mailliard JA. Levamisole and fluorouracil for adjuvant therapy of resected colon carcinoma. *N Engl J Med* 322:352–358, 1990.
30. Thornes RD, and Lynch G. Combination of cimetidine with other drugs for treatment of cancer. Letter to the Editor. *N Engl J Med* 308(10):591, 1983.
31. Stewart T. *The Interferon System*. New York: Academic Press, 1979.
32. Lengyel P. Biochemistry of interferons and their actions. *Ann Ref Biochem* 51:251, 1982.
33. Giacomini P, Aguzzi A, Pestka S, Fisher PB, and Ferrone S. Modulation by recombinant DNA leukocyte (alpha) and fibroblast (beta) interferons of the expression and shedding of HLA- and tumor-associated antigens by human melanoma cells. *J Immunol* 133(3):1649–1655, 1984.
34. Carrel S, Schmidt-Kessen A, and Giuffrè L. Recombinant interferon-gamma can induce the expression of HLA-DR and -DC on DR-negative melanoma cells and enhance the expression of HLA-ABC and tumor-associated antigens. *Eur J Immunol* 15:118–123, 1985.
35. Wadler S, Einzig AI, Dutcher JP, Ciobanu N, Landau L, and Wiernik PH. Phase II trial of recombinant alpha-2b-interferon and low-dose cyclophosphamide in advanced melanoma and renal cell carcinoma. *Am J Clin Oncol* 11(1):55–59, 1988.
36. Sayers TJ, Mason AT, and Ortaldo JR. Regulation of human natural killer cell activity by interferon-gamma: Lack of a role in interleukin 2-mediated augmentation. *J Immunol* 136(6):2176–2180, 1986.
37. Kirkwood JM, and Ernstoff MS. Therapeutic option with recombinant interferons: Lessons drawn from studies of human melanoma. *Semin Oncol* 13:48, 1986.
38. Krown SE, Burk MW, Kirkwood JM, Kerr D, Morton DL, and Oettgen HF. Human leukocyte (alpha) interferon in metastatic malignant melanoma: The American Cancer Society phase II trial. *Cancer Treat Rep* 68:5:723–726, 1984.
39. Creagan ET, Ahmann DL, Green SJ, Long HJ, Frytak S, O'Fallon JR, and Itri LM. Phase II study of low-dose recombinant leukocyte A interferon in disseminated malignant melanoma. *J Clin Oncol* 2(9):1002–1005, 1984.
40. Creagan ET, Ahmann DL, Green SJ, Long HJ, Rubin J, Schutt AJ, and Dziewanowski ZE. Phase II study of recombinant leukocyte A interferon (rIFN-alpha A) in disseminated malignant melanoma. *Cancer* 54(12):2844–2849, 1984.
41. Coates A, Rallings M, Hersey P, and Swanson C. Phase II study of recombinant alpha *2*-interferon in advanced malignant melanoma. *J Interferon Res* 6:1–4, 1986.
42. Hersey P, Hasic E, MacDonald M, Edwards A, Spurling A,

Coates AS, Milton GW, and McCarthy WH. Effects of recombinant leukocyte interferon (rIFN-alpha a) on tumor growth and immune responses in patients with metastatic melanoma. *Br J Cancer* 51(6):815–826, 1985.
43. Legha SS, Papadopoulos NE, Plager C, Ring S, Chawla SP, Evans LM, and Benjamin RS. Clinical evaluation of recombinant interferon alfa-2a (Roferon-a) in metastatic melanoma using two different schedules. *J Clin Oncol* 5(8):1240–1246, 1987.
44. Elsasser-Beile U, and Drews H. Interferon in the treatment of malignant melanoma. Results of clinical studies. *Fortschr Med* 105(21):401, 1987.
45. Steiner A, Wolf C, and Pehamberger H. Comparison of the effects of three different treatment regimens of recombinant interferons (r-IFN alpha, r-IFN gamma, and r-IFN-alpha + cimetidine) in disseminated malignant melanoma. *J Cancer Res Clin Oncol* 113:459–465, 1987.
46. Kirkwood JM, Ernstoff MS, Davis CA, Reiss M, Ferraresi R, and Rudnick SA. Comparison of intramuscular and intravenous recombinant alpha-2 interferon in melanoma and other cancers. *Ann Intern Med* 103(1):32–36, 1985.
47. Dorval T, Palangie T, Jouve M, Garcia-Giralt E, Israel L, Falcoff E, Schwab D, and Pouillart P. Clinical phase II trial of recombinant DNA interferon (interferon alfa 2b) in patients with metastatic malignant melanoma. *Cancer* 58(2):215–218, 1986.
48. Robinson WA, Mughal TI, Thomas MR, Johnson M, and Spiegel RJ. Treatment of metastatic malignant melanoma with recombinant interferon alpha-2. *Immunobiol* 172:275–282, 1986.
49. Sertoli MR, Bernengo MG, Ardizzoni A, Brunetti I, Falcone A, Vidili MG, Cusimano MP, Appino A, Doveil G, Fortini C, and Rosso R. Phase II trial of recombinant alpha-2b interferon in the treatment of metastatic skin melanoma. *Oncology* 46(2):96–98, 1989.
50. Creagan ET, Ahmann DL, Long HJ, Frytak S, Sherwin SA, and Chang MN. Phase II study of recombinant interferon-gamma in patients with disseminated malignant melanoma. *Cancer Treat Rep* 71(9):843–844, 1987.
51. Perez R, Lipton A, Harvey HA, Simmonds MA, Romano PJ, Imboden SL, Giudice G, Downing MR, and Alton NK. A phase I trial of recombinant human gamma interferon (IFN-g_{4A}) in patients with advanced malignancy. *J Biol Response Modif* 7:309–317, 1988.
52. Ernstoff MS, Trautman T, Davis CA, Reich SD, Witman P, Balser J, Rudnick S, and Kirkwood JM. A randomized phase I/II study of continuous versus intermittent intravenous interferon gamma in patients with metastatic melanoma. *J Clin Oncol* 5(11):1804–1810, 1987.
53. Kirkwood JM, Logan TF, Vlock DR, and Ernstoff MS. Biological response modifiers in the therapy of metastatic melanoma. In: Rumke P (ed.), *Therapy of Advanced Melanoma. Pigment Cells. Vol. 10.* Basel, Switzerland: Karger, 1990, 105–140.
54. Osanto S, Jansen R, Naipal AMIH, Gratama J-W, Van-Leeuwen A, and Cleton FJ. In vivo effects of combination treatment with recombinant interferon-gamma and -alpha in metastatic melanoma. *Int J Cancer* 43:1001–1006, 1989.
55. Kurzrock R, Rosenblum MG, Quesada JR, Sherwin SA, Itri LM, and Gutterman JU. Phase I study of a combination of recombinant interferon-alpha and recombinant interferon-gamma in cancer patients. *J Clin Oncol* 4:1677, 1986.
56. Ernstoff MS, Nair S, Bahnson RB, Miketic LM, Banner B, Gooding W, Day R, Whiteside T, Hakala T, and Kirkwood JM. Sequential administration of recombinant DNA-produced interferons: A phase IA trial of combination rIFN gamma and rIFN alpha in patients with metastatic renal cell carcinoma. *J Clin Oncol* 8:1637–1649, 1990.
57. Talpaz M, Plager C, Quesada J, Benjamin R, Kantarjian H, and Gutterman J. Difluoromethylornithine and leukocyte interferon: A phase I study in cancer patients. *Eur J Cancer Clin Oncol* 22(6):685–689, 1986.
58. Budd GT, Osgood B, Barna B, Boyett JM, Finke J, Medendorp SV, Murthy S, Novak C, Sergi J, Tubbs R, and Bukowski RM. Phase I clinical trial of interleukin 2 and alpha-interferon: Toxicity and immunologic effects. *Cancer Res* 49:6432–6436, 1989.
59. Rosenberg SA, Lotze MT, Young JC, Linehan WM, Seipp C, Calabro S, Karp SE, Sherry RM, Steinberg S, and White DE. Combination therapy with interleukin-2 and alpha-interferon for the treatment of patients with advanced cancer. *J Clin Oncol* 7(12):1863–1874, 1989.
60. Lee KH, Talpaz M, Rothberg JM, Murray JL, Papadopoulos N, Plager C, Benjamin R, Levitt D, and Gutterman J. Concomitant administration of recombinant human interleukin-2 and recombinant interferon-alpha 2a in cancer patients: A phase I study. *J Clin Oncol* 7:1726–1732, 1989.
61. Sznol M, Mier JW, Sparano J, Gaynor ER, Weiss GR, Margolin KA, Bar MH, Hawkins MJ, Atkins MB, Dutcher JP, Fisher RI, Boldt DH, Doroshow JH, Louie A, and Aronson FR. A phase I study of high-dose interleukin-2 in combination with interferon-alpha-2b. *J Biol Response Modif* 9:529–537, 1990.
62. Bukowski RM, Murthy S, Sergi J, Budd TG, McKeever S, Medendorp SV, Tubbs R, Gibbson V, and Finke J. Phase I trial of continuous infusion recombinant interleukin-2 and intermittent recombinant interferon-alpha-2a: Clinical effects. *J Biol Response Modif* 9:538–545, 1990.
63. Whitehead RP, Figlin R, Citro ML, Pfile J, Morton D, Patel D, Jones G, and Levitt D. A phase II study of concomitant recombinant human interleukin-2 (IL-2) and recombinant interferon alpha-2a (alpha-IFN) in patients with disseminated malignant melanoma. *Proc Amer Soc Clin Oncol* 9:281–#1088, 1990, Abstract.
64. Goey SH, Monson JRT, Stahel RA, Calabresi F, Mertelsmann R, Holdener EE, and Stoter G. A multicenter study of human recombinant interleukin-2 (IL2) and alfa-2a interferon (aIFN) in metastatic melanoma. *Proc Amer Soc Clin Oncol* 9:185–#3922, 1990, Abstract.
65. Krigel RL, Padavic-Shaller KA, Rudolph AR, Litwin S, Konrad M, Bradley EC, and Comis RL. A phase I study of recombinant interleukin 2 plus recombinant beta-interferon. *Cancer Res* 48:3875–3881, 1988.
66. Redman BG, Flaherty L, Chou T-H, AL-Katib A, Kraut M, Martino S, Chen B, Kaplan J, and Valdivieso M. A phase I trial of recombinant interleukin-2 combined with recombinant interferon-gamma in patients with cancer. *J Clin Oncol* 8:1269–1276, 1990.
67. McLeod GR, Thomson DB, and Hersey P. Recombinant interferon alfa-2a in advanced malignant melanoma. A phase I-II study in combination with DTIC. *Int J Cancer Suppl.* 1:31–35, 1987.
68. Kirkwood JM, and Ernstoff MS. The role of interferons in the management of melanoma. In: Nathanson L (ed.), *Management of Advanced Melanoma.* New York: Churchill Livingstone, Inc., 1986, 209.
69. Abdi EA, McPherson TA, and Tan YH. Combination of fibroblast interferon (HuIFN beta), carboxamide (DTIC), and cimetidine for advanced malignant melanoma. *J Biol Response Modif* 5:423–428, 1986.
70. Falkson CI, Falkson G, and Falkson HC. Improved results with the addition of recombinant interferon alpha-2b to dacarbazine in the treatment of patients with metastatic

malignant melanoma. *Proc Am Assoc Cancer Res* 31:199–#1185, 1990, Abstract.
71. von Wussow P, Block B, Hartmann F, and Deicher H. Intralesional interferon-alpha therapy in advanced malignant melanoma. *Cancer* 61(6):1071–1074, 1988.
72. Ruggiero V, Latham K, and Baglioni C. Cytostatic and cytotoxic activity of tumor necrosis factor on human cancer cells. *J Immunol* 138(8):2711–2717, 1987.
73. Kull FC, Jacobs S, and Cuatrecasa P. Cellular receptor for 125I-labeled tumor necrosis factor specific binding, affinity labeling, and relationship to sensitivity. *Proc Natl Acad Sci U S A* 82:5756–5760, 1985.
74. Darzynkiewicz Z, Williamson B, Carswell EA, and Old LJ. Cell cycle-specific effects of tumor necrosis factor. *Cancer Res* 44:83–90, 1984.
75. Laster SM, Wood JG, and Gooding LR. Tumor necrosis factor can induce both apoptic and necrotic forms of cell lysis. *J Immunol* 141(8):2629–2634, 1986.
76. Salmon SE, Young L, Scuderi P, and Clark B. Antineoplastic effects of tumor necrosis factor alone and in combination with gamma-interferon on tumor biopsies in clonogenic assay. *J Clin Oncol* 5(11):1816–1821, 1987.
77. Kaushansky K, Broudy VC, Harlan JM, and Adamson JW. Tumor necrosis factor-alpha and tumor necrosis factor-beta (lymphotoxin) stimulate the production of granulocyte-macrophage colony-stimulating factor, macrophage colony-stimulating factor, and IL-1 in vivo. *J Immunol* 141:3410–3415, 1988.
78. Mace KF, Ehrke MJ, Hori K, Maccubbin DL, and Mihich E. Role of tumor necrosis factor in macrophage activation and tumoricidal activity. *Cancer Res* 48:5427–5432, 1988.
79. Ostensen ME, Thiele DL, and Lipsky PE. Cachexin/tumor necrosis factor-alpha enhances cytolytic activity of human natural killer cells. *J Immunol* 138:4185–4191, 1987.
80. Klebanoff SJ, Vadas MA, Harlan JM, Sparks LH, Gamble JR, Agosti JM, and Waltersdorph AM. Stimulation of neutrophils by tumor necrosis factor. *J Immunol* 136:4220–4225, 1986.
81. Scheurich P, Thomas B, Ucer U, and Pfizenmaier K. Immunoregulatory activity of recombinant human tumor necrosis factor (TNf)-alpha: Induction of TNF receptors on human T cells and TNF-alpha-mediated enhancement of T cell responses. *J Immunol* 138:1786–1790, 1987.
82. Collins T, Lapierre LA, Fiers W, Strominger JL, and Pober JS. Recombinant human tumor necrosis factor increases mRNA levels and surface expression of HLA-A, B antigens in vascular endothelial cells and dermal fibroblasts in vitro. *Proc Natl Acad Sci U S A* 83:446–450, 1986.
83. Vilcek J, Palombella VJ, Henriksen-DeStefano D, Swenson C, Feinman R, Hiral M, and Tsujimoto M. Fibroblast growth enhancing activity of tumor necrosis factor and its relationship to other polypeptide growth factors. *J Exp Med* 163:632–643, 1986.
84. Goodwin JS, and Ceuppens J. Regulation of the immune response by prostaglandins. *J Clin Immunol* 3:295, 1983.
85. Ferri WA, Bahnson R, Hakala T, Schwentker F, Banner B, Downs MA, Nadler P, and Ernstoff MS. Phase I trial of intravesical recombinant human tumor necrosis factor (rHuTNF) in patients with superficial transitional cell carcinoma (TCC) or carcinoma in situ (CIS) of the urinary bladder. *Proc Amer Soc Clin Oncol* 9:153–#595, 1990, Abstract.
86. Reichman B, Markman M, Ianotti N, Hakes T, Hoskins W, Rubin S, Jones W, Almadrones L, and Lewis JL, Jr. Phase I trial of intraperitoneal (IP) recombinant tumor necrosis factor (rTNF). *Proc Amer Soc Clin Oncol* 8:64–#249, 1989, Abstract.
87. Lienard D, Delmotte JJ, Renard N, Ewalenko P, and Lejeune FJ. High dose recombinant tumor necrosis factor-alfa in combination with interferon-gamma and melphalan in isolation perfusion of the limbs for melanoma and sarcoma. *J Clin Oncol* 10:52–60, 1992.
88. Sacchi M, Snyderman CH, Heo DS, Johnson JF, d'Amico F, Herberman RB, and Whiteside TL. Local adoptive immunotherapy of head and neck cancer xenografts in nude mice with lymphokine-activated killer cells and inteleukin-2. *Cancer Res* 50:3113–3118, 1990.
89. Margolin KA, Rayner AA, Hawkins MJ, Atkins MB, Dutcher JP, Fisher RI, Weiss GR, Doroshow JH, Jaffe HS, Roper M, Parkinson DR, Wiernik PH, Creekmore SP, and Boldt DH. Interleukin-2 and lymphokine-activated killer cell therapy of solid tumors: Analysis of toxicity and management guidelines. *J Clin Oncol* 7(4):486–498, 1989.
90. Gaynor ER, Weiss GR, Margolin KA, Aronson FR, Sznol M, Demchak P, Grima KM, Fisher RI, Boldt DH, Doroshow JH, Bar MH, Hawkins MJ, Mier JW, and Caliendo G. Phase I study of high-dose continuous-infusion recombinant interleukin-2 and autologous lymphokine-activated killer cells in patients with metastatic or unresectable malignant melanoma and renal cell carcinoma. *J Natl Cancer Inst* 82:1397–1402, 1990.
91. Klempner MS, Noring R, Mier JW, and Atkins MB. An acquired chemotactic defect in neutrophils from patients receiving interleukin-2 immunotherapy. *N Engl J Med* 322(14):959–965, 1990.
92. Staunton MR, Scully MC, Le Boit PE, and Aronson FR. Life-threatening bullous skin eruptions during Interleukin-2 therapy. *J Natl Cancer Inst* 83(1):56–57, 1991.
93. Mulé JJ, Shu S, Schwarz SL, and Rosenberg SA. Adoptive immunotherapy of established pulmonary metastases with LAK cells and recombinant interleukin-2. *Science* 225:1487–1489, 1984.
94. Lafreniere R, and Rosenberg SA. Adoptive immunotherapy of murine hepatic metastases with lymphokine activated killer (LAK) cells and recombinant interleukin 2 (rIL2) can mediate the regression of both immunogenic and nonimmunogenic sarcomas and an adenocarcinoma. *J Immunol* 135:4273–4280, 1985.
95. Mulé JJ, Shu S, and Rosenberg SA. The anti-tumor efficacy of lymphokine-activated killer cells and recombinant interleukin 2 in vivo. *J Immunol* 135(1):646–652, 1985.
96. Rosenberg SA, Lotze MT, Yang JC, Aebersold PM, Linehan WM, Seipp CA, and White DE. Experience with the use of high-dose inteleukin-2 in the treatment of 652 cancer patients. *Ann Surg* 210:474–485, 1990.
97. Parkinson DR, and Lotzova E. Interleukin-2, killer cells and cancer therapy: an overview. *Nat Immun Cell Growth Regul* 9:237–241, 1990.
98. Atkins MB, Gould JA, Allegretta M, Li JJ, Dempsey RA, Rudders RA, Parkinson DR, Reichlin S, and Mier JW. Phase I evaluation of recombinant interleukin-2 in patients with advanced malignant disease. *J Clin Oncol* 4(9):1380–1391, 1986.
99. Thompson JA, Lee DJ, Lindgren CG, Benz LA, Collins C, Levitt D, and Fefer A. Influence of dose and duration of infusion of interleukin-2 on toxicity and immunomodulation. *J Clin Oncol* 6:669–678, 1988.
100. Sosman JA, Kohler PC, Hank JA, Moore KH, Bechhofer R, Storer B, and Sondel PM. Repetitive weekly cycles of interleukin-2. II. Clinical and immunologic effects of dose, schedule, and addition of indomethacin. *J Natl Cancer Inst* 80:1451–1461, 1988.
101. Richards JM, Bajorin DF, Vogelzang NJ, Houghton AN, Seigler HF, Sell K, Zeffrin J, and Levitt D. Treatment of

metastatic melanoma with continuous intravenous (CIV) IL2 ± LAK cells: A randomized trial. *Proc Amer Soc Clin Oncol* 9:279–#1080, 1990, Abstract.

102. Kohler PC, Hank JA, Moore KH, Storer B, Bechhofer R, Hong R, and Sondel PM. Phase I clinical trial of recombinant interleukin-2: A comparison of bolus and continuous intravenous infusion. *Cancer Invest* 7(3):213–223, 1989.
103. Paciucci PA, Bhardwaj S, Odchimar R, Glidewell O, and Holland JF. Immunotherapy for metastatic cancer with recombinant interleukin-2 (rIL2) by continuous infusion with and without adoptive cell transfer. *Proc Amer Soc Clin Oncol* 7:163–#630, 1988, Abstract.
104. Creekmore SP, Harris JE, Ellis TM, Braun DP, McMannis JD, Cohen II, Bhoopalam N, Jassak PF, Cahill MA, Canzoneri CL, and Fisher RI. Phase I/II trial of recombinant interleukin-2 by 24-hr continuous infusion—an Illinois Cancer Council trial. *Proc Amer Soc Clin Oncol* 6:244–#960, 1987, Abstract.
105. Dutcher J, Gaynor E, Boldt DH, Doroshow J, Rayner AA, Sznol M, and Mier J. Phase II study of high dose intravenous continuous infusion (IVCI) interleukin-2 (IL2) and lymphokine activated killer (LAK) cells in patients (PTS) with metastatic melanoma (MM). *Proc Amer Soc Clin Oncol* 87:2827–#1097, 1987, Abstract.
106. Rubin JT, Elwood LJ, Rosenberg SA, and Lotze MT. Immunohistochemical correlates of response to recombinant interleukin-2-based immunotherapy in humans. *Cancer Res* 49:7086–7092, 1989.
107. Mitchell MS, Kempf RA, Harel W, Shau H, Boswell WD, Lind S, and Bradley EC. Effectiveness and tolerability of low-dose cyclophosphamide and low-dose intravenous interleukin-2 disseminated melanoma. *J Clin Oncol* 6(3):409–424, 1988.
108. Lindemann A, Hoeffken K, Schmidt RE, Diehl V, Kloke O, Gamm H, Hayungs J, Oster W, Boehm M, Franks CR, Herrmann F, and Mertelsmann R. A multicenter trial of interleukin-2 and low-dose cyclophosphamide in highly chemotherapy-resistant malignancies. *Cancer Treat Rev* 16 (Suppl A):53–57, 1989.
109. Stoter G, Shiloni E, Gundersen S, Cleton FJ, Iacobelli S, Bijman JTh, Palmer P, Franks CR, and Rodenhuis S. Alternating recombinant human interleukin-2 and dacarbazine in advanced melanoma. A multicentric phase II study. *Cancer Treat Rev* 16:59–63, 1989.
110. Stoter G, Shiloni E, Aamdal S, Cleton FJ, Iacobelli S, Bijman JT, Palmer P, Franks CR, and Rodenhuis S. Sequential administration of recombinant human interleukin-2 and dacarbazine in metastatic melanoma. A multicentre phase II study. *Eur J Cancer Clin Oncol* 25:S41–S43, 1989.
111. Flaherty L. The combination of recombinant interleukin-2 and dacarbazine (DTIC) in metastatic malignant melanoma. *Cancer Treat Rev* 16 (Suppl. A):65–66, 1989.
112. Flaherty LE, Redman BG, Chabot GG, Martino S, Gualdoni SM, Heilbrun LK, Valdivieso M, and Bradley EC. A phase I-II study of dacarbazine in combination with outpatient interleukin-2 in metastatic malignant melanoma. *Cancer* 65(11):2471–2477, 1990.
113. Flaherty L, Robinson W, Redman B, Gonzales R, Martino S, Kraut M, Valdivieso M, and Rudolph A. A phase II study of Dacarbazine (DTIC), Cisplatin (DDP), and outpatient interleukin-2 (IL-2) (RIDD-2) in metastatic malignant melanoma (M.M.M.). *Proc Amer Soc Clin Oncol* 9:187–#723, 1990, Abstract.
114. Atkins M, Demchak P, Mier J, Robert N, Gould J, and Sznol M. Phase II study of alternating interleukin-2 (IL2) and cisplatin (cisDDP) with WR-2721 in metastatic melanoma. *Proc Amer Soc Clin Oncol* 8:287–#280, 1980, Abstract.
115. Atkins M, Demchak P, Mier J, Robert N, and Sznol M. Phase II study of alternating interleukin-2 (IL2) and cisplatin (CDDP) with WR-2721 (WR) in metastatic melanoma. *Proc Amer Soc Clin Oncol* 9:186–#719, 1990, Abstract.
116. Redman BG, Flaherty L, Chou T-H, Nakeff A, Pillote K, and Kaplan J. Sequential dacarbazine/cisplatin and IL-2 in metastatic melanoma: Immunologic effects of therapy. *J Immunother* 10:147–151, 1991.
117. Griffith KD, Read EJ, Carrasquillo JA, Carter CS, Yang JC, Fisher B, Aebersold P, Packard BS, Yu MY, and Rosenberg SA. In vivo distribution of adoptively transferred indium-111-labeled tumor infiltrating lymphocytes and peripheral blood lymphocytes in patients with metastatic melanoma. *J Natl Cancer Inst* 81:1709–1717, 1989.
118. Dutcher JP, Creekmore S, Weiss GR, Margolin K, Markowitz AB, Roper M, Parkinson D, Ciobanu N, Fisher RI, Boldt DH, Doroshow JH, Rayner AA, Hawkins M, and Atkins M. A phase II study of interleukin-2 and lymphokine-activated killer cells in patients with metastatic malignant melanoma. *J Clin Oncol* 7:477–485, 1989.
119. Cascinelli N, Belli F, Marchini S, Marolda R, Prada A, Sciorelli G, Villani F, Gambacorti-Passerini C, Galazka A, and Parmiani G. A phase II study of the administration of recombinant interleukin 2 (rIL-2) plus lymphokine activated killer (LAK) cells in stage IV melanoma patients. *Tumori* 75:233–244, 1989.
120. Stahel RA, Sculier JP, Jost LM, Delforge A, Bron D, Gmur J, Oelz O, Sauter C, Stryckmans P, and Klastersky J. Tolerance and effectiveness of recombinant interleukin-2 (r-met Hu IL-2 [ala-125]) and lymphokine-activated killer cells in patients with metastatic solid tumors. *Eur J Cancer Clin Oncol* 25(6):965–972, 1989.
121. West WH. Continuous infusion recombinant inteleukin-2 (rIL-2) in adoptive cellular therapy of renal carcinoma and other malignancies. *Cancer Treat Rev* 16:83–89, 1989.
122. Rayner AA, Lionetto R, and Atkins MB. Phase II trial of Interleukin-2 bolus priming followed by continuous infusion with lymphokine activated killer cells (IL-2/LAK) in metastatic melanoma. *Proc Amer Soc Clin Oncol* 7:246, 1988, Abstract.
123. Hoon DSB, Ando I, Sviland G, Tsuchida T, Okun E, Morton DL, and Irie RF. Ganglioside GM2 expression on human melanoma cells correlates with sensitivity to lymphokine-activated killer cells. *Int J Cancer* 43:857–862, 1989.
124. Nair S, Ernstoff MS, Whiteside TL, Miketic L, Vlock DR, Gemperlein M, Bahnson R, Herberman RB, and Kirkwood JM. Adoptive immunotherapy with adherent LAK (ALAK) cells. *Proc Amer Soc Clin Oncol* 9:200–#775, 1990, Abstract.
125. Spiess PJ, Yang JC, and Rosenberg SA. In vivo antitumor activity of tumor-infiltrating lymphocytes expanded in recombinant interleukin-2. *J Natl Cancer Inst* 79:1067–1075, 1987.
126. Rosenberg SA, Packard BS, Aebersold PM, Solomon D, Topalian SL, Toy ST, Simon P, Lotze MT, Yang JC, Seipp CA, Simpson C, Carter C, Bock S, Schwartzentruber D, Wei JP, and White DE. Use of tumor-infiltrating lymphocytes and interleukin-2 in the immunotherapy of patients with metastatic melanoma. A preliminary report. *N Engl J Med* 319(25):1676–1680, 1988.
127. Whiteside TL, Jost LM, and Herberman RB. Tumor-infiltrating lymphocytes: Potential and limitations to their use for cancer therapy. *Crit Rev Oncol Hematol* 12:25–47, 1992.
128. Sondel PM, Sosman JA, Hank JA, Kohler PC, Storer B. Tumor infiltrating lymphocytes and interleukin-2 in melanomas (letter). *N Engl J Med* 320:1418–1420, 1989.

129. Kradin Rl, Lazarus DS, Dubinett SM, Gifford J, Grove B, Kurnick JT, Preffer FI, Pinto CE, Davidson E, Callahan RJ, and Strauss HW. Tumor-infiltrating lymphocytes and interleukin-2 in treatment of advanced cancer. *Lancet* 18:577–580, 1989.
130. Oldham RK, Dillman RO, Birch R, Barth N, Cohen RJ, Minor DR, Maleckar J, Yannelli J, and West WH. Treatment of advanced cancer with interleukin-2 (rIL-2) and tumor derived activated cells (TDAC). *Proc Am Assoc Cancer Res* 31:268–#1587, 1990, Abstract.
131. Aebersold P, Hyatt C, Johnson S, Hines K, Korcak L, Sanders M, Lotze M, Topolian S, Yang J, and Rosenberg SA. Lysis of autologous melanoma cells by tumor infiltrating is associated with clinical response. *J Natl Cancer Inst* 83:932–937, 1991.
132. Fisher B, Packard BS, Read EJ, Carrasquillo JA, Carter CS, Topalian SL, Yang JC, Yolles P, Larson SM, and Rosenberg SA. Tumor localization of adoptively transferred indium-111 labeled tumor-infiltrating lymphocytes in patients with metastatic melanoma. *J Clin Oncol* 7(2):250–261, 1989.
133. Rosenberg SA, Aebersold P, Cornetta K, Kasid A, Morgan RA, Moen R, Karson EM, Lotze MT, Yang JC, Topalian SL, Merino MJ, Culver K, Miller AD, Blaese RM, and Anderson WF. Gene transfer into humans—Immunotherapy of patients with advanced melanoma, using tumor-infiltrating lymphocytes modified by retroviral gene transduction. *N Engl J Med* 323:570–578, 1990.
134. Dillman RO, Oldham RK, Birch R, Barth NM, Cohen RJ, Minor DR, Maleckar J, Yannelli J, West W, National Biotherapy Study Group: Treatment of melanoma with interleukin-2 (IL-2) and tumor derived activated cells (TDAC). *Proc Amer Soc Clin Oncol* 9:276–#1069, 1990, Abstract.
135. Kavakami Y, Rosenberg SA, and Lotze MT. Interleukin-4 promotes the growth of tumor-infiltrating lymphocytes cytotoxic for human autologous melanoma. *J Exp Med* 168:2183–2191, 1988.
136. Mukherji B, Guha A, Chakraborty NG, Sivanandham M, Nashed AL, Sporn JR, and Ergin MT. Clonal analysis of cytotoxic and regulatory T cell responses against human melanoma. *J Exp Med* 169:1961–1976, 1989.
137. Chakraborty NG, Twardzik DR, Sivanandham M, Ergin MT, Hellstrom KE, and Mukherji B. Autologous melanoma-induced activation of regulatory T cells that suppress cytotoxic response. *J Immunol* 145(7):2359–2364, 1990.
138. Topalian SL, Kasid A, and Rosenberg SA. Immunoselection of a human melanoma resistant to specific lysis by autologous tumor-infiltrating lymphocytes. *J Immunol* 144(11): 4487–4495, 1990.
139. Logan T, Kirkwood J, Wolmark N, Whiteside T, Elder E, Vlock D, Ernstoff M, Dexter L, Posner M, and Herberman R. Pilot study of in vitro sensitized (IVS) T cells in adoptive transfer therapy of cancer. *Proc Amer Soc Clin Oncol* 9:188–#726, 1990, Abstract.
140. Bystryn J-C, Jacobsen S, Harris M, Roses D, Speyer J, and Levin M. Preparation and characterization of a polyvalent human melanoma antigen vaccine. *J Biol Response Modif* 5:211–224, 1986.
141. Bystryn J-C, Dugan M, Oratz R, Speyer J, Harris MN, and Roses DF. Vaccine immunotherapy of human malignant melanoma: Relationship between method of immunization, immunogenicity, and tumor progression. In Metzgar RS and Mitchell MS (eds.), *Human Tumor Antigens and Specific Tumor Therapy*. New York: Alan R. Liss, Inc., 1989, 307–315.
142. Dugan M, Oratz R, Harris MN, Roses DF, Speyer J, Golomb F, Henn M, and Bystryn J-C. Delayed tumor progression in melanoma pts with cellular immune response to melanoma vaccine. *Clin Res* 36:495A, 1988, Abstract.
143. Hollinshead A, Arlen M, Yonemoto R, Cohen M, Tanner K, Kundin WD, and Scherrer J. Pilot studies using melanoma tumor-associated antigens (TAA) in specific-active immunochemotherapy of malignant melanoma. *Cancer* 49:1387–1404, 1982.
144. Livingston PO, Natoli EJ, Calves MJ, Stocker E, Oettgen HF, and Old LJ. Vaccines containing purified GM2 ganglioside elicit GM2 antibodies in melanoma patients. *Proc Natl Acad Sci U S A* 84:2911–2915, 1987.
145. Jones PC, Sze LL, Liu PY, Morton DL, and Irie RF. Prolonged survival for melanoma patients with elevated IgM antibody to oncofetal antigen. *J Natl Cancer Inst* 66:249–254, 1981.
146. Vlock DR, DerSimonian R, and Kirkwood JM. Prognostic role of antibody reactivity to melanoma. *J Clin Invest* 77(4):1116–1121, 1986.
147. Mitchell MS, Kan-Mitchell J, Kempf RA, Harel W, Shau H, and Lind S. Active specific immunotherapy for melanoma: Phase I trial of allogeneic lysates and a novel adjuvant. *Cancer Res* 48:5883–5893, 1988.
148. Mitchell MS. Active specific immunotherapy of melanoma: clinical results and correlates. *Biotechnology Therapeutics* 1(2):163–179, 1989.
149. Wallack MK, Steplewski Z, and Koprowski H. A new approach in active specific immunotherapy. *Cancer* 39:560–564, 1977.
150. Wallack MK, Bash JA, Leftheriotis E, Seigler H, Bland K, Wanebo H, and Balch C. Positive relationship of clinical and serological responses to vaccinia melanoma oncolysate. *Arch Surg* 122:1460–1463, 1987.
151. Seigler HF, Cox E, Mutzner F, Shepherd L, Nicholson E, and Shingleton WW. Specific active immunotherapy for melanoma. *Ann Surg* 190(3):366–372, 1979.
152. Morton DL, Foshag LJ, Nizze JA, Gupta RK, Famatiga E, Hoon DSB, and Irie RF. Active specific immunotherapy in malignant melanoma. *Semin Surg Oncol* 5:420–425, 1989.
153. Berd D, Maguire HC, Jr., McCue P, and Mastrangelo MJ. Treatment of metastatic melanoma with an autologous tumor-cell vaccine: clinical and immunologic results in 64 patients. *J Clin Oncol* 8(11):1858–1867, 1990.
154. Fearon ER, Itaya T, Hunt B, Vogelstein B, and Frost P. Induction in a murine tumor of immunogenic tumor variants by transfection with a foreign gene. *Cancer Res* 48:2975–2980, 1988.
155. Fearon ER, Pardoll DM, Itaya T, Golumbek P, Levitsky HI, Simons JW, Karasuyama H, Vogelstein B, and Frost P. Interleukin-2 production of tumor cells bypasses T helper function in the generation of an antitumor response. *Cell* 60:397–403, 1990.
156. Kawamura H, Rosenberg SA, and Berzofsky JA. Immunization with antigen and interleukin 2 in vivo overcomes Ir gene low responsiveness. *J Exp Med* 162:381–386, 1985.
157. Hellstrom I, Brown JP, and Hellstrom KE. Workshop on monoclonal antibodies of human melanoma-associated antigens: Findings of the Seattle Group. *Hybridoma* 1:266, 1982.
158. Herlyn D, Wettendorff M, Schmoll E, Iliopoulos D, Schedel I, Dreikhausen U, Raab R, Ross AH, Jaksche H, Scriba M, and Koprowski H. Anti-idiotype immunization of cancer patients: Modulation of the immune response. *Proc Natl Acad Sci U S A* 84:8055–8059, 1987.
159. Lichtin A, Iliopoulos D, Guerry D, Elder D, Herlyn D, and Steplewski Z. Therapy of melanoma with an anti-mela-

noma ganglioside monoclonal antibody: A possible mechanism of a complete response. *Proc Amer Soc Clin Oncol* 7:247, 1988, Abstract.

160. Sobol RE, Dillman RO, and Smith DJ. In: Mitchell MF, and Oettgen HF (eds.), *Hybridomas in Cancer Diagnostics and Treatment.* New York: Raven Press, 1982, 192–206.
161. Oldham RK, Thurman GB, Talmadge JE, Stevenson HC, and Foon KA. Lymphokine, monoclonal antibody, and other biological response modifiers in treatment of cancer. *Cancer* 54:2795–2806, 1984.
162. Houghton AN, Mintzer D, Cordon-Cardo C, Welt S, Fliegel B, Vadhan S, Carswell E, Melamed MR, Oettgen HF, and Old LJ. Mouse monoclonal IgG3 antibody detecting G_{D3} ganglioside: A phase I trial in patients with malignant melanoma. *Proc Natl Acad Sci U S A* 82:1242–1246, 1985.
163. Goodman GE, Beaumier P, Hellstrom I, Fernyhough B, and Hellstrom K-E. Pilot trial of murine monoclonal antibodies in patients with advanced melanoma. *J Clin Oncol* 3(3):340–352, 1985.
164. Dippold WG, Bernhard H, and Dienes HP. Treatment of patients with malignant melanoma by monoclonal antiganglioside antibodies. *Eur J Cancer Clin Oncol* 24:S65, 1988.
165. Vadhan-Raj S, Cordon-Cardo C, Carswell E, Mintzer D, Dantis L, Duteau C, Templeton MA, Oettgen HF, Old LJ, and Houghton AN. Phase I trial of mouse monoclonal antibody against G_{D3} ganglioside in patients with melanoma: Induction of inflammatory response at tumor sites. *J Clin Oncol* 6(10):1636–1648, 1988.
166. Cheung N-K, Lazarus H, and Niraldi FD. Ganglioside GD2 specific monoclonal antibody 3F8: A phase I study in patients with neuroblastoma and malignant melanoma. *J Clin Oncol* 5:1430, 1987.
167. Larson SM, Carrasquillo JA, and Krohn KA. Localization of 131I-labeled p97-specific Fab fragments in human melanomas as a basis for radiotherapy. *J Clin Invest* 72:2101, 1983.
168. Larson SM, Carrasquillo JA, McGuffin RW, Krohn KA, Ferens JM, Hill LD, Beaumier PL, Reynolds JC, Hellstrom KE, and Hellstrom I. Use of I-131 labeled, murine Fab against a high molecular weight antigen of human melanoma: Preliminary experience. *Radiology* 155:487–492, 1985.
169. Larson SM. Lymphoma, melanoma, colon cancer: Diagnosis and treatment with radiolabeled monoclonal antibodies. The 1986 Eugene P. Pendergrass New Horizons Lecture. *Radiology* 165:297–304, 1987.
170. Spitler LE, Del Rio M, Khentigan A, Wedel NI, Brophy NA, Miller LL, Harkonen WS, Rosendorf LL, Lee HM, and Mischak RP. Therapy of patients with malignant melanoma using a monoclonal antimelanoma antibody-ricin A chain immunotoxin. *Cancer Res* 47:1717–1723, 1987.
171. Spitler LE, von Wussow P, Carey RW, Borden E, Benjamin RS, Oratz R, Tseng A, Jr, Mastrangelo M, Ernstoff MS, and Scannon PJ. Therapy of patients with malignant melanoma with a monoclonal antimelanoma antibody ricin A chain immunotoxin: Phase II study results. 1998, unpublished work.
172. Wong JH, Irie RF, Morton DL. Human monoclonal antibodies: prospects for the therapy of cancer. *Semin Surg Oncol* 5:448–452, 1989.
173. Irie RF, Sze LL, and Saxton RE. Human antibody to OFA-2, a tumor antigen produced in vitro by Epstein-Barr virus transformed human B-lymphoid cell lines. *Proc Natl Acad Sci U S A* 79(18):5666–5670, 1982.
174. Katano M, Jien M, and Irie RF. Human monoclonal antibody to ganglioside GD2-inhibited human melanoma xenograft. *Eur J Cancer Clin Oncol* 20:1053–1059, 1984.
175. Irie RF, and Morton DL. Regression of cutaneous metastatic melanoma by intralesional injection with human monoclonal antibody to ganglioside GD2. *Proc Natl Acad Sci U S A* 83:8694–8698, 1986.
176. Irie RF, Matsuki T, and Morton DL. Human monoclonal antibody to ganglioside GM2 for melanoma treatment. *Lancet* April:786–787, 1989.
177. Queen C, Schneider WP, Selick HE, Payne PW, Landolfi NF, Duncan JF, Adalovic NM, Levitt M, Junghans RP, and Waldmann TA. A humanized antibody that binds to the interleukin-2 receptor. *Proc Natl Acad Sci U S A* 86:10029–10033, 1989.
178. Caulfield MJ, Barna B, Murphy S, Tubbs R, Sergi J, Medendorp S, and Bukowski RM. Phase Ia-Ib trial of an anti-G_{D3} monoclonal antibody in combination with interferon-alpha in patients with malignant melanoma. *J Biol Response Modif* 9:319–328, 1990.
179. Bajorin DF, Chapman PB, Wong G, Coit DG, Kunicka J, Dimaggio J, Cordon-Cardo C, Urmacher C, Dantes L, Templeton MA, Liu J, Oettgen HF, and Houghton AN. Phase I evaluation of a combination of monoclonal antibody R24 and interleukin-2 in patients with metastatic melanoma. *Cancer Res* 50:7490–7495, 1990.
180. Titus JA, Perez P, Kaubisch A, Garrido MA, and Segal DM. Human K/natural killer cells targeted with hetero-cross-linked antibodies specifically lyse tumor cells in vitro and prevent tumor growth in vivo. *J Immunol* 139(9):3153–3158, 1987.
181. Starling JJ, Maciak RS, Hinson NA, Hoskins J, Laguzza BC, Gadski RA, Strand J, Rittmann-Grauer L, DeHerdt SV, Bumol TF, and Moore RE. In vivo selection of human tumor cells resistant to monoclonal antibody-vinca alcaloid immunoconjugates. *Cancer Res* 50:7634–7640, 1990.
182. Cardinali M, Uchino R, and Chung S. Interaction of fibrinogen with murine melanoma cells: Covalent association with cell membranes and protection against recognition by lymphokine-activated killer cells. *Cancer Res* 50:8010–8016, 1990.
183. Oh S-K, Kim S-H, and Walker JE. Interference with immune response at the level of generating effector cells by tumor-associated haptoglobin. *J Natl Cancer Inst* 82:934–940, 1990.
184. Sarna GP, Figlin RA, and Pertcheck M. Phase II study of betaseron (Beta ser^{17}-interferon) as treatment of advanced malignant melanoma. *J Biol Response Modif* 6:375–378, 1987.
185. Schoof DD, Gramolini BA, Davidson DL, Massaro AF, Wilson RE, and Eberlein TJ. Adoptive immunotherapy of human cancer using low-dose recombinant interleukin-2 and lymphokine-activated killer cells. *Cancer Res* 48:5007–5010, 1988.
186. Bystryn J-C, Oratz R, Harris MN, Roses DF, Golomb FM, and Speyer JL. Immunogenicity of a polyvalent melanoma antigen vaccine in humans. *Cancer* 61:1065–1070, 1988.
187. Oratz R, Speyer JC, Wernz H, Hochster H, Meyers M, Mischak R, and Spitler LE. Antimelanoma monoclonal antibody-ricin A chain immunoconjugate (XMMME-001-RTA) plus cyclophosphamide in the treatment of metastatic malignant melanoma: Results of a phase II Trial. *J Biol Response Modif* 9(4):345–354, 1990.

Chapter 30

RADIATION THERAPY OF MALIGNANT MELANOMA

Brian O'Sullivan, Richard Tsang

INTRODUCTION

Traditional beliefs about melanoma have viewed it as a disease resistant to radiotherapy. Nevertheless, the paradox exists that radiation oncologists are frequently asked to consider radiotherapy for melanoma, often under unfavorable clinical circumstances where cure is less likely, such as recurrent and metastatic disease. These circumstances, where the benefits of other treatment modalities have generally been exhausted, have tended to uphold the long standing dogma of radioresistance, which finds its roots in the older literature prior to the era of modern radiation techniques.[1] In spite of the use of radiotherapy in such adverse situations, a growing body of evidence has emerged contesting the traditional view. While not all the historical literature supported the "myth" of radioresistance, it was not until the 1970s that laboratory melanoma cell lines were observed to display broad shouldered but relatively low D_0 survival curves. These findings may explain the poor results using conventional fractionated radiotherapy as standard treatment in all cases of melanoma. These concepts and the methods, indications and results of treatment of cutaneous melanoma with radiotherapy in various situations will be the subject of this chapter. This review will not discuss ocular or mucosal melanomas, nor will it emphasize the management of cerebral metastases, which are described in other chapters in this volume. In general, similar radiotherapy principles will apply in these different clinical situations.

CLINICAL SENSITIVITY OF MELANOMA TO RADIATION

Statements about the outcome of malignant melanoma after radiation therapy require a description of the end point being assessed. Radioresponsive tumors demonstrate visible regression following treatment. On the other hand, radiotherapy may have succeeded in sterilizing all clonogenic tumor cells, but any persisting stromal masses and sterilized cells may result in the illusion of an incompletely regressed tumor and may be equated with failure to respond to the treatment and hence mistaken as radioresistant. Radiobiology teaching currently emphasizes cellular radioresistance with failure of irradiation to sterilize clonogenic cells being paramount, but other factors may also operate. For example, the cell loss factor, the host's response to remove sterilized cells and stromal debris, is an important component of the assessment of the clinical response and could be misinterpreted as clinical radioresistance otherwise. Lack of recognition to factors such as the prominent desmoplastic stromal reaction in melanoma[2] have contributed to the impression of a slow and perhaps incomplete response to radiation even if clonogenic tumor cells are completely sterilized.

THE RADIOBIOLOGIC BASIS OF RADIOTHERAPY

Melanoma is unusual among malignant tumors in its biologic response to therapeutic radiation. This may have contributed to the previous misconception that melanomas are "radioresistant" and may provide a rationale for the use of high fraction size in the therapy of these tumors. In order to facilitate the discussion, an initial description of some basic principles of radiobiology is required.

The relationship between cell survival and radiation dose is often represented by a cell-survival curve (Fig. 30-1). Since radiation in a particular dose kills a certain proportion rather than a fixed absolute number of cells, the best chance to cure a tumor locally occurs when there is the smallest number of clonogenic cells present for therapeutic radiation. In clinical practice, examples of this include the situation of a small primary tumor or a postoperative field where the bulk of tumor has been removed surgically and the intent of treatment is to sterilize microscopic residuum. This principle generally underlies the use of adjuvant radiation therapy for cancer and, as will be discussed later, may be considered in selected situations when radiotherapy may be integrated into a combined modality approach in the treatment of malignant melanoma.

One method of characterizing a cell survival curve is illustrated in Fig. 30-1, where the cell-surviving fraction is plotted on a logarithmic scale and radiation dose on a linear scale. For radiation with *low energy transfer* (X-rays), there is an initial shoulder at low doses, and a straighter portion with higher doses. Traditionally, two parameters are used to describe this curve: *n* is the extrapolation number, obtained by extrapolating the straight portion of the curve to the Y-axis (zero dose) and D_0 reflects the slope of the final straight portion of the curve and is the dose required to reduce the cell surviving fraction to 37 percent (e^{-1}). The extrapolation number *(n)* is important because it reflects the size of the "shoulder" of the cell survival curve. Curves with large shoulders will tend to have large values of *n* (see Figs. 30-1 and 30-3). Mechanistically, the initial shoulder on a survival curve is attributed to repair of sublethal radiation damage (possibly as a result of enzymatic and other cellular mechanisms), which result in a higher level of cell survival than would occur if there would have been no repair processes. Therefore, a large shoulder means that the target cells have a large capacity to repair sublethal radiation damage. Since a conventional course of fractionated radiotherapy usually consists of repeated small individual doses in the range of 2 to 3 Gy,* small changes in the shape of the shoulder region of the survival curve will be magnified in the final level of cell kill achieved (Fig. 30-2). Most radiation oncologists would define *conventional* fractionation as daily administration of 1.8 to 2.5 Gy doses, given 5 days a week. The use of higher doses per fraction, in the range of 3 to 10 Gy, given less frequently than 5 days a week, is termed *hypofractionation.* It has been documented that melanoma cell lines grown in vitro and melanoma xenografts grown in mice often display cell survival curves that have large initial

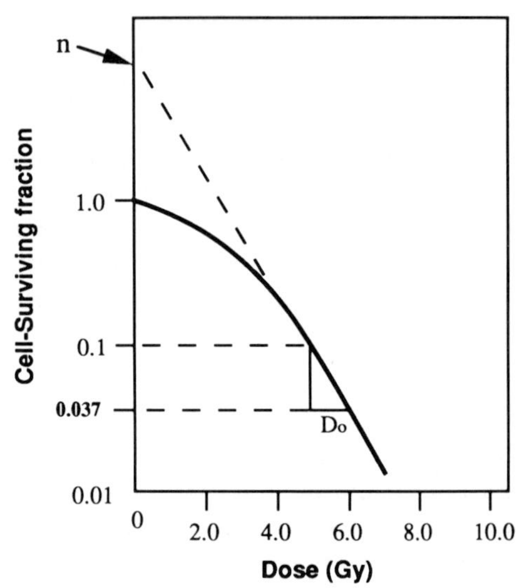

FIG. 30-1. Schematic representation of a cell-survival curve, with cell-surviving fraction plotted on a logarithmic scale, and radiation dose on a linear scale. D_0 is the dose that reduces cell survival to 37 percent in the final straight portion of the curve. The extrapolation number (n) reflects the size of the initial shoulder of the curve, obtained by extending the straight portion of the curve back to zero radiation dose (dashed line).

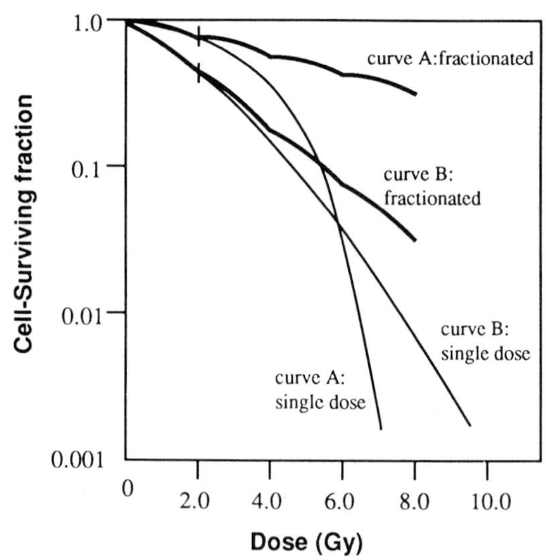

FIG. 30-2. Hypothetical cell-survival curves, showing the effects of fractionated irradiation in a curve with a large shoulder (curve A, seen in some melanoma cell lines), relative to a curve with a small shoulder (curve B, typical of other solid tumor cell lines). With repeated low doses of 2 Gy, the level of cell kill achieved in A is much less than that in B, due to the magnifying effect of the shoulder region by fractionation (see text). The situation is reversed if large dose per fraction (> 6 Gy) is used, with more cell-kill obtained in A than B. Current terminology according to the linear-quadratic equation would describe curve A having a smaller α/β value compared to curve B.[14]

*The Gray (Gy) is the SI unit of Absorbed Dose; 1 Gy = 100 cGy = 100 rad.

shoulders[3–8] in comparison with other tumor cell lines. This may be the radiobiologic basis of the poorer tumor response rates observed in the clinic when conventional low-fraction-size treatments were given compared to hypofractionation with fraction sizes above 4 to 6 Gy. However, there are also reports in the literature that document high tumor response rates using conventional low-fraction-size radiotherapy.[9,10] While it is erroneous to assume that all melanoma cell lines have large initial shoulders in their survival curves, the extent to which this phenomenon translates into an explanation for the degree of clinical response is unknown. McBride et al[11] studied eight melanoma cell lines recently and found four with large initial shoulders (Fig. 30-3A *n* ranging from 4.6 to 40), with the remainder (Fig. 30-3B) having small shoulders with $n \leq 1.5$. In addition, they found karyotypic changes on chromosome number 7 in all four of the cell lines with large shoulders, which were absent in three out of the four cell lines with small initial shoulders. These preliminary data point to a genetic or epigenetic basis in radiation response, a phenomenon that has been correlated with biologic aggressiveness in metastatic disease.[12]

A more recent model to describe a cell-survival curve is the linear quadratic equation, where survival fraction $= \exp(-\alpha D - \beta D^2)$ (D is the radiation dose and α and β are parameters in the model that dictate the shape of the curve). A detailed account of this model is beyond the scope of this discussion, but interested readers are referred to some excellent reviews on this topic both of a general nature[13] and more specifically to malignant melanoma.[14,15]

While the importance of the contribution of the "broad shoulder" of the melanoma survival curve to the radiation response of this tumor is recognized, attention to the "intrinsic radiosensitivity" of melanoma cells is also helpful. Radiobiologists use this term to denote the inherent radiosensitivity of the tumor, distinguishing it from the radiosensitivity that can be modified by other biologic processes such as oxygenation, repair, and cell cycle position. The

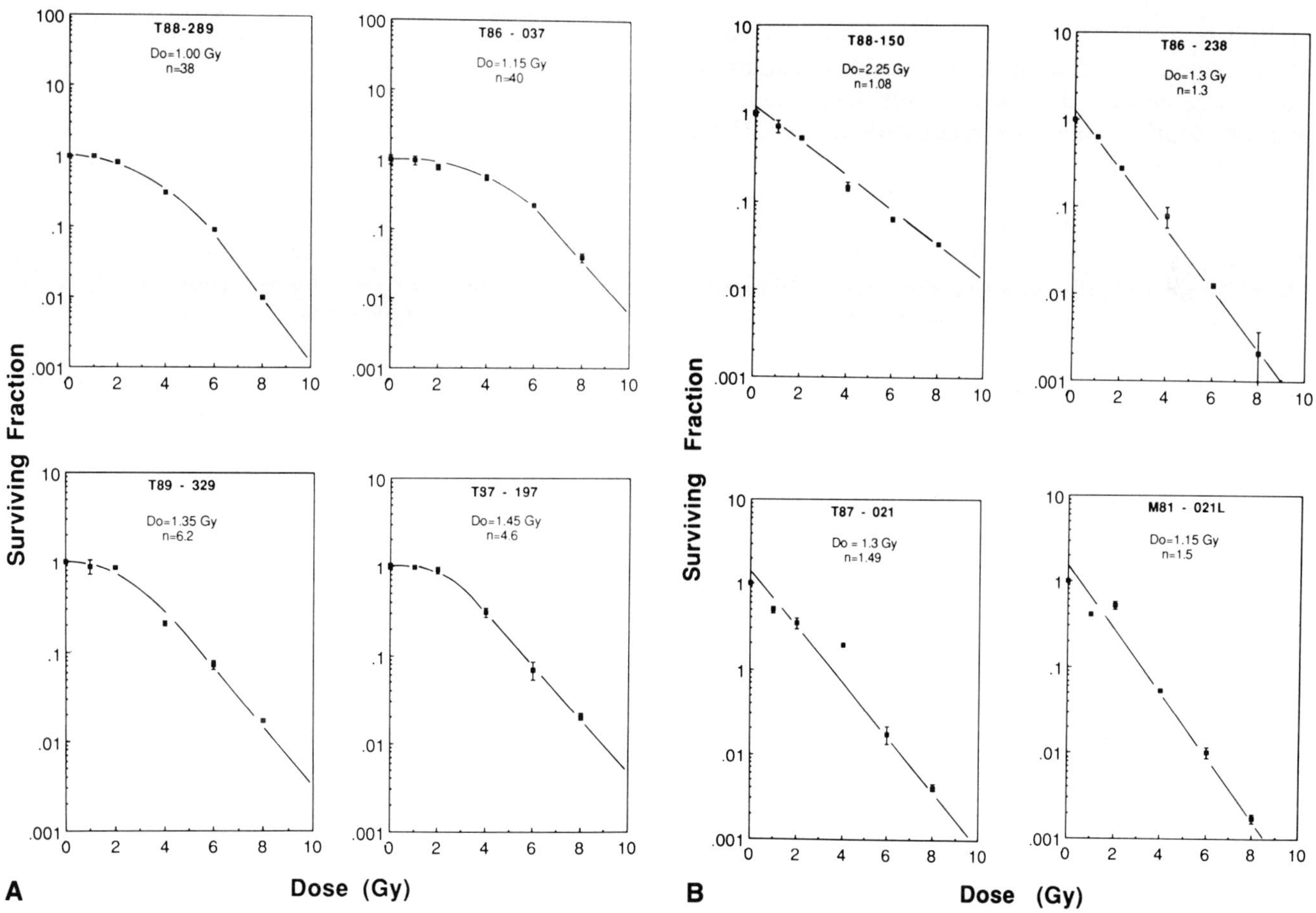

FIG. 30-3. (A) Cell-survival curves of four melanoma cell lines with large initial shoulders. Note they all possess high extrapolation numbers (n over 2). (B) Cell-survival curves of four melanoma cell lines with little or no initial shoulders. Note their small extrapolation numbers (n less than 2). From McBride et al.,[11] used with permission.

frequently used yardstick for intrinsic radiosensitivity has been the surviving fraction at a radiation dose of 2 Gy (SF_2). Figure 30-4 shows the SF_2 of human tumor cell lines from the published literature summarized by Deacon et al.[16] and plotted against five clinical groups, A to E, in decreasing order of radioresponsiveness. Group E has the highest mean SF_2 of .518, and 18 out of the 25 points in this category are melanoma cell lines. These data contrast with the more radioresponsive tumor cell lines in groups A (neuroblastomas, myelomas), B (small cell lung carcinoma), C (cervix and bladder), and D (colorectal, squamous cell carcinoma of lung), with mean SF_2 values of .187, .218, .460, and .428, respectively. However, it should be noted that a large degree of variation of radioresponsiveness exists in each of the categories, with possibly even more intertumoral heterogeneity of radioresponsiveness for human tumors in situ. Therefore, it would be desirable to develop in vitro techniques to assess radiosensitivity as a basis for selecting radiotherapy for individual patients. This area is currently the focus of active study.[17,18]

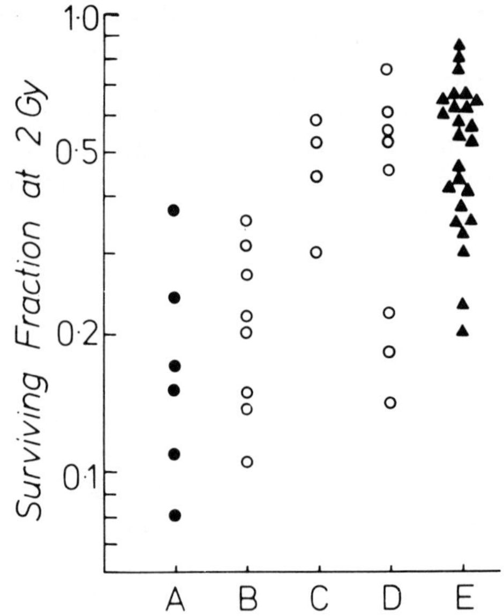

FIG. 30-4. The surviving fraction at 2 Gy (SF_2), used as a measure of intrinsic radiosensitivity, plotted against tumor cell type ranked from A through to E according to their degree of radioresponsiveness. For example, category A includes tumors generally regarded as radioresponsive (myeloma, neuroblastoma), while category E includes tumors generally regarded as radioresistant (glioblastoma, malignant melanoma). Note the large variation of SF_2 between and within categories. From Deacon et al.,[16] used with permission.

RADIOTHERAPY TECHNIQUE

A detailed description of the principles of radiation therapy is beyond the scope of this discussion, but more in-depth reviews are readily available[19–21] for the interested reader.

In devising a radiation treatment plan, most centers apply the guidelines of the International Commission on Radiation Units and Measurements (ICRU) and initially identify the "target volume," which is the volume of tissue containing the tumor that should receive the prescribed radiation dose, to an accuracy of ± 5 percent. In the last 30 years, there have been dramatic improvements in technology that made various forms of radiation available to suit the need. An example is the development of megavoltage linear accelerators that have superior depth dose characteristics compared with orthovoltage X-rays or gamma rays from ^{60}Co, allowing treatment of deep seated tumors with less complications. For superficial skin lesions, soft X-rays have been used traditionally and are still commonly utilized. Electron beams generated from linear accelerators have special depth dose characteristics that makes them ideal for the treatment of superficial skin or subcutaneous lesions and are also commonly used.[22]

An important issue is the optimal radiation dose for the therapy of melanoma and, in particular, the optimal dose per fraction for this disease.[23] As has been discussed earlier, evidence exists in melanoma cell lines to support the efficacy of both high and low dose per fraction approaches.[4,16,24] In the clinical situation, the trend has been to support higher doses per fraction schedules[25–35] but without universal consistency in the reports of all authors.[9,10,36–38] The recent randomized trial by the Radiation Therapy Oncology Group (RTOG) in patients with metastatic disease showed no detectable difference in response between 2.5 Gy fractions delivered 5 days a week to total dose of 50 Gy compared to 8.0 Gy fractions delivered once weekly to a total of 32 Gy.[39] Both regimens are unconventional in so far as they are aggressive courses administered in a shorter treatment time than is standard practice for most tumor sites in many centers and, while going a considerable way towards addressing the controversy, may not fully resolve it. The 8.0 Gy per fraction regimen is similar to an approach, to be described next, that we employ in Toronto but the RTOG utilizes one additional fraction for a higher total dose (32 Gy versus 24 Gy). The RTOG authors suggested a slight increase in late complications in the 8 Gy per fraction arm of the trial[39] and the study has been the subject of cautious editorial comment for that reason.[37] Excellent discussions on the clinical data relating to the controversy about the use of conventional versus high dose per fraction radiotherapy are available and should be consulted for further reference.[24,37,40]

CLINICAL APPLICATIONS OF RADIOTHERAPY

A review of the modern literature provides reports of treatment of melanoma with radiotherapy in a variety of different clinical circumstances. These include primary radical radiotherapy as curative management,[41–44] adjuvant preoperative and post surgical treatment to the primary site,[45] adjuvant treatment for lymph node bearing regions or for unresectable lymph node bearing areas,[46,47] and palliative treatment most usually for metastatic disease.[48,49]

Primary Radical Management

LENTIGO MALIGNA AND LENTIGO MALIGNA MELANOMA

Lentigo maligna (LM), or Hutchinson's melanotic freckle, is a flat pigmented lesion usually found in actinically damaged skin of elderly people and is considered as the precursor of lentigo maligna melanoma (see Chapter 9). It generally grows slowly in a horizontal direction and is commonly located on the face. X-ray therapy has been used in Europe for many years as a primary treatment, using the Miescher technique, although the traditional treatment in North America has been surgical excision. The Miescher technique uses high doses of soft X-rays (10–20 keV) from a contact therapy machine, delivering surface doses of 20 Gy once weekly for four to five treatments. These low energy X-rays penetrate tissues poorly, attenuating to 50 percent of the prescribed dose after traversing 1 mm of tissue. Harwood and Cummings have summarized this European experience showing an over 95 percent control rate for LM.[50] In Toronto, Harwood et al., from the Princess Margaret Hospital (P.M.H.) have advocated radiotherapy for selected cases of LM and LM melanoma.[40,41,51] They reported excellent control rate of LM after irradiation, with seven out of eight lesions treated between 1958 and 1977 controlled,[51] and 18 out of 20 lesions controlled in a further update.[43] We have continued to follow some of these patients and have recently updated our experience to 1988. Thirty-six lesions (all proven LM with biopsy) in 34 patients were diagnosed and treated with irradiation from 1968 to 1988. The P.M.H. technique uses slightly more penetrating X-rays, usually with maximum energy of 100 or 125 keV (Figs. 30-5–30-7). The most commonly used doses are 35 Gy in 5 daily treatments over 1 week, or 45 Gy in 10 daily treatments over 2 weeks. Of 36 lesions treated in this manner, 32 were controlled with irradiation alone (88.9 percent), with a median follow-up duration of 6 years. Three lesions not controlled by irradiation were successfully treated by surgical excision at a later time. Two of these showed invasive melanoma (both Clark's level II) when excised. Thus, the overall control rate approached 100 percent. One patient had residual pigmentation at 4 months from the time of radiotherapy, was lost to follow-up, and was counted as a treatment failure. It should be stressed that the pigmentation of LM may take 12 to 18 months to disappear, and it is unclear whether that particular patient's lesion would eventually have been controlled if the patient had been followed for a longer time. The overall cosmetic result is excellent, although most patients develop a mild degree of skin pallor and atrophy, with a minority developing pigmentation or telangiectasia several years after radiation as a late skin effect. Patients with repigmentation were carefully evaluated, frequently with

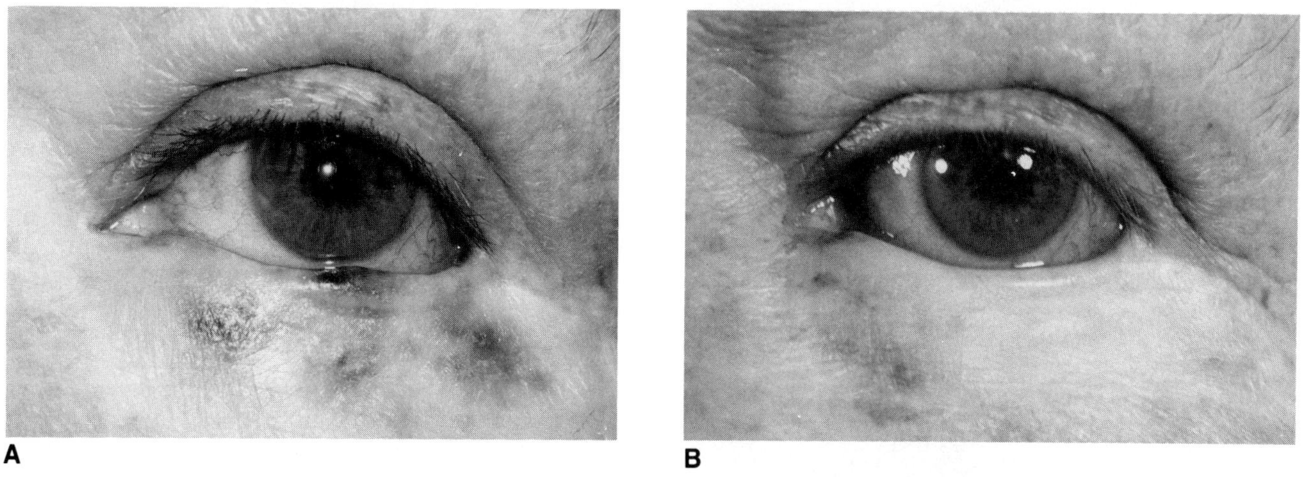

FIG. 30-5. (A) A 67-year-old woman with recurrence of malignant melanoma involving the left lower eyelid, after multiple surgical procedures previously for lentigo maligna melanoma. After this photograph was taken, she was treated by local radiotherapy, 45 Gy in 10 daily fractions over 2 weeks. (B) Same patient 4 years after radiotherapy, free of malignant melanoma. Note mild skin pallor with atrophy, secondary to radiotherapy.

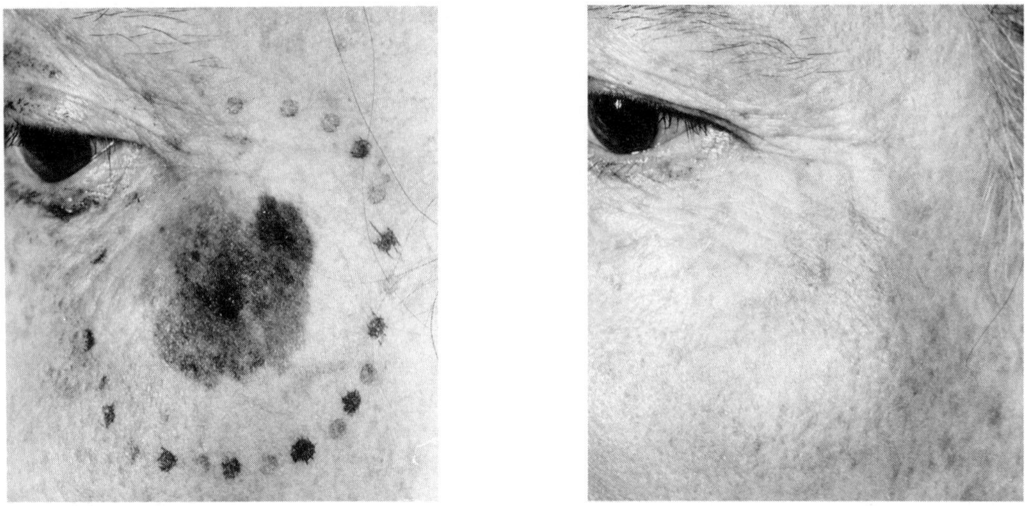

FIG. 30-6. (A) Lentigo maligna of the left cheek in a 54-year-old man, before irradiation with superficial X-rays (HVL .7 mm Aluminium, maximum energy 100 kV) to a dose of 45 Gy in 10 daily fractions over 2 week. The dotted marks outline the circular radiation field. Note the proximity of the lesion to the eye. (B) Same patient 5 months after irradiation, showing complete resolution of lentigo maligna.

a biopsy to rule out recurrent LM or invasive melanoma. No patients developed uncontrolled primary or metastatic melanoma, and no patients died of disease or from treatment. Because LM often involve large areas of skin in the facial areas of elderly patients, we believe irradiation remains a good treatment option and provides an excellent alternative to surgery in certain clinical circumstances. Typical situations include large lesions close to the eye where major reconstruction may be required to yield a satisfactory cosmetic result. However, it should be appreciated that the late skin effects from radiation are often slowly progressive in nature, manifested by increasing hyper- or hypopigmentation, skin atrophy, and telangiectasia 5 or more years after treatment, as illustrated in Fig. 30-7.

The Princess Margaret Hospital results of radiation therapy as primary treatment for lentigo maligna melanoma (LMM) were previously reported by Harwood.[41–43] Up to the middle of 1982, 23 of 25 lesions treated with irradiation achieved local control. An update of the outcome of 17 patients treated from 1968 to 1988 showed that 14 remained controlled locally (82 percent), with a median follow-up

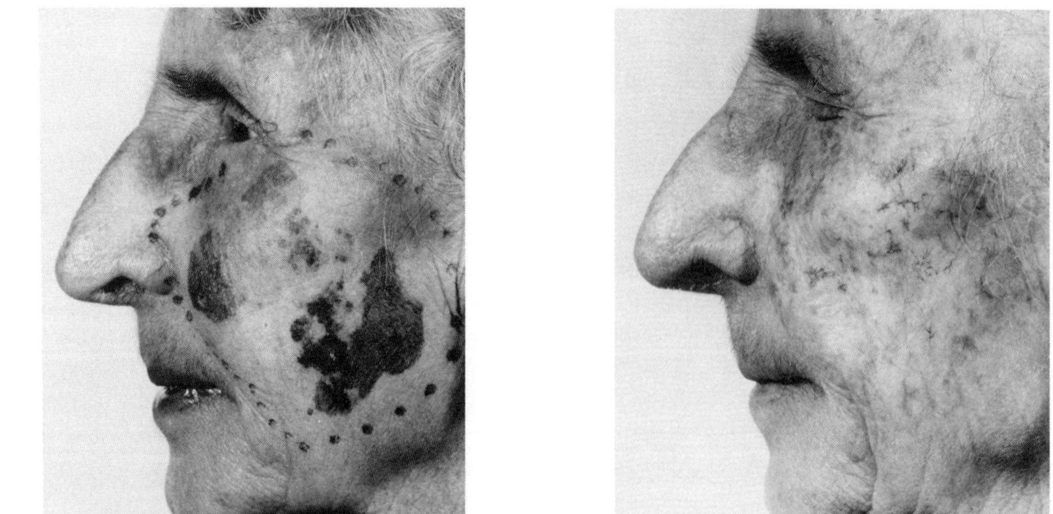

FIG. 30-7. (A) An extensive lentigo maligna involving a large portion of the left cheek of an elderly woman. The area marked by dots was treated to 45 Gy in 15 daily fractions over 3 weeks. From Harwood,[41] used with permission. (B) Appearance 5 years after radiotherapy. There was no recurrence of lentigo maligna, but a moderate degree of radiation-induced changes were evident, with skin pallor, atrophy, and telangiectasia.

time of 4 years. Of the three patients not controlled, one was due to residual disease 4 months after radiotherapy, and he eventually died of an unrelated locally extensive squamous carcinoma of the oral cavity. One patient recurred with lentigo maligna 7 years after radiotherapy and was successfully treated by surgical excision. The third patient recurred locally with a level V melanoma 4 years after radiation and was also successfully salvaged by surgery. Of the 17 patients, one subsequently developed regional nodal disease in the neck that was successfully treated by a neck dissection, and another patient developed distant metastases which were eventually fatal.

SUPERFICIAL SPREADING AND NODULAR MELANOMA

The literature contains a variety of reports over a time period spanning more than 30 years for radiotherapy as the primary treatment of superficial spreading melanoma (SSM) and nodular melanoma (NM). While surgical treatment has continued to provide the mainstay of management, radiotherapy is felt to possess advantages either alone or in combination with surgery in certain circumstances. Generally these include the elderly or debilitated patient and anatomic locations where the extent of surgery required is unacceptable or unjustified for functional or cosmetic reasons or where the risks of the surgical procedure outweigh its potential benefits. Pre-operative radiotherapy has also been used with claims of either improved control or alternatively may permit more conservative surgery than would otherwise be appropriate.[45] The concept of combining conservative surgery and postoperative radiotherapy has also been attractive as previously reported from Toronto in SSM and NM.[50] In SSM six out of six cases treated with irradiation following biopsy or local excision for the primary were controlled at the local site following treatment. In an earlier time period Dickson reported the results of 121 patients with NM treated with radiotherapy following local excision.[52] The results at 5 years demonstrated 41 percent disease-free survival, which compared favorably to those of wide local excision and was superior to local excision alone (20 percent disease-free survival) in similar patients treated in the same time period. A more recent series of patients at P.M.H. confirmed these findings and demonstrated a local control rate of 88 percent (15 of 17 patients) with a radiation schedule employing a dose per fraction of 4 Gy or greater, administered as the initial management after local excision, frequently in patients with microscopic residuum.[44] This radiotherapy technique is similar to that used by Dickson in the earlier report. In contrast, only 25 percent of patients (3 of 12) achieved local control when the dose per fraction was less than 4 Gy in the more recent P.M.H. series. In recent years an altered referral pattern, coinciding largely with improvement in surgical technique, has resulted in fewer cases treated in this manner.

The results for primary local management should be interpreted in the light of the retrospective nature of the data and the realization that selection factors frequently determine that patients in surgical and radiotherapy series are not generally comparable. On the other hand, any bias that may exist is usually towards treating the less fit patients with radiotherapy and utilizing surgery where possible in lesions that are clearly resectable. In addition, most experts now accept that radiotherapy is capable of sterilizing residual disease at the local site and provides an attractive alternative to major surgery in appropriate clinical situations. This does not imply that radiotherapy provides superior treatment outcome to radical surgery, but rather may optimize the treatment strategy without compromising local control or survival.

Management of Regional Disease

There is no dispute about the place of surgery as the principal modality in the management of clinically involved nodal disease in malignant melanoma. What is less clear is the role of radiation treatment as an adjunctive measure to prevent subsequent relapse within the regional surgical field after excision of involved nodal tissues by limited surgical procedures or by formal node dissection. While the latter is generally regarded as the optimal approach, this may not be feasible or appropriate in the varied presentations of primary or recurrent melanoma with regional nodal disease. Patients in this situation may be compromised by virtue of their age, medical condition, or the extent of the disease and may not be realistic candidates for radical surgery; alternatively, they may be afflicted by disease that is either difficult or impossible to resect completely by a major resection without significant functional sequelae. While judgment is required to define the extent of appropriate surgical intervention, the justification for a radical surgical approach is even less compelling if the patient also has distant metastases. Nevertheless, the problem of uncontrolled regional disease is frequently distressing and a realistic attempt to achieve control is reasonable in patients judged to be at significant risk for future relapse or who have active disease but are unsuitable candidates for surgery.

At the Princess Margaret Hospital, Toronto, we have maintained a philosophy of administering high dose per fraction radiotherapy (24 Gy in three equal fractions over a period of 21 days and so called "0-7-21 Fractionation") in patients deemed to be at high risk for relapse after surgery for clinically involved nodal disease or where further surgery is not indicated. This fractionation regimen was originally reported for use with hyperbaric oxygen therapy[53] and is similar to that of the RTOG[39] discussed earlier but P.M.H. uses three instead of four fractions and hence 25 percent reduction in total dose. This may explain the relative absence of specific radiation-related adverse sequelae (see the following). The program is well suited to the treatment of melanoma since it administers high dose per fraction radiotherapy to large volumes of tissue such as the axilla, supraclavicular fossa, and ilio-inguinal regions while being well tolerated and relatively simple to administer with minimal time expenditure by the patient. Our dose specification has restricted the maximum tissue dose at any point within the volume to 8.25 Gy per fraction thereby eliminating the significant soft tissue morbidity noted with the original 10 Gy fractionation regimen.[53] Initial results for this approach in 51 cases with regional disease have previously been described.[47] Since then further cases provide a series of 170 patients treated between January 1979 and December 1988. The indications for radiotherapy included gross (visible or palpable) disease for which definitive surgery was felt not to be indicated, or disease that was residual after an attempted resection. Other indications comprised known microscopic residual disease based on the surgical or pathology reports irrespective of other findings, disease greater than 3 cm in size completely replacing the resected node, multiple nodes (three or more) involved by melanoma in the specimen, and histologic evidence of penetration of the lymph node capsule. All these features were believed to be significant risk factors for recurrence within the surgical field.[47]

The 5-year actuarial relapse-free-rates in the irradiated field were 87 percent for those patients with microscopically complete resections, 67 percent for those with microscopic residuum, and 17 percent for those with gross disease. In the sub-group with gross disease, 14 of 58 patients (24 percent) achieved complete disappearance of disease, while 17 were not evaluable for response to radiotherapy due to inadequate assessment of tumor size before or after treatment or due to loss of follow-up after irradiation. All nonevaluable cases, partial responders, and stable or progressive disease are deemed to have failed treatment and are reflected in the 5-year disease-free rate. Despite these strict criteria, 11 of the 14 complete responders, or 17 percent of the 58 cases with gross disease, remained disease-free at the irradiated site until the date of last assessment or death. While this assessment is confounded by the high risk of metastatic failure whereby patients may have insufficient opportunity to develop an "in-field" recurrence, certain of these patients with gross residual disease became long-term survivors of this program. The range of follow-up for the 14 cases is 5 to 97 months with six disease-free patients having been followed beyond 50 months, some with substantial bulk disease prior to irradiation. Similar observations have been made by Creagan and colleagues from the Mayo Clinic in the management of locally advanced disease.[54]

The "0-7-21 fractionation" approach was well tolerated in this group of patients (see case report, Fig. 30-8). Soft tissue fibrosis or induration within the treatment field occurred in 46 percent but was asymptomatic. Limb edema was observed in 34 percent but was mild or transient in most. Six patients suffered severe toxicity, which in four cases included skin breakdown, severe edema, or nerve entrapment. All four had massive uncontrolled tumor at the irradiated site, which could also have explained these observations, while two of these cases also underwent further interventions with chemotherapy, hyperthermia, and aggressive surgery prior to the onset of the complications. The remaining two patients had toxicity related to the radiotherapy alone. Both cases were middle-aged females who received treatment to the inguinal regions where the hip joint was also included in the high dose volume. Both cases required total hip replacement for subsequent femoral head collapse. While other cases were successfully treated by the same technique to this region, we now shield the femoral and humeral heads from the beams wherever possible for the third and final treatment fraction of a course and have seen no further cases of joint damage.

Our policy of elective nodal irradiation in high-risk cases has not been compared prospectively to surgery as a single modality. The Mayo Clinic published a randomized study of radiation as a post-surgical adjuvant after lymphadenectomy, which suggested a survival advantage for this approach compared to lymphadenectomy alone, but the difference was felt to be due to imbalance between the treatment groups.[55] On the other hand, the number of cases entered was small (27 in one arm and 29 in the other), and such statistical inferences are likely to be less valid than if the data set had been larger. Furthermore, the study attempted to enter all cases with nodal disease irrespective of prognostic factors for regional control. Inclusion of low risk cases in this manner may be expected to dilute a treatment effect if the number of high risk cases is small. Of importance also was the choice of radiotherapy dose in this study, which employed a low dose per fraction of 1.78 Gy, a 3 to 4 week rest midway through the treatment course where no treatment was administered, and a low total dose of 50 Gy, particularly

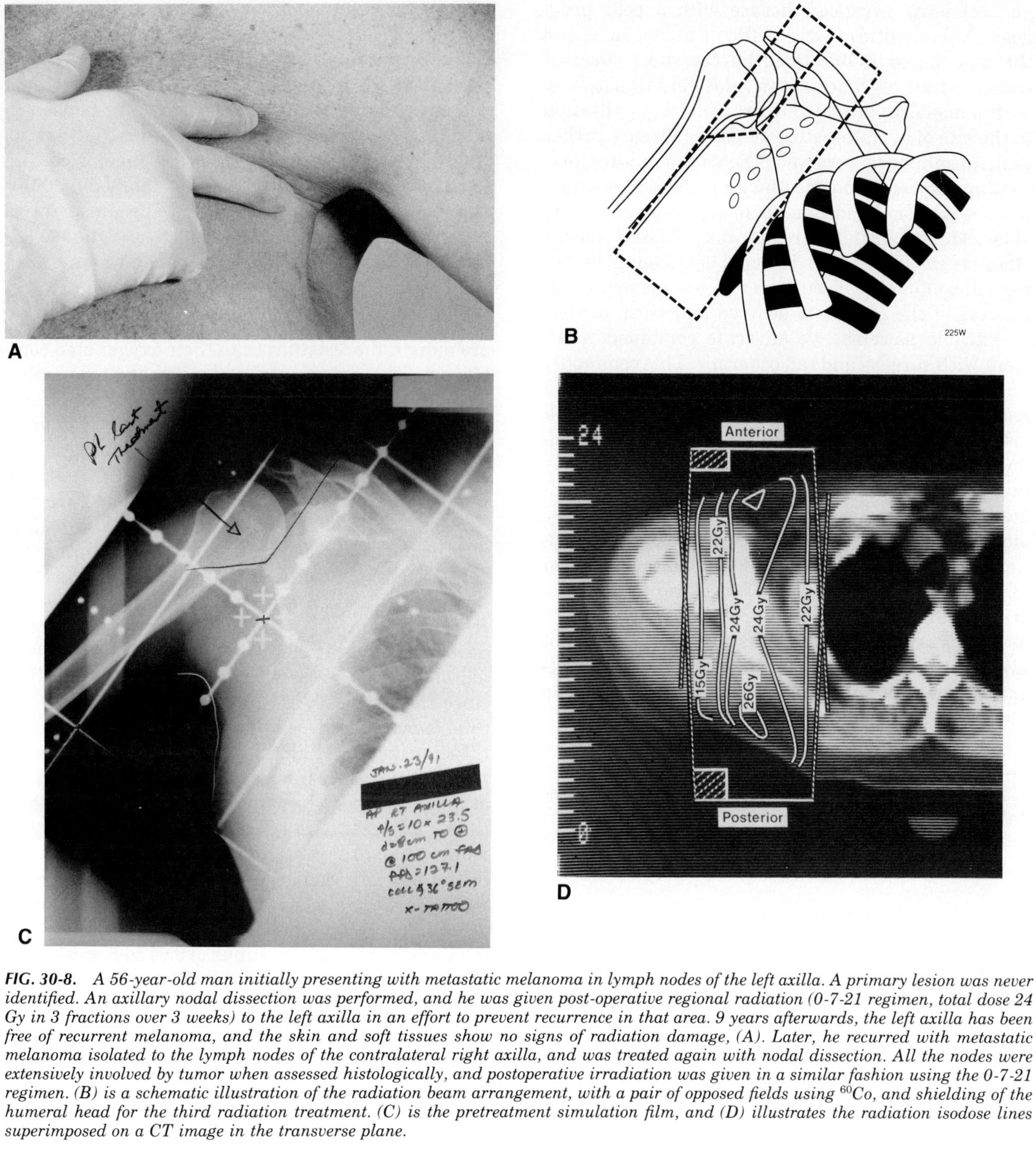

FIG. 30-8. *A 56-year-old man initially presenting with metastatic melanoma in lymph nodes of the left axilla. A primary lesion was never identified. An axillary nodal dissection was performed, and he was given post-operative regional radiation (0-7-21 regimen, total dose 24 Gy in 3 fractions over 3 weeks) to the left axilla in an effort to prevent recurrence in that area. 9 years afterwards, the left axilla has been free of recurrent melanoma, and the skin and soft tissues show no signs of radiation damage, (A). Later, he recurred with metastatic melanoma isolated to the lymph nodes of the contralateral right axilla, and was treated again with nodal dissection. All the nodes were extensively involved by tumor when assessed histologically, and postoperative irradiation was given in a similar fashion using the 0-7-21 regimen. (B) is a schematic illustration of the radiation beam arrangement, with a pair of opposed fields using* ^{60}*Co, and shielding of the humeral head for the third radiation treatment. (C) is the pretreatment simulation film, and (D) illustrates the radiation isodose lines superimposed on a CT image in the transverse plane.*

when one takes account of the "split" in the course and the low fraction size which are well known to degrade the biological effect of radiation on tumor kill.[56,57]

We have continued to advocate a policy of conventional surgical management for regional disease in melanoma. We do not recommend adjuvant radiotherapy in this situation for routine use but feel that it has a role in selected cases. These include cases where appropriate surgery cannot be performed or where residual disease remains after surgery, and our approach has been to continue to administer the treatment according to the principles previously described.

Management of Metastatic Disease

The treatment of metastatic disease with radiotherapy in melanoma is unrewarding. Patients in general have advanced disease with a poor prognosis. Therapeutic effect is difficult to measure, and the assessment is disturbed by the short survival from the time of treatment in relatively ill patients, with a modality intended to provide local palliation to the site of symptomatic metastatic disease rather than to influence survival. The common sites presenting for radiation treatment include the brain, the osseous skeleton, lymph node metastases, and skin nodules. While the reader may wish to consult other references[58–62] for additional detail on this topic, we will confine the discussion to a few principles. In general, if the goal is to achieve long-term control in suitable patients, we advocate combined treatment with surgery and radiotherapy. This commonly occurs with brain involvement where surgical resection of a solitary lesion is generally advised followed by conventional palliative radiotherapy regimens of relatively short duration,[63] such as 20 Gy in 5 fractions or 30 Gy in 10 fractions. These regimens have the advantage of being well tolerated by most anatomic regions while combining the potential advantage of a relatively high dose per fraction (3 Gy to 4 Gy per fraction). This also follows the principles and recommendations of other authors[64,65] for the treatment of brain disease. Surgery is not always realistic or appropriate in other sites of metastatic disease, and similar radiation regimens to those noted are employed as single modality for palliation. In general, the high dose per fraction regimen (0-7-21) described for the management of regional disease is not appropriate for most other palliative indications, because it is above the tolerance of structures frequently located in the target volume, which may include the brain or spinal cord.

COMBINING RADIOTHERAPY WITH OTHER MODALITIES

Radiotherapy and Chemotherapy

Reports of chemotherapy agents used as a radiosensitizer in combination with radiotherapy have not been particularly encouraging in malignant melanoma. Dewit et al.[66] treated 25 patients with metastatic disease with radiation (6 fractions of 6 Gy over 6 weeks) and *cis*-platinum (weekly infusions of 20–40 mg/m^2) and found that only three out of eight patients obtained sustained local control of over 6 months. Severe and disabling subcutaneous fibrosis was observed in two out of the eight patients, possibly due to the radiation enhancing effect of *cis*-platinum on connective tissue. Stewart et al.[67] treated 18 patients with brain metastases with a combination of intravenous *cis*-platinum administered weekly and whole brain irradiation to 30 Gy in 12 fractions administered over a period of 2.5 weeks. The median survival was 10 weeks, and few patients experienced neurologic improvement. *Cis*-platinum contributed significantly to treatment toxicity including, in particular, nausea and vomiting. Another study of 30 patients with metastatic lesions treated by radiotherapy and 5-fluorouracil reported a response rate of 70 percent (complete response 10 percent) lasting from 3 to 13 months.[68] There are no randomized studies that provide evidence that a combined modality approach is superior to radiotherapy alone in improving the chances of local control, and the meager clinical data that is available is difficult to interpret.

Hypoxic Cell Sensitizers and Radiotherapy

Since it is well established that hypoxic tumor cells are more radioresistant than their oxygenated counterparts, the presence of a significant proportion of hypoxic tumor cells in a tumor may contribute to radioresistance in clinical radiotherapy. This forms the rationale for the use of hyperbaric oxygen as a radiosensitizer. A report on this type of treatment in malignant melanoma[69] gave a response rate of 57 percent (13 out of 23 lesions improved), although no direct comparison can be made with irradiation under normobaric conditions. Another strategy has been to use drugs that mimic the action of oxygen, thereby restoring radiosensitivity in the hypoxic tumor cells. Several prototypic compounds (for example, misonidazole) have been developed and have been utilized since the early 1970s, mostly in various epithelial solid tumors.[70] There is experimental evidence that these drugs have radiosensitizing effects in human melanoma grown in athymic mice.[71] Investigators at Mount Vernon Hospital, England, have found high tumor concentrations of the drug Ro 03-8799 (pimonidazole) in several human melanomas,[72] and the initial clinical studies were reported to be encouraging.[73] Of their seven patients treated for recurrent disease with pimonidazole and radiation doses of 50 to 56 Gy in 20 to 21 fractions over 4 to 5 weeks, five achieved sustained regression. The authors suggest that this approach merits further study.

Radiotherapy and Hyperthermia

Combination of irradiation and hyperthermia as a treatment for cancer is attractive because radioresistant hypoxic tumor cells remain sensitive to heat, and there is also evidence that heat has radiosensitizing effects. Nonrandomized studies comparing hyperthermia and radiation with radiation alone suggest a higher tumor control rate with the combined approach.[74–76] In metastatic malignant melanoma, Kim et al.[77] reported a tumor control rate of 75 percent with the combined approach, compared to 46 percent with radiation alone; an observation similar to that of other authors.[76,78] While the role of hyperthermia has not been proven in a randomized trial, it should retain a palliative role as an adjunct to radiotherapy. Realistically, it should be the subject of controlled protocols designed to determine the precise indications and techniques for its administration.

OTHER INNOVATIVE APPROACHES OF RADIOTHERAPY

High L.E.T. Radiation

Because X-rays utilized in conventional radiotherapy are *sparsely-ionizing,* investigators have also examined more *densely ionizing* radiation modalities, such as neutrons or other heavy particles in the treatment of cancer. These types of radiation with high *linear energy transfer* (L.E.T.) are more lethal because they deposit their energy densely over the tract traveled, making it more likely to damage the target structures (DNA) in cells. This physical phenomenon is manifested by absence of the initial shoulder on the cell survival curve for fast neutrons, because the majority of radiation-induced damage even at low doses cannot be repaired. This may be particularly advantageous for melanomas that tend to have broad shoulders on their cell-survival curves, as previously discussed.

Blake et al.[79] reported a complete response rate of 71 percent using fast neutrons (7.5 meV) in melanoma, although complications were noted in 22 percent, consisting generally of severe subcutaneous fibrosis due to high absorption of neutrons by hydrogen-rich adipose tissue. In contrast, Tsunemoto et al. reported a much lower response rate of approximately 30 percent.[80] These results and the absence of a control group make it difficult to draw conclusions on fast neutron therapy.

Other types of particles (for example, pions) have been utilized in treating superficial metastatic melanoma,[81] but their role in relation to conventional X-rays have not been evaluated.

Targeted Radiotherapy

This interesting approach utilizes radiolabeled compounds that are selectively taken up by tumors and not by normal tissues. Monoclonal antibodies have been used for this purpose. Larson et al. reported on the use of ^{131}I-labeled Fab fragments specific to the p97 glycoprotein expressed by human melanoma cells[82] in 33 patients with advanced malignant melanoma, with acceptable toxicity. Much experimental and clinical work are underway to try and optimize either radioimmunotherapy[83,84] or targeted radiotherapy,[85] although they should still be limited to defined investigative protocols.

Another innovative approach termed Boron Neutron Capture Therapy (BNCT), is undergoing investigation in several centers.[86–89] This uses low energy (about 0.025 eV) neutrons, and relies on the "capture" of these thermal neutrons by a stable isotope of Boron, ^{10}B, previously administered and concentrated by the tumor. This reaction leads to the formation of ^{11}B, which instantly fissions, producing an α particle (helium nuclei) and ^{7}Li. These heavy particles deposit densely ionizing radiation with an extremely short path length of 10 to 14 μm, approximately the diameter of one cell. Preliminary results of this therapy are encouraging,[88] although it is too soon to fully evaluate its effectiveness in the primary treatment of melanoma, and little published data exist for the treatment of metastatic disease.

CONCLUSIONS

This review discusses the uses of radiation therapy in the management of malignant melanoma. Information is presented from the clinical literature showing that this disease is not radioresistant and certain radiobiologic principles and data are presented that may explain the unfavorable reports in the previous literature. Furthermore, while radiotherapy will continue to be used for the palliative management of melanoma, indications also exist where radiotherapy provides options in the curative treatment of this disease. In general, these are in the areas of adjuvant treatment in addition to surgery for high-risk cases or where major ablative surgery is not feasible or appropriate. Indications for the use of radiotherapy as a sole radical treatment modality are also presented. Finally, more recent strategies for delivering radiotherapy and for integrating it with other nonsurgical cancer treatment modalities are described.

REFERENCES

1. Adair FE. Treatment of melanoma. *Surg Gynecol Obstet* 62:406–409, 1936.
2. McGovern BJ, and Murad TM. Pathology of melanoma. In: Balch CM, Milton GW, Shaw HM, and Soong S (eds.), Cutaneous Melanoma: Clinical Management and Treatment Results Worldwide. Philadelphia, PA: Lippincott; 1985:29–53.
3. Dewey DL. The radiosensitivity of melanoma cells in culture. *Br J Radiol* 44:816–817, 1971.
4. Rofstad EK. Radiation biology of malignant melanoma. *Acta Radiol* 25:1–10, 1986.
5. Rofstad EK, and Brustad T. Radioresponsiveness of human melanoma xenografts given fractionated irradiation in vivo—relationship to the initial slope of the cell survival curve in vitro. *Radiother Oncol* 9:45–56, 1987.
6. Rofstad EK, and Brustad T. Broad-shouldered survival curves of a human melanoma xenograft. *Acta Radiol Oncol* 20(4):261–265, 1981.
7. Trott KR, von Lieven H, Kummermehr J, Skopal D, Lukacs S, and Braun-Falco O. The radiosensitivity of malignant melanomas. Part I: Experimental studies. *Int J Radiat Oncol Biol Phys* 7:9–13, 1981.
8. Weichselbaum RR, and Little JB. The differential response of human tumors to fractionated radiation may be due to a post-irradiation repair process. *Br J Cancer* 46:532–537, 1982.

9. Lobo PA, and Liebner EJ. Radiotherapy in the management of malignant melanoma. *Int J Radiat Oncol Biol Phys* 7:21–26, 1981.
10. Trott KR, von Lieven H, Kummermehr J, Skopal D, Lukacs S. Brauno-Falco O, and Kellerer A. The radiosensitivity of malignant melanomas. Part II: Clinical studies. *Int J Radiat Oncol Biol Phys* 7:15–20, 1981.
11. McBride H, Stea B, Hill A, and Trent J. Possible relationship between chromosome alterations and in vitro cellular radiosensitivity of human malignant melanoma. *Int J Radiat Oncol Biol Phys* 19:349–355, 1990.
12. Trent JM, Meyskens FL, Salmon S, Ryschon K, Leong SPL, Davis JR, and McGee DL. Relation of cytogenetic abnormalities and clinical outcome in metastatic melanoma. *N Engl J Med* 322:1508–1511, 1990.
13. Williams MV, Denekamp J, and Fowler JF. A review of α/β ratios for experimental tumors: Implications for clinical studies of altered fractionation. *Int J Radiat Oncol Biol Phys* 11:87–96, 1985.
14. Bentzen SM, Overgaard J, Thames HD, Overgaard M, Vejby Hansen P, von der Maase H, and Meder J. Clinical radiobiology of malignant melanoma. *Radiother Oncol* 16:169–182, 1989.
15. Overgaard J. The role of radiotherapy in recurrent and metastatic malignant melanoma: A clinical radiobiological study. *Int J Radiat Oncol Biol Phys* 12:867–872, 1986.
16. Deacon J, Peckham MJ, and Steel GG. The radioresponsiveness of human tumours and the initial slope of the cell survival curve. *Radiother Oncol* 2:317–323, 1984.
17. Peters LJ, Brock WA, Chapman JD, and Wilson G. Predictive assays of tumor radiocurability. *Am J Clin Oncol* 11(3):275–287, 1988.
18. West CML, Davidson SE, and Hunter RD. Evaluation of surviving fraction at 2 Gy as a potential prognostic factor for the radiotherapy of carcinoma of the cervix. *Int J Radiat Biol* 56(5):761–765, 1989.
19. Glasgow GF, Sampiere VA, and Purdy JA. External beam dosimetry and treatment planning. In: Perez CA and Brady LW (eds.), Principles and Practice of Radiation Oncology. Philadelphia, PA: JB Lippincott Co., 1987:159–198.
20. Hellman S. Principles of radiation therapy. In: Devita VT, Hellman S, and Rosenberg SA (eds.), *Cancer, Principles and Practice of Oncology*. Philadelphia, PA: JB Lippincott Co., 1989:247–275.
21. O'Sullivan B, and Sutcliffe SB. The toxicity of radiotherapy. *Clin Oncol* 4(3):485–509, 1985.
22. Overgaard J. Radiation treatment of malignant melanoma. *Int J Radiat Oncol Biol Phys* 6:41–44, 1980.
23. Wheldon TE. Optimal fractionation for the radiotherapy of tumour cells possessing wide-shouldered survival curves. *Br J Radiol* 52:417–418, 1979.
24. Fowler JF. Radioresponsiveness of malignant melanoma to fractionated irradiation [letter]. *Int J Radiat Oncol Biol Phys* 10:439–441. 1984.
25. Adam JS, Habeshaw T, and Kirk J. Response rate of malignant melanoma to large fraction irradiation. *Br J Radiol* 55:605–607, 1982.
26. Doss LL, and Memula N. The radioresponsiveness of melanoma. *Int J Radiat Oncol Biol Phys* 8:1131–1134, 1982.
27. Habermalz, HJ. Irradiation of malignant melanoma: Experience in the past and present. *Int J Radiat Oncol Biol Phys* 7:131–133, 1981.
28. Habermalz H, and Fischer JJ. Radiation therapy of malignant melanoma. Experience with high individual treatment doses. *Cancer* 38:2258–2262, 1976.
29. Katz HR. The results of different fractionation schemes in the palliative irradiation of metastatic melanoma. *Int J Radiat Oncol Biol Phys* 7:907–911, 1981.
30. Khan MS, and Ross WM. Management of malignant melanoma: A retrospective analysis of 182 patients. *Clin Radiol* 35:151–154, 1984.
31. Konefal JB, Emami B, and Pilepich MV. Malignant melanoma: Analysis of dose fractionation in radiation therapy. *Radiology* 164:607–610, 1987.
32. Overgaard J, Overgaard M, Vejby Hansen P, and von der Maase H. Some factors of importance in the radiation treatment of malignant melanoma. *Radiother Oncol* 5:183–192, 1986.
33. Overgaard J, von der Maase, and Overgaard M. A randomized study comparing two high-dose per fraction radiation schedules in recurrent or metastatic malignant melanoma. *Int J Radiat Oncol Biol Phys* 11:1837–1839, 1985.
34. Strauss A, Dritschilo A, Nathanson L, and Piro AJ. Radiation therapy of malignant melanomas: an evaluation of clinically used fractionation schemes. *Cancer* 47:1262–1266, 1981.
35. Vlock DR, Kirkwood JM, Leutzinger C, Kapp DS, and Fishcher JJ. High-dose fraction radiation therapy for intracranial metastases of malignant melanoma. *Cancer* 49:2289–2294, 1982.
36. Konefal JB, Emami B, and Pilepich MV. Analysis of dose fractionation in the palliation of metastases from malignant melanoma. *Cancer* 61:243–246, 1988.
37. Trott KR. The optimal radiation dose per fraction for the treatment of malignant melanomas. *Int J Radiat Oncol Biol Phys* 20:905–907, 1991.
38. Ziegler JC, and Cooper JS. Brain metastases from malignant melanoma: Conventional vs. high-dose-per-fraction radiotherapy. *Int J Radiat Oncol Biol Phys* 12:1839–1842, 1986.
39. Sause WT, Cooper JS, Rush S, Ago CT, Cosmatos D, Coughlin CT, Janjan N, and Lipsett J. Fraction size in external beam radiation therapy in the treatment of melanoma. *Int J Radiat Oncol Biol Phys* 20:429–432, 1991.
40. Rounsaville MC, Cantril ST, Fontanesi J, Vaeth JM, and Green JP. Radiotherapy in the management of cutaneous melanoma: Effect of time, dose, and fractionation. *Front Radiat Ther Oncol* 22:62–78, 1988.
41. Harwood AR. Conventional fractionated radiotherapy for 51 patients with lentigo maligna and lentigo maligna melanoma. *Int J Radiat Oncol Biol Phys.* 9:1019–1021, 1983.
42. Harwood AR. Conventional radiotherapy in the treatment of lentigo maligna and lentigo maligna melanoma. *J Am Acad Dermatol* 6:310–316, 1982.
43. Harwood AR. Melanomas of the head and neck. *J Otolaryngol* 12:64–69, 1983.
44. Harwood AR, Dancuart F, Fitzpatrick PJ, and Brown T. Radiotherapy in nonlentiginous melanoma of the head and neck. *Cancer* 48:2599–2605, 1981.
45. Benediktsdottir K, Edenholm M, Lindholm Å, Mårtensson B, Ståhl L, and Zotterlund B. Pre-operative irradiation of malignant melanoma. A multifactorial analysis of survival. *Acta Radiol Oncol* 23(5):315–320, 1984.
46. Ang KK, Byers RM, Peters LJ, Maor MH, Wendt CD, Morrison WH, Hussey DH, and Goepfert H. Regional radiotherapy as adjuvant treatment for head and neck malignant melanoma. Preliminary results. *Arch Otolaryngol Head Neck Surg* 116:169–172, 1990.
47. Johanson CR, Harwood AR, Cummings BJ, and Quirt I. 0-7-21 Radiotherapy in nodular melanoma. *Cancer* 51:226–232, 1983.
48. Rate WR, Solin LJ, and Turrisi AT. Palliative radiotherapy for metastatic malignant melanoma: Brain metastases, bone metastases, and spinal cord compression. *Int J Radiat Oncol Biol Phys* 15:859–864, 1988.

49. Salmi R, and Holsti P. Effects of Roentgen irradiation on human melanoma metastases in the skin. *Acta Oncologica* 26(1):37–40, 1987.
50. Harwood AR, and Cummings BJ. Radiotherapy for malignant melanoma: A re-appraisal. *Cancer Treatment Rev* 8:271–282, 1981.
51. Dancuart F, Harwood AR, and Fitzpatrick PJ. The radiotherapy of lentigo maligna and lentigo maligna melanoma of the head and neck. *Cancer* 45:2279–2283, 1980.
52. Dickson RJ. Malignant melanoma. A combined surgical and radiotherapeutic approach. *Am J Roent Genol* 79:1063–1070, 1958.
53. Hurley RA, Richter W, and Torrens L. The results of radiotherapy with high pressure oxygen in carcinoma of the pharynx, larynx and oral cavity. *Br J Radiol* 45:98–109, 1972.
54. Creagan ET, Woods JE, Cupps RE, and O'Fallon JR. Radiation therapy for malignant melanoma of the head and neck. *Am J Surg* 138:604–606, 1979.
55. Creagan ET, Cupps RE, Ivins JC, Pritchard DJ, Sim FH, Soule EH, and O'Fallon JR. Adjuvant radiation therapy for regional node metastases from malignant melanoma. *Cancer* 42:2206–2210, 1978.
56. Amdur RJ, Parsons JT, Mendenhall WM, Million RR, and Cassisi NJ. Split-course versus continuous-course irradiation in the postoperative setting for squamous cell carcinoma of the head and neck. *Int J Radiat Oncol Biol Phys* 17:279–285, 1989.
57. Overgaard J, Hjelm-Hansen M, Vendelbo Johansen L, and Andersen AP. Comparison of conventional and split-course radiotherapy as primary treatment in carcinoma of the larynx. *Acta Oncologia* 27:147–152, 1988.
58. Carella RJ, Gelber R, Hendrickson F, Berry HC, and Cooper JS. Value of radiation therapy in the management of patients with cerebral metastases from malignant melanoma. *Cancer* 45:679–683, 1980.
59. Cooper JS. Radiotherapy of malignant melanoma. *Dermatol Clin* 3(2):341–350, 1985.
60. Cooper JS, and Carella R. Radiotherapy of intracerebral metastatic malignant melanoma. *Radiology* 134:735–738, 1980.
61. Habeshaw T, and Wheldon TE. Malignant melanoma: The role of radiotherapy. *Clin Oncol* 3:571–596, 1984.
62. Hellriegel W. Radiation therapy of primary and metastatic melanoma. *Ann N Y Acad Sci* 100, 131–141, 1963.
63. Hagen NA, Cirrincione C. Thaler HT, and DeAngelis LM. The role of radiation therapy following resection of single brain metastasis from melanoma. *Neurology* 40:158–160, 1990.
64. Choi KN, Withers HR, and Rotman M. Intracranial metastases from melanoma: Clinical features and treatment by accelerated fractionation. *Cancer* 56:1–9, 1985.
65. Choi KN, Withers HR, and Rotman M. Metastatic melanoma in brain: Rapid treatment or large dose fractions. *Cancer* 56:10–15, 1985.
66. Dewit L, Bartelink H, and Rumke P. Concurrent cis-diamminedichloroplatinum (II) and radiation treatment for melanoma metastases: A pilot study. *Radiother Oncol* 3:303–309, 1985.
67. Stewart DJ, Feun LG, Maor M, Leavens M, Burgess MA, Benjamin RS, and Bodey GP Sr. Weekly cisplatin during cranial irradiation for malignant melanoma metastatic to brain. *J Neuro-Oncol* 1(1):49–51, 1983.
68. Klausner JM, Gutman M, Rozin RR, Lelcuk S, Chaitchik S, and Inbar M. Conventional fractionation radiotherapy combined with 5-fluorouracil for metastatic malignant melanoma. *Am J Clin Oncol* 10(5):448–450, 1987.
69. Sealey R. Hockly J, and Shepstone B. The treatment of malignant melanoma with cobalt and hyperbaric oxygen. *Clin Radiol* 25:211–215, 1974.
70. Dische S. Chemical sensitizers for hypoxic cells: A decade of experience in clinical radiotherapy. *Radiother Oncol* 3:97–115, 1985.
71. Rofstad EK, and Brustad T. The radiosensitizing effect of metronidazole and misonidazole (Ro-07-0582) on a human malignant melanoma grown in the athymic mutant nude mouse. *Br J Radiol* 51:381–386, 1978.
72. Dische S, Saunders MI, Dunphy EP, Bennett MH, Des-Rochers C, Stratford MRL, Minchington AI, and Orchard RA. Concentrations achieved in human tumors after administration of misonidazole, SR-2508 and Ro 03-8799. *Int J Radiat Oncol Biol Phys* 12:1109–1111, 1986.
73. Dische S. Radiotherapy using the hypoxic cell sensitizer Ro 03-8799 in malignant melanoma. *Radiother Oncol* 10:111–116, 1987.
74. Arcangeli G, Benassi M, Cividalli A, Lovisalo GA, and Mauro F. Radiotherapy and hyperthermia. Analysis of clinical results and identification of prognostic variables. *Cancer* 60:950–956, 1987.
75. Enami B, Perez CA, Konefal J, Pilepich MV, Leybovich L. Straube W, Von Gerichten D, and Hederman MA. Thermoradiotherapy of malignant melanoma. *Int J Hyperthermia* 4:373–381, 1988.
76. Gonzalez D, Van Dijk JDP, Blank LECM, and Rumke PH. Combined treatment with radiation and hyperthermia in metastatic malignant melanoma. *Radiother Oncol* 6:105–113, 1986.
77. Kim JH, Hahn EW, and Ahmed SA. Combination hyperthermia and radiation therapy for malignant melanoma. *Cancer* 50:478–482, 1982.
78. Overgaard J, and Overgaard M. Hyperthermia as an adjuvant to radiotherapy in the treatment of malignant melanoma. *Int J Hyperthermia* 3:483–501, 1987.
79. Blake PR, Catterall M, and Errington RD. Treatment of malignant melanoma by fast neutrons. *Br J Surg* 72:517–519, 1985.
80. Tsunemoto H, Morita S, and Mori S. Characteristics of malignant melanoma cells in the treatment with fast neutrons. *Pigment Cell Res* 2:372–378, 1989.
81. Kligerman MM, West G, Dicello J, Sternhagen CJ, Barnes JE, Loeffler RK, Dobrowolski, Davis HT, Bradbury JN, Lane TF, Petersen DF, and Knapp EA. Initial comparative response to peak pions and x-rays of normal skin and underlying tissue surrounding superficial metastatic nodules. *Am J Roentgenol* 126:261–267, 1976.
82. Larson SM, Carrasquillo JA, Krohn KA, Brown JP, McGuffin RW, Ferens JM, Graham MM, Hill LD, Beaumier PL, Hellstrom KE, and Hellstrom I. Localization of ^{131}I-labeled p97-specific Fab fragments in human melanoma as a basis for radiotherapy. *J Clin Invest* 72:2101–2114, 1983.
83. Kwok CS, Crivici A, MacGregor WD, and Unger MW. Optimization of radioimmunotherapy using human malignant melanoma multicell spheroids as a model. *Cancer Res* 49:3276–3281, 1989.
84. Lamki LM, Zukiwski AA, Shanken LJ, Legha SS, Benjamin RS, Plager CE, Salk DF, Schroff RW, and Murray JL. Radio imaging of melanoma using ^{99m}Tc-labeled Fab fragments reactive with a high molecular weight melanoma antigen. *Cancer Res* 50(3, supp):904s–908s, 1990.
85. Link EM, and Carpenter RN. ^{211}At-methylene blue for targeted radiotherapy of human melanoma xenografts: Treatment of micrometastases. *Cancer Res* 50:2963–2967, 1990.

86. Barth RF, Soloway AH, and Fairchild RG. Boron neutron capture therapy of cancer. *Cancer Res* 50:1061–1070, 1990.
87. Hersey P. Preclinical and Phase I studies of monoclonal antibodies in melanoma: Application to boron neutron capture therapy of melanoma. *Pigment Cell Res* 2:264–272, 1989.
88. Mishima Y, Ichihashi M, Hatta S, Honda C, Yamamura K, and Nakagawa T. New thermal neutron capture therapy for malignant melanoma: Melanogenesis—seeking ^{10}B molecule—melanoma cell interaction from in vitro to first clinical trial. *Pigment Cell Res* 2:226–234, 1989.
89. Tamat SR, Moore DE, Patwardhan A, and Hersey P. Boronated monoclonal antibody 225.28S for potential use in neutron capture therapy of malignant melanoma. *Pigment Cell Res* 2:278–280, 1989.

Chapter 31

MANAGEMENT OF PRIMARY MUCOSAL MELANOMA

Jan H. Wong and Donald L. Morton

INTRODUCTION

Early in fetal development, melanocytes break away from the neural crest, and by 4 to 6 weeks of fetal gestation, they migrate to their final destination in the skin, uveal tract, meninges, or ectodermal mucosa.[1,2] Although most melanocytes are found at the dermoepidermal junction of the skin, melanocytes have been documented in the mucosa of the respiratory, digestive, and urogenital tracts. Laidlaw and Cahn[3] demonstrated that melanocytes, which are presumed to be the cells of origin of mucosal melanomas, are a normal and consistent constituent of the oral mucosa, not only of Blacks and other dark skin races but also of Caucasians with fair skin and blue eyes.

Epidemiology and Etiology

Melanomas arising from the mucosa of the respiratory, digestive, or urogenital tracts are unusual. The actual incidence of mucosal melanoma is difficult to determine accurately in part because it occurs infrequently and is difficult to define, and in part because it is usually reported by tertiary care centers to which patients are referred. The reported incidence of mucosal melanoma ranges from 0.2 to 8 percent of all melanomas; mucosal melanomas represent approximately 1 percent of all melanomas treated by the staff of the John Wayne Cancer Institute.[4] The incidence may vary by race, with a higher incidence of certain lesions in Oriental,[5–7] Indian,[8] and Black[9] populations.

It is often extremely difficult to determine whether a mucosal melanoma is a primary or metastatic lesion, because cutaneous melanoma may metastasize widely, including to the mucous membranes. In 1953, Allen and Spitz[10] suggested that to consider a melanoma in mucous membranes a primary lesion, there must be histological evidence of overlying or lateral junctional changes. Although this is considered the most reasonable evidence of the primary nature of a mucosal melanoma, junctional changes adjacent to an identified mucosal melanoma are not always present. Ulceration, which is not uncommon in these lesions, may destroy these histologic changes. In this setting, it is critical to discount the possibility of a primary cutaneous lesion prior to diagnosing a primary mucosal melanoma. Patients with a history of cutaneous or ocular melanoma or nevi that have regressed should be considered to have metastatic melanoma rather than primary mucosal melanoma.

Although ultraviolet radiation has been strongly established as an etiologic agent for cutaneous melanoma, the etiological agent(s) responsible for mucosal melanoma is (are) unknown. The potential role of carcinogens in the development of mucosal melanoma is unclear, although the use of known carcinogens such as tobaccos and bechtel nuts has been noted in Indian populations with a higher incidence of oral and anal melanoma.[11] The frequent development, or pre-existence for several years, of melanosis in Japanese and Indian patients with oral melanoma suggests that radial proliferation of melanocytes associated with mucosal melanoma may be important in the development of melanoma.[7,8]

MELANOMA OF THE HEAD AND NECK MUCOSA

Melanoma arising in the oral, pharyngeal, and nasopharyngeal mucosa most commonly occurs in men, with a peak incidence in the sixth decade of life.[12,13] Mucosal melanosis is frequently encountered adjacent to oral melanoma[7] and may exist for a considerable period of time prior to diagnosis. Oral pigmentation is common in Blacks and is usually considered physiological. Oral pigmentation is also found to varying degrees in other ethnic groups. For this reason, differentiation between benign and malignant lesions may be difficult. These tumors are usually nodular in shape, with irregular erythematous borders, and often may be ulcerated. However, a significant number may be clinically innocent in appearance. Tumors arising in the nasopharynx are most commonly polypoid in character, often friable, and bleed. Bleeding or the presence of a mass are the most frequent symptoms prompting medical consultation for melanoma arising in the head and neck mucosa. Painful lesions are relatively infrequent.

In most series, mucosal melanoma of the head and neck has a distinct pattern of occurrence. Oral melanomas most commonly occur on the upper jaw.[13] The hard palate is the most frequent site of involvement, followed by the alveolar ridge and soft palate. Mucosal melanoma arising from the buccal mucosa or from the floor of the mouth is distinctly unusual. Intranasal melanomas are not infrequent in Blacks. They occur frequently on the anterior septum, less commonly on the inferior turbinates, and most infrequently on the middle turbinates and floor of the nasal cavity.[12,14] Paranasal sinus melanoma is exceedingly rare, but the paranasal sinus is also an uncommon site of metastases from cutaneous melanoma.

Natural History

Melanomas arising from mucosa of the oral, pharyngeal, or nasopharyngeal cavities are believed to be particularly aggressive lesions. The 5-year survival is approximately 20 percent, with a range of less than 5 percent[12] to 29 percent.[15] Regional node metastases are not infrequent and have been reported in approximately 50 percent of patients with melanoma of the head and neck mucosa, although Shah et al.[16] and Iverson and Robins[17] have reported regional node metastases to be far less common. In contrast to cutaneous melanoma, for which the original three-stage system has important prognostic implications, the difference in survival of patients with apparently localized head and neck mucosal melanomas and those with regionally metastatic disease is not striking.[16,18] Approximately 10 percent of patients with melanoma of the head and neck mucosa will present with evidence of metastatic disease at the time of diagnosis.[16,18,19]

Treatment

The standard recommendation for the treatment of mucosal melanoma of the head and neck is radical resection of the primary. The nature of the surgical procedure depends on the site and extent of the primary lesion. This could include partial or radical maxillectomy for lesions in the nasal cavity, paranasal sinus, or hard palate. The capability of immediate prosthetic rehabilitation minimizes severe postoperative defects. Appropriate radical resection is generally recommended for melanoma of the floor of the mouth. Treatment of nasal melanoma may involve removal of the mucosa, septum, and lateral nasal wall via a lateral rhinotomy.[20]

The efficacy, and therefore the necessity, of immediate node dissection in the absence of clinically suspicious disease is as unclear for mucosal melanoma as it is for cutaneous melanoma. Far less data is available to guide the therapy for mucosal melanoma than for cutaneous melanoma. The limited experience in even large series of mucosal melanoma of the head and neck has prevented direct comparison of treatment alternatives. Hoyt et al. noted that the major factor in the failure of mucosal melanoma of the head and neck is not regional disease but local recurrence.[18] In the presence of clinically detectable disease, neck dissection is generally recommended, although the impact on survival may be minimal. Hoyt et al.[18] and Shah et al.[16] noted little difference in the survival of patients whose disease was confined to the primary site and those who presented with regional metastases.

Comparative analysis of the treatments of patients with mucosal melanoma of the head and neck,[11] suggests that surgery with immediate node dissection produced results similar to those resulting from surgery with postoperative radiation therapy. In the primary treatment of mucosal melanoma of the head and neck, radiation therapy alone was inferior to surgery, although it should be recognized that patients treated primarily with radiation therapy alone were not generally considered surgical candidates because of the extent of disease and/or status of the patient.

MELANOMA OF THE ESOPHAGUS

Primary melanoma arising in the mucosa of the esophagus is an extremely rare condition. Metastatic melanoma of the esophagus is far more common. Although clinically not detectable in the majority of patients, esophageal disease is evident at autopsy in approximately 3 percent of patients with disseminated melanoma.[21] De La Pava et al.[22] have convincingly demonstrated melanocytes in the basal layer of the esophageal epithelium, indicating the potential for primary melanoma of the esophagus. The first histologically confirmed case of primary melanoma of the esophagus was reported in 1952.[23] Since then, there have been reports of approximately 50 other patients with primary melanoma of the esophagus. Primary melanoma of the esophagus has been reported in children,[24] but it is most common in the sixth and seventh decades of life. As previously discussed, the demonstration of junctional changes at the tumor site is considered absolute evidence of the primary origin of the tumor.

The predominant symptom of patients with primary melanoma of the esophagus is dysphagia, which is often associated with substernal pain. Weight loss is almost a uniform occurrence. Bleeding from primary melanoma of the esophagus is unusual. Grossly, these lesions are almost uniformly polypoid in appearance[25] and often pigmented. The distal third of the esophagus is the most common site of involvement.

Natural History

Metastatic involvement of periesophageal lymph nodes and/or of the viscera is common at the time of diagnosis. Like cutaneous melanoma, primary melanoma of the esophagus can metastasize widely, essentially to all organ sites. The median survival of this group of patients is extremely short, and long-term survival is extremely unusual; the majority of patients succumb to recurrent or persistent disease within months of the original diagnosis. Only one patient has been reported to have had prolonged survival following resection: Pomeranz and Garlock[26] reported a patient with primary melanoma of the esophagus who appeared to be well more than 6 years following resection of disease.

TREATMENT

Esophagectomy with primary reconstruction is considered the only potentially curative treatment for primary melanoma of the esophagus. Despite an aggressive surgical approach, however, the prognosis remains poor. A significant number of patients will not be candidates for resection because of regional or distant metastatic disease, but they may be candidates for palliative local radiation to relieve symptoms of dysphagia associated with the tumor.

MELANOMA OF THE GALLBLADDER

Approximately 12 patients with primary melanoma arising in the gallbladder have been reported.[27–32] Although there is some question whether primary melanoma of the gallbladder exists, Breathnach[33] has described the presence of melanocytes in the gallbladder. Melanocytes are presumably the cells of origin of primary melanoma of the gallbladder. The absence of pathologic material has made it difficult to characterize the histologic patterns of primary melanoma of the gallbladder. Microscopic pigmentation appears to be a uniform finding. Junctional changes have also been described. Like primary melanoma of the esophagus, primary melanoma of the gallbladder often appears polypoid, large (up to 8 cm in diameter), and pigmented.[32] This is in contrast to metastatic melanoma to the gallbladder, which usually is only a few millimeters in diameter.[34]

Symptoms associated with primary melanoma of the gallbladder may be related to biliary obstruction and inflammation, with right upper quadrant tenderness, which may be typical of acute cholecystitis or associated with symptoms of metastatic disease. There have been reports of neurologic symptoms secondary to brain metastases and hematemesis from ulcerating duodenal metastases.

Natural History

Patients commonly have metastatic involvement at the time they are diagnosed with primary melanoma of the gallbladder. Cholecystitis is uniformly invasive at the time of diagnosis, which is most commonly an incidental finding at the time of cholecystectomy. Long-term survival in this setting is unusual, with most patients dead of tumor within 2 to 3 years, although two patients have been reported to have survived beyond 5 years.[35]

Treatment

Cholecystectomy has resulted in the only long-term survival in patients with primary melanoma of the gallbladder. The extent of disease in the majority of patients with primary melanoma of the gallbladder lends itself to only systemic therapy or palliative supportive therapy at the time of diagnosis.

PRIMARY MELANOMA OF THE ANORECTUM

Approximately 36 new cases of anorectal melanoma are diagnosed annually in the United States.[36] Although substantially more frequent than melanoma of other mucosal sites and the third most common melanoma following melanoma of the skin and eye, anorectal melanoma is still a rare neoplasm, far less common than epidermoid carcinoma of the anus.

A controversy exits whether melanomas can arise in the mucosa of the rectum[37] or whether the tumors are actually extensions from a primary anal melanoma. Based on pathologic examination of 15 cases of primary melanoma of the anorectum, Morson and Volkstädt[38] suggested that these tumors appear to arise from the squamous epithelial lining of the anal canal just proximal to the anal valves. Quan et al.[39] found that the majority of anorectal melanoma arose from the anal skin or from the mucocutaneous junction, and that if the rectal mucosa was involved, it was only by upward extension of the tumor. However, the demonstration of melanocytes in rectal mucosa by electron microscopy[40] suggests that primary melanoma can arise in the rectum.

Anorectal melanomas demonstrate junctional changes that confirm the primary origin. Often, however, overlying ulceration will destroy this histological finding. Again, it should be cautioned that autopsy studies document an approximately 14 percent incidence of large bowel and rectal metastases from cutaneous melanoma.[21]

The majority of patients with anorectal melanoma present with rectal bleeding, which is often associated with a painful mass. A change in bowel habits and weight loss, suggestive of extensive local or metastatic disease, and a history of symptomatic hemorrhoids are common presenting complaints. Pigmented changes in the tumor are common and obvious in the majority of patients. Grossly, the tumors are often polypoid, ulcerated, and may prolapse through the anus.

Natural History

Anorectal melanoma is a particularly virulent tumor, which is generally detected late and associated with poor survival.[41–51] Eight to sixty-nine percent of patients with anorectal melanoma demonstrate nodal metastases, either to mesenteric lymph nodes or inguinal nodes.[24,37] Approximately 8 percent of patients present with distant metastases at the time of diagnosis.[37] Primary melanoma of the anorectum tends to be an extremely invasive lesion, with the primary tumor ranging from 0.5 mm to greater than 2 cm in thickness.[37] The overall 5-year survival of patients with resectable primary melanoma of the anorectum varies from 7 to 20 percent. Wanebo et al.[37] demonstrated a relationship between tumor thickness and survival in 26 patients with anorectal melanoma.

Treatment

The choice of primary treatment of anorectal melanoma is controversial. Abdominal-perineal resection, at times in combination with radiation therapy, has been associated with the longest survival; the only 5-year survivors reported by Chiu et al.,[52] Quan et al.,[39] and Wanebo et al.[37] were those who had undergone abdominal-perineal resection. An aggressive surgical approach has not, however, demonstrated a statistically significant benefit.[11] Local, wide excision of the primary lesions has achieved survival results comparable to those that result from abdominal-perineal resection. However, local recurrences appear to be more common following local wide excision than following abdominal-perineal resection. Wanebo[37] has suggested that abdominal-perineal resection should be reserved for those patients with small, thin lesions, the only potentially curable anorectal melanomas. There is, however, little data to support this recommendation. Because of the virulent nature of anorectal melanoma, in the majority of cases the realistic goal of therapy is palliation by means of conservative surgery.[53]

PRIMARY MELANOMA OF THE VAGINA

Vaginal melanoma accounts for approximately 0.5 percent of all melanomas. Benign melanosis of the vagina occurs in approximately 3 percent of women,[54] and a similar percentage of patients demonstrate melanocytes. Vaginal melanoma has been associated with benign melanosis[55] as well as with multifocal melanosis, which may be located some distance from the primary lesion.[56–59]

Vaginal melanomas are most commonly tumors elevated above the normal vaginal mucosa and are often polypoid in appearance. At presentation, the tumors are usually 2 to 3 cm but may be as large as 8 cm in diameter. They are commonly associated with overlying ulceration of the mucosa and most commonly occur in the lower half of the vagina, without predilection for any wall of the vagina.[11] The majority of cases, however, will have lateral junctional changes,[60] indicating the primary nature of the tumor. This leads to the most common presenting symptom, vaginal bleeding or a vaginal discharge, usually in postmenopausal women. Other presenting complaints include pelvic pain, or a vaginal mass.[61]

Natural History

Like all mucosal melanomas, vaginal melanoma is viewed as an aggressive tumor with a poor prognosis. Regional adenopathy is unusual. Chung et al. reported 19 patients with melanoma of the vagina who had a median time to recurrence of 9 months and a 5-year survival of 21 percent following primary treatment.[61] Five-year survival is distinctly unusual in this disease.[62–64] Norris and Taylor[60] reported a median survival of only 10 months. Local recurrences are common following primary treatment, as is regional node metastasis. At autopsy, the liver, lungs, pelvic peritoneum, pancreas and spleen, as well as periaortic, pelvic, and mediastinal lymph nodes are commonly involved with metastatic melanoma.[59]

Treatment

The treatment of primary melanoma of the vagina is generally considered to be surgery. The extent of surgery has varied from wide local excision to radical vaginectomy, with superficial inguinal node dissection and/or pelvic node dissection. It is unclear, however, whether extensive surgical resection improves local control or actuarial survival. Analysis of case reports[11] suggests that the median survival of patients undergoing only wide local excision was similar to that of those undergoing radical resection. One patient treated with local radioactive isotope therapy has survived 5 years,[65] but the only long-term survivors have been treated by radical surgical excision of the lesion, suggesting that surgery might be the treatment of choice. As with all mucosal melanomas, however, the absence of significant numbers of patients has prevented direct comparisons of various treatment alternatives.

SUMMARY

Primary melanoma arising in mucous membranes is an unusual clinical entity. Despite the rarity of these lesions, a number of points regarding the diagnosis, natural history, and treatment appear to be justified:

1. Cutaneous melanoma may metastasize to essentially all organ systems, and the histological diagnosis of primary mucosal melanoma is difficult. Therefore, it is critical to exclude the possibility that the mucosal lesion represents a metastatic lesion.
2. Most primary mucosal melanomas appear to be diagnosed relatively late in the natural history of the disease, at a time when distant metastatic disease is likely. As in cutaneous melanoma, tumor thickness may have some prognostic significance, although this is unclear from currently available data.
3. Even in tertiary referral centers, experience with primary melanoma arising in mucous membranes is limited. For this reason, no comparative analysis of the different approaches to the management of these lesions has been performed. Therefore, optimal treatment has yet to be defined. Studies of the natural history of the majority of these lesions suggests that these tumors are diagnosed late in the course of disease and that the primary consideration in therapy should be local regional therapy directed at local control with wide local excision.

REFERENCES

1. Weston JA. The migration and differentiation of neural crest cells. *Adv Morphog* 8:41–114, 1970.
2. Le Douarin N. Migration and differentiation of neural crest cells. *Curr Top Dev Biol* 61:31, 1980.
3. Laidlaw GF, and Cahn LR. Melanoblasts in the gum. *J Dent Res* 12:534–537, 1932.
4. Wong JH, Cagle LA, Storm FK, and Morton DL. Natural history of surgically treated mucosal melanoma. *Am J Surg* 154:54–57, 1987.
5. Mori W. Geographic pathology of malignant melanoma in Japan. In: McGovern VJ, and Russell (eds.), *International Pigment Cell Conference* (8th, 1972: Sydney, NSW) *Mechanisms in Pigmentation.* (series, *Pigment Cell, vol 1.*) Basel and New York: Karger, 1973, 246–254.
6. Mori W. A geo-pathological study on malignant melanoma in Japan. *Pathol Microbiol (Basel)* 37:169–180, 1971.
7. Takagi M, Ishikawa G, and Mori W. Primary malignant melanoma of the oral cavity in Japan with special reference to mucosal melanosis. *Cancer* 34:358–370, 1974.
8. Sampat MB, and Sirsat MV. Malignant melanoma of the skin and mucous membranes in Indians. *Int J Cancer* 3:228–254, 1966.
9. Trodahl JN, and Sprague WB. Benign and malignant melanocytic lesions of the oral mucosa. An analysis of 135 cases. *Cancer* 25:812–823, 1970.
10. Allen AC, and Spitz S. Malignant melanoma: A clinicopathologic analysis of the criteria for diagnosis and prognosis. *Cancer* 6:1–45, 1953.
11. Presant CA. Malignant melanoma of mucosal sites. IN: Constanzi JJ (ed.) *Malignant Melanoma.* Boston: Martinus Nijohoff, 1982, vol 1, 55–83.
12. Martin H, and Moore ES. Melanoma of the upper respiratory tract and oral cavity. *Cancer* 8:1167–1176, 1955.
13. Chaudry AP, Hampel A, and Gorlin RJ. Primary malignant melanoma of the oral cavity. A review of 105 cases. *Cancer* 11:923–927, 1958.
14. Pearlman K. Malignant melanoma of the nasal mucous membrane. *J Laryngol Otol* 93:1003–1009, 1979.
15. Catlin D. Mucosal melanoma of the head and neck. *Am J Roentgenol Radium Ther Nucl Med* 99:809–816, 1967.
16. Shah JP, Huvos AG, and Strong EW. Mucosal melanoma of the head and neck. *Am J Surg* 134:531–535, 1977.
17. Iverson K, and Robins RE. Mucosal malignant melanoma. *Am J Surg* 139:660–664, 1980.
18. Hoyt DJ, Jordan T, and Fisher SR. Mucosal melanoma of the head and neck. *Arch Otolaryngol Head Neck Surg* 115:1096–1099, 1989.
19. Bartkowski SB, Panas M, Wilczanska H, and Dubiel-Bigaj M. Primary malignant melanoma of the oral cavity. A review of 20 cases. *Am J Surg* 148:362–366, 1984.
20. Harrison DFN. Malignant melanomata arising in the nasal mucous membrane. *J Laryngol Otol* 90:993–1005, 1976.
21. Einhorn LH, Burgess MA, Vallejos C, Bodey GP Sr, Gutterman J, Mavligit G, Hersh EM, Luce JK, Frei E III, Freireich EJ, and Gottlieb JA. Prognostic correlation and response to treatment in advanced metastatic malignant melanoma. *Cancer Res* 34:1995–2004, 1974.
22. De La Pava S, Nigogosyan G, Pickren JW, et al. Melanosis of the esophagus. *Cancer* 16:48–52, 1963.
23. Garfinkle JM, and Cahan WG. Primary melanocarcinoma of the esophagus. First histological proved case. *Cancer* 5:921–926, 1952.
24. Basque GJ, Boline JE, and Holyoke JB. Malignant melanoma of the esophagus: First reported case in a child. *Am J Clin Pathol* 53:609, 1970.
25. Biagham DLC, Chadsey LC, Ramchaud S, and Doris PJ. Primary melanocarcinoma of the esophagus. *Can Med Assoc J* 105:607–610, 1971.
26. Pomeranz A, and Garlock JH. Primary melanomacarcinoma of the esophagus. *Ann Surg* 42:296–301, 1955.
27. Rosenthal SR. Primary melanocarcinoma of the gallbladder. *Am J Cancer* 15:2288–2300, 1931.
28. Thayer KH, Williams OO, and Rowed D. Malignant melanoma of the gall bladder. Report of a case and review of the literature. *Arizona Med* 12:15, 1955.
29. Walsh TS Jr. Primary melanoma of the gallbladder with

cervical metastasis and survival. First histologically proved case. *Cancer* 9:518, 1956.
30. Jones CH. Malignant melanoma of the gallbladder. *J Pathol Bacteriol* 81:423–430, 1961.
31. Raffensperger EC, Brason FW, and Triano G. Primary melanoma of the gallbladder. *Dig Dis* 8:356, 1963.
32. Peison B, and Rabin L. Malignant melanoma of the gallbladder. Report of three cases and review of the literature. *Cancer* 37:2448, 1976.
33. Breathnach AS. Normal and abnormal melanin pigmentation of the skin. In: Wolman M (ed.), *Pigments in Pathology* vol 1. New York: Academic Press, 1969, 355.
34. Willis RA. The spread of tumours in the human body. 2nd ed. London: Butterworth and Co, 1952, 219.
35. Mills SE, and Cooper PH. Malignant melanoma of the digestive system. *Pathol Annu* 18, part 2:1–26, 1983.
36. Scotto J, Fraumeni JF Jr, and Lee JAH. Melanoma of the eye and other non-cutaneous sites: Epidemiologic aspects. *J Natl Cancer Inst* 56:489, 1976.
37. Wanebo HJ, Woodruff JM, Farr GH, and Quan SH. Anorectal melanoma. *Cancer* 47:1891–1900, 1981.
38. Morson BC, and Volkstädt H. Malignant melanoma of the anal canal. *J Clin Pathol* 16:126–132, 1963.
39. Quan SHQ, White JE, and Diddish MR. Malignant melanoma of the anorectum. *Dis Colon Rectum* 2:275–283, 1959.
40. Werdin C, Limas C, and Knodell RB. Primary malignant melanoma of the rectum. Evidence for origination from rectal mucosal melanocytes. *Cancer* 61:1364–1370, 1988.
41. Braastad FW, Dockerty MB, and Dixon CF. Melanoepithelioma of the anus and rectum. *Surgery* 25:82–85, 1949.
42. Chulani HL. Anal malignant melanoma: Report of a case. *Dis Colon Rectum* 20:517–520, 1977.
43. Dukes C, and Bussey HJR. Sarcoma and melanoma of the rectum. *Br J Cancer* 1:30–37, 1947.
44. Gupta S, and Rastogi BL. Metastatic and melanoma presenting as double intassusception of the small bowel. *Am J Protocol* 28:49–57, 1977.
45. Harrison EG, Beahrs OH, and Hill JR. Anal and perianal malignant neoplasms: Pathology and treatment. *Dis Colon Rectum* 9:255–267, 1966.
46. Husa A, and Hocherstedt K. Anorectal malignant melanoma. A report of 14 cases. *Acta Chir Scand* 140:68-72, 1974.
47. Quan SH, White JE, and Deddish MR. Malignant melanoma of the anorectum. *Dis Colon Rectum* 2:275–283, 1959.
48. Raven RW. Anorectal malignant melanoma. *Royal Society of Medicine, Proceedings* 41:469–474, 1918.
49. Remigo PA, Der BK, and Fosberg RT. Anorectal melanoma: Report of two cases. *Dis Colon Rectum* 19:350–356, 1976.
50. Sinclair DM, Hannah G, McLaughlin IS, Patrick RS, Slavin G, and Neville AM. Malignant melanoma of the anal canal. *Br J Surgery* 57:808–811, 1957.
51. Singh W, and Madaan TR. Malignant melanoma of the anal canal. *Am J Protocol* 27:49-55, 1976.
52. Chiu YS, Unni KK, and Beart RW Jr. Malignant melanoma of the anorectum. *Dis Col Rectum* 23:122–124, 1980.
53. Garnick M, and Lokich JJ. Primary malignant melanoma of the rectum: Rational for conservative surgical management. *J Surg Oncol* 10:529–531, 1978.
54. Nigogosyan G, De La Pava S, and Pickren JW. Melanoblast in vaginal mucosa: Origin for primary malignant melanoma. *Cancer* 17:912–913, 1964.
55. Ehrman RC, Younge PA, and Lerch VL. Exfoliative cytology and histogenesis of early primary malignant melanoma of vagina. *Acta Cytol* 6:245–254, 1962.
56. Batasakis JG, and Dito WR. Primary malignant melanoma of the vagina. *Obstet Gynecol* 20:109–111, 1962.
57. DasGupta TK, Bowden L, and Berg J. Malignant melanoma of unknown primary origin. *Surg Gynecol Obstet* 117:341–346, 1963.
58. Mullaney J. Primary melanoma of the vagina. *J Pathol Bacteriol* 81:473–480, 1961.
59. Hasumi K, Sakamoto G, Sugano H, Kasuga T, and Masubuchi K. Primary malignant melanoma of the vagina. Study of four autopsy cases with ultrastructural findings. *Cancer* 42:2675–2686, 1978.
60. Norris HJ, and Taylor HB. Melanomas of the vagina. *Am J Clin Pathol* 46:420–426, 1966.
61. Chung AF, Murray CJ, Flannery JT, Woodruff JM, and Lewis JL. Malignant melanoma of the vagina—report of 19 cases. *Obstet Gyn* 55:720–727, 1980.
62. Ariel IM. Malignant melanoma of the vagina: Report of a successfully treated case. *Obstet Gynecol* 17:222, 1961.
63. Casa PF, Picena J, and Garcia CG: Malignant melanoma of the vagina, with a review of the literature. *Surg Gynecol Obstet* 94:159, 1952.
64. Mino RA, Mino UH, and Livingstone RG. Primary malignant melanoma of the vagina with a review of the literature. *Am J Obstet Gynecol* 56:325, 1948.
65. Ariel IM. Five year cure of a primary malignant melanoma of the vagina by local radioactive isotope therapy. *Am J Obstet Gynecol* 82:405, 1961.

Chapter 32

PRIMARY OCULAR MELANOMAS

Devron H. Char

INTRODUCTION

Melanoma can involve the eyelid, orbit, optic nerve, conjunctiva, uveal tract, retina and the vitreous.[1] Approximately 9 percent of melanomas occur in the eye.[2] The most common primary ocular melanomas arise in the vascular support structure, the uveal tract; they account for about 80 percent of primary adult eye tumors. Conjunctival melanoma is uncommon and accounts for approximately 2 percent of eye malignancies.[3,4] The ratio of uveal to conjunctival melanomas is approximately 40:1.[5]

Approximately 80 percent of uveal melanomas arise in the choroid, a structure between the sclera and the retina; 10 percent of melanomas involve the iris, and the remainder the ciliary body. Most uveal melanoma patients present because of visual symptoms; conjunctival melanomas usually are discovered when a pigmented spot is noted.

EPIDEMIOLOGY

The incidence of uveal melanoma is about 7.5/1,000,000/year in the United States; about 1500 new cases are seen yearly. There is a strong racial predilection; whites are tenfold more likely than darker skinned races to develop this tumor.[4] Iris melanomas are more frequent in light than dark colored irises.[6,7] The mean age of uveal melanoma diagnosis is in the seventh decade of life; less than 2 percent of patients are diagnosed prior to the age of 20 years old.[8] Sun exposure has been implicated in uveal melanoma development.[6,7,9] In a case-control study of 407 patients a 7.2 relative risk for uveal melanoma in men was associated with welding burn, ocular sunburn, or snow blindness ($p < 0.001$).[9]

The rarity of conjunctival melanoma has precluded the development of similar epidemiologic data. In conjunctival squamous cell carcinoma, viruses are important in the pathophysiology; however, no etiologic agents or consistent genetic aberrations have been described for ocular melanomas.[10]

DIAGNOSIS

Clinical Presentations

CONJUNCTIVAL MELANOMA

Conjunctival melanomas arise from the epithelium; approximately 75 percent develop from an area of primary acquired melanosis.[11] Conjunctival nevi often have cystic inclusions, while melanomas are almost always solid. The malignancy can be focal or diffuse; the latter is usually due to malignant transformation of a diffuse primary acquired melanosis. Simulating lesions include normal racial pigmentation, subconjunctival foreign bodies, nevi, chronic conjunctival inflammation, and pigmentation from the chronic use of eye drops.[1]

UVEAL MELANOMA

Most uveal melanomas develop in the choroid and are not visible without an ophthalmoscope. Pain is uncommon; pain is a presenting symptom in less than 1 percent of cases. Usually distortion of the overlying retinal photoreceptors, either by the growing mass or an exudative retinal detachment produces diminished visual acuity, visual field loss, or distortion of vision. These symptoms are not specific, and patients are often referred with the diagnosis of a retinal detachment. Less frequently, other findings can include unilateral cataract tumor penetration through the sclera, intense inflammation, or dilated vessels on the episcleral surface of the eye. Rarely patients can have either ocular or oculodermal melanosis (nevus of Ota) and a uveal melanoma.

Clinically it is almost impossible to differentiate a very small uveal melanoma from an atypical nevus.[1] As melanomas enlarge they usually become globular in shape, produce a secondary exudative retinal detachment, and may break through the retina into a mushroom shape configuration. Approximately 30 percent of melanomas are amelanotic, and establishing the correct diagnosis in such cases can be impeded by history. As many as 15 percent of patients have had other nonocular systemic malignancies.[12]

A number of lesions can simulate a uveal melanoma; Table 32-1 lists some of these entities. Four of the most common differential diagnoses are atypical nevi, metastatic tumors to the uvea, hemorrhagic uveal lesions, and rhegmatogenous retinal detachment.

TABLE 32-1
LESIONS THAT SIMULATE CHOROIDAL MELANOMA

CHOROIDAL NEOPLASMS	***RETINAL PIGMENT EPITHELIAL PROCESSES***
Choroidal nevus	Retinal pigment hyperplasia
Choroidal metastasis	Retinal pigment epithelial hypertrophy
Choroidal hemangioma	Retinal pigment epithelial adenocarcinoma
Choroidal osteoma	
Choroidal neurilemmoma	***INFLAMMATORY PROCESSES***
Choroidal neurofibroma	Posterior scleritis
Peripheral melanocytoma	Posterior uveitis
Benign lymphoid tumor	
Choroidal hemangiopericytoma	***MISCELLANEOUS***
Choroidal leiomyoma	Hemorrhagic retinal detachment
	Retinoschisis with hemorrhage
HEMORRHAGIC PROCESSES	Staphyloma
Involutional macular degeneration	Intraocular foreign body granuloma
Extramacular disciform lesion	Massive retinal gliosis
Ruptured arteriolar macroaneurysm	Acquired retinal hemangioma
Localized choroidal detachment/hemorrhage	Retinal glioma

Diagnostic Evaluation

CONJUNCTIVAL MELANOMA

There is no adverse prognostic effect of an incisional biopsy, although it may be difficult to histologically differentiate conjunctival melanomas from nevi.[13,14] Analysis in an eye pathology laboratory is the most effective means to establish the diagnosis.[14] Conjunctival nevi almost never involve the palpebral conjunctiva or fornix.[15] Intralesional cysts are clinically helpful to differentiate benign and malignant pigmented tumors.

In neither conjunctival nor uveal melanoma are the staging classifications of Breslow or Clark applicable.[16] In general, focal, bulbar conjunctival melanomas less than 1 mm thick have a very low tumor-related mortality. Overall, approximately 20 percent of conjunctival melanoma patients develop metastatic disease, and the pattern of dissemination is similar to cutaneous melanoma.[11,12,17,18] In conjunctival melanomas over 1.5 mm thick, especially those that are diffuse and involve the palpebral conjunctiva, prognosis is worse. Table 32-2 lists important conjunctival melanoma prognostic factors.

UVEAL MELANOMA

Historically almost 20 percent of eyes enucleated with a diagnosis of a uveal melanoma contained a simulating lesion on histologic evaluation.[19] Over 99 percent of uveal melanomas that require therapy are now correctly diagnosed in major ocular oncology units with noninvasive, multimodality techniques including ophthalmoscopy, ultrasonography, and fluorescein angiography.[1,20] In an analysis of diagnostic efficacy, an experienced observer had over 95 percent accuracy with ophthalmoscopy alone; adding ultrasonography increased diagnostic accuracy to over 98 percent.[20] We have not removed an eye with the clinical diagnosis of a uveal melanoma that was not confirmed histologically in over 12 years.

In atypical lesions, fine needle aspiration biopsy (FNAB) can correctly differentiate melanomas from simulating conditions. A number of investigators have used this technique in various ocular oncologic dis-

TABLE 32-2
CONJUNCTIVAL MELANOMA: PROGNOSTIC PARAMETERS FOR TUMOR-RELATED MORTALITY

	FORNIX/ CARUNCULAR INVOLVEMENT	*DIFFUSE INVOLVMENT*	*BULBAR INVOLVEMENT ONLY*	*THICKNESS < 1.75*	*THICKNESS > 1.8*
Silver et al.	8/10	10/15	1/9	0/16	12/12
Jaffrey et al.	7/10	2/6	1/21	2/18	8/16[1]
Liesegang et al.	2/8		2/20		6/6[1]
Crawford	4/4			3/10	4/5
Folberg et al.		8/25	9/63[2]		36/94[2]

[1] >2.0 mm
[2] >1.6 mm

eases.[21–24] A 25-gauge needle is passed through either a trans-scleral or trans-vitreal route to sample the tumor; there have been no reports of tumor dissemination or significant morbidity.[25] In a masked study, an excellent correlation between the melanoma cell type on FNAB and standard histology was noted.[25,26] We have assessed DNA content, morphometric data, and cell cycling on fine needle biopsies.[25,26]

A systemic evaluation is usually indicated in uveal melanoma patients who require ocular treatment. There are a few caveats to the accuracy of such evaluations. (1) Less than 2 percent of patients will present with simultaneously detectable uveal melanoma and metastases; many patients with large uveal melanomas have micrometastatic disease, undetected at initial ocular diagnosis.[1] (2) In uveal melanoma patients an initial evaluation should include a physical examination, chest roentengram, and serum lactic dehydrogenase and glutyml transpeptidase. If any of these are positive, further evaluation is indicated. The pattern of uveal melanoma dissemination differs from cutaneous melanoma.[27] Over 60 percent of uveal melanoma metastases are first detected in the liver; 25 percent initially present with subcutaneous lesions. Pleural or parenchymal lung involvement is initially noted in less than 10 percent, and bone or central nervous system metastases are the first sign of widespread disease in less than 2 percent of patients.[27]

Almost 50 percent of patients with metastases to the eye present to their ophthalmologist prior to the discovery of the primary neoplasm; this is uncommon in women with breast carcinoma; however, in lung or renal choroidal metastases, eye symptoms and findings almost always predate the diagnosis of the primary tumor.[28] In such patients, plasma carcinoembyronic antigen assay is useful since it is elevated above 10 ng/ml in over 50 percent of patients with choroidal metastases but not in primary uveal melanomas.[29]

MANAGEMENT

Conjunctival Melanoma

Tumor rarity precludes definitive statements on the relative efficacies of treatment modalities.[1] Thin (< 1.5 mm thick), focal tumors located on the bulbar conjunctiva rarely metastasize. In contrast, diffuse tumors over 1.8 mm thick that involve the fornix and caruncle have over 80 percent tumor-related mortality (Table 32-2). The behavior of conjunctival melanoma is unpredictable, and we have removed several lesions more than 10 years ago that were > 3 mm thick and the patients remain alive. The pattern of metastases is similar to cutaneous melanoma; however, a few cases of intraconjunctival metastases have been reported.[30]

Primary acquired melanosis was first described by Reese.[31] Unilateral conjunctival epithelial pigmentation develops in middle-aged individuals, and there is approximately a 20 percent incidence of malignant degeneration.[31] Management of these patients has been controversial. Many investigators initially suggested close follow-up without intervention unless there was pigment spread, increased vascularity, or documented growth. Folberg and colleagues described histologic features that identify lesions that undergo malignant degeneration, although sometimes this determination is difficult.[11,32] Most clinicians now biopsy such lesions, and if histologic features demonstrate malignant potential, many will treat them with cryotherapy.[33,34] Usually melanomas that develop in association with clinical primary acquired melanosis are diffuse, and rarely they also involve the eyelid and sinuses.[35]

The choice of therapy for conjunctival melanoma usually is predicated on the tumor area. We use surgical excision with frozen section control and adjunctive cryotherapy for most melanomas.[1,32] The tumor is resected, if necessary, with a partial thickness sclerectomy. Margins are monitored with frozen sections, and adjunctive cryotherapy is delivered to both the base and resection margins. A large conjunctival area is removed, and inflammation occurs with freezing so the defect is covered with either autologous conjunctiva or buccal mucous membrane.

Orbital or orbital-sinus exenteration is usually not performed. In diffuse, bulky melanomas that have destroyed visual potential and are painful, there is almost always micrometastatic disease. Disfiguring surgical approaches are usually indicated only when local tumor destruction has mandated their use to debulk the area for patient comfort.

There are a number of reports of brachytherapy or external beam radiation.[36,37] Surgery and cryotherapy have over 98 percent local control for focal lesions. When a melanoma is diffuse and involves both the superior and inferior bulbar and palpebral conjunctiva, there is little chance of retention of a useful eye with either surgery or radiation. While radiation can sterilize such a neoplasm, damage to lacrimal ductules and goblet cells results in a dry, painful eye, and eventually an anterior exenteration is usually required. Similarly, when such diffuse lesions are resected with mucosal replacement, a dry, painful, nonfunctional eye is a common sequela.

Uveal Melanoma Therapies

The treatment of uveal melanoma has been controversial for over 120 years.[38–41] The goals of uveal melanoma therapies are to decrease both ocular morbidity and tumor-related mortality.

ENUCLEATION

Indications for enucleation include: patient request after informed consent, a melanoma in a blind, painful eye, a melanoma too large for alternative therapy, recurrent tumor after alternative therapy, and melanomas in eyes with neovascularization. The prognosis after enucleation is dependent on patient age, largest tumor diameter, anterior margin of the tumor, local extrascleral extension, and histology. Patients over 60 years old, those with tumors over 15 mm in diameter, melanomas that cross the ocular equator, tumors with epithelioid cells, those with increased DNA content (hyperploidy), or those with a wide variation in nucleolar area (1/SDNA) are associated with a worse prognosis.[1]

The efficacy of adjuvant therapy is uncertain. In a small prospective study, the use of a methanol extracted residue of BCG did not decrease metastases.[42] In an uncontrolled study of 20 cases, multiple agent chemotherapy appeared to decrease metastases.[43]

In 1977, we initiated a phase I-II study of 20 Gy of pre-enucleation irradiation in poor risk uveal melanomas.[44] In a 10-year retrospective study, this adjunctive therapy has not been effective. Twenty Gy of radiation altered the reproductive integrity of melanomas; there was both diminished tissue culture propagation as well as decreased cell cycling.[44] Unfortunately, survival was worse after pre-enucleation radiation. The retrospective control group chosen had similar size tumors enucleated by the same surgeon. The reasons for poorer survival in the adjunct radiation group are unclear. Other groups have also noted no better survival after pre-enucleation radiation.[45,46] While there is a national trial to study this protocol in a prospective randomized manner, it is doubtful that positive results will be obtained.[47]

ALTERNATIVE THERAPIES

Vision-saving alternative treatments have been attempted since 1911.[48,49] Uveal melanoma radiation was first used in the 1920s.[50,51] A number of radiobiologic issues remain unresolved. The radiation dose and delivery schedule necessary to destroy the reproductive integrity of uveal melanoma is poorly delineated. Historically, 100 gray equivalents (GyE) were used; however, we noted no difference in survival, control, or complication rates with 50, 60, 70, or 80 GyE of helium ion irradiation.[52]

The goal of radiation is to destroy the reproductive integrity of the uveal melanoma. Successfully irradiated larger tumors are not completely obliterated. Tumors studied several years after treatment in eyes enucleated because of late therapeutic complications showed complete loss of melanoma cell reproductive integrity.[53]

Two types of radiation have been used to treat uveal melanomas, brachytherapy (radioactive plaques) and charged particle (proton and helium ion) irradiation.[1] All brachytherapy approaches require placement and removal of a radioactive plaque from the scleral surface of the tumor. Historically,[60] cobalt was used; however, most treatments are now done with a lower energy, ^{125}I sources.[54–57] ^{125}I can be partially focused using a 0.2 mm gold seed carrier to minimize both orbital radiation and lateral scatter. All brachytherapy produce a radiation gradient from the scleral surface to the tumor apex. As thicker tumors are treated, there is exponentially more scleral and lateral dose spread with a higher incidence of radiation damage.

Charged particles (helium ions and protons), have extremely sharp distal and lateral focus; helium ion dose diminishes from 90 percent to less than 10 percent in under 2.3 mm.[1] Unfortunately, there is almost a 70 percent entrance dose. Potential advantages of charged particles, as compared with brachytherapy, include better focusability, no radiation exposure to medical personnel, the need for only one surgical procedure, significantly less secondary strabismus, a uniform radiation dose to the sclera and tumor, the ability to treat larger tumors, and a lower local failure rate.

There are some disadvantages with charged particles. Only five uveal melanoma charged particle treatment centers exist and the entrance beam results in more anterior segment complications than with ^{125}I radioactive plaques.[58]

It is difficult to summarize uveal melanoma radiation results since studies are not randomized, different size and location melanomas have been treated, and follow-up varies in different centers. Approximately 4000 uveal melanomas have been irradiated; most tumors treated with brachytherapy have been relatively small (< 10 mm in diameter and < 5 mm thick) and located in the posterior choroid.[1] Larger tumors have been treated with helium ions and protons. In over 1500 cases that have been irradiated with charged particles, about 90 percent of eyes have been retained; the 5-year tumor-related mortality has been 20 percent.[59,60]

Radiation visual results depend on patient age, tumor size, and proximity to visually vital structures. Unfortunately, almost 50 percent of uveal melanomas are located within 3 mm of either the optic nerve or fovea. In order to avoid a marginal miss, even with particles, such eyes receive a destructive radiation dose to these structures.[58] Approximately half of helium ion or ^{125}I plaque patients with > 20/50 vision retain it 3 years after therapy; overall, about one-third of treated patients have this level of final visual acuity in.[58–60] Tumor size, especially thickness, is an independent visually prognostic parameter.[60,61] Tumors greater than 5 mm thick have a 5.3-fold increased chance of poor vision, as compared with melanomas less than 3 mm thick.[61]

Prognostically important parameters in irradiated patients are similar to enucleated cases; survival has correlated with age, largest tumor diameter, and anterior tumor location.[1] In a recent study, we obtained 100 percent follow-up on patients irradiated with helium ions more than 5 years ago; the 5-year tumor-related mortality in tumors less than 16 mm in diameter and less than 8 mm thick was 10 percent.[59] A number of retrospective studies have compared survival after radiation and enucleation. There is no evidence to suggest better survival with enucleation.[62–64] One study purported to show worse survival after cobalt plaque radiation; however, when appropriate statistical analysis was performed no difference was observed.[65–66]

There is a National Eye Institute clinical trial prospectively randomizing patients with tumors less than 16 mm in diameter and less than 8 mm thick to either enucleation or ^{125}I radioactive plaque therapy (COMS).[47] Many such eyes, especially those containing tumors that are less than 5 mm thick and are more than 5 mm from the nerve or the fovea retain excellent vision; overall > 94 percent of eyes with tumors < 16 mm in diameter and < 8 mm thick did not require enucleation in the combined Boston and San Francisco experience.[58,60,61] It is ethically difficult to justify randomization to enucleation in such cases. There is no data to suggest better survival after eye removal.[64] It is doubtful that, if a difference in survival exists, it could be detected in a reasonable time frame. Even if a 50 percent difference (that is, 5 percent or 20 percent survival with enucleation as compared with 10 percent we observed with radiation) was to be detected, insufficient numbers of patients could be accrued in 5 years to detect such a treatment effect. In fact, that study hopes to detect even a smaller difference.[47] If a difference in the metastatic rate exists, it is small; to detect a small treatment effect, it is imperative that therapy at each institution is almost identical. While local tumor control failure is almost identical in Boston and San Francisco (approximately 4 percent), in many centers participating in the trial, enucleation because of tumor regrowth or progression has been reported as high as 40 percent.[52,56,65,67]

Multiple etiologies account for posttreatment ocular morbidity. In tumors adjacent to the optic nerve or fovea, direct radiation vascular damage is a major cause of visual loss. In both a phase I-II and a prospective randomized dynamically balanced study comparing helium ion versus ^{125}I brachytherapy, more anterior segment complications were seen with helium and more strabismus and posterior segment complications with ^{125}I radioactive plaques.[58] Intrinsic tumor factors and cytokines released from immune/inflammatory cells are also important in post-treatment eye damage. Patients have had macular edema, optic nerve neovascularization, and neovascular glaucoma prior to uveal melanoma treatment.[68] The inflammatory-immunologic component responsible for ocular morbidity is incompletely understood, and many cytokines can promote both neovascularization and inflammation.[69]

Most enucleations after radiation are required because of morbidity. Larger tumors are at greater risk for enucleation.[59] Over 80 percent of enucleated eyes after helium ion therapy had good tumor control, but sufficient treatment complications to require removal. In long-term follow-up after helium ion or proton irradiation, there appears to be less than a 4 percent local recurrence rate.[59,60] The incidence of tumor regrowth may be slightly higher after brachytherapy; Karlsson and co-worker estimated a 12 percent five-year recurrence rate after cobalt plaques.[67] In our randomized projective plaque/particle study, there was significantly better local control with helium ions (unpublished data). As discussed, enucleation is highly influenced by the experience and expertise of the treating center.

A number of different approaches are being studied to decrease the radiation ocular morbidity. We have an ongoing prospective randomized dynamically balanced study comparing ^{125}I plaques with helium ion irradiation.[58] In short term follow-up, it appears that the survival and enucleation rates are similar. There was significantly more neovascular glaucoma, epiphora, and lash loss after helium ion treatment. Vitreous hemorrhage, secondary strabismus, and radiation retinopathy are more common after ^{125}I plaque therapy.[58] Additional follow-up will be necessary to delineate complication rates and assess which patients will be better treated with a given modality.

A second approach to reduce radiation complications has been to use hyperthermia with a lower radiation dose. There are a number of unsolved problems with hyperthermia.[70–73] The relative thermal enhancement ratio is unknown for human uveal melanoma, and the optimum timing of heat in relation to radiation is unclear.[74] Clinical studies have been initiated in a number of institutions including our own.[75,76] Human uveal melanoma hyperthermia treatment data are difficult to interpret. As an example, promising results were reported with hyperthermia combined with a decreased mean radiation dose of approximately 70 Gy.[76] As previously discussed, we have less than a 4 percent incidence of failure of local tumor control when 70 Gy alone is used. Such studies illustrate acceptable morbidity but cannot demonstrate hyperthermia efficacy.

A third alternative to decrease ocular morbidity is to resect uveal neoplasms, obviating the need for ionizing radiation. The indications, contraindications, and efficacy of eyewall resection remain unclear. There is a paucity of long-term follow-up data, and many reports are difficult to interpret.[77–79] In a number of series, as many as 40 percent of resected melanomas were benign on histologic examination.[80,81]

The resection of uveal melanomas is technically difficult and has a high incidence of complications.[1,82,83] Approximately 30 percent of eyes have required enucleation.[81,82] The rate of eye removal appears to be higher than that observed in similarly sized irradiated tumors.[1]

Major questions remain unresolved for local tumor resection. (1) What is the optimum size and tumor location for this treatment? Most surgeons believe that tumors over 15 mm in diameter are better treated with radiation or enucleation. (2) There is a much higher incidence of incomplete tumor resection than radiation marginal miss.

A few investigators have attempted internal surgical resection after laser tumor ablation.[84] In neurosurgery while the tumor volume is diminished with this approach, there is incomplete tumor destruction.[85] In an animal eye tumor model treated with high-energy argon, eight of 11 tumors regrew.[86] Thus, internal resection is worrisome since viable tumor cells may exit through the 19 gauge opening in eye.

Photocoagulation is most useful for small, growing tumors either contiguous or just nasal to the optic nerve or those within 3 mm of the fovea.[87–89] Most reports of photochemotherapy have emphasized failures.[90,91]

There is a paucity of data on the relative efficacies of alternative uveal melanoma therapies. What are current indications for radiation, surgery, or laser? Approximately 20 percent of eyes require enucleation. Most eyes can be salvaged.

In many eyes the choice of radiation modality is probably not critical. Eyes with melanomas 5 to 8 mm thick that are 4 to 6 mm from the optic disc or fovea are likely to have a better visual outcome with particles than with plaques.

In patients with tumors less than < 10 mm thick that involve the fovea or are contiguous with the optic nerve, long-term visual outcome after radiation will be poor. In patients who wish to retain such an eye, radioactive plaques offer the advantage of less cosmetic complications (lash loss, conjunctival telangiectasia, and so on) and a lower incidence of neovascular glaucoma than particle treatment. A potential caveat to this statement is that the local failure rate is higher with plaques than charged particles. Larger tumors (> 16 mm in largest diameter or > 10 mm thickness) are better managed with particle irradiation.

The role of surgical resection is uncertain, because there is a long learning curve with the technique and a higher incidence of both incomplete removal of tumor and eye loss. In patients with large anterior tumors, if surgical resection is successful, this approach may offer a better visual outcome. Photocoagulation is currently indicated in less than 5 percent of uveal melanoma patients.

UVEAL MELANOMA METASTASES

A major clinical challenge in uveal melanoma management is to prevent and treat metastatic disease. At least three issues require further resolution. (1) To delineate patients at high risk to develop metastatic disease, (2) to detect micrometastatic disease when the systemic tumor burden is small, and (3) to design treatment strategies to prevent or destroy micrometastases.

Historically, almost all melanoma patients died from metastases.[38–41] Better survival has been observed because of earlier diagnosis. Patients with tumors less than 10 mm in diameter and less than 3 mm thick have a 5-year tumor-related mortality less than 5 percent.[1] Most tumor mortality has occurred in older patients with large diameter, thicker tumors that involve both anterior and posterior uvea.

Detection of early uveal melanoma metastases is difficult. Probably most patients who develop metastases have them prior to the discovery of the uveal tumor. Clinically, detectable metastases is discovered at the time of ocular tumor diagnosis in less than 2.5 percent of uveal melanoma patients.[1] Radionucleide imaging with murine monoclonal antibodies directed toward melanoma-associated antigens has a detection rate for tumors < 1 cm^2 of approximately 41 percent.[92,93] The incidence of false positive and false negative results is too high for clinical use.[94–96]

A number of systemic treatment approaches are being investigated for metastatic uveal melanoma. Historically, metastatic uveal melanoma survival has been dismal.[97] Using single or combination chemotherapy, less than 25 percent of patients had a partial remission. In metastatic uveal melanoma to the liver, hepatic arterial chemoembolization has shown some promise.[98] In cutaneous metastatic melanoma, a combination of interleukin-2 (IL-2) with lymphocyte activated killer (LAK) cells has also shown promise; however, results with uveal melanoma metastases continue to be dismal.[99] Newer approaches using tumor infiltrating lymphocytes are experimental.[100,101] (See Chap. 29.)

Other options include newer chemotherapy combinations and the use of monoclonal antibodies conjugated with various toxins. Newer chemotherapy trials are still not sufficiently mature to comment on the efficacy of these agents for uveal melanoma metastases. Monoclonal antibody therapies have yet to show definite effect in this disease.[102–104]

REFERENCES

1. Char DH. Clinical Ocular Oncology. New York: Churchill-Livingstone, 1990.
2. Osterlind A. Trends in incidence of ocular malignant melanoma in Denmark 1943–1982. *Int J Cancer* 40:161–164, 1987.
3. Keller AZ. Histology, survivorship and related factors in the epidemiology of eye cancers. *Am J Epidemiol* 97:386–393, 1973.
4. Scotto J, Fraumeni JF Jr, and Lee JA. Melanomas of the eye and other non-cutaneous sites: Epidemiologic aspects. *J Natl Cancer Inst* 56:489–491, 1976.
5. Ash JE. Epibulbar tumors. *Am J Ophthalmol* 33:1203–1219, 1950.
6. Tucker MA, Shields JA, Hartge P, Augsburger J, Hoover RN, and Fraumeni JF. Sunlight exposure as risk factor for intraocular malignant melanoma. *N Engl J Med* 313:789–792, 1985.
7. Gallagher RP, Elwood JM, Rootman J, Spinelli JJ, Gill GB, Threlfall WJ, and Birdsell JM. Risk factors for ocular melanoma: Western Canada melanoma study. *J Natl Cancer Inst* 74:775–778, 1985.
8. Egan KM, Seddon JM, Glynn RJ, Gragoudas ES, and Albert DM. Epidemiologic aspects of uveal melanoma. *Surv Ophthalmol* 32:239–251, 1988.
9. Holly EA, Aston DA, Char DH, Kristiansen JJ, and Ahn DK. Uveal melanoma in relation to ultraviolet light exposure and host factors. *Cancer Res* 50:5773–5777, 1990.
10. McDonnell JM, Mayer AJ, and Martin WJ. DNA of human papillomavirus type 16 in dysplastic and malignant lesions of the conjunctiva and cornea. *N Engl J Med* 320:1442–1446, 1989.
11. Folberg R, McLean IW, and Zimmerman LE. Malignant melanoma of the conjunctiva. *Hum Pathol* 16:136–143, 1985.
12. Kindy-Degnan N, Char DH, and Kroll SM. Coincident systemic malignant disease in uveal melanoma patients. *Can J Ophthalmol* 24:204–206, 1989.
13. Everall JD and Dowd PM. Diagnosis, prognosis, and treatment of melanoma. *Lancet* 2:286–289, 1977.
14. Jay B. Naevi and melanomata of the conjunctiva. *Br J Ophthalmol* 49:169–204, 1965.
15. Folberg R, Jakobiec FA, Bernardino VB, and Iwamoto T. Benign conjunctival melanocytic lesions. *Ophthalmology* 96:436–461, 1989.
16. Jakobiec FA, Folberg R, and Iwamoto T. Clinicopathologic characteristics of premalignant malignant melanocytic lesions of the conjunctiva. *Ophthalmology* 96:147–166, 1989.
17. Stefani FH. A prognostic index for patients with malignant melanoma of the conjunctiva. *Graefe's Arch Clin Exp Ophthalmol* 224:580–582, 1986.
18. Jeffrey IJM, Lucas DR, McEwan C, and Lee WR. Malignant melanoma of the conjunctiva. *Histopathology* 10:363–378, 1986.
19. Ferry AP. Lesions mistaken for malignant melanoma of the posterior uvea: A clinical pathologic analysis of 100 cases with ophthalmoscopically visible lesions. *Arch Ophthalmol* 72:463–469, 1964.
20. Char DH, Stone RD, Irvine AR, Crawford JB, Hilton GF, Lonn LI, and Schwartz A. Diagnostic modalities in choroidal melanoma. *Am J Ophthalmol* 89:223–230, 1980.
21. Char DH, and Miller TR. Fine needle biopsy in retinoblastoma. *Am J Ophthalmol* 97:686–690, 1984.
22. Augsburger JJ, Shields JA, Folberg R, et al. Fine needle aspiration biopsy in the diagnosis of intraocular cancer. Cytologic-histologic correlations. *Ophthalmology* 92:39–49, 1985.
23. Czerniak B, Woyke S, Domagala W, and Krzysztolik Z. Fine Needle aspiration cytology of intraocular malignant melanoma. *Acta Cytol.* 27:157–165, 1983.
24. Glasgow BJ, Brown HH, Zargoza AM, and Foos RY. Quantitation of tumor seeding from fine needle aspiration of ocular melanomas. *Am J Ophthalmol.*
25. Char DH, Kroll SM, Stoloff A, Kaleta-Michaels S, Crawford JB, Miller TR, Howes EL Jr, and Ljung B-M. Cytomorphometry of uveal melanomas: Fine needle aspiration biopsy versus standard histology. *Anal Quant Cytol Histol* 13:293–299, 1991.
26. Char DH, Miller T, Ljung B-M, Howes E, and Stoloff A. Fine needle aspiration biopsy in uveal melanoma. *Acta Cytologica* 33:599–605, 1989.
27. Char DH. Metastatic choroidal melanoma. *Am J Ophthalmol* 86:76–80, 1978.
28. Ferry AP, and Front RL. Carcinoma metastatic to the eye and orbit. I. A clinicopathologic study of 227 cases. *Arch Ophthalmol* 92:276–286, 1974.
29. Michelson JB, Felberg NT, and Shields JA. Evaluation of metastatic cancer to the eye. Carcinoembryonic antigen and gamma glutamyl transpeptidase. *Arch Ophthalmol* 95:692–694, 1977.
30. Jakobiec FA, Buckman G, Zimmerman LE, LaPiana FG, Levine MR, Ferry AP, and Crawford JB. Metastatic melanoma within and to the conjunctiva. *Ophthalmology* 96:999–1005, 1989.
31. Reese AB. Precancerous and cancerous melanosis of the conjunctiva. *Am J Ophthalmol* 39:96–100, 1955.
32. Jakobiec FA, Folberg R, and Iwamoto T. Clinicopathologic characteristics of premalignant malignant melanocytic lesions of the conjunctiva. *Ophthalmology* 96:147–166, 1989.
33. Brownstein S, Jakobiec FA, Wilkinson RD, Lombardo J, and Jackson WB. Cryotherapy for precancerous melanosis (a typical melanocytic hyperplasia) of the conjunctiva. *Arch Ophthalmol* 99:1224–1231, 1981.
34. Jakobiec FA, Brownstein S, Albert W, Schwarz F, and Anderson R. The role of cryotherapy in the management of conjunctival melanoma. *Ophthalmology* 89:502–515, 1982.
35. Robertson DM, Hungerford JB, and McCartney AL. Malignant melanomas of the conjunctiva, nasal cavity, and paranasal sinuses. *Am J Ophthalmol* 108:440–442, 1989.
36. Lederman M. Radiotherapy of cancerous and precancerous melanosis. *Tr Ophthalmol Soc UK* 78:147–164, 1958.
37. Lommatzsch TK. Beta-ray treatment of malignant epibulbar melanoma. *Albrecht v. Graefes Arch Klin Ophthalmol* 209:111, 1978.
38. Fuchs E. Das Sarcom des Uvealtractus. Vienna: Braumuller, 1882.
39. Jaensch PA. Die Prognose der Enukleation beim Melanosarkom der Uvea. *Klin Mbl Augenheilk* 84:649–662, 1930.

40. Lawford JB, and Collins ET. Sarcoma of the uveal tract, with notes of one hundred and three cases. *Lond Ophthalmic Hosp Rep* 13:104, 1891.
41. Von Hippel E. Zur Prognose der Uvealsarkome. *Arch f Ophthalmol* 124:206, 1930.
42. McLean IW, Berd D, Mastrangelo MJ, et al. A randomized study of methanol-extraction residue (MER) of bacillus Calmette-Guerin as postsurgical adjuvant therapy of uveal melanoma. *Am J Opthalmol* 110:522–526, 1990.
43. Sellami M, Weil M, Dhermy P, et al. Adjuvant chemotherapy in ocular melanoma. Study of 20 cases. *Oncology* 43:221, 1986.
44. Char DH, Phillips TL, Andejeski Y, Crawford JB, and Kroll S. Failure of preenucleation radiation to decrease uveal melanoma mortality. *Am J Ophthalmol* 106:21, 1988.
45. Bornfeld N, Huser U, Sauerwein W, et al. Praoperative Bestrahlung vor Enukleation bei malignem Melanom der Uvea. *Klin Mbl Augenheilk* 194:252, 1989.
46. Kreissig I, Rohrbach M, and Lincoff H. Irradiation of choroidal melanomas before enucleation? *Retina* 9:101, 1989.
47. Robertson DM. A Rationale for comparing radiation to enucleation in the management of choroidal melanoma (editorial). *Am J Ophthalmol* 108:448, 1989.
48. Zirm E. Uber endobulbare Operationen. *Arch Augenheilk* 69:233, 1911.
49. Raubitschek E. Uber Iristumoren. *Klin Monastbl Augenheilkd* 52:683, 1914.
50. Schubert F. Operation eines "Leucosarkoms" der choroididea mit Erhaltung des Auges: Dauerheilung. *Wien Klin Wochenschr* 38:677–678, 1925.
51. Moore RF. Choroidal sarcoma treated by the intraocular insertion of radon seeds. *Br J Ophthalmol* 14:145, 1930.
52. Kindy-Degnan N, Char DH, Castro JR, Kroll S, Stone RD, Quivey JM, Phillips TL, and Irvine AR. Effect of various doses of radiation for uveal melanoma on regression, visual acuity, complications, and survival. *Am J Ophthalmol* 107:114–120, 1989.
53. Char DH, Huhta K, and Waldman F. DNA cell cycle studies in uveal melanoma. *Am J Ophthalmol* 107:65–72, 1989.
54. Sealy R, Buret E, Cleminshaw H, et al. Progress in the use of iodine therapy for tumours of the eye. *Br J Radiol* 53:1052, 1980.
55. Robertson DM, Earle J, and Anderson JA. Preliminary observations regarding the use of iodine-125 in the management of choroidal melanoma. *Trans Ophthalmol Soc UK* 103:155, 1983.
56. Bosworth JL, Packer S, Rotman M, et al. Choroidal melanoma: I-125 plaque therapy. *Radiology* 169:249, 1988
57. Stallard HB. Malignant melanoblastoma of the choroid. *Bibl Ophthalmol* 75:16, 1968.
58. Char DH, Castro JR, Quivey JM, et al. Uveal melanoma radiation. ^{125}I brachytherapy versus helium ion irradiation. *Ophthalmology* 96:1708–1715, 1989.
59. Char DH, Castro JR, Kroll SM, et al. Five year follow-up of helium ion therapy for uveal melanoma. *Arch Ophthalmol* 108:209–214, 1990.
60. Gragoudas ES, Seddon JM, Egan K, et al. Long-term results of proton beam irradiated uveal melanomas. *Ophthalmology* 94:349, 1987.
61. Seddon JM, Gragoudas ES, Polivogianis L, et al. Visual outcome after proton beam irradiation of uveal melanoma. *Ophthalmology* 93:666, 1986.
62. Adams KS, Abramson DH, Ellsworth RM, Haik BG, Bedford M, Packer S, Seddon J, Albert D, and Polivogianis L. Cobalt plaque versus enucleation for uveal melanoma. Comparison of survival rates. *Br J Ophthalmol* 72:494–497, 1988.
63. Augsburger JJ, Gamel JW, Lauritzen K, and Brady LW. Cobalt-60 plaque radiotherapy vs. enucleation for posterior uveal melanoma. *Am J Ophthalmol* 109:585–592, 1990.
64. Seddon JM, Gragoudas ES, Egan KM, Glynn RJ, Howard S, Fante RG, Albert DM, et al. Relative survival rates after alternative therapies for uveal melanoma. *Ophthalmology* 97:769–777, 1990.
65. Gass JD. Comparison of prognosis after enucleation vs. cobalt 60 irradiation of melanomas. *Arch Ophthalmol* 103:916, 1985.
66. Seddon JM, Polivogianis L, Gragoudas ES, et al. Enucleation vs. cobalt 60 irradiation of melanomas. *Arch Ophthalmol* 104:175, 1986.
67. Karlsson UL, Augsburger JJ, Shields JA, et al. Recurrence of posterior uveal melanoma after ^{60}Co episcleral plaque therapy. *Ophthalmology* 96:382, 1989.
68. Cappin JM. Malignant melanoma and rubeosis iridis. Histopathological and statistical study. *Br J Ophthalmol* 57:815, 1973.
69. Dinarllo GA and Mier JW. Lymphokines. *N Engl J Med* 317:940, 1987.
70. Perez CA, Gillespie B, Pajak T, et al. Quality assurance problems in clinical hyperthermia and their impact on therapeutic outcome: A report by the radiation therapy oncology group. *Int J Radiation Oncol Biol Phys* 16:551, 1989.
71. Scrivastava PN, Saylor TK, Matloubieh AY, et al. Hyperthermia thermometry evaluation: Criteria and guidelines. *Int J Radiation Oncol Biol Phys* 14:327, 1988.
72. Barbe MF, Tytell M, Gower DJ, and Welch WJ. Hyperthermia protects against light damage in the rat retina. *Science* 241:1817–1820, 1988.
73. Braakman R, Van der Valk P, Van Delft JL, et al. The effects of ultrasonically induced hyperthemia and experimental tumors in the rabbit eye. *Invest Ophthalmol Vis Sci* 30:835, 1989.
74. Meyer JL, Van Kersen I, and Hahn GM. Tumor responses following multiple hyperthermia and X-ray treatments: Role of thermotolerance at the cellular level. *Cancer Res* 46:5691, 1986.
75. Coleman DJ, Lizzi FL, Burgess SEP, et al. Ultrasonic hyperthermia and radiation in the management of intraocular malignant melanoma. *Am J Ophthalmol* 101:635, 1986.
76. Finger PT, Packer S, Paglione RW, et al. Thermoradiotherapy of choroidal melanoma. *Ophthalmology* 96:1384, 1989.
77. Kara GB. Excision of uveal melanomas: a 15-year experience. *Trans Am Acad Ophthalmol Otolaryngol* 36:997, 1979.
78. Muller HK. Die Partielle Ausschneidung von Iris und Ciliarkorper. *Doc Ophthalol* 26:279, 1969.
79. Vail DT. Iridocyclectomy. A review. *Am J Ophthalmol* 71:161, 1971.
80. Linnic LF. Surgical treatment of melanomas of the iris, ciliary body and choroid. In: Lommatzsch PK, and Blodi FC (eds.), *Intraocular Tumors*. Berlin: Akademie Verlag, 1983, 409–416.
81. Peyman GA, Schulman J, and Raichand M. Diagnosis and therapeutic surgery of the uvea—part two: Results. *Ophthal Surg* 18:310, 1987.
82. Foulds WS, Damato BE, and Burton RL. Local resection versus enucleation in the management of choroidal melanoma. *Eye* 1:676, 1987.
83. Shields JA, and Shields CL. Surgical approach to lamellar sclerouvectomy for posterior uveal melanoma. The 1986 Schoenberg Lecture. *Ophthalmic Surg* 19:774, 1988.
84. Peyman GA and Charles H. Internal eye wall resection in the management of uveal melanoma. *Can J Ophthalmol* 23:220, 1988.

85. Edwards MSB, Boggan JE, and Fuller TA. The laser in neurological surgery. *J Neurosurg* 59:555, 1983.
86. Jaffe GJ, Mieler WF, Burke JM, et al. Photoablation of ocular melanoma with I-argon endolaser. *Arch Ophthalmol* 107:113, 1989.
87. Folk JC, Weingeist TA, Coonan P, et al. The treatment of serous macular detachment secondary to choroidal melanomas and nevi. *Ophthalmology* 96:547, 1989.
88. Jalkh AE, Trempe CL, Nasrallah FP, et al. Treatment of small choroidal melanomas with photocoagulation. *Ophthal Surg* 19:738, 1988.
89. Shields JA, Glazer LC, Mieler WF, Shields CL, and Gottlieb MA. Comparison of xenon arc and argon laser photocoagulation in the treatment of choroidal melanomas. *Am J Ophthalmol* 109:647–655, 1990.
90. Panagopoulos JA, Svitra PP, Puliafito CA, et al. Photodynamic therapy for experimental intraocular melanoma using chloroaluminum sulfonated phthalocyanine. *Arch Ophthalmol* 107:886, 1989.
91. Tse DT, Dutton JJ, Weingeist TA, et al. Hematoporphyrin photoradiation therapy for intraocular and orbital malignant melanoma. *Arch Ophthalmol* 102:833, 1984.
92. Cheung N-KV, Lazarus H, Miraldi FD, et al. Ganglioside G_{D2} specific monoclonal antibody 3F8: A phase I study in patients with neuroblastoma and malignant melanoma. *J Clin Oncol* 5:1430, 1987.
93. Goldenberg DM. Targeting of cancer with radiolabeled antibodies. *Arch Pathol Lab Med* 112:580, 1988.
94. Salk D and the Multicenter Study Group. Technetium-labeled monoclonal antibodies for imaging metastatic melanoma: results of a multicenter clinical study. *Sem Oncol* 15:608, 1988.
95. Bomanji J, Nimmon CC, Hungerford JL, Solanki K, Granowska M, and Britton KE. Ocular radioimmunoscintigraphy: sensitivity and practical considerations. *J Nucl Med* 29:1038–1044, 1988.
96. Tullo AB, Dodd CL, Noble JL, et al. Correspondence: Ocular Melanoma. *Br J Ophthalmol* 73:771, 1989.
97. Char DH. Metastatic choroidal melanoma. *Am J Ophthalmol* 86:76, 1978.
98. Mavligit GM, Charnsangavej C, Carrasco H, et al. Regression of ocular melanoma metastatic to the liver after hepatic arterial chemoembolization with cisplatin and polyvinyl sponge. *JAMA* 260:974, 1988.
99. Rosenberg SA, Lotze MT, and Mule JJ. New approaches to the immunotherapy of cancer using interleukin-2. *Ann Int Med* 108:853, 1988.
100. Kawakami Y, Rosenberg SA, and Lotze MT. Interleukin 4 promotes the growth of tumor-infiltrating lymphocytes cytotoxic for human autologous melanoma. *J Exp Med* 168:2183, 1988.
101. Kiyohara T, Taniguchi K, Kubota S, et al. Induction of lymphokine-activated killer-like cells by cancer chemotherapy. *J Exp Med* 168:2355, 1988.
102. Natali PG, Bigotti A, Nicotra MR, et al. Analysis of the antigenic profile of uveal melanoma lesions with anti-cutaneous melanoma-associated antigen and anti-HLA monoclonal antibodies. *Cancer Res* 49:1269, 1989.
102. Mitchell MS, Kempf RA, Harel W, et al. Effectiveness and tolerability of low-dose cyclophosphamide and low-dose intravenous interleukin-2 disseminated melanoma. *J Clin Oncol* 6:409, 1988.
104. Furukawa KS, Furukawa K, Real FX, et al. A unique antigenic epitope of human melanomas carried on the common melanoma glycoprotein gp^{95}/p^{97}. *J Exp Med* 169:585, 1989.

Chapter 33

APPRAISAL OF CLINICAL STUDIES

N. Cascinelli, F. Belli, R. Bufalino, and M. Santinami

INTRODUCTION

Treatment of cutaneous melanoma remains one of the most complex problems in surgical oncology. The variety of the biological, immunological, clinical, and surgical problems related to this disease explains the large number of studies conducted in the past years or are ongoing. Some aspects of these therapies are actually well defined and worldwide standardized. However, many other areas remain unsolved and opened to further studies.

TREATMENT OF PRIMARY TUMOR

Usually for primary melanoma a wide excision with 3 to 5 cm margins around the tumor was considered mandatory. The excision included the subcutaneous fat and usually the fascia covering underlying muscle. In the last few years many authors[1,2] have questioned the need for a wide excision. Several studies published till now have not clarified the situation because the number of patients studied were small[3,4] and patients were not randomized and consequently biases were introduced by the investigators. Any comparative analysis in which the groups are not randomized may be subject to patient selection and/or environmental system biases. These biases may be only partially controlled by analysis techniques and mathematical modeling since the environmental biases cannot be corrected by statistical techniques. Through prospective determination of control groups on the basis of randomization, it is possible to control such biases within a trial. Only a well-designed study may be appropriate to be representative of a larger population. The use of a minimal number of exclusion criteria is desirable to ensure that the study may be representative.

There is also a lack of precision in terminology in the exact definition of local recurrence, resulting in difficulty to determine whether the reappearance of a neoplasm close to the scar is really due to a failure of surgical therapy. The practical question that must be asked is whether it is useful or an over treatment to perform a classic wide excision. The question is a difficult one to answer. To evaluate whether or not to consider a narrow excision as the treatment of choice for a thin melanoma, the WHO Melanoma Programme conducted a prospective randomized clinical trial.[5] In order to ensure the feasibility, its design was as simple as possible. The two issues which were evaluated were (a) up to what thickness of the melanoma may a narrow excision be adequate and (b) what is the safe width of a narrow excision. Melanomas of up to 2 mm were considered for narrow excision because up to this thickness lesions have good prognosis. The choice of minimum safe width was more complicated and advocated from few millimeters[6,7] to 2 cm.[2,8] It was decided to choose 1 cm margin, measured by the surgeons at the time of operation primarily because of ease of closure without skin graft following excision of this width. Two groups of patients were randomized to either "narrow excision" or "wide excision." Stratification was done by institution. Altogether, 612 patients were entered in the study. There were 305 patients entered in the "narrow excision" group and 307 patients entered in the "wide excision" group. The mean follow-up period was 55 months.

The survival curve results of both groups is shown in Fig. 33-1. Results[5] have shown that a narrow excision, 1 cm from the neoplasm, is certainly a safe procedure for melanoma up to 2 mm thick, and probably the indication could be extended to melanomas thicker than 2 mm.

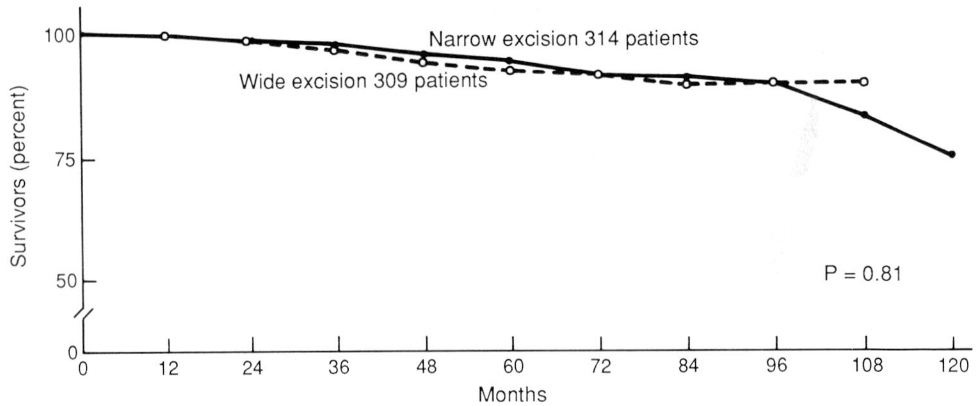

FIG. 33-1. Trial 10—Overall Survival of 612 evaluable patients according to type of treatment

TREATMENT OF REGIONAL NODES

The necessity to perform a regional node dissection in the presence of palpable lymph nodes is well accepted. Much more controversial is the role of an elective node dissection. The rationale for performing an elective node dissection is based on the fact that melanoma usually metastasizes sequentially in lymph nodes and afterwards in distant sites, and that some particular subgroups of melanoma patients have a high probability of developing regional node metastases, such as thick lesions by Breslow's measurement[9] or in some particular primary site like the trunk or head and neck.[10]

The principal studies supporting benefit from the elective node dissection are from the reports by Balch[9,11] and Milton.[12] These studies were carried out on homogeneous groups of patients submitted for surgical treatment and were very well standardized because they were performed at the same institutions by a selected group of surgeons. Moreover, the statistical analysis was very carefully done. However, the results were not accepted universally because the studies were not randomized. Using a control group without randomization requires an assumption that both the control and the treatment groups are identical regarding all important prognostic variables related to melanoma and/or it is possible to correct for any of such differences. The randomization method gives the possibility to statistically analyze data without any special assumption. The difficulty of analysis without randomization is shown by the fact that other retrospective studies have been published with different conclusions.[13–18] The reason for these contradictory results is related to the difficulty of comparing different series of patients if results are not collected from randomization and to the fact that a surgeon's selection of treatment may introduce biases into the study that are difficult to identify a-posteriori.

Randomized studies[19–21] did not show any benefit related to immediate node dissection in any subgroup of patients considered. In the WHO study,[20,21] a total of 267 patients were submitted to wide excision of the primary lesion and immediate node dissection, and 286 to wide excision of the primary lesion only. Delayed node dissections were performed when clinically evident regional node metastases occurred. Figure 33-2 shows that the survival curves for the two groups are superimposable. Elective regional node dissection did not improve survival even when subgroups of patients were evaluated according to the presence or absence of a previous biopsy, sex, age, and site of origin (upper and lower extremity).

A second trial, carried out at the Mayo Clinic[19] confirmed that there is no difference in the survival of patients with Stage I melanoma, whether immediate (i.e., prophylactic) or delayed (i.e., therapeutic) node dissection is performed.

These studies provide convincing evidence that prophylactic node dissection has not proven to be of any value in the treatment of patients with Stage I melanoma, since it does not improve survival and its usefulness as a staging procedure has not yet been determined, due to lack of uniformly effective adjuvant therapy at the present time (see Chap. 26).

The criticisms made of these studies were mainly based on the observation that there was a predominance of female patients and that in the two major studies[21] dealt only with melanoma of the extremities. The rationale for the lack of benefit from immediate (or elective) node dissection is based on the observation that metastatic spread of melanoma does not always follow the pattern of primary-lymph nodes-distant site. Data from WHO Melanoma Register[22] show that among Stage I patients who relapsed, 51 percent had recurrences in regional nodes, while 18

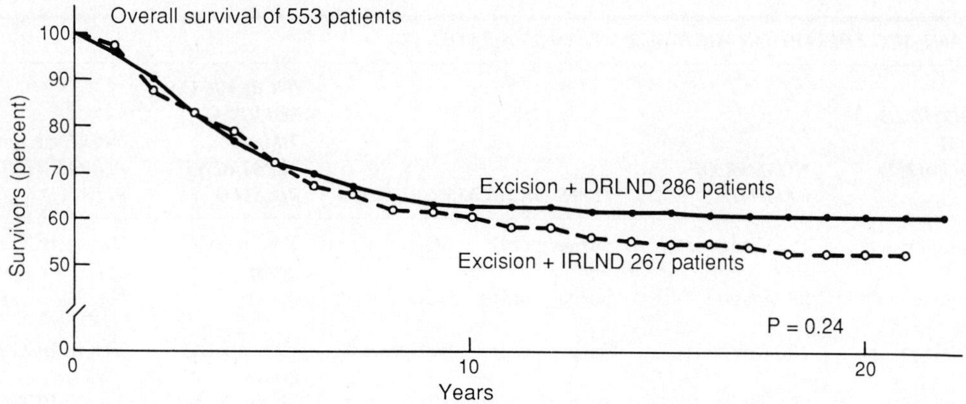

FIG. 33-2. Trial 1—Evaluation of the efficacy of elective nodes dissection on limbs melanoma with clinically uninvolved regional nodes, Stage I

percent relapsed first at distant site and 31 percent in both.

The debate over elective node dissection is complex and is not resolved completely.[23]

It may be concluded that, taking into consideration the fact that a node dissection has postoperative morbidity,[24] there is a good reason for caution against routine "prophylactic lymphadenectomy." There is good agreement that immediate node dissection is not indicated in all melanoma patients. Regarding prophylactic lymphadenectomy, there appears to be two groups of investigators. One who is in favor of the wait-and-see policy agrees to perform an elective node dissection only in patients with melanoma at high risk of recurrence (thickness > 2.00 mm) when these patients may not be regularly followed every 3 months. The other who is in favor of elective node dissection recommends this procedure in patients with melanoma of intermediate thickness (between 1.50 mm and 4.00 mm).

To resolve the dilemma regarding elective node dissection, there are two randomized trials active at present: one being carried out by the WHO Melanoma Programme, aided at answering the question whether or not an elective node dissection may be of benefit for patients with a melanoma of the trunk thicker than 1.50 mm, stratified by sex, the other being carried out by the Intergroup Melanoma Committee in the United States aimed at answering the question of whether or not elective node dissection should be recommended for a melanoma with an intermediate thickness (1.50–4.00 mm) at any site.

ADJUVANT SYSTEMIC THERAPY

Overall risk for Stage II patients to be affected by microscopic metastases at distant sites is high and ranges up to 80 to 85 percent. For this reason in the last 20 years a great number of studies and clinical trials have been set in order to evaluate the beneficial effects of an adjuvant treatment in high-risk Stage I and Stage II melanoma patients.

In spite of many theoretical considerations, all the trials of chemotherapy with single or multiple agents, by and large, have not shown substantial benefit in treating melanoma patients with high risk for relapse.[25–27] The WHO Melanoma Programme Trial 6 based on a four arms randomization (DTIC, BCG, DTIC + BCG, surgery only) with 761 Stage I and II patients, the survival has not improved in treated groups compared to control groups following systemic adjuvant therapy in melanoma patients.[28] (See Chapters 26 and 29.)

Because of the specific immunogenic activity of melanoma, a number of clinico-immunologic studies were performed on melanoma patients reporting a sporadic beneficial effect obtained utilizing immunotherapy alone as adjuvant after surgery for high-risk melanoma patients.[29–31]

Morton and co-workers pioneered the use of the bacillus Calmette-Guerin (BCG) in the treatment of malignant melanoma. Based on the observations of tumor regression after intralesional injection of BCG in 90 percent of injected lesions and 17 percent of uninjected lesions, numerous studies of adjuvant immunotherapy following surgical resection have been undertaken.[29] Later, Gutterman and associates from M.D. Anderson Hospital reported a nonrandomized study in 1973 in which there was an apparent survival benefit from BCG immunotherapy for recurrent malignant melanoma.[30] One of the most adequate study on adjuvant immunotherapy after radical surgery in Stage II patients was conducted by Eilber and Morton from UCLA on 126 patients from 1971 to 1975.[31] At two years, the incidence of metastases in the patients treated with BCG was one half of the control group. Because of the promising results using BCG adjuvant immunotherapy in these nonrandomized trials, prospective randomized trials were

TABLE 33-1
EFFECT OF ADJUVANT BCG THERAPY ON HIGH-RISK MELANOMA PATIENTS

AUTHOR	RANDOMIZED OR NOT RANDOMIZED TRIAL	NUMBER OF PATIENTS	TYPES OF TREATMENT		INCREASE ON SURVIVAL TIME TREATMENT RELATED	INCREASE ON DISEASE-FREE PERIOD TIME TREATMENT RELATED
Eilber (1976)	Not randomized	126 (Stage II)	Surgery only	BCG	Yes in GCG group	Yes in BCG group
ECOG (1979)	Randomized	98 (Stage I + II)	Surgery only	OCG	No	No
UCLA (1981)	Randomized	139 (Stage II)	Surgery only	BCG vaccine	Yes in BCG group	Yes in BCG group
Paterson (1981)	Randomzied	153 (Stage I)	Surgery only	BCG	Slight increase in BCG group	Yes in BCG group
Fisher (1981)	Randomized	181 (Stage I + II)	Surgery only/BCG	BCG vaccine/MeCCNU	No	No

ried out in a number of institutions in an attempt to reproduce these results.[32–34]

Some of the reports on this topic confirmed the initial observations of Morton and Eilber but many other authors did not observe objective improvement with this type of adjuvant treatment (Table 33-1). However, several clinical studies[35] have confirmed the susceptibility of melanoma to the immunotherapy. (See Chapter 29 for details.)

Another immunostimulating agent, Interferon (IFN) has been introduced as therapeutic mean in melanoma patients at different stages. The rationale for application of interferon in the treatment of melanoma is based on the evidence suggesting that this tumor exhibits antigens capable of stimulating a host immune response. Agents that act as immunomodulators or that enhance the expression of tumor antigens may have greater therapeutic potential than agents with only direct cytotoxic activities. Many studies suggest that IFN may manifest all three types of antineoplastic function. In fact, IFN administered alone to patients with metastatic melanoma, has already achieved meaningful results in some series of patients.[36,37] Thus, the rationale exists for a trial design in which IFN would be administered to individuals with melanoma at high risk for relapse, who may be most sensitive to the antiproliferative and immunomodulatory effects of this agent, and able to tolerate it for protracted periods of time.

This approach is under current investigation in two cooperative group studies in the United States that are adopting different schemes of therapy (Eastern Cooperative Oncology Group (ECOG) and North Central Oncology Group (NCOG)), but conclusive data are not available.

On this basis of rationale, the WHO Melanoma Programme has activated a new trial, (clinical trial #15), to evaluate the effect of adjuvant treatment with recombinant IFN-α in patients with nodal metastases from cutaneous melanoma as these patients are at high risk for relapse locally and at distant sites. This is an open randomized multicentric study designed to evaluate the efficacy of adjuvant recombinant IFN-α2A treatment. The aim of this study is to evaluate the toxicity and tolerance of chronic three times a week therapy with rIFN-α2A and to evaluate the efficacy of an adjuvant therapy with rIFN-α2A in patients at high risk for relapse after radical surgery. Simultaneously, biological data regarding immunomodulation activity on each patient will be monitored. Each patient will be closely evaluated to monitor immunologic activities and lymphocytic phenotype before and during the treatment. Correlating clinical and laboratory data is one of the more interesting goals of this study.

To be eligible for this study, patients must undergo radical lymphadenectomy and have histologically proven metastatic lymph node. Patients with positive lymph nodes are randomized to control group (follow-up observation only) or to treated group where patients receive recombinant IFN-α2A 3 million I.U. subcutaneously three injections per week starting 30 to 35 days after lymphadenectomy till appearance of clinical or radiologically detectable disease or maximum period of 2 years.

To reduce the bias in this multicentric study, patients are randomized through a central data center rather than providing the treatment assignment in sealed envelopes and an ad hoc computerized randomization system is designed to ensure that the balance of prognostic criteria inside each treatment arm is guaranteed for each patient entry. Taking into account the effect of various prognostic factors, stratification is used at the time of randomization by institution. These stratification factors include clinically detectable metastatic nodes, number of positive nodes, and extension of the tumor through lymph node capsule (Fig. 33-3). These three criteria

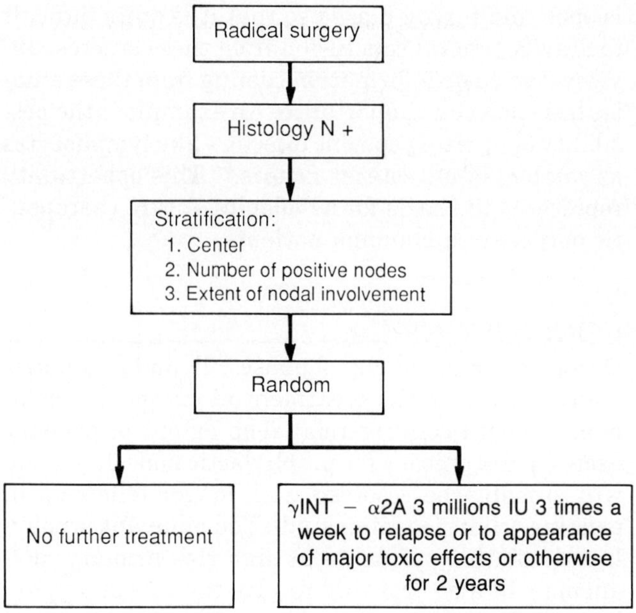

FIG. 33-3. Design of WHO melanoma program clinical trial #15 to evaluate effect of adjuvant γINF α2A on stage II melanoma.

are the most important prognostic factors in Stage II melanoma patients (see Chapter 12). All patients will be closely monitored for side effects and tolerance as well as for quality of life during treatment. In absence of major toxicity, the treatment will be continued for 2 years.

TREATMENT OF IN TRANSIT METASTASIS

The ideal treatment for in transit metastasis is by isolated perfusion of the involved limb. The appearance of so-called "in transit" metastases occurs in 13 to 20 percent of cases of melanoma and is directly correlated with Breslow's thickness: in practice these metastases are absent for melanoma up to 1 mm thickness and starting from 1.5 mm the percentage noticeably increase. This event has a broad impact on prognosis as demonstrated by a 10-year overall survival of 16.3 percent.

Prophylactic isolation perfusion with high doses of melphalan also has been used for preventing recurrences and improving survival following treatment of primary melanoma. This treatment procedure appears to be the most complete, as it involves the entire disease extremity. In addition, in the case of lymph node recurrence, therapeutic lymph node dissection can be performed at the time of isolation perfusion. Recurrence rates of less than 2 percent and an increase in the 5-year survival from 70 to 95 percent have been reported with prophylactic isolation perfusion in high-risk melanoma of the extremities (Table 33-2).[38–43] However, there are some controversies regarding the effectiveness of prophylactic isolation perfusion as some authors claim that recurrence and survival rates are similar to the results of conventional surgery.

To resolve these problems, there appears to be justification for a phase III randomized clinical trial, as a mean of obtaining a definite answer. On this basis the WHO Melanoma Programme, the EORTC, and the NAPG (North American Perfusion Group) decided to perform a study concerning this issue. This multicentric trial includes all patients at Stage I with a Breslow's thickness more than 1.5 mm. Results of these trials will be available in 3 or 4 years. At present, the choice between the policies mentioned is left to the experience and judgement of clinicians.

TREATMENT OF METASTASES

Treatment of metastases from cutaneous melanoma remains unsatisfactory. Many drugs have been utilized in the treatment of metastatic melanoma but objective responses are extremely poor.[44,45] To date, dacarbazine remains the most active drug with a mean response rate of 23 percent.[44] Several studies with single or multiple drug schedule have produced unconvincing results. However, some encouraging response has been obtained by the treatment of melanoma metastases by cytotoxic lymphocytes

TABLE 33-2
ADJUVANT PERFUSION—STAGE I

AUTHOR	NUMBER OF PATIENTS	CONTROL	RANDOMIZED	RESULTS
Rege et al.[38]	30	Yes	No	Significant improvement of survival in perfused patients
Sugarbaker and McBride[39]	199	None	No	83% survival at 5 years
Davis et al.[40]	72	None	No	90% at least 5 years
Schraffordt Koops et al.[41]	132	None	No	78% survival at 5 years (normotherma)
W.H.O./EORTC/NAPG[42]	404[a]	Yes	Yes	No data available[a]
Krementz[43]	381	No	None	80% survival at 10 years

[a]Patient accrual still open.

associated with a specific growth factor, interleukin-2 (IL-2).[46–52] (See Chapter 29.)

Initially, phase I study was conducted to evaluate maximum tolerable dose on patients with disseminated melanoma no longer amenable to treatment but with a life expectancy of over 12 weeks but not having received other treatment in previous 4 weeks.[50] Phase II studies for possible antitumor activity of IL-2 followed these phase I studies. The end points for these phase II studies were the response rate and toxicity.[48,51] Some interesting but not homogeneous data emerged also in studies when IL-2 has been utilized alone or in combination with IFN or DTIC.[53] (See Table 33-3.) Currently, two types of activated lymphocytes are mainly available for adoptive immunotherapy: lymphokine activated killer cells (LAK cells) and tumor infiltrating lymphocyte (TIL cells). In the first case, the source of lymphocytes is the peripheral blood. The source of the TIL cells is a tumor mass surgically removed from the patient. Modality of treatment, biological specificity, and cell characteristic are different in these two types of adoptive immunotherapy.

Some authors have reported very intriguing results with these modalities of therapy, obtaining 20 to 25 percent response with LAK cells associated with IL-2[46–49] treatments and up to 60 percent of remissions (CR + PR) in the TIL plus IL-2 schedule.[52] (See Table 33-3.)

All these phase II studies are nonrandomized with all patients receiving the same treatment. This may be a critical point since the selection of patients is open and highly biased so that it is quite difficult to draw a general conclusion from these studies. anyway, the basic information coming from these studies has enormous importance. An example is the possibility of utilizing specific effectors like lymphocytes as carriers of anticancer factors.[54] This opportunity represents the basis for developing future therapeutic options in melanoma patients.

CONCLUSIONS

Despite the multiplicity of phase I, II, and III studies, many aspects of the treatment of cutaneous melanoma remain controversial. The extent of primary excision and efficacy for prophylactic node dissection will probably be resolved with longer follow-up in existing trials. Ongoing studies on adjuvant prophylactic isolation perfusion in high-risk primary melanoma will also probably resolve the role of prophylactic isolation perfusion. However, management of occult metastasis or overt metastasis by systemic therapy will be more difficult to resolve. Introduction of innovative route of administration and newer agent may improve the outcome. On the other hand, biological response modifier and immunomodulator are showing optimism in control of systemic disease. Adoptive immunotherapy, although plagued with serious side effects, shows remarkable promise for treatment of metastatic melanoma. Integrated biological and clinic studies such as WHO melanoma trial #16 will be most helpful in resolving many unanswered questions on treatment of this disease.

TABLE 33-3
INFLUENCE OF INTERLEUKIN ALONE OR IN COMBINATION THERAPY ON METASTATIC MELANOMA

TYPE OF TREATMENT	NUMBER OF PATIENTS	COMPLETE RESPONSE	PARTIAL RESPONSE	PERCENT RESPONSE	AUTHOR
IL-2	37	0	9	24	Rosenberg, 1989
IL-2	10	0	5	50	West, 1987
IL-2	33	0	3	9	Richards, 1990
IL-2	15	0	0	0	Thompson, 1985
IL-2/LAK	48	4	6	21	Rosenberg, 1989
IL-2/LAK	26	6		23	Weidmann, 1988
IL-2/LAK	42	0	6	14	Rayner, 1988
IL-2/LAK	39	0	1	3	Dutcher, 1989
IL-2/LAK	31	0	4	13	Ghosh, 1989
IL-2/LAK	35	0	2	6	Richards, 1990
IL-2/LAK + DTIC	25	2	4	24	West, 1989
IL-2 + IFN	15	1	2	20	Lee, 1989
IL-2 + IFN	14	0	0	0	Whitehead, 1990
IL-2 + DTIC	13	0	5	38	Flaherty, 1988
IL-2 + DTIC	18	5		28	Bergmann, 1988
IL-2 + DTIC	18	1	4	28	Stoter, 1989
IL-2 + DTIC	30	4	6	33	Papadopoulos, 1990
IL-2 + CTX (low doses)	24	1	5	25	Mitchell, 1988
IL-2 + TIL	15	1	8	60	Rosenberg, 1988

From Lopez et al. in IL Melanoma. Monduzzi Editors (1990)[53]

REFERENCES

1. Elias EG, Didolkar MS, Joel IP, Formeister JF, Valenzuela LA, Pickren IL, and Moore RH. A clinico pathological study of prognostic factors in cutaneous malignant melanoma. *Surg Gynecol Obstet* 144:327–329, 1977.
2. Everall JD, and Dowd PM. Diagnosis, prognosis and treatment of melanoma. (A review). *Lancet* ii:286–289, 1977.
3. Breslow A, and Macht SD. Optimal size of resection margin for this cutaneous melanoma. *Surg Gynecol Obstet* 145:691–692, 1977.
4. Day CL Jr, Mihm MC, Sober AJ, Fitzpatrick TB, and Malt RA. Narrower margins for clinical stage I malignant melanoma. *N Engl J Med* 306:479–482, 1982.
5. Veronesi U, Cascinelli N, Adamus J, Balch C, et al. Thin stage I primary cutaneous malignant melanoma—Comparison of excision with margins of 1 or 3 cm. *N Engl J Med* 318:1159–1162, 1988.
6. Ackerman A, and Scheiner AM. How wide and deep is wide and deep enough? A critique of surgical practice in excisions of primary cutaneous malignant melanoma. *Hum Pathol* 14:743–744, 1983.
7. Bagley FH, Cady B, Lee A, and Legg MA. Changes in clinical presentation and management of malignant melanoma. *Cancer* 47:2126–2134, 1981.
8. Hansen MG, and McCarten AB. Tumor thickness and lymphocyte infiltration in malignant melanoma of the head and neck. *Am J Surg* 128:557, 1974.
9. Balch CM. Surgical management of regional lymph nodes in cutaneous melanoma. *J Am Acad Dermatol* 3:511, 1980.
10. Urist MM, Balch CM, Soong S-j, Milton GW, Shaw HM, McGovern VJ, Murad TM, McCarthy WH, and Maddox WA. Head and neck melanoma in 536 clinical stage I patients: A prognostic factors analysis and results of surgical treatment. *Ann Surg* 200:769–775, 1984.
11. Balch CM, Soong S-j, Milton GW, Shaw HM, McGovern VJ, Murad TM, McCarthy WH, and Maddox WA. A comparison of prognostic factors and surgical results in 1786 patients with localized (Stage I) melanoma treated in Alabama, U.S.A., and New South Wales, Australia. *Ann Surg* 196:677–684, 1982.
12. Milton GW, Shaw HM, McCarthy WH, Pearson L, Balch CM, and Soong S-j. Prophylactic lymph nodes dissection in clinical stage I cutaneous malignant melanoma: Results of surgical treatment in 1319 patients. *Br J Surg* 69:108–111, 1982.
13. Conrad FG. Treatment of malignant melanoma: Wide excision alone vs lymphadenectomy. *Arch Surg* 104:587–593, 1972.
14. Goldsmith HS, Shah JP, and Kim DH. Prognostic significance of lymph node dissection in the treatment of malignant melanoma. *Cancer* 26:606–609, 1970.
15. Gumporp SL, and Harris MN. Results of regional lymph node dissection for melanoma. *Ann Surg* 179:105–108, 1974.
16. McCarthy JG, Haagensen CD, and Herter, FP. The role of groin dissection in the management of the lower extremity. *Ann Surg* 179:156–159, 1974.
17. Moore GE, and Gerner RE. Malignant melanoma. *Surg Gynecol Obstet* 132:427–436, 1971.
18. Veronesi U, and Cascinelli N. Margins of resection of malignant melanomas that are less than the hitherto conventional "wide and deep" margins are not advisable as yet. *Am J Dermatopathol* 7:123–126, Supplement, 1985.
19. Sim FH, Taylor WF, Ivins JC, Pritchard DJ, and Soule EH. A prospective randomized study of the efficacy of routine elective lymphadenectomy in management of malignant melanoma: Preliminary results. *Cancer* 41:948, 1978.
20. Veronesi U, Adamus J, Bandiera DC, Brennhovd IO, Caceres E, Cascinelli N, Claudio F, Ikonopisov RL, Javorskj VV, Kirov S, Kulakowski A, Lacour J, LeJeune F, Mechl Z, Morabito A, Rodé I, Sergeev S, van Slooten E, Szczygiel K, Trapeznikov NN, and Wagner RI. Delayed regional lymph node dissection in stage I melanoma of the skin of the lower extremities. *Cancer* 49:2420–2430, 1982.
21. Veronesi U, Adamus J, Bandiera DC, Brennhovd IO, Caceres E, Cascinelli N, Claudio F, Ikonopisov RL, Javorskj VV, Kirov S, Kulakowski A, Lacour J, LeJeune F, Mechl Z, Morabito A, Rodé I, Sergeev S, van Slooten E, Szczygiel K, Trapeznikov NN, and Wagner RI, and W.H.O. Collaborating Centers for Evaluation of Methods of Diagnosis and Treatment of Melanoma. Inefficacy of immediate node dissection in Stage I melanoma of the limbs. *N Engl J Med* 297:627–630, 1977.
22. Cascinelli N, Preda F, Vaglini M, Orefice S, Bufalino R, Morabito A, Nava M, and Santinami M. Metastatic spread of stage I melanoma of the skin. *Tumori,* 69:449–452, 1983.
23. Balch CM, Cascinelli N, Milton GW, and Sim FH. Elective lymph nodes dissection: Pros and cons. In: Balch C and Milton GW (eds.), *Cutaneous Melanoma: Clinical Management and Treatment Results Worldwide.* Philadelphia: J. B. Lippincott, 1985, 131–157.
24. Urist MM, Maddox WA, Kennedy JE, and Balch CM. Patient risk factors and surgical morbidity after regional lymphadenectomy in 204 melanoma patients. *Cancer* 51:2152–2156, 1983.
25. Czarnetski BM, Macher E, Berendt H, et al. Current status of melanoma chemotherapy and immunotherapy. Recent Results *Cancer Res* 80:264–268, 1982.
26. Hill GJ, Moss SE, Golomb FM, et al. DTIC and combination therapy for melanoma: III DTIC (NSC 45388) surgical adjuvant study COG protocol 7040. *Cancer* 47:2556, 1981.
27. Macher E, LeJeune F, Kleeberg U, et al. A randomized study on DTIC Levamisole and placebo as adjuvant treatment of high risk stage I primary melanoma. First International Conference on Skin Melanoma. Venice, May 6–9, 200, 1985.
28. Veronesi U, Adamus J, et al. A Randomized trial of adjuvant chemotherapy and immunotherapy in cutaneous melanoma. *N Engl J Med* 307:913–916, 1982.
29. Morton DL, Eilber FR, Malmgren RA, et al. Immunological factors which influence response to immunotherapy in malignant melanoma. *Surgery* 68:158, 1970.
30. Gutterman JU, McBride C, Freireich EJ, et al. Active immunotherapy with BCG for recurrent malignant melanoma. *Lancet* 814:1208–1212, 1973.
31. Eilber FR, Morton DL, Holmes EC, et al. Adjuvant immunotherapy with BCG in the treatment of regional lymph node metastases from malignant melanoma. *N Engl J Med* 294:237–240, 1976.
32. Cunningham TT, Schoenfeld D, Nathanson L, et al. A controlled ECOG study of adjuvant therapy in patients with stage I and II malignant melanoma. In program and Abstracts of the Second International Conference on the Adjuvant Therapy of Cancer. Tucson, March 1979.
33. Lawrence B, Lipton A, Harvey H, et al. Corynebacterium parvum vs. BCG as adjuvant immunotherapy for stage I and II malignant melanoma. In program and Abstracts of the Second International Conference on the Adjuvant Therapy of Cancer. Tucson, March 1979.
34. Morton DL, and Eilber FR. Adjuvant therapy for sarcomas and melanomas. In program and Abstracts of the Second International Conference on the Adjuvant Therapy of Cancer. Tucson, March 1981.
35. Cascinelli N, Rumke P, Mackie R, et al. The significance of

conversion of skin reactivity of efficacy of bacillus Calmette-Guerin (BCG) vaccinations given immediately after radical surgery in stage II melanoma patients. *Cancer Immunol Immunother* 28:282–286, 1989.

36. Hawkins MJ, McCune CS, Speyer JL, et al. Recombinant alpha (2) interferon (IFN alpha (2)) (SCH 30550) in patients with metastatic malignant melanoma (MMM): An ECOG pilot study. *Proc Am Soc Clin Oncol* 3:51, 1984 (abstract C-195).
37. Robinson WA, Kirkwood J, Harvey H, et al. Effective use of recombinant human alpha-2 interferon (IFN-alpha 2) in metastatic malignant melanoma: A comparison of two regiments. *Proc Am Soc Clin Oncol* 3:60, 1984 (abstract C-234).
38. Rege VB, Leone LA, Soderberg CH Jr, Coleman GV, Robidoux HJ, Fiyman R, and Brown J. Hyperthermic adjuvant perfusion chemotherapy for stage I malignant melanoma of the extremities with literature review. *Cancer* 52:2033–2039, 1983.
39. Sugarbaker EV, and McBride CM. Survival and regional disease control after isolation perfusion for invasive stage I melanoma of the extremities. *Cancer* 37:188–198, 1976.
40. Davis CD, Ivins JC, and Soule EH. Mayo Clinic experience with isolated perfusion for invasive malignant melanoma of the extremities. In: Melanomas: Basic Properties and Clinical Behaviour. Proceedings of the Ninth International Pigment Cell Conference, Houston, Texas, 1975. New York: S. Karger, Vol. II:379, 1976.
41. Schraffordt Koops H, Beekhuis H, Oldhoff J, Oosterhuis JW, van der Ploeg E, and Vermey A. Local recurrence and survival in patients with (Clark level IV/V and over 1.5 mm thickness) stage I malignant melanoma of the extremities after regional perfusion. *Cancer* 48:1952, 1981.
42. W.H.O. Collaborating Centre for Evaluation of Methods of Diagnosis and Treatment of Melanoma—EORTC Malignant Melanoma Cooperative Group—North America Perfusion Group: A randomized trial on prophylactic isolation perfusion for stage I high risk (> 1.5 mm thickness) malignant melanoma of the limbs. Protocol of ongoing trial.
43. Krementz ET. Regional perfusion. Current sophistication, what next? *Cancer* 57:416–432, 1986.
44. Luce JK. Chemotherapy of melanoma. *Semin Oncol* 2:179, 1975.
45. Cascinelli N, Belli F, Testori A, and Bajetta E. Il trattamento medico del melanoma cutaneo disseminato. From: Atti del Novantesimo Congresso della Società Italiana di Chirurgia, Roma, 23–27, Ottobre 1988. Edizioni Luigi Pozzi s.r.l. Roma.
46. Lotze MT, Chang AE, Seipp CA, et al. High-dose recombinant interleukin-2 in the treatment of patients with disseminated cancer. *J Am Med Wom Assoc* 256:3117, 1986.
47. Rosenberg SA. Cancer therapy with interleukin-2: Immunologic manipulations can mediate the regression of cancer in humans (editorial). *J Clin Oncol* 6:403, 19--.
48. Rosenberg SA, Lotze MT, Muul LM, et al. A progress report on the treatment of 157 patients with advanced cancer using lymphokine activated killer cells and interleukin-2 alone. *N Engl J Med* 316:889, 1987.
49. Rosenberg SA. Lymphokine activated killer cells: A new approach to the immunotherapy of cancer. *J Natl Cancer Inst* 75:595, 1985.
50. Marolda R, Belli F, Prada A, et al. A phase I study of recombinant interleukin-2 in melanoma patients. Toxicity and clinical effects. *Tumori* 73:575–584, 1987.
51. Cascinelli N, Belli F, Marchini S, et al. A phase II study of the administration of recombinant interleukin-2 (rIL-2) plus lymphokine activated killer (LAK) cells in stage IV melanoma patients. *Tumori* 75:233–244, 1989.
52. Steven A, Rosenberg PhD. et al. Use of tumor-infiltrating lymphocytes and interleukin-2 in the immunotherapy of patients with metastatic melanoma. *N Engl J Med* 319:25, 1976.
53. Lopez M, Carpano S, Di Lauro L, and Vici P. Chemioterapia e terapia biologica del melanoma in fase avanzata. In: Battelli T, Cascinelli N, Pilone A, Delprete S, Rossini S, Silva RR (eds.) *Il Melanoma,* Vol. XII, Corso Nazionale di Aggiornamento in Oncologia 1990-92, Ancona 3 novembre 1990; p. 145, 1990.
54. Yang CJ, and Rosenberg SA. Update or adoptive cellular immunotherapy with LAK cells and TIL. Proceedings Int. Conference on Biology Treat. of Melanoma and other cancers. Newcastle, NSW Australia, p. 14, September 1990.

Chapter 34

STATISTICAL ANALYSIS AND DATA MANAGEMENT

Stefan Suciu

INTRODUCTION

In the last two decades, clinical trials have played an increasingly important role in testing new ideas in cancer research. In the field of malignant melanoma, questions like the value of lymph node dissection, isolation perfusion, immunotherapy and chemotherapy have been raised. Most of the questions deal with increasing the duration of survival, decreasing the toxicity, or improving the quality of life of patients receiving new treatments or treatment strategies. For instance, some questions, like elective lymph node dissection, may be seen as the value of immediate treatment versus delayed treatment after an eventual recurrence. Should the isolation perfusion be performed in Stage I or IIb melanoma patients immediately, after a wide excision, or should the perfusion be proposed after local or regional recurrence?

Most cancer clinical trials need large data sets. The expected treatment differences are generally of low to medium magnitude. Therefore, one needs a large number of patients to be entered in phase III clinical trials in order to detect such differences with sufficient statistical power. Careful data collection and adequate statistical analyses are required in order to be able to draw reliable conclusions in a reasonable period of time. The emphasis will be placed on the way different clinical trials should be designed, conducted, analyzed, and therefore, what the prerequisites are in terms of data management (form design, frequency of sending the forms, etc.). Specific issues related to malignant melanoma clinical trials will be presented. Some examples from the EORTC Data Center experience will be given in order to better understand certain problems, like the number of patients required, protocol design, prognostic factors, end-points, univariate and multivariate analyses. For more technical details refer to the cited references.

PHASE III CANCER CLINICAL TRIALS

Cancer clinical trials represent a scientific tool for the investigation of new treatment modalities. The literature related to the methodology of conducting and analyzing cancer clinical trials is quite large.[1–6] Some of the more important aspects, and specifically those related to phase III clinical trials in melanoma, are as follows.

Design

The design of a clinical trial is the key aspect in determining its success. A poorly designed trial has a low chance to be conducted properly and to be finally successful.

PATIENT POPULATION

In any phase III clinical trial one should carefully define the patient population for whom the treatment(s) are targeted. A too particular or restricted patient population may be harmful for the clinical trial. One should aim to have a broad selection criteria, as broad as possible from an ethical and a practical point of view. If one group of institutions would prefer to enter patients with tumors having a Breslow thickness between 0.76 and 2 mm, and other centers prefer to enter only patients with a tumor thickness ranging from 1.01 to 3 mm, the protocol should allow patients with a tumor thickness from 0.76 to 3 mm to be entered and not to restrict the inclusion to tumors from 1.01 to 2 mm. In this way each center continues its own policy, the entry rate will be higher and the chance to finish the trial will be higher. One important point not to forget in such a trial, like in most clinical trials, is to stratify the randomization by center: in each center an approximately equal number of patients will receive the treatments required by the protocol. A good balance of the treatment arms within each center avoids a possible bias due to the institution effect (due to patient selection and/or different treatment results in centers). One should not forget that the aim of any clinical trial is to avoid systematic biases, and to compare treatment effects based on groups of patients as comparable as possible (where the treatment has been allocated randomly), and not two or more groups of patients with different prognoses, where the treatment choice has been decided following extensive examinations and accordingly to numerous prognostic factors.

NUMBER OF TREATMENT ARMS

Very often a trial represents a compromise between several individuals coming from different teams, centers, and so on. Generally, a clinical trial takes 1 to 3 years to be started, several years for patient inclusion, and several more years to reach the required number of "events" (deaths, etc.). This requires an important amount of time, efforts, and costs from a considerable number of people (physicians, nurses, data managers, statisticians, computer analysts, etc.). Therefore, the questions to be asked by a trial should be very important for the medical community, in order to be considered and incorporated in a clinical trial. The temptation to add several treatment arms in a clinical trial in order to ask several questions (should one drug or several drugs be added, for how long a period of time, at what dose) is quite high. However, as the number of patients and the other resources are limited, it is, for the moment, unrealistic to think that a clinical trial may answer the question "what is the best treatment for each particular patient?" What a clinical trial, or several clinical trials asking the same question, may do is just to try to answer the question what is the treatment which, on the average, gives the best results in a particular group of patients included in a trial according to the selection criteria defined in the proposal. There is no magic formula to determine the optimum number of treatment arms that a clinical trial should contain. As mentioned, this should be based on the potential patient population, the end point to be considered in the trial, the expected magnitude of the difference between the results of the treatment arms and the size of the two possible errors for drawing a conclusion, alpha and beta (see following).

The simplest clinical trial contains two arms: one control arm (accepted by the medical community) and one "experimental" arm. This arm may represent a new treatment strategy or a modification of the "usual" treatment. As the new arm may result in either better or in worse results than that obtained applying the control arm, one should foresee enough patients in order to detect such differences.

ALPHA AND BETA

The statistician involved in the design of a clinical trial specifies the minimum number of patients to be included per treatment arm, and therefore in the trial, based on the difference which may be reasonably expected with the particular treatments under study and given the size of the two errors: the alpha ("false positive" error: probability of declaring—based on the sample of patients treated in the trial—the new treatment to be better than the control given that there is no true difference between the treatment results in the whole potential population), and beta ("false negative" error: probability of declaring—based on the sample of patients treated in the trial—the two treatments to be equivalent given that in fact there is a real difference between the treatment results in the whole potential population). The statistical power (= 1 − beta) is just the probability to detect a difference between two treatment arms in a clinical trial when in fact there is a real difference between the treatment results in the whole potential population. Very often, alpha is taken as 5 percent (chance to unduly declare a new treatment to be superior to the control arm when in fact there is no difference) and beta as 20 percent, that is, the statistical power equals 80 percent (chance to detect a true difference).

NUMBER OF PATIENTS AND EVENTS

There are tables[7] giving the total number of events to be reported and the total number of patients to be entered according to different values of the expected difference, alpha and beta. Of course, the smaller the value of these parameters, the larger the number of events (or end points) to be observed and, therefore, the larger the total number of patients to be entered. If for all patients entered in the trial, the end point will be reached in a reasonable period of time, which is the case in advanced stages, then the total number of patients required will be equal to the total number of events required. If this is not the case, which generally happens in the early cancer stages, the total number of patients should be increased by a certain factor. If in high-risk Stage 1 melanoma of the limbs, the expected survival at 5 years after wide excision is only 65 percent, and one would like to increase by 10 percent the survival to 75 percent by adding isolation perfusion, then the next table gives the total number of patients to be entered and the total number of deaths to be observed according to alpha (5% or 1%) and the statistical power (80%, 90%, and 95%).

For instance, in order to detect a significant (alpha = 5%) difference with 80 percent chance between the two treatment arms (65% versus 75% at 5 years) then a total of 663 patients should be entered and 198 patients should be followed until death. Of interest, one may notice that the number of endpoints to be reached (198 deaths) is just 663 × 30 percent: indeed, 30 percent is the expected death rate at 5 years in this trial, because one may expect to have a survival rate of 65 percent in one arm, and 75 percent in the other.

FACTORIAL DESIGN

Generally, one should avoid "octopus" trials with a large number of treatment arms. For example, a three-treatment arm trial (one control and two new treatments), necessitates not only 50 percent more patients than a two-arm study (with the same assumptions of the treatment differences to be detected), but additionally, one should increase[5] by 23 percent the total number required, in order to keep the alpha at the 5 percent level and to be able to detect a significant difference in the worst case where the results for one arm are in the middle of the results of the two other arms. For instance, if one should enter 100 patients per treatment arm in a two-arm study, in a three-arm study one should enter 300 × 1.23 = 369 patients. Therefore, such inefficient studies should be avoided as much as possible.

On the contrary, a 2 × 2 factorial design should be applied whenever possible. Let's consider a trial studying the value of isolation perfusion (IP) in high-risk Stage 1 and 2 limb melanoma patients after wide excision. Approximately 1000 patients are required to answer the question of the value of isolation perfusion with an alpha of 1 percent and a beta of 20 percent. It would be worthwhile to add a second question concerning postsurgery treatment with interferon (IFN) by using a factorial design. For example, a 2 × 2 factorial design as outlined in Table 34-2 could be considered.

This design allows the data to be used "twice," once for assessing the effectiveness of IP (whether the patients receive subsequent IFN or not) and once for assessing the efficacy of IFN (whether the patients receive IP or not) after surgery—wide excision (WE). In addition to the efficiency of such a design (approximately the same number of patients is needed to answer two questions instead of one), the inference from such a trial might be more convincing (IFN is useful or harmful, according to whether after IP is used or not, and vice-versa, IP is of any use after WE, according to whether IFN is used or not as an adjuvant treatment). The final estimate of the efficacy of IFN, and therefore, the final decision, will be based on the average efficacy of IFN added to WE ± IP (this is done by stratifying retrospectively for the treatment scheme WE only or WE + IP). This is appropriate, unless a *qualitative interaction* (which seems very unlikely) exists between the postsurgery treatment scheme (IP or no IP) and IFN, for example, a positive effect (e.g., +10%) if no IP has been performed and a negative one (e.g., −10%) if IP has been performed. *Quantitative interactions* are more likely to occur in clinical trials. This means that the magnitude of effectiveness of IFN may be different whether IP has been performed or not. For example a 12.5 percent benefit in favor of IFN (if no IP previously performed) and a 7.5 percent benefit in the other one (if IP previously performed). This leads to an average benefit of 10 percent. Therefore, the same general conclusion will apply (a benefit in using IFN)

TABLE 34-1
SAMPLE SIZE CALCULATION: AN EXAMPLE

Difference in survival at 5 years to be detected: from 65% to 75%

	STATISTICAL POWER FOR ALPHA = 5%		
	80%	*90%*	*95%*
Number of patients randomized	660	887	1093
Number of deaths	198	266	328

	STATISTICAL POWER FOR ALPHA = 1%		
	80%	*90%*	*95%*
Number of patients randomized	987	1252	1500
Number of deaths	296	376	450

TABLE 34-2
EXAMPLE OF A 2 × 2 FACTORIAL DESIGN AFTER WIDE EXCISION

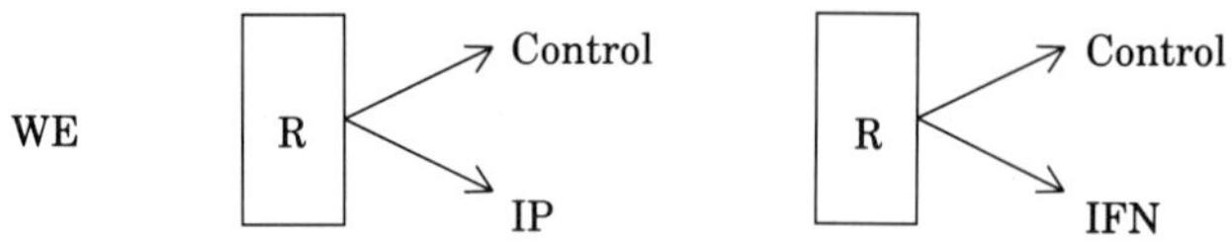

R = Randomization

just as if one had drawn the conclusion from the use of one treatment scheme, WE without IP or WE with IP. One should also remember that in any multicenter clinical trial the conclusions are based on an average treatment effect, based on the results obtained by different institutions, in different categories of prognostic factors, and so forth.

Randomization

A key issue in phase III clinical trials is the randomization procedure. Such trials are carried out in order to answer a specific question concerning the relative efficacy and/or side effects of two or more treatments. They should be randomized since it is only through a random assignment of the treatments that one can eliminate systematic biases in the treatment comparisons. A centralized randomization, by telephone call or by a computerized network, is to be preferred to randomization by envelopes or by some other unrealistic method such as: day of admission to the ward (even day: treatment 1, or odd day: treatment 2), patient's sex (male: treatment 1, or female: treatment 2), and so on. The randomization (pure randomization, block size, minimization technique[8]) should be done in such a way that the physician, when calling the Data Center, will be unable to predict with certainty the next treatment for any particular patient. The lack of predictability of the treatment arm is the basis of any good randomization technique.

Prognostic Factors

The issue of prognostic factors for melanoma is discussed extensively.[9] In any randomized clinical trial, it is very important to compare "like to like." It is essential to know that the important prognostic factors are well balanced in the treatment arms so that one actually compares the treatment policies and not groups of patients with different prognoses. The randomization tends to balance the distribution of the prognostic factors in the different treatment groups. However, it does not guarantee, for all factors, a good balance, during the whole duration of the trial. This is especially true in the case of the pure randomization technique: a good balance of different factors in the treatment arms is obtained only in "on the average," after entering a considerable number of patients into the trial. A method like the "minimization technique"[8] allows one to prospectively stratify patients according to one or more prognostic factors, thus assuring a balance for those particular factors in the treatment groups, and this during the whole period the protocol is open to entry.

The prognostic factors literature is quite extensive in the field of melanoma.[10–17] Tables 34-3 and 34-4 represent just a brief and nonexhaustive summary of those factors influencing the prognosis in different stages of this disease.

These factors, being of prognostic importance, should be collected prospectively in cancer clinical trials. From a *data-management* point of view, all these variables should be contained in the case report forms (CRF) along eventually with other information: the patient's weight, height, surface area (necessary to check the dose of chemotherapy for instance), precise information on the localization and measurability of lesion(s), and so on, depending on the stage of disease and type of protocol. In an isolation perfusion trial, the dose of Melphalan is given according to the limb volume in which the tumor is localized and the flow is based on the volume of this limb. All information collected on the CRFs should be carefully checked and if inconsistent or erroneous data are reported, it is mandatory to obtain the correct answer from the local investigator.

A *pathology review committee* may be of great help in the process of collecting correct data. The pathology review of slides may help to better determine the Breslow thickness for instance, which is the most important prognostic factor in Stage 1 melanoma. Figures 34-1 and 34-2 show the prognosis of

TABLE 34-3
SOME PROGNOSTIC FACTORS IN STAGE 1 MALIGNANT MELANOMA

Sex	Ulceration
Age	Histogenetic type
Localization	Mitotic activity
Lymph node dissection	Clark grade
(Number of + nodes)	Breslow thickness

TABLE 34-4
SOME PROGNOSTIC FACTORS IN STAGES 2 TO 3 MALIGNANT MELANOMA

Extent of progression (number) and type:
- local
- in transit metastases
- regional lymph nodes
- metastases: cutaneous, visceral, brain

Previous treatment(s): type and last administration
Time elapsed from Stage 1 to Stages 2 to 3

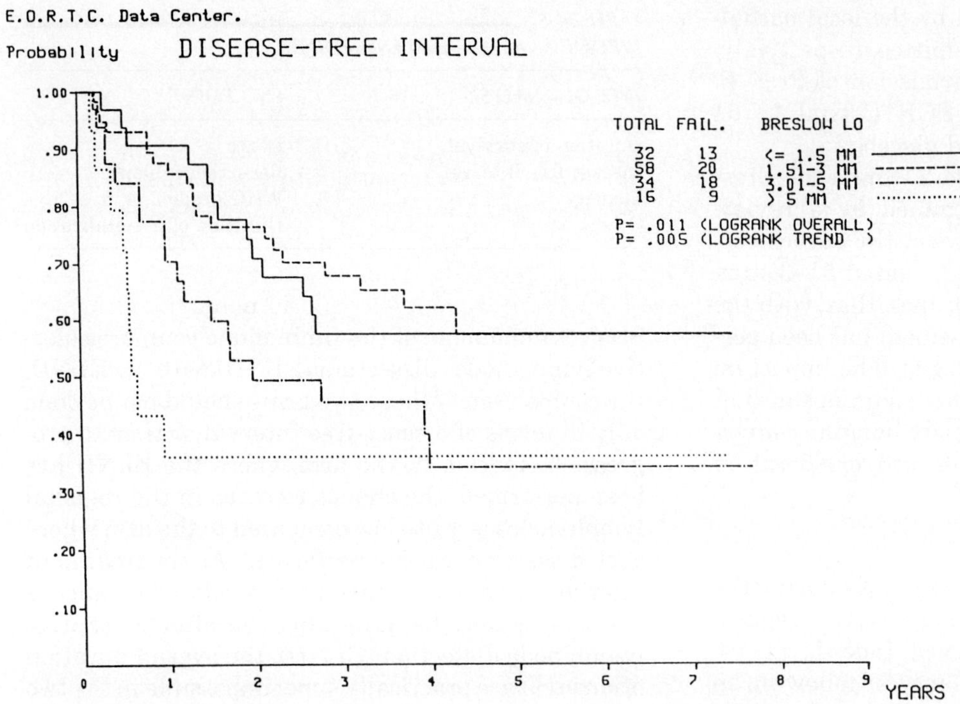

FIG. 34-1. Disease free interval according to the Breslow thickness assessed by the local pathologist: Breslow < 1.5 mm (——), 1.5 mm < Breslow ≤ 3.0 mm (------), 3.0 mm < Breslow ≤ 5.0 mm (·-·-·-·-·-), Breslow > 5.0 mm (······); logrank test gives P = .011.

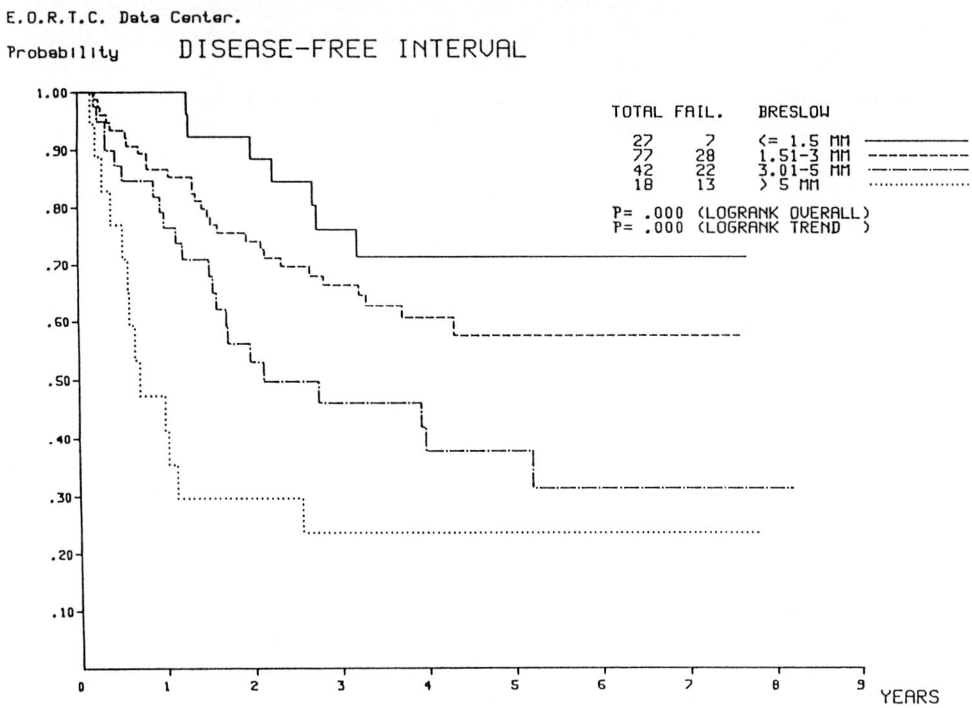

FIG. 34-2. Disease free interval according to the Breslow thickness assessed by the pathological reviewer: Breslow < 1.5 mm (——), 1.5 mm < Breslow ≤ 3.0 mm (------), 3.0 mm < Breslow ≤ 5.0 mm (·-·-·-·-·-), Breslow > 5.0 mm (······); logrank test gives P < .001.

the Breslow thickness assessed by the local pathologist and pathology review committee, respectively. Data are provided with the permission of Prof. F. Lejeune, study coordinator of EORTC trial 18761 comparing DTIC, levamisol and placebo.[18]

One may see that in Fig. 34-2, where the Breslow thickness has been determined by a review committee, the separation between the curves corresponding to four groups (≤1.5 mm, 1.51–3 mm, 3.01–5 mm and >5 mm) is wider than that, with the same cutpoints, where the assessment has been performed only by the local pathologist. The impact on the treatment comparison was not enormous in that particular trial, but one may easily imagine contradictory results whether one takes into consideration one measurement or another.

Conduct

All patients have to be followed regularly during the study until progression and death, and this regardless of the treatment arm assigned. Indeed, it is essential to have the same frequency of follow-up in both treatment groups, otherwise a serious bias may be introduced by reporting progressions earlier in one arm than in the other one. The treatment comparison in terms of time to progression will favor that arm where the follow-up is less frequent. However, from a medical point of view, such an arm may be disadvantaged in terms of duration of survival, especially if the salvage treatment, applied earlier after recurrence, may be effective.

END POINT

The end point of the study has to be as objective as possible. In advanced melanoma patients, treatment comparisons are very often made in terms of response rate, after one or several courses of a specific treatment or combined treatments. Changes in measurable or evaluable lesions are generally assessed using the WHO system,[19] comprising categories such as complete response, partial response, no change, progression. Duration of response, time to progression, duration of survival are also assessed. For adjuvant trials, after surgery, the time to recurrence or disease free interval, and duration of survival after surgery are important end points (See Table 34-5).

Since these end points (lack of response, progression, recurrence) occur prior to death, they are surrogate end points for survival. A study may use these end points in order to perform a treatment comparison only if: these end points are clearly related with duration of survival, they are appearing before death, and if the duration of survival post that particular end point does not change significantly according to the initial treatment. For instance, in Stage 1 melanoma of the limb, if one compares elective lymph nodes dissection (ELND) with No ELND, the comparison of these two arms should not be done only in terms of disease-free interval or time to progression. Indeed, in the arm where the ELND has been performed, the chance to recur in the regional lymph nodes is quite low compared to the arm where such dissection was not performed. As the treatment after local regional recurrence or isolated cutaneous metastases may be quite effective after a curative lymph node dissection (CLND), the overall duration of survival are practically superimpossible in the two arms of immediate ELND versus No ELND followed by CLND in case of specific recurrence. These were in fact the results of a study conducted by the WHO melanoma group.[20] The treatment evaluation may be based on a surrogate end point, especially if such an end point is highly predictive for the duration of survival: for instance the time of distant metastases.

TABLE 34-5
TYPE OF ANALYSIS AND END POINT

TYPE OF ANALYSIS	*END POINT*
Duration of survival	Death
Disease free interval	Recurrence/relapse
Toxicity	WHO grade 3, 4, 5
Other	Duration of hospitalization

From a *data-management* point of view one should ask on the CRFs not only the response to therapy (in case of advanced stages), the time and the type of recurrence, but also the date and cause of death and the latest examination date. If a particular end point is used (for instance time to local or regional recurrence) one should ask on the CRFs not only the time and the type of the first recurrence but also the subsequent recurrences (time and type). Indeed, in a trial where one would like to assess the value of isolation perfusion (IP) on the loco–regional relapse, and No ELND is performed, approximately 50 percent of first recurrences will be reported in the lymph nodes, which implies that the other types of recurrences will be "masked" by that particular type of recurrence. Therefore, it is mandatory to ask on the CRFs each type of end point, that is, the date of each type of recurrence, with a brief description of the salvage treatment applied (wide excision, CLND, IP, etc.). Thus, one may be in the position to explain an eventual difference between two treatment policies in terms of the time to first progression or time to loco-regional progression, a small difference in terms of time to distant metastases, and almost no difference in terms of duration of survival (an example of a "progress report" from an EORTC melanoma study is given in Table 34-6).

TABLE 34-6
AN EORTC CASE REPORT FORM USED IN THE EORTC TRIAL 18832

EORTC MMCG TRIAL 18832 N.A.P.G. TRIAL 1 WHO TRIAL No 15 — Pg 1 of 1

PROGRESS REPORT FORM 3

INSTRUCTIONS: *The purpose of this form is to follow patients who have been put "off-study" in order to analyse their duration of survival. Please complete this form EVERY 6 MONTHS AFTER PATIENT HAS GONE OFF-STUDY and send it to the EORTC DATA CENTER, 83 Av. E. Mounier, 1000 Brussels.*
Please leave blank any box for which the requested information is not applicable.

Patient (or code): ______ Birthdate: ______ Chart No.: ______

Institution: ______ Responsible Physician: ______

1 | 1 | 8 | 8 | 3 | 2 | | _ _ _ _ | | _ _ _ | | _ _ _ | | _ _ _ | | _ _ | | 1 | 3 | 1 | _ | _ |

22 |__| Survival status: 1 = alive, 2 = dead, 3 = lost to follow-up/unknown

23 |__|__| |__|__| |__|__| Date of death or last known to be alive

29 |__| Cause of death (if applicable)
1 = Malignant disease
2 = Toxicity
3 = Infection
4 = Cardiovascular disease
5 = Other associated chronic disease, specify: ______
8 = Other: ______

30 | 30 to 37 leave blank |

SUBSEQUENT TREATMENT GIVEN SINCE LAST FOLLOW-UP

38 |__| Local treatment
1 = None
2 = Wide excision only
3 = Wide excision + isolation-perfusion (Melphalan)
4 = Wide excision + isolation-perfusion (other)
5 = Other: ______

39 |__| Systemic treatment
1 = None
2 = DTIC only
3 = DTIC + other drugs, specify: ______
4 = Other chemotherapy regimen, specify: ______
5 = Immunotherapy, specify: ______
6 = Immunotherapy + Chemotherapy, specify: ______
7 = Other, specify: ______

FIRST OCCURRENCE OF:

40 |__|__| |__|__| |__|__| Date of FIRST local recurrence

46 |__|__| |__|__| |__|__| Date of FIRST occurrence of in transit metastases

52 |__|__| |__|__| |__|__| Date of FIRST occurrence of regional lymph node metastases

58 |__| Regional lymph nodes surgery performed?: 1 = no, 2 = yes

59 |__|__| |__|__| |__|__| Date of FIRST occurrence of distant metastases

Investigator comments: ______

______

65 |__|__| |__|__| |__|__| DATE Signature: ______

The follow-up should be the same in both arms. However, it may be more frequent during the period of high risk of recurrence/progression or of occurrence of toxicity. As a general rule, the frequency of sending the CRFs should coincide with the patient's visit at the hospital in order to be able to collect reliable data. For instance, if the usual visit frequency is six times during the first year, four times during the second year, and two times yearly thereafter, the CRFs should be sent at the same rate.

Analysis

When treatments are compared, an objective end point should be used (as mentioned). In many trials, the most reliable and most convincing results may be drawn from duration of survival analyses. In the last two decades, the literature dealing with "duration of survival" analyses has had an impressive expansion. However, the most appropriate methods are not always used to compare treatment groups because they are not easy to explain to clinicians. The comparisons of the percentage of patients still alive at a fixed point in time after randomization or of the median survival are not always reliable and do not have adequate statistical power; however, these methods are still used because they are easy to summarize and present.

UNIVARIATE ANALYSIS

In order to compare the outcome of two or more treatment groups in terms of the duration of survival, the "usual" *statistical tests*[1,2,4,5] are recommended. The logrank test gives the same weight to the differences occurring during the time between two or more survival curves, whereas the generalized Wilcoxon test gives more weight to early differences appearing after randomization. These tests allow one to compare the death rates per time unit in two or more treatment groups following randomization. In each treatment arm all the follow-up information is used, such as in the well-known Kaplan-Meier method[1,2,4,5] used for calculating the percentage of patients still alive after randomization. The logrank test, or any similar test, is very convenient to stratify a posteriori in order to adjust for prognostic factors.[4,5] Since such statistical tests are based on the observed and the expected number of deaths in each treatment group,[4] they may be summarized in terms of the reduction of the death rate per unit time (year for example).

MULTIVARIATE ANALYSIS

In order to assess the relative importance of several variables that appeared to be of prognostic importance as well as of the treatment arm, multivariate analyses should be done. In this manner it is possible to adjust for any imbalances of prognostic factors that may exist on the treatment arms, and to obtain a more reliable estimate of the treatment difference. The most popular model is Cox's proportional hazards model,[21] which represents the multivariate version of the logrank test. This model represents a very sensitive method to detect factors that have a constant influence (over time) on the outcome, that is, the instantaneous risk of death (in case of an analysis of duration of survival). Several other models exist, nonparametric or parametric, like the Weibull. However, modeling is not an easy task, although many user friendly statistical analysis packages exist. The aim of using the models is to determine risk groups having different prognoses. Using risk groups one may better describe the patient population entered in a protocol, one may even adjust the therapy, for example, by increasing its intensity in poor prognosis patients (larger margin in case of surgery, isolation perfusion after wide excision, higher intensity of chemotherapy or immunotherapy, etc.). However, any model derived from one series should be validated using other trials having a similar patient population and treatment(s). Generally, it is recommended to have simple models which do not over fit the data coming from one particular series, and variables that are easily measured and reliable, not necessitating a special lab to perform a particular assessment.

INTENT TO TREAT

The treatment groups should be compared according to the "intent to treat" principle.[1–6,22] All patients should be included in the analyses of treatment efficacy and kept in the treatment group originally allocated by randomization. Thus, when one treatment strategy is better than another, it may be recommended to all other patients having the same or similar characteristics as those included in the clinical trial. Of course, one should also record the patient's compliance in order to see how many patients actually received treatment according to the protocol. In advanced melanoma stages, one should record all patients who started therapy whether they interrupted or not the course of treatment, for any reason (e.g., early progression and/or toxicity, etc.), otherwise, the treatment results may be seriously biased.

Meta-Analysis

Too often the results from one particular trial are not strong enough in order to reach a conclusion. This might be due to too few patients, too short a follow-up and so one. One solution is to pool all trials (published or not) asking the same kind of question. Conclusions based on several trials are generally more reliable than those coming only from one trial and the generalization of the results to a larger patient population is more reliable. Meta-analyses have been performed in early breast cancer,[23] in colorectal cancer,[24] several others are in process: lung cancer, acute lymphoblastic leukemia, Hodgkin disease, advanced prostatic cancer, but none is foreseen in melanoma.

When one is doing a meta-analysis or an overview analysis, one should consider the trials with good methodological background (randomization, data collection, etc.). The overall comparison between the treatment arms is done using the trial as an a posteriori stratification factor. This allows one to adjust the treatment comparisons for an eventual difference between the trials in terms of duration of follow-up, patient characteristics, or for other differences of known or unknown origin. Adjustment of the treatment comparison by the study will result in "summing" the treatment differences from each of these studies, giving a larger weight to studies having a greater number of patients and events. The adjusted treatment comparison, therefore, represents a weighted average of the differences observed in two or more clinical trials, each trial having its own particularities (patient population, follow-up, second-line treatment, etc.) and showing a certain difference between the treatment groups. At no time are patients in one study compared to patients in another study.

When pooling the data from different trials, the temptation to search for possible interactions between the prognostic factors and the treatment results is quite high. As clinical trials are performed in order to see what is the mean effect of one treatment in comparison to another, it would be very surprising that the same difference would exist between the treatments in all subgroups of patients (male versus female, young versus old patients, low versus high Breslow thickness, etc.). One may search for treatment differences in specific subgroups, having an a priori hypothesis formulated before undertaking analyses (for example, "the magnitude of difference between the treatment results is greater in one subgroup than in another"). One should not blindly carry out the treatment comparisons in too many different subgroups. Just due to chance it is very possible that one will find that in one subgroup one treatment group is significantly better than the other treatment group, and in another subgroup the reverse happens.

The meta-analysis process requires "raw data" for each group. Generally, one asks for each randomized patient, eligible or not, the birth date, sex, date of randomization, randomized treatment, date of first relapse/recurrence, type of such relapse/recurrence, date of death and cause of death or the date of the last follow-up. This process is not an easy one, due to the heterogeneity of the data collection systems (computers, data management systems, case report forms, etc.). However, generally from each data base one should be able to extract this kind of information without many difficulties. The way of categorizing the questions, and therefore the trials, in order to obtain a consensus of the all participating members of the meta-analysis might represent a problem. This step should be overcome before starting the analyses, and one should not give the possibility to any member to withdraw from the meta-analysis once the results have been obtained and the subsequent conclusions are derived.

Drawing Conclusions

When making a decision concerning the choice of treatment, one should pay attention not only to the P-values given by the statistical tests, but also to the size of the treatment differences. For example, one may obtain a very significant P-value when analyzing data from several large trials, in which thousands of patients have been entered, when in fact the difference in efficacy between the two treatments is very small and not worthwhile from a medical point of view. Confidence intervals should be constructed in order to judge the magnitude of the difference. Additionally, a cost-benefit analysis should take into consideration not only the objective benefit of one treatment strategy in comparison to another, but also the cost and the toxicity (objective and subjective) of the two strategies. For instance, when one is asking the question of the value of isolation perfusion after wide excision in Stage 1 melanoma patients, one should take into consideration not only the treatment results in terms of disease-free interval but also the results in terms of toxicity (IP adds toxicity) and duration of survival (those who had local and/or regional relapses without having had an initial IP may have effective salvage treatment: IP or ELND ± WE). Only the present EORTC/WHO/NAPG clinical trial[25] asks this question, because sufficient patients have been planned to be recruited in this trial and additional data concerning the treatment toxicity and the subsequent treatment after relapse are collected.

CONCLUSIONS

Cancer clinical trials represent an important tool in clinical research. Many ideas and hopes have been tested and there are still important questions such as the value of isolation perfusion (subquestions: duration of IP, optimal temperature, type of chemotherapy, addition of immunotherapy);

immunotherapy (interferons, etc.); elective lymph node dissection in head and neck melanoma, the most conservative surgical procedure (1, 2, or 3 cm margin); and so on, are yet to be answered. One should not expect major breakthroughs from these large scale randomized trials. However, a small fraction gained in terms of survival represents an important number of lives saved. Therefore, one must correctly design the clinical trials which might recruit hundreds if not thousands of patients. Combining the question in a 2 by 2 factorial design represents an elegant way, as the WHO did when it asked what is the value of chemotherapy (DTIC) and immunotherapy (BCG) after wide excision in high-risk Stage I and Stage II melanoma.[26] A good cooperation between the clinicians, the statisticians, and the data managers is necessary in order to prospectively collect the data, to follow the patients in the treatment arms of a trial at the same frequency. The assessment of the end points (response, relapse or recurrence, death) should be based on objective criteria and one should carefully record toxicities and different types of recurrences, the different time patterns of these relapses, and to briefly record an eventual subsequent treatment. As many trials may be seen as immediate versus delayed treatment in case of relapse, such information is essential in order to be able to explain an eventual difference between the treatment groups in terms of disease free interval and no, or small differences in terms of duration of survival. Appropriate univariate and multivariate analyses should be used in order to detect small, but meaningful treatment differences. All patients, even those considered as "inevaluable" due to an early termination of the protocol (cause: treatment progression, toxicity, protocol violations), should be reported and included in the analyses in order to have reliable inferences from clinical trials by properly applying the "intent to treat" principle. The conclusions of these trials should always balance the treatment efficacy and the corresponding toxicity (early and/or delayed), in order to fully inform the medical readers, as well as future patients, about the risk and hopes of any treatment strategy. Finally, even if no definite conclusion can be drawn from a randomized trial, one should be ready to share the data with other cooperative groups which have asked a similar, but not necessarily the same question, in order to perform a meta-analysis.

ACKNOWLEDGMENTS

The author wishes to thank Denis Thomas, Data Manager of the EORTC Melanoma Cooperative Group at the EORTC Data Center, for the fruitful discussions in the data management field of melanoma trials.

REFERENCES

1. Muenz LR. Comparing survival distributions: A review for Nonstatisticians. I. *Cancer Invest* 1:455–466, 1983.
2. Muenz LR. Comparing survival distributions: A review for Nonstatisticians. II. *Cancer Invest* 1:537–545, 1983.
3. Peto R, Pike MC, Armitage P, Breslow NE, Cox DR, Howard SV, Mantel N, McPherson K, Peto J, and Smith PG. Design and analysis of randomized clinical trials requiring prolonged observation on each patient. I. Introduction and Design. *Br J Cancer* 34:585–612, 1976.
4. Peto R, Pike MC, Armitage P, Breslow NE, Cox DR, Howard SV, Mantel N, McPherson K, Peto J, and Smith PG. Design and analysis of randomized clinical trials requiring prolonged observation on each patient. II. Analysis and Examples. *Br J Cancer* 35:1–39, 1977.
5. Buyse M, Staquet M, and Sylvester R, (eds.). *Cancer Clinical Trials: Methods and Practice.* Oxford: England, Oxford University Press, 1984.
6. Buyse ME. Potential and pitfalls of randomized clinical trial in cancer research. *Cancer Surv* 8:91–105, 1989.
7. Machin D, and Campbell MJ. *Statistical Tables for the Design of Clinical Trials.* Oxford: Blackwell Scientific Publications, 1987.
8. Pocock S. Allocation of patients to treatment in clinical trials. *Biometrics* 35:183–197, 1979.
9. Mc Carthy WH. The influence of prognostic factors in melanoma management. In FJ Lejeune, Chaudhui PK, Das Gupta TK (eds.), *Malignant Melanoma, Medical and Surgical Management.* New York: McGraw-Hill, 1993, Chap. 14.
10. Day CL, Mihm MC, Sober AJ, Harris MN, Kopf AW, Fitzpatrick TB, Lew RA, Harrist TJ, At AL, Friedman RJ, and Mintzis MM. Prognostic factors for melanoma patients with lesions 0.76–1.69 mm thickness. An appraisal of "thin" level IV lesions. *Ann Surg* 195:30–34, 1982.
11. Day CL, Mihm MC, Lew RA, Harris MN, Kopf AW, Fitzpatrick TB, Harrist TJ, At AL, Friedman RJ, Mintzis MM, and Sober AJ. Prognostic factors for patients with clinical stage I melanoma of intermediate thickness (1.51–3.99 mm). A conceptual model for tumor growth and metastasis. *Ann Surg* 195:35–43, 1982.
12. Day CL, Lew RA, Mihm MC, Sober AJ, Harris MN, Kopf AW, Fitzpatrick TB, At AL, Friedman RJ, Mintzis MM, and Grier RW. A multivariate analysis of prognostic factors for melanoma patients with lesions > 3.65 mm in thickness. The importance of revealing alternative Cox models. *Ann Surg* 195:44–49, 1982.
13. McLeod GR. Factors influencing prognosis in malignant melanoma. In Ariel MA (ed.), *Progress in Clinical Cancer.* Orlando: Grune and Stratton, 1975, vol V, 177–182.
14. Johnson OK Jr, Emrich LJ, Karakousis CP, Rao U, and Greco WR. Comparison of prognostic factors for survival and recurrence in malignant melanoma of the skin, clinical stage I. *Cancer* 55:1107–1117, 1985.
15. Callery C, Cochran AJ, Roe DJ, Rees W, Nathanson SD, Benedetti JK, Elashoff RM, and Morton DL. Factors prognostic for survival in patients with malignant melanoma spread to the regional lymph nodes. *Ann Surg* 196:69–75, 1981.
16. Balch CM, Soong SJ, Murad TM, Ingalls AL, and Maddox WA: A multifactorial analysis of melanoma. III. Prognostic factors in melanoma patients with lymph nodes metastases (stage III). *Ann Surg* 193:377–389, 1981.
17. Shaw HM, Balch CM, S-J Soong, Milton GW, and McCarthy WH. Prognostic histopathological factors in malignant melanoma. *Pathology,* 17:271–274, 1985.
18. Lejeune P, Macher E, Klebeerg U, Rumke P, Prade M, Thomas D, and Suciu S. An assessment of DTIC versus levamisole

or placebo in the treatment of high risk stage I patients after surgical removal of a primary melanoma of the skin. A phase III adjuvant study. EORTC Protocol 18761. *Eur J Cancer Clin Oncol,* 24:S81–S90, 1988.

19. WHO Offset Publication No. 48. *WHO Handbook for Reporting Results of Cancer Treatment.* World Health Organization, Geneva, 1979.
20. Veronesi U, Adamus J, Bandiera DC, Brennhodh IO, Caceres E, Cascinelli N, Claudio F, Ikonopisov RL, Javorskj VV, Kirov S, Kulakoowski A, Lacour J, Lejeune F, Mechl Z, Morabito A, Rodé I, Sergeev S, van Slooten E, Szczygiel K, Trapeznikov NN, and Wagner RI. Inefficacy of immediate node dissection in stage I melanoma of the limbs. *N Engl J Med* 297:627–630, 1977.
21. Christensen E. Multivariate survival analysis using Cox's regression model. *Hepatology* 7:1346–1358, 1987.
22. Simon R, and Wittes RE. Methodologic guidelines for reports of clinical trials. *Cancer Treat Rep* 69:1–3, 1985.
23. Early Breast Cancer Trialists' Collaborative Group (prepared by Collins R, Gray R, Henderson C, Peta R). Effects of adjuvant tamoxifen and of cytotoxic therapy on mortality in early breast cancer. An overview of 61 randomized trials among 28,896 women. *N Engl J Med* 319:1681–1692, 1988.
24. Buyse M, Zeleniuch-Jacquotte A, and Chalmers TC: Adjuvant therapy of colorectal cancer. Why we still don't know. *JAMA* 259:3571–3578, 1988.
25. EORTC Protocol 18832, NAPG Protocol 1, WHO Trial No. 15. *A randomized trial on prophylactic isolation perfusion for stage I high risk (> 1.5 mm thickness) malignant melanoma of the limbs.*
26. Veronesi U, Adamus J, Aubert C, Bajetta E, Beretta G, Bonadonna G, Bufalino R, Cascinelli N, Cocconi G, Durand J, De Marsillac J, Ikonopisov RL, Kiss B, Lejeune F, MacKie R, Madej G, Mulder H, Mechl Z, Milton GW, Morabito A, Peter H, Priario J, Paul E, Rumke P, Sertoli R, and Tomin R. A randomized trial of adjuvant chemotherapy and immunotherapy in cutaneous melanoma. *N Engl J Med* 307:913–916, 1982.

Index

Page numbers followed by *f* indicate illustrations.
Page numbers followed by *t* indicate tables.